Modern Vascular Surgery
Volume 6

Modern Vascular Surgery

Volume 6

Edited by
John B. Chang

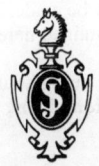

Springer-Verlag
New York Berlin Heidelberg London Paris
Tokyo Hong Kong Barcelona Budapest

John B. Chang, MD, FACS
Long Island Vascular Center
Roslyn, NY 11576 USA

With 239 Illustrations in 253 Parts

Library of Congress Cataloging-in-Publication Data
Modern vascular surgery, Volume 6 / [edited by] John B. Chang.
    p. cm.
  Includes bibliographical references and index.
  ISBN-13:978-1-4612-7616-6
  1. Blood-vessels—Surgery—Congresses.   2. Blood-vessels—
Diseases—Congresses.   I. Chang, John B.
  [DNLM: 1. Vascular Surgery—congresses. WG 170 M6895 1994]
RD598.5.M6376   1994
617.4'13—dc20
DNLM/DLC
for Library of Congress   93-38113

Printed on acid-free paper.
© 1994 Springer-Verlag New York Inc.

Production coordinated by Laura Carlson; manufacturing supervised by Jacqui Ashri.
Typeset by Asco Trade Typesetting Ltd., Hong Kong.

9 8 7 6 5 4 3 2 1

ISBN-13:978-1-4612-7616-6   e-ISBN-13:978-1-4612-2632-1
DOI: 10.1007/978-1-4612-2632-1

This book is dedicated to all my residents, interns, and medical students, who have been an endless source of inspiration, education, and commitment.

As I am sincerely grateful to those teachers who have guided me in my professional and personal life, it is my commitment and duty to inspire and guide our future generations so that the legacy of our noble profession will continue to inspire generation after generation.

I have been blessed to be a member of this noble profession, providing me with boundless inner satisfaction.

I salute you all.

John B. Chang, MD, FACS

Contents

Contributors xv
Introduction xxv
About the Editor xxvi

I NEWER CONCEPTS IN VASCULAR SURGERY

1 Arterial Reconstruction of the Lower Extremities 3
   Yoshihiko Kubo, Tadahiro Sasajima, Kazutomo Goh,
   Masashi Inaba, Yuichi Izumi, and Nobuyoshi Azuma

2 Development of Modern Vascular Surgery in Korea 24
   Yong Kak Lee

3 A Novel Approach to Preventing Intimal Hyperplasia:
   Inhibition of Smooth Muscle Cell Migration with Enalapril .. 28
   Eric T. Choi, Niraj Sehgal, Shaping Sun, Jeffrey Trachtenberg,
   Una S. Ryan, and Allan D. Callow

4 Involvement of Calpain in the Development of
   Myonephropathic Metabolic Syndrome (MNMS) 41
   Yoshifumi Tsuji, Ei-ichi Shiba, and Jun-ichi Kambayashi

II ANESTHESIA IN VASCULAR SURGERY

5 Anesthesia and Perioperative Cardiac Risk in Vascular
   Surgery Patients 51
   Thomas R. Eide

III ANGIOGRAPHY

6 Brachial Approach for Lower Limb Arteriography 67
   Seok Kil Zeon, Soo Jhi Suh, Won Hyun Cho, Ki Yong Chung, and
   You-Sah Kim

7 Angiographic and Doppler Evaluation of Profunda Femoris
   Artery Runoff 77
   Hiroshi Yasuhara, Hiroshi Shigematsu, Toshiyuki Kubo, Takashi
   Komiyama, and Tetuichiro Muto

IV CAROTID ARTERY SURGERY

8 Endarterectomy and Reimplantation for Carotid Stenosis ... 85
   Rudolph G. Vanmaele, Paul E. Van Schil, Marianne G.
   De Maeseneer, Philippe Lehert, and Robin F. Van Look

V CARDIAC HEMODYNAMICS

9   Effect of Acute Normovolemic Hemodilution on Blood
    Coagulation 99
    Zsolt A. Varga, Jill C. Locke-Edmunds, Peter M. Lamont, Roger N.
    Baird, and John F. Thompson

10 Percutaneous Bidirectional Femoral Artery Cannulation for
    Extended Extracorporeal Circulatory Support 110
    Hiroshi Matsuura, Xi Ming Yang, James D. Fonger,
    Gabriel S. Aldea, and Richard J. Shemin

11 Plain Chest Radiographic Assessment of Cardiac Tamponade
    in Patients with Penetrating Chest Injury Using Vascular
    Pedicle Width Measurements 118
    Felisberto M. Soriano and Romulo G. Vea

12 Incidence and Anatomy of the Posterior Gastric Artery and
    Its Surgical Importance 132
    You-Sah Kim, Seok Kil Zeon, Wansik Yu, and Il Woo Whang

13 Coronary Artery Bypass Surgery with Right Gastroepiploic
    Artery 138
    Thay-Hsiung Chen

14 Inferior Epigastric Artery for Coronary Bypass 145
    Hendrick B. Barner

15 Significant Decrease in Mortality in Surgery for Ventricular
    Septal Defect with Serious Pulmonary Hypertension by Use
    of Vasodilators 150
    Liu Zong-gui, Liu Wei-gong, Ju Ming-da, Zhang Wei-lian,
    Yan Jing-xue, and Liang Ji-he

VI AORTOILIAC OCCLUSIVE DISEASE

16 Early Functional Outcome After Treatment of Chronic
    Aortoiliac Occlusive Disease 159
    Young Wook Kim, Thomas C. Park, Jae Seok Choi, and Soo Il
    Chang

17 Intrapleural Preperitoneal Route of Axillofemoral and
    Axilloiliac Bypass for the Treatment of Leg Ischemia or
    Stenotic/Obstructive Lesion of the Aorta 166
    Nobuyuki Nakajima, Shigeyasu Takeuchi, Masahisa Masuda,
    Mitsuru Nakaya, and Narutsugu Adachi

VII AORTIC DISSECTION

18 Follow-up of Aortic Dissection with Thrombosed False
    Lumen 175
    Nobuhiko Mukohara, Kyoichi Ogawa, Tatsuro Asada, Masami
    Nishiwaki, Tetsuya Higami, and Takaki Sugimoto

VIII   AORTIC ANEURYSM

19   Evolution of Treatment of Aortic Aneurysms   187
        Denton A. Cooley

20   Abdominal Aortic Aneurysm with Perianeurysmal Fibrosis:
        An Analysis of 27 Cases in 1,004 AAAs Treated in a Single
        Vascular Center   194
        Mikael Bitsch, Jørgen E. Lorentzen, and Torben V. Schroeder

21   Vasospasm and Ruptured Aneurysmal Surgery   201
        Hwan Hung Chung

22   Aneurysm of the Abdominal Aorta Associated with
        Aortocaval Fistula: A Case Report   206
        Duck Jong Han and Young Soon Hyun

23   Management of Coronary Disease in Patients with
        Abdominal Aortic Aneurysm   213
        J. Ernesto Molina, Fredy Abed, and Michael G. Petty

24   Management of Thoracoabdominal Aneurysm and Difficult
        Aneurysmal Problems of the Aorta   219
        Samuel R. Money and Larry H. Hollier

25   Inflammatory Abdominal Aortic Aneurysms   226
        Hiroshi Ouchi, Masataka Ichiki, Kichiya Okuyama, and Shuzo
        Kamioki

26   Inflammatory Aneurysms of the Abdominal Aorta   238
        Keishu Yasuda, Makoto Sakuma, Yoshiro Matsui, and
        Tatsuzo Tanabe

27   Treatment of Consumption Coagulopathy Complicated with
        Abdominal Aortic Aneurysm   248
        Haruo Aramoto, Hiroshi Shigematsu, Toshiyuki Kubo, and
        Tetsuichiro Muto

28   Abdominal Aortic Aneurysms and Surgical Management . . .   257
        Takeshi Ueyama

IX   AORTIC SURGERY

29   Clinical Application of Deep Hypothermia and Total
        Circulatory Arrest for Treatment of Aortic Disease   269
        Wan Ki Baek and Hyuk Ahn

30   Results of Concomitant Renal Artery Reconstruction in
        Abdominal Aortic Surgery   278
        Masashi Inaba, Tadahiro Sasajima, Yoshihiko Kubo, Yuhichi
        Izumi, and Kazutomo Goh

31   Complications Following Aortic Reconstructive Surgery   286
        Jang Sang Park, Wook Kim, and Yong Bok Koh

32   Cardiovascular Changes After Infrarenal Aortic Cross-
     Clamping in Clinical and Animal Studies 296
     Kazuro Sugi, Akira Furutani, Takayuki Kuga, Kentaro Fujioka,
     Hidetoshi Tuboi, and Kensuke Esato

33   Surgical Management of Aortoiliac Occlusive Disease 306
     John B. Chang

  X ILIOFEMORAL OCCLUSIVE DISEASE

34   Treatment of Iliofemoral Stenosis and Occlusion by Means of
     Modified Gianturco Expandable Metallic Stents 337
     Byung Suk Roh, See Sung Choi, Seon Kwan Juhng, Chang Guhn
     Kim, and Jong Jin Won

 XI ARTERIAL ANEURYSM

35   A Profile of Peripheral Arterial Aneurysms in South India .. 347
     Booshanam V. Moses, Stanley John, R. David Sadhu, and Sunil
     Agarwal

XII ARTERITIS

36   Surgical Treatment of Takayasu's Arteritis: Report of Clinical
     Experience of 27 Patients 359
     Yong Bok Koh, Seung Nam Kim, Hae Myung Chun, and In Chul
     Kim

37   Characteristic Angiographic Findings of Thromboangiitis
     Obliterans 370
     Choong Ki Park, Bum Gyu Ahn, and Chang Sig Choi

XIII CONGENITAL VASCULAR DEFECTS

38   Surgical Treatment of Congenital Vascular Defects 383
     Stefan Belov

XIV FEMORAL POPLITEAL ARTERY DISEASE

39   Clinical Review of 49 Cases of Lower Limb Ischemic
     Disease 401
     Byung Jun So and Kwon Mook Chae

40   Current Status of the Surgical Treatment of Chronic Arterial
     Occlusive Disease in Japan 409
     Yoshio Mishima

41   Long-Term Results of Arterial Bypass in the
     Femoropopliteal Region 415
     Sohei Suzuki, Masayuki Shimizu, Masahiko Tanaka, Shinji
     Nomura, and Hisaaki Koie

42 Reevaluation of Effectiveness of Low-Dose Warfarin as
    Antithrombotic Therapy After Vascular Reconstruction 424
    Joonghee Kang, Masato Sakon, and Jun-ichi Kambayashi

43 Percutaneous Transluminal Angioplasty and Segmentally
    Enclosed Thrombolysis for Femoropopliteal Occlusions 430
    Bo Jørgensen and Jørn Dalsgaard Nielsen

44 Results of Surgical Treatment of Multivessel Disease in the
    Lower Limb 441
    Roy Vargese, A.N. Kosencov, and Yury V. Belov

45 Late Complications Following Surgery for Popliteal Artery
    Entrapment Syndrome 445
    Takehisa Iwai, Shoji Sato, Yoshinori Inoue, Noriaki Takiguchi, and
    Mitsuo Endo

XV   TIBIAL PERONEAL OCCLUSIVE DISEASE

46 Tibial Revascularization Under Transmicroscopic
    Technique 455
    Masayasu Yokokawa, Masaki Tomikawa, Takeshi Ueyama, and
    Keiichi Yamamoto

47 Clinical Review of Adjunctive Arteriovenous Fistula with
    Tibial and Peroneal Reconstruction for Extensive Occlusive
    Arterial Disease of Lower Extremity 461
    Yong Bok Koh, Cho Hyun Park, Jong Man Won, and Chang Joon
    Ahn

XVI   ACUTE ARTERIAL OCCLUSION

48 Results of Treatment of Acute Arterial Occlusion 469
    Takashi Komiyama, Hiroshi Shigematsu, Hiroshi Yasuhara, and
    Tetsuichiro Muto

XVII   AMPUTATION

49 Should Chemical Sympathectomy Precede Below-Knee
    Amputation? 477
    Leonid Lantsberg and Mark Goldman

XVIII   VASCULAR GRAFTS

50 Increased Resistance to Staphylococcal Graft Infection by
    Rifampicin Impregnation of Gelatin-Sealed Dacron 483
    John P. Fletcher, J. Avramovic, J. Kenny, and F. Sardelic

51 Involvement of Growth Factors in Pseudointimal
    Hyperplasia Analyzed by Synthetic Somatostatin Analogues   488
    Jun-ichi Kambayashi, Suguru Shibuya, and Makoto Watase

52 Experimental Evaluation of a New Compliant Biological
    Arterial Substitute 495
    Armin Welz, G. Murrmann, S. Grenzner, R. Triefenbach, and
    M. Beyer

XIX VENOUS SYSTEM

53 A New Valvuloplasty for Primary Deep Venous
    Insufficiency 507
    Katsushi Akemoto and Takeshi Ueyama

54 Homolateral Long Saphenous Vein as a Valvulated Graft for
    Reflux Treatment of Deep Venous Postthrombotic Disease   515
    J.M. Cardon, A. Joyeaux, D. Noblet, M.M. Faye, and P. Bousquet

55 Local Gas Analysis in Patients with Venous Ulcers 523
    Živan V. Maksimović, Tomislav Jovanović, Slobodanka Dukić, and
    Siniša Jagodić

56 Local Lactate and Pyruvate Values Prior to and Following a
    Shearing Operation for Venous Ulcers 528
    Živan V. Maksimović, Veljko Djukić, Djordje Radak, and Tomislav
    Javanović

57 Ablative Surgery Versus Sclerotherapy in the Treatment of
    Vein Disease 535
    George M. Robb

58 Functional Evaluation of the Venocuff Sleeve in the Primary
    Great Saphenous Varicose Vein 539
    Bo Yang Suh, Dong Kweon Suh, and Koing Bo Kwun

XX PULMONARY EMBOLISM

59 Genetic Predisposition to Pulmonary Embolism Following
    Deep Vein Thrombosis 549
    Tomio Kawasaki, Jun-ichi Kambayashi, and Yoshio Uemura

XXI PORTOSYSTEMIC SHUNT

60 Transjugular Intrahepatic Portosystemic Shunt 561
    Jae Hyung Park, Joon Koo Han, Jin Wook Chung, and Man
    Chung Han

61 Effectiveness of Portal Vein Arterialization During an
    Emergency Situation in Partial Liver Transplantation 569
    Masahiko Yamaguchi, Kaoru Kumada, Hiroshi Higashiyama,
    Taisuke Morimoto, and Kazue Ozawa

XXII ANGIOACCESS

62 Factors Influencing the Patency of Arteriovenous Fistulae in
Patients with Chronic Renal Failure 577
W.H. Cho, Y.S. Kim, and H.C. Kim

63 Arteriovenous Fistula for Hemodialysis: Early Failure or
Complications According to Different Criteria for Patient
Selection and Surgical Procedures 587
Yu Seun Kim, Soo Ho Choo, and Kiil Park

Index 593

Contributors

Fredy Abed, MD, Department of Surgery, Hospital Herrera Llerandi, Guatemala City, Guatemala

Narutsugu Adachi, MD, Department of Cardiovascular Surgery, National Cardiovascular Center, Osaka, Japan

Sunil Agarwal, MS, Lecturer in Surgery, Department of Surgery, Christian Medical College and Hospital, Vellore, South India

Bum Gyu Ahn, MD, Department of Radiology, Chunchon Sacred Heart Hospital, School of Medicine, Hallym University, Kangwon-Do, Chunchon, Korea

Chang Joon Ahn, MD, Department of Surgery, Kangnam St. Mary's Hospital, Catholic University Medical College, Seoul, Korea

Hyuk Ahn, MD, Department of Thoracic and Cardiovascular Surgery, College of Medicine, Seoul National University Hospital, Seoul, Korea

Katsushi Akemoto, MD, Department of Cardiovascular Surgery, National Hospital of Kanazawa, Kanazawa, Ishikawa, Japan

Gabriel S. Aldea, MD, Department of Cardiothoracic Surgery, Boston University Medical Center, Boston, Massachusetts, USA

Haruo Aramoto, MD, First Department of Surgery, University of Tokyo, Tokyo, Japan

Tatsuro Asada, MD, Department of Cardiovascular Surgery, Hyogo Brain and Heart Center, Himeji, Japan

J. Avramovic, MB, BS, FRACS, Department of Surgery, Westmead Hospital, Sydney, New South Wales, Australia

Nobuyoshi Azuma, MD, First Department of Surgery, Asahikawa Medical College, Asahikawa, Japan

Wan Ki Baek, MD, Department of Thoracic and Cardiovascular Surgery, Sejong General Hospital, Puchon, Kyunggi-do, Korea

Roger N. Baird, MD, Consultant Surgeon and Honorary Clinical Lecturer in Surgery, Bristol Royal Infirmary, Bristol, United Kingdom

Hendrick B. Barner, MD, Professor of Cardiothoracic Surgery, Albert Einstein College of Medicine; Chief, Division of Cardiothoracic Surgery, The Heart Institute, Long Island Jewish Medical Center, New Hyde Park, New York, USA

Stefan Belov, MD, PhD, Former Chief, Department of Thoracic Surgery, Clinic of Thoracic and Cardiovascular Surgery, Sofia, Bulgaria; Professor of Surgery, Consultant and Lecturer, Center for Haemodynamic Disturbances and Vascular Defects, Hamburg, Germany; Center for Diagnostics and Treatment of Vascular Malformations, Milan, Italy

Yury V. Belov, MD, Professor, Department of Coronary and Vascular Surgery, National Research Center of Surgery, Moscow, Russia

M. Beyer, MD, Department of Surgery, Ulm University Hospital, Ulm, Germany

Mikael Bitsch, MD, Registrar, Department of Vascular Surgery, Rigshospitalet, Copenhagen, Denmark

P. Bousquet, MD, Clinique de Franciscaines, Nimes, France

Allan D. Callow, MD, PhD, Department of Surgery, Washington University School of Medicine, St. Louis, Missouri, USA

Jean-Marie Cardon, MD, Clinique de Franciscaines, Nimes, France

Kwon Mook Chae, MD, Department of General Surgery, Wonkwang University Hospital, I-Ri City, Cheonbuk, Korea

John B. Chang, MD, Director, Long Island Vascular Clinic, Roslyn, New York; Associate Clinical Professor of Surgery, Albert Einstein College of Medicine, Bronx, New York, USA

Soo Il Chang, MD, Professor of Surgery, Kyungpook National University Hospital, Taegu, Korea

Thay-Hsiung Chen, MD, Department of Thoracic and Cardiovascular Surgery, Cathay General Hospital, Taipei, Taiwan, ROC

Won Hyun Cho, MD, PhD, Associate Professor of Surgery, Department of General Surgery, Keimyung University School of Medicine, Taegu, Korea

Chang Sig Choi, MD, Department of Surgery, Chunchon Sacred Heart Hospital, School of Medicine, Hallym University, Chunchon, Kangwon-Do, Korea

Eric T. Choi, MD, Department of Surgery, Washington University School of Medicine, St. Louis, Missouri, USA

Jae Seok Choi, MD, Resident in Surgery, Kyungpook National University Hospital, Taegu, Korea

See Sung Choi, MD, Department of Radiology, Wonkwang University School of Medicine, Cheonbuk, Korea

Soo Ho Choo, MD, Chief Resident, Yonsei University College of Medicine; Department of Surgery, Severance Hospital, Seoul, Korea

Hae Myung Chun, MD, Department of Surgery, Kangnam St. Mary's Hospital, Catholic University Medical College, Seoul, Korea

Hwan Yung Chung, MD, Professor and Chairman, Department of Neurosurgery, Hanyang University School of Medicine, Inchun, Korea

Jin Wook Chung, MD, Department of Radiology, Seoul National University, College of Medicine, Seoul, Korea

Ki Yong Chung, MD, PhD, Professor of Surgery, Department of General Surgery, Keimyung University School of Medicine, Taegu, Korea

Denton A. Cooley, MD, Surgeon-in-Chief, Texas Heart Institute; Clinical Professor of Surgery, Unversity of Texas Medical School, Houston, Texas, USA

Marianne G. De Maeseneer, MD, Division of Vascular Surgery, Antwerp University Hospital and Medical School, Edegem, Belgium

Veljko Djukić, MD, PhD, Department of Vascular Surgery, University Clinical Centre, Institute for Cardiovascular Diseases, Belgrade, Yugoslavia

Slobodanka Dukić, MD, Institute for Microbiology, Belgrade Faculty for Medicine, Belgrade, Yugoslavia

Thomas R. Eide, MD, Clinical Director, Department of Anesthesiology, Long Island Jewish Medical Center, New Hyde Park, New York, USA

Mitsuo Endo, MD, First Department of Surgery, School of Medicine, Tokyo Medical and Dental University, Tokyo, Japan

Kensuke Esato, MD, First Department of Surgery, Yamaguchi University of Medicine, Ube, Yamaguchi, Japan

M. M. Faye, MD, Clinique de Franciscaines, Nimes, France

John P. Fletcher, MD, MS, FRACS, FRCS, DDU, Associate Professor of Surgery, University of Sydney, Chairman, Division of Surgery, Westmead Hospital, Sydney, New South Wales, Australia

James D. Fonger, MD, Associate Professor of Surgery, Division of Cardiac Surgery, Johns Hopkins University, Baltimore, Maryland; Department of Cardiothoracic Surgery, Boston University Medical Center, Boston, Masssachusetts, USA

Kentaro Fujioka, MD, First Department of Surgery, Yamaguchi University of Medicine, Ube, Yamaguchi, Japan

Akira Furutani, MD, First Department of Surgery, Yamaguchi University of Medicine, Ube, Yamaguchi, Japan

Kazutomo Goh, MD, First Department of Surgery, Asahikawa Medical College, Asahikawa, Japan

Mark Goldman, MD, Consultant General and Vascular Surgeon, Department of Surgery, East Birmingham Hospital, Birmingham, United Kingdom

S. Grenzner, MD, Department of Surgery, Ulm University Hospital, Ulm, Germany

Duck Jong Han, MD, Department of Surgery, College of Medicine, Ulsan University, Seoul, Korea

Joon Koo Han, MD, Department of Radiology, Seoul National University College of Medicine, Seoul, Korea

Man Chung Han, MD, Department of Radiology, Seoul National University College of Medicine, Seoul, Korea

Tetsuya Higami, MD, Department of Cardiovascular Surgery, Hyogo Brain and Heart Center, Himeji, Japan

Hiroshi Higashiyama, MD, Second Department of Surgery, Kyoto University, Kyoto, Japan

Larry H. Hollier, MD, FACS, FACC, Clinical Professor of Surgery, Louisiana State University Medical Center and Tulane University Medical Center; Chairman, Department of Surgery, Ochsner Clinic and Alton Ochsner Medical Foundation, New Orleans, Louisiana, USA

Young Soon Hyun, MD, Department of Surgery, College of Medicine, Ulsan University, Seoul, Korea

Masataka Ichiki, MD, Associate Director of the Department of Surgery, Sendai Hospital of East Japan Railway Company, Sendai, Japan

Masashi Inaba, MD, First Department of Surgery, Asahikawa Medical College, Asahikawa, Japan

Yoshinori Inoue, MD, First Department of Surgery, School of Medicine, Tokyo Medical and Dental University, Tokyo, Japan

Takehisa Iwai, MD, Associate Professor, First Department of Surgery, School of Medicine, Tokyo Medical and Dental University, Tokyo, Japan

Yuhichi Izumi, MD, First Department of Surgery, Asahikawa Medical College, Asahikawa, Japan

Tomislav Jovanović, MD, PhD, School of Medicine, Institute for Physiology, Belgrade, Yugoslavia

Liang Ji-he, Department of Cardiothoracic Surgery, Xi-Jing Hospital, Xi'an, Shaanxi Province, PR China

Yan Jing-xue, Department of Cardiothoracic Surgery, Xi-Jing Hospital, Xi'an, Shaanxi Province, PR China

Siniša Jagodić, MD, Institute for Cardiovascular Diseases; Department of Vascular Surgery, University Clinical Centre, Belgrade, Yugoslavia

Stanley John, MD, Professor, Head of the Department of Thoracic and Cardiovascular Surgery, Christian Medical College and Hospital, Vellore, South India

Bo Jørgensen, MD, Departments of Clinical Physiology/Nuclear Medicine and Thoracic and Vascular Surgery, Skejby Hospital, University of Aarhus, Aarhus N., Denmark

Tomislav Jovanović, MD, PhD, Institute for Physiology, Belgrade Faculty for Medicine, Belgrade, Yugoslavia

Andre Joyeaux, MD, Clinique de Franciscaines, Nimes, France

Seon Kwan Juhng, MD, Department of Radiology, Wonkwang University, School of Medicine, Chonbuk, Korea

Jun-ichi Kambayashi, MD, PhD, Associate Professor, Vascular Surgery Service, Second Department of Surgery, Osaka University Medical School, Osaka, Japan

Shuzo Kamioki, MD, Director of the Department of Surgery, Sendai Hospital of East Japan Railway Company, Sendai, Japan

Joonghee Kang, MD, Second Department of Surgery, Osaka University Medical School, Osaka, Japan

Tomio Kawasaki, MD, PhD, Assistant Professor, Vascular Surgery Service, Second Department of Surgery, Osaka University Medical School, Osaka, Japan

J. Kenny, MB, ChB, Department of Surgery, Westmead Hospital, Sydney, New South Wales, Australia

Chang Guhn Kim, MD, Department of Radiology, Wonkwang University, School of Medicine, Chonbuk, Korea

H.C. Kim, MD, Department of Internal Medicine, Keimyung University, School of Medicine, Taegu, Korea

In Chul Kim, MD, Department of Surgery, Kangnam St. Mary's Hospital, Catholic Univerity Medical College, Seoul, Korea

Seung Nam Kim, MD, Department of Surgery, Kangnam St. Mary's Hospital, Catholic University Medical College, Seoul, Korea

Wook Kim, MD, Department of Surgery, Kangnam St. Mary's Hospital, Catholic University Medical College, Seoul, Korea

You-Sah Kim, MD, PhD, Professor, Department of Surgery, Keimyung University School of Medicine, Taegu, Korea

Young Wook Kim, MD, Assistant Professor of Surgery, Kyungpook National University Hospital, Taegu, Korea

Yu Seun Kim, MD, Assistant Professor, Yonsei University College of Medicine, Department of Surgery, Severance Hospital, Seoul, Korea

Yong Bok Koh, MD, Professor, Department of Surgery, Kangnam St. Mary's Hospital, Catholic University Medical College, Seoul, Korea

Hisaaki Koie, MD, Professor, First Department of Surgery, Hirosaki University School of Medicine, Hirosaki City, Aomori Prefecture, Japan

Takashi Komiyama, MD, First Department of Surgery, University of Tokyo, Tokyo, Japan

A.N. Kosencov, PhD, Lecturer, Department of Coronary and Vascular Surgery, National Research Center of Surgery, Moscow, Russia

Toshiyuki Kubo, MD, First Department of Surgery, University of Tokyo, Tokyo, Japan

Yoshihiko Kubo, MD, Professor and Chairman, First Department of Surgery, Asahikawa Medical College, Asahikawa, Japan

Takayuki Kuga, MD, First Department of Surgery, Yamaguchi University of Medicine, Ube, Yamaguchi, Japan

Kaoru Kumada, MD, Department of Surgery, Showa University, Yokohama, Japan

Koing Bo Kwun, MD, FACS, Professor, Department of Surgery, Yeungnam University College of Medicine, Taegu, Korea

Peter M. Lamont, MD, Consultant Surgeon and Honorary Clinical Lecturer in Surgery, Bristol Royal Infirmary, Bristol, United Kingdom

Leonid Lantsberg, MD, Senior Surgeon, Department of General and Vascular Surgery, Soroka Medical Center; Lecturer in Surgery, Ben-Gurion University of the Negev, Israel

Yong Kak Lee, MD, PhD, FACS, President, Korean Vascular Surgery Society; Director and President, Inha University Medical Center, Seoul, Korea

Philippe Lehert, DR IR, PhD, Facultes Universitaires de Mons, Mons, Belgium

Jill C. Locke-Edmunds, DMS, Department of Surgery, University of Bristol, Bristol Royal Infirmary, Bristol, United Kingdom

Jørgen E. Lorentzen, MD, Consultant and Chief of Vascular Surgery, Department of Vascular Surgery, Rigshospitalet, Copenhagen, Denmark

Živan V. Maksimović, MD, PhD, Assistant Professor, Department of Vascular Surgery, University Clinical Centre, Institute for Cardiovascular Diseases, Belgrade, Yugoslavia

Masahisa Masuda, MD, First Department of Surgery, Chiba University School of Medicine, Chiba, Japan

Yoshiro Matsui, MD, Department of Cardiovascular Surgery, Hokkaido University School of Medicine, Sapporo, Japan

Hiroshi Matsuura, MD, Department of Cardiothoracic Surgery, Boston University Medical Center, Boston, Massachusetts, USA

Ju Ming-da, MD, Department of Cardiothoracic Surgery, Xi-Jing Hospital, Xi'an, Shaanxi province, PR of China

Yoshio Mishima, MD, Professor and Chairman, Department of Surgery, Tokyo Medical and Dental University, Tokyo, Japan

J. Ernesto Molina, MD, PhD, Department of Surgery, Division of Cardiovascular and Thoracic Surgery, University of Minnesota, Minneapolis, Minnesota

Samuel R. Money, MD, Fellow in Vascular Surgery, Department of Surgery, Ochsner Clinic and Alton Ochsner Medical Foundation, New Orleans, Louisiana, USA

Taisuke Morimoto, MD, Second Department of Surgery, Kyoto University, Kyoto, Japan

Booshanam V. Moses, MD, Professor of Surgery, Head of the Department of Surgery, Christian Medical College and Hospital, Vellore, South India

Nobuhiko Mukohara, MD, Department of Cardiovascular Surgery, Hyogo Brain and Heart Center, Himeji, Japan

G. Murrmann, MD, Department of Surgery, Ulm University Hospital, Ulm, Germany

Tetsuichiro Muto, MD, First Department of Surgery, University of Tokyo, Tokyo, Japan

Nobuyuki Nakajima, MD, First Department of Surgery, Chiba University School of Medicine, Chiba, Japan

Mitsuru Nakaya, MD, Department of Cardiovascular Surgery, National Cardiovascular Center, Osaka, Japan

Jørn Dalsgaard Nielsen, MD, Department of Internal Medicine, Thrombosis Research Center, Bispebjerg Hospital, University of Copenhagen, Copenhagen, Denmark

Masami Nishiwaki, MD, Department of Cardiovascular Surgery, Hyogo Brain and Heart Center, Himeji, Japan

Daniel Noblet, MD, Clinique de Franciscaines, Nimes, France

Shinji Nomura, MD, First Department of Surgery, Hirosaki University School of Medicine, Hirosaki City, Aomori Prefecture, Japan

Kyoichi Ogawa, MD, Department of Cardiovascular Surgery, Hyogo Brain and Heart Center, Himeji, Japan

Kichiya Okuyama, MD, Associate Director of the Department of Surgery, Sendai Hospital of East Japan Railway Company, Sendai, Japan

Hiroshi Ouchi, MD, Director of the Hospital, Sendai Hospital of East Japan Railway Company, Sendai, Japan

Kazue Ozawa, MD, Second Department of Surgery, Kyoto University, Kyoto, Japan

Cho Hyun Park, MD, Department of Surgery, Kangnam St. Mary's Hospital, Catholic University Medical College, Seoul, Korea

Choong Ki Park, MD, Department of Radiology, Chunchon Sacred Heart Hospital, School of Medicine, Hallym University, Chunchon, Kangwon-Do, Korea

Jae Hyung Park, MD, Department of Radiology, Seoul National University College of Medicine, Seoul, Korea

Jang Sang Park, MD, PhD, Department of Surgery, Kangnam St. Mary's Hospital, Catholic University Medical College, Seoul, Korea

Kiil Park, MD, Professor of Surgery, Yonsei University College of Medicine; Department of Surgery, Severance Hospital, Seoul, Korea

Thomas C. Park, MD, Vascular Surgery Fellow, Oregon Health Sciences University, Portland, Oregon, USA

Michael G. Petty, RN, Division of Cardiovascular and Thoracic Surgery, University of Minnesota, Minneapolis, Minnesota

Djordje Radak, MD, PhD, Department of Vascular Surgery, University Clinical Centre, Institute for Cardiovascular Diseases, Belgrade, Yugoslavia

George M. Robb, MD, Vein Clinic, New Westminster, British Columbia, Canada

Byung Suk Roh, MD, Department of Radiology, Wonkwang University School of Medicine, Chonbuk, Korea

Una S. Ryan, PhD, Department of Surgery, Washington University School of Medicine, St. Louis, Missouri, USA

R. David Sadhu, MD, Department of Surgery, Christian Medical College and Hospital, Vellore, South India

Masato Sakon, MD, Second Department of Surgery, Osaka University Medical School, Osaka, Japan

Makoto Sakuma, MD, Department of Cardiovascular Surgery, Second Department of Surgery, Hokkaido University School of Medicine, Sapporo, Japan

F. Sardelic, MB, BS, Department of Surgery, Westmead Hospital, Sydney, New Sourh Wales, Australia

Tadahiro Sasajima, MD, First Department of Surgery, Asahikawa Mcdical College, Asahikawa, Japan

Shoji Sato, MD, First Department of Surgery, School of Medicine, Tokyo Medical and Dental University, Tokyo, Japan

Torben V. Schroeder, MD, DMSc, Professor of Surgery, University of Copenhagen; Consultant in Surgery, Department of Vascular Surgery, Rigshospitalet, Copenhagen, Denmark

Niraj Sehgal, Department of Surgery, Washington University School of Medicine, St. Louis, Missouri, USA

Richard J. Shemin, MD, Department of Cardiothoracic Surgery, Boston University Medical Center, Boston, Massachusetts, USA

Ei-ichi Shiba, MD, Second Department of Surgery, Osaka University School of Medicine, Osaka, Japan

Suguru Shibuya, MD, Research Fellow, Second Department of Surgery, Osaka University Medical School, Osaka, Japan

Hiroshi Shigematsu, MD, First Department of Surgery, University of Tokyo, Tokyo, Japan

Masayuki Shimizu, MD, First Department of Surgery, Hirosaki University School of Medicine, Hirosaki City, Aomori Prefecture, Japan

Byung Jun So, MD, Department of Surgery, Wonkwang University Hospital, I-Ri City, Cheonbuk, Korea

Felisberto M. Soriano, Jr., MD, Department of Surgery, San Juan De Dios Hospital, Manila, Phillipines

Kazuro Sugi, MD, First Department of Surgery, Yamaguchi University of Medicine, Ube, Yamaguchi, Japan

Takaki Sugimoto, MD, Department of Cardiovascular Surgery, Hyogo Brain and Heart Center, Himeji, Japan

Bo Yang Suh, MD, FACS, Professor, Department of Surgery, Yeungnam University College of Medicine, Taegu, Korea

Dong Kweon Suh, MD, Department of Surgery, Yeungnam University College of Medicine, Taegu, Korea

Soo Jhi Suh, MD, PhD, Professor of Radiology, Department of Radiology, Keimyung University School of Medicine, Taegu, Korea

Shaping Sun, MMS, Department of Surgery, Washington University School of Medicine, St. Louis, Missouri, USA

Sohei Suzuki, MD, Assistant Professor, First Department of Surgery, Hirosaki University School of Medicine, Hirosaki City, Aomori Prefecture, Japan

Shigeyasu Takeuchi, MD, First Department of Surgery, Chiba University School of Medicine, Chiba, Japan

Noriakai Takiguchi, MD, First Department of Surgery, School of Medicine, Tokyo Medical and Dental University, Tokyo, Japan

Tatsuzo Tanabe, MD, Department of Cardiovascular Surgery, Second Department of Surgery, Hokkaido University School of Medicine, Sapporo, Japan

Masahiko Tanaka, MD, First Department of Surgery, Hirosaki University School of Medicine, Hirosaki City, Aomori Prefecture, Japan

John F. Thompson, MD, Lecturer in Surgery and Honorary Senior Registrar in Surgery, Bristol Royal Infirmary, Bristol, United Kingdom

Masaki Tomikawa, MD, Department of Surgery, Toyama Medical and Pharmaceutical University, Toyama, Japan

Jeffrey Trachtenberg, MD, Department of Surgery, Washington University School of Medicine, St. Louis, Missouri, USA

R. Triefenbach, MD, Department of Surgery, Ulm University Hospital, Ulm, Germany

Yoshifumi Tsuji, MD, Second Department of Surgery, Osaka University School of Medicine, Osaka, Japan

Hidetoshi Tuboi, MD, First Department of Surgery, Yamaguchi University of Medicine, Ube, Yamaguchi, Japan

Yoshio Uemura, MD, PhD, Research Fellow, Vascular Surgery Service, Second Department of Surgery, Osaka University Medical School, Osaka, Japan

Takeshi Ueyama, MD, Department of Surgery, Toyama Medical and Pharmaceutical University Toyama; Department of Cardiovascular Surgery, National Hospital of Kanazawa, Kanazawa, Japan

Robin F. Van Look, MD, Division of Vascular Surgery, Antwerp University Hospital and Medical School, Edegem, Belgium

Rudolph G. Vanmaele, MD, PhD, FICA, Chief, Division of Vascular Surgery, Antwerp University Hospital and Medical School, Edegem, Belgium

Paul E. Van Schil, MD, Department of Vascular Surgery, Antwerp University Hospital and Medical School, Edegem, Belgium

Zsolt A. Varga, MD, Assistant Professor, Department of Cardiovascular Surgery, Semmelweis Medical University, Budapest, Hungary

Roy Vargese, MS, Department of Coronary and Vascular Surgery, National Research Center of Surgery, Moscow, Russia

Romulo G. Vea, MD, Department of Radiology, San Juan De Dios Hospital, Manilla, Philippines

Makoto Watase, MD, PhD, Research Fellow, Division of Vascular Surgery, Yale University School of Medicine, New Haven, Connecticut, USA

Zhang Wei-lian, MD, Department of Thoracic and Cardiovascular Surgery, Xi-jing Hospital, Xi'an, Shaanxi Province, PR of China

Liu Wei-yong, MD, Department of Thoracic and Cardiovascular Surgery, Xi-jing Hospital, Xi'an, Shaanxi Province, PR of China

Armin Welz, MD, Department of Surgery, Ulm University Hospital, Ulm, Germany

Il Woo Whang, MD, Professor, Department of Surgery, Kyungpook National University School of Medicine, Taegu, Korea

Jong Jin Won, MD, Department of Radiology, Wonkwang University School of Medicine, Chonbuk, Korea

Jong Man Won, MD, Department of Surgery, Kangnam St. Mary's Hospital, Catholic University Medical College, Seoul, Korea

Masahiko Yamaguchi, MD, Second Department of Surgery, Kyoto University, Kyoto, Japan

Keiichi Yamamoto, MD, Department of Surgery, Toyama Medical and Pharmaceutical University, Toyama, Japan

Xi Ming Yang, MD, PhD, Department of Cardiothoracic Surgery, Boston University Medical Center, Boston, Massachusetts, USA

Keishu Yasuda, MD, Chairman, Professor of Surgery, Department of Cardiovascular Surgery, Hokkaido University School of Medicine, Sapporo, Japan

Hiroshi Yasuhara, MD, First Department of Surgery, University of Tokyo, Tokyo, Japan

Masayasu Yokokawa, MD, Department of Surgery, Toyama Medical and Pharmaceutical University, Toyama, Japan

Wansik Yu, MD, Associate Professor, Department of Surgery, Kyungpook National University School of Medicine, Taegu, Korea

Seok Kil Zeon, MD, PhD, Professor of Radiology, Department of Radiology, Keimyung University School of Medicine, Taegu, Korea

Liu Zong-gui, MD, Associate Professor, Department of Thoracic and Cardiovascular Surgery, Xi-jing Hospital, Xi'an, Shaanxi Province, PR of China

Introduction

For many years I have been very fortunate to have the opportunity to meet leading scholars from around the world at the international vascular symposia. I am indebted to many outstanding teachers, surgeons, physicians, and students through the years. This book is based upon the presentations made at the International Vascular Symposium held in October 1992. We moved our International Vascular Symposium to Seoul, South Korea, where we met with many outstanding scholars from all over the world, including East and West. There are many different vascular disease entities which we are not familiar with in the United States. Therefore, I truly believe that the scientific podium offered a panoramic view of international vascular surgical practices, in both the basic and clinical arenas.

I extend my sincere appreciation to my many friends at our institution for their support. Also, my special appreciation goes to my long-time friends, Denton Cooley, MD, Larry Hollier, MD, Yoshio Mishima, MD, and so many others. My sincere gratitude goes to the members of the Korean Vascular Society, particularly President Yong Kak Lee, MD. My personal thanks go to Ms. Ann J. Boehme, who has been exceptionally loyal to me in helping to put together this wonderful academic symposium. I thank the members of my staff at the Long Island Vascular Center for their continuing support and unselfish work to support my academic duties. My special thanks go to Ms. Eileen Moran Zanini, my executive secretary, who for over a decade has helped in many aspects of my work and in developing this book. My sincere appreciation and love go to my dear wife and lifetime friend, Lucy J. Chang, MD, for her strong support and understanding through the years.

John B. Chang, MD, FACS

About the Editor

John B. Chang, MD, FACS

Director
Long Island Vascular Center
Roslyn, New York

President
International College of Angiology

Editor-in-Chief
International Journal of Angiology

Founding Chairman
Board of Directors
Asian Vascular Society

Chairman
Vascular Surgery Section
International College of Surgeons
USA Section

Program Chairman
6th International Vascular Symposium

Chairman
Department of Surgery
Chief, Division of Vascular Surgery
Little Neck Community Hospital
Little Neck, New York

Attending Vascular Surgeon
St. Francis Hospital
Roslyn, New York

Former and Founding Director
Division of Vascular Surgery
Department of Surgery
Long Island Jewish Medical Center
New Hyde Park, New York

Consultant
Department of Surgery
Long Island Jewish Medical Center
New Hyde Park, New York

Associate Professor of Clinical Surgery
Albert Einstein College of Medicine
Bronx, New York

I
Newer Concepts in Vascular Surgery

1
Arterial Reconstruction of the Lower Extremities

YOSHIHIKO KUBO, TADAHIRO SASAJIMA, KAZUTOMO GOH,
MASASHI INABA, YUICHI IZUMI, AND NOBUYOSHI AZUMA

Introduction

Although the recent advances in arterial reconstructive surgery have been steady and remarkable, there still remain several tall hurdles to overcome. One problem is suitable graft material for small-caliber arteries. Another is its biological behavior in human tissue.

Between 1976 and 1992 we performed about 1,500 arterial reconstructions of the lower extremities with occlusive lesions due to arteriosclerosis obliterans (ASO) or thromboangiitis obliterans (Table 1.1). Here, the operative results obtained mainly from patients with ASO are discussed, focusing especially on the pathologic changes of the grafts that have occurred in the follow-up period and our clinical strategy against them.

Data were analyzed in accordance with the recommendations made by the Ad Hoc Committee of the International Society of Cardiovascular Surgery in 1986.[1]

Aortoiliac Region

Patients

The age of the patients with the disease in this region becomes higher as the severity of the symptom progresses. Patients older than 70 years constitute only 39% of patients with grade II disease. On the other hand, the percentage of patients in this age group in the population with grade III or IV disease is as high as 59% (Table 1.2).

Operative Strategy

The lesions recognized in ASO patients tend to be multiple. Like others,[2] our previous studies suggested that more favorable long-term results could

TABLE 1.1. Procedures for peripheral arterial reconstruction during the past 17 years in Asahikawa Medical College.

Procedure	No.
Aortoiliac	224
Aortofemoral	457
Femoropopliteal	307
Femorocrural	183
Femoroplantar	24
Extraanatomical	162
Renal, visceral	110
Carotid, vertebral	7
Upper extremities	16
Others	14
Total	1,504

TABLE 1.2. Distribution of patients' age and the grade of the disease. Older patients tend to present with more severe disease.

Fontaine	Total cases	Over 70 years old
II	223	87 (39.0%)
III and IV	92	54 (58.7%)
	315	141 (44.8%)

be obtained by more complete revascularization. An aggressive policy to reconstruct all distal lesions as much as technically possible has been maintained when aortoiliac revascularization has been attempted. The graft of choice in this region has been a Dacron prosthesis.

Operative Results

The operative mortality was 2.7%. The overall cumulative primary patency rate of 457 aortofemoral bypasses at 10 years was 82.8%, and the secondary patency rate reached as high as 96.5%. Major complications encountered in this region were anastomotic aneurysm in the femoral artery in 3.9%, outflow occlusion in 2.8%, and graft infection in 1.2%. These rates are almost comparable to those in other reports.[3]

Bioprosthesis in the Infrainguinal Region

In the infrainguinal region, there are still problems to be solved. First of all, there is no graft material comparable to the autogenous vein. Many vascular substitutes, including bioprostheses as well as synthetic grafts, have been developed since Dr. Voorhees' new concept.

Operative Strategy

For patients without suitable vein grafts, with poor vein grafts, or in whom the need for coronary artery reconstruction is likely, the human umbilical cord vein homograft, Biograft, developed by Dr. Dardik, has been used as the graft of second choice.[4] The graft was implanted with the proximal anastomosis on the femoral artery and the distal anastomosis on the above-knee popliteal artery, the below-knee popliteal artery, and the crural artery.

Operative Results

The overall 5-year primary patency rate is 36%, and the secondary patency rate is 47%. These low patency rates were largely influenced by the poor results in the group of patients whose distal anastomosis had to be on the popliteal artery below the knee or the crural artery. The 5-year primary and secondary patency rates were 32% and 48%, respectively, in the patients with femoropopliteal bypass below the knee, and 8% in those with femorocrural bypass. On the contrary, the 5-year primary and secondary cumulative patency rates in those with femoro-popliteal bypass above the knee are 65% and 72%, respectively.

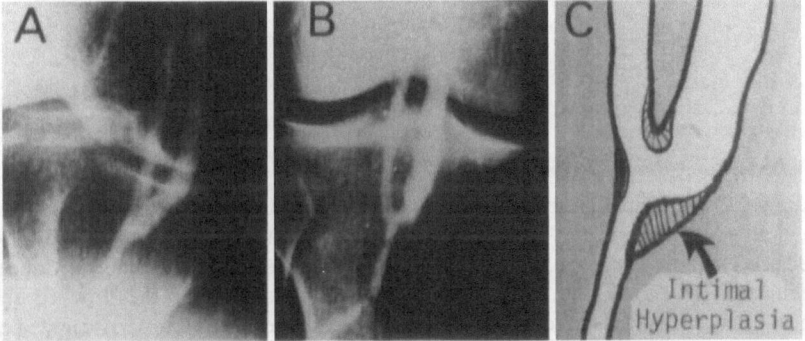

FIGURE 1.1. Intimal hyperplasia is noted at the toe and the heel of the anastomosis 16 months after operation in a 67-year-old patient who has received Biograft for femoropopliteal bypass.

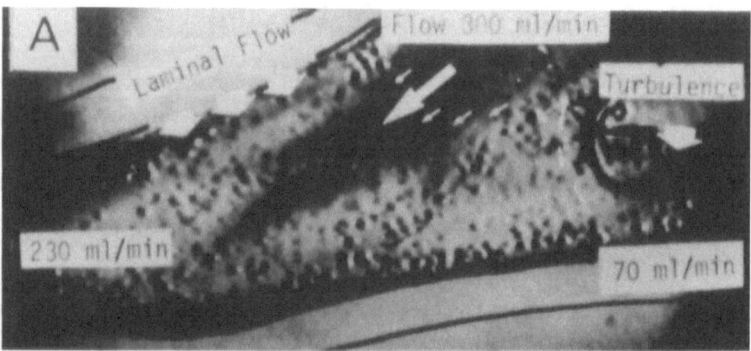

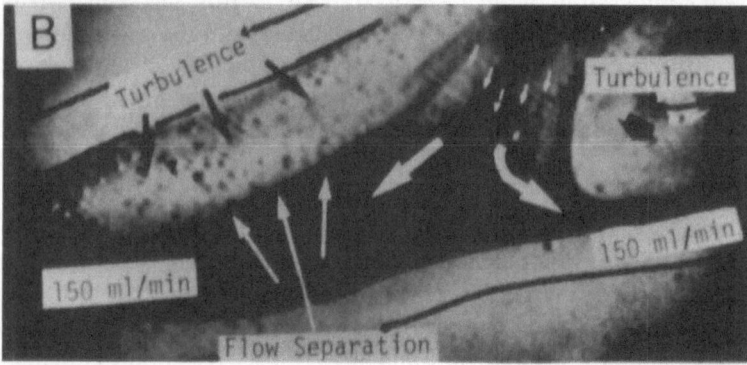

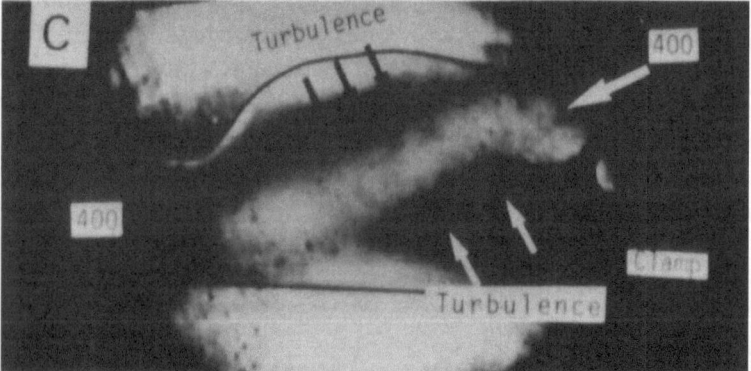

FIGURE 1.2. Experimental model of flow distribution at the distal anastomosis. (A) Total inflow of 300 mL/min is divided into 230 mL/min to the toe and 70 mL/min to the heel. The flow to the toe is a nice laminar flow, whereas that to the heel produces turbulence. (B) When the total flow is divided equally, both the flow to the toe and that to the heel cause turbulence. (C) When the recipient artery is occluded at the heel, the flow forward still generates turbulence if the anastomosis is shaped in a wrong way, like a cobra head.

From these results we conclude that Biograft could be used in this region as an alternative graft to autogenous veins, like other small-caliber prostheses.

Pathological Findings

In clinical observations we have noted that Biograft failure is mainly caused by progressive stenosis at the site of anastomosis due to intimal hyperplasia. The anastomotic intimal hyperplasia has a tendency to occur at the toe and the heel of the distal anastomosis (Fig. 1.1).

The location of progressive hyperplasia corresponds fairly well with the site where turbulence is generated and flow separation happens in an in vitro flow distribution model. Fig. 1.2 shows the generation of turbulence and flow separation at the anastomotic site. These become significant if the proximal flow rate increases compared to the distal flow or if the anastomosis is shaped in the wrong way, like a cobra's head.

In animal experiments, anastomotic intimal hyperplasia similar to the clinical pathology was produced in our model after 1 year of observation. A significant anastomic intimal hyperplasia was observed, and the hyperplastic tissue was separated from the internal surface of the Biograft, with coagula filling between them (Fig. 1.3).

From these observations, we speculated that separation of the hyperplastic

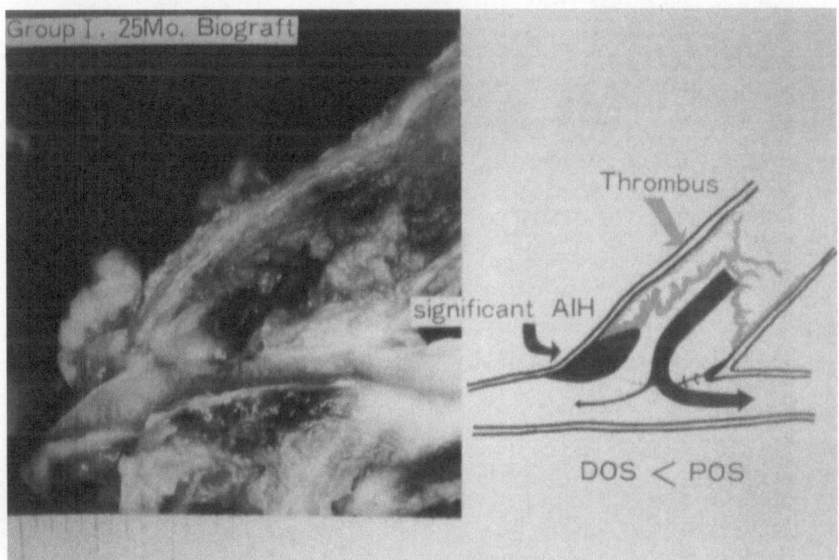

FIGURE 1.3. Biograft at the distal anastomosis taken out 1 year after implantation. Anastomotic intimal hyperplasia (AIH) and thrombus formation in the graft are shown.

pannus from the internal surface of the Biograft at the anastomotic sites would be due to the incapability of the pannus to anchor to the internal surface. This is the main cause of anastomotic intimal hyperplasia and graft failure of Biograft.[5]

Fig. 1.4 shows aneurysm formation of Biograft 7 years after implantation. Degradation of the bioprosthesis in human tissue could not be avoided.[6]

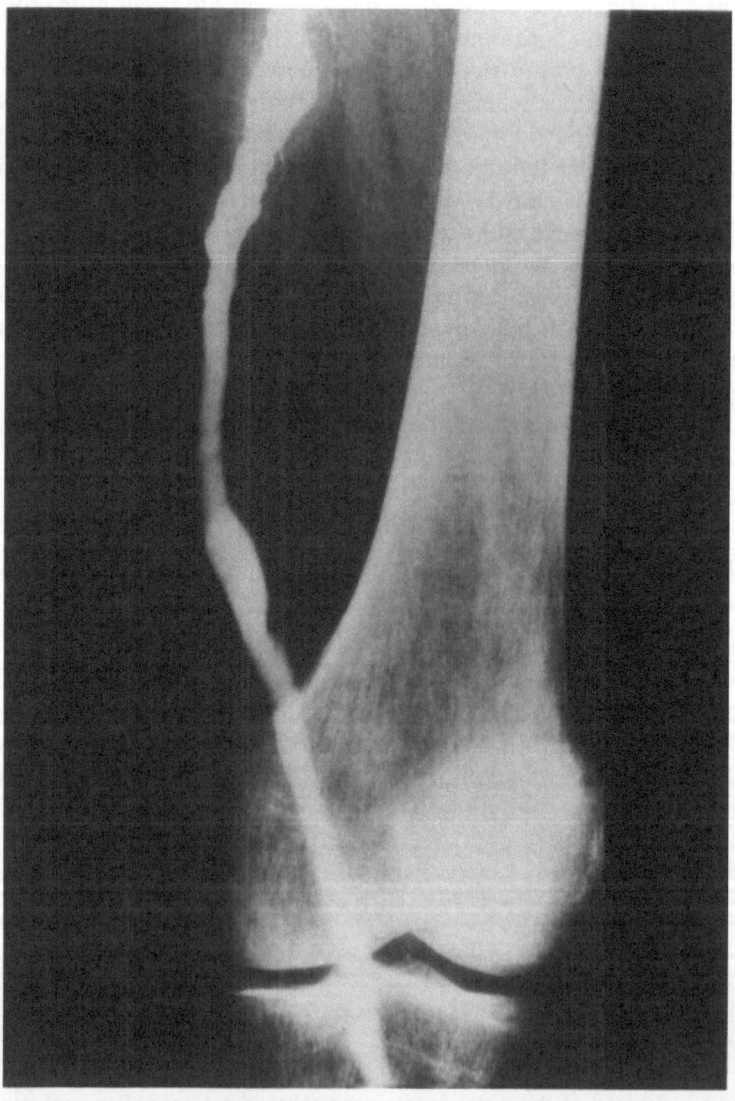

FIGURE 1.4. Aneurysm in Biograft 7 years after implantation.

Autogenous Vein Grafts in the Infrainguinal Region

Autogenous saphenous vein introduced by Dr. Kunlin, is still the graft of choice for arterial reconstruction in the infrainguinal region. However, even autogenous vein should suffer pathological changes from the environment in the long term following surgery.

Operative Strategy

Since 1980 we have performed femoropopliteal bypass with a reversed saphenous vein graft in 163 limbs of 154 patients. Five years later, we started to use in situ vein grafts in comparable regions and patients. Up to 116 in situ vein grafts have been used so far. Both reversed vein and in situ vein grafts were used in almost identical procedures; they were anastomosed between the femoral and the popliteal artery below the knee or the crural artery.

Operative Results

The operative mortality was 2.6%. The cumulative primary and secondary patency rates of 86 reversed-vein grafts in femoropopliteal below-knee bypass at 5 years were 76.5% and 94.7%, respectively (Fig. 1.5). The cumulative primary and secondary patency rates of 81 in situ vein grafts in femoropopliteal below-knee bypass were 68.7% and 92.9%, respectively, at 5 years (Fig. 1.6). The secondary patency rate of the in situ vein grafts is fairly comparable to that of reversed-vein grafts. However, the primary patency rate at 5

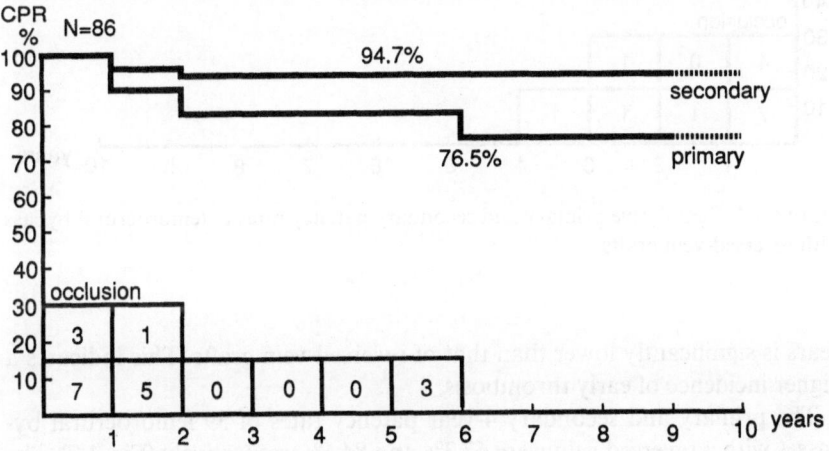

FIGURE 1.5. Cumulative primary and secondary patency rates of femoropopliteal below-knee bypass with reversed saphenous vein grafts.

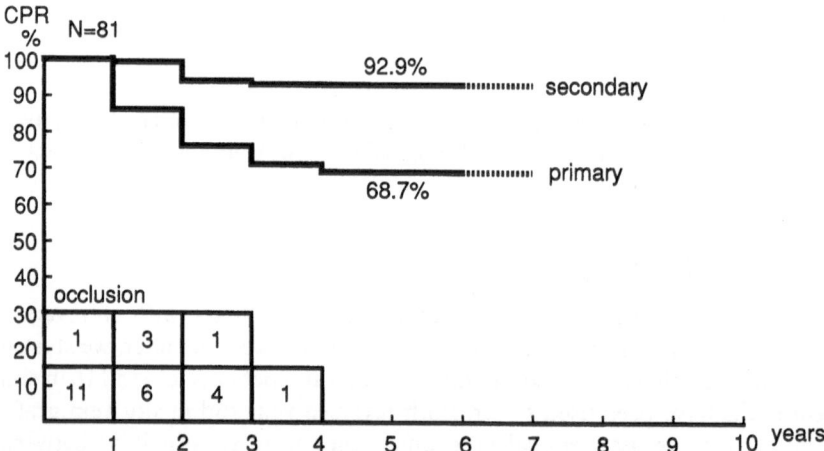

FIGURE 1.6. Cumulative primary and secondary patency rates of femoropopliteal below-knee bypass with *in situ* vein grafts.

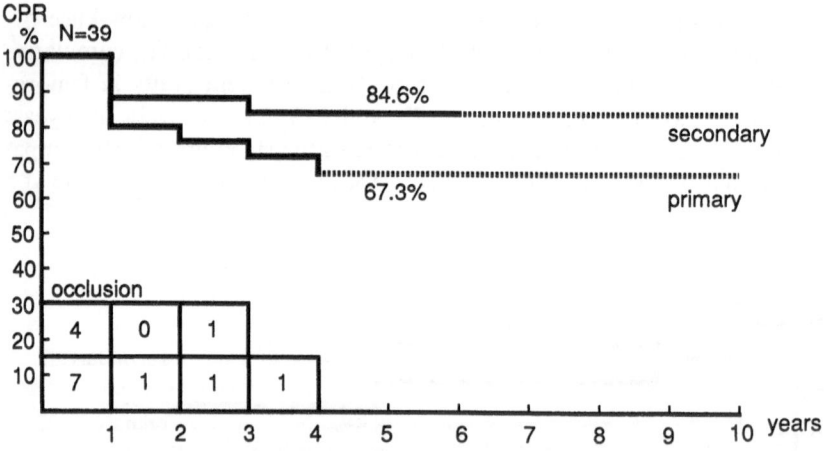

FIGURE 1.7. Cumulative primary and secondary patency rates of femorocrural bypass with reversed-vein grafts.

years is significantly lower than that of reversed-vein grafts. This indicates a higher incidence of early thrombosis.

The primary and secondary 4-year patency rates of 39 femorocrural by-passes with a reversed vein were 67.3% and 84.6%, respectively (Fig. 1.7). The primary and secondary cumulative patency rates of 34 femorocrural bypasses with *in situ* veins were 86.3% and 92.9%, respectively (Fig. 1.8). There is no statistically significant difference between the two vein grafts in the 4-year

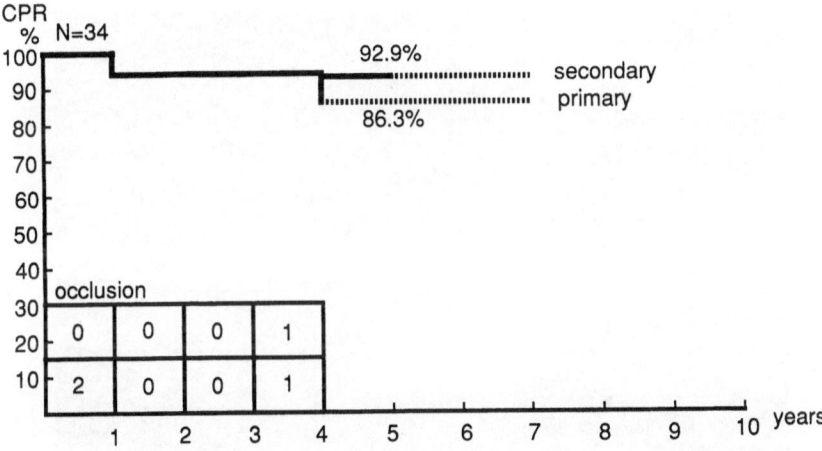

FIGURE 1.8. Cumulative primary and secondary patency rates of femorocrural bypass with in situ vein grafts.

patency rates, although a tendency toward better results in patients with *in situ* vein grafts was noted.

At present, no difference in long-term results can be recognized between reversed and *in situ* vein grafts.[7]

The cumulative limb salvage rate for patients with grade III and IV disease who underwent bypass procedures with vein grafts was 84.9% at 5 years and 80.5% at 8 years. Fig. 1.9 is a postoperative arteriogram showing a patent saphenous vein graft that has been bypassed to the common plantar artery. The patient was a 59-year-old man who had already lost his fifth toe from a severe ischemic condition of the right foot. The ulcer was completely covered by the skin 3 months later (Fig. 1.10). From experiences like this case, we consider that the distal limits of satisfactory revascularization with autogenous vein grafts are the common and proximal medial or lateral plantar arteries.

Pathological Findings

To make the graft function for a long time after implantation, it is essential to understand the behavior of the graft material in human tissue. Usually the major part of early graft failure is caused by inappropriate operative technique and the poor quality of the vein graft. The incidence of these has become very low.

Fig 1.11 is a scanning electron microscope finding showing a sound endothelial layer on a reversed-vein intima immediately after harvesting during operation. The upper picture in Fig. 1.12 demonstrates the internal surface of a reversed-vein graft 3 hours after implantation in a dog. Almost complete disappearance of endothelial cells from the surface except in the area near the

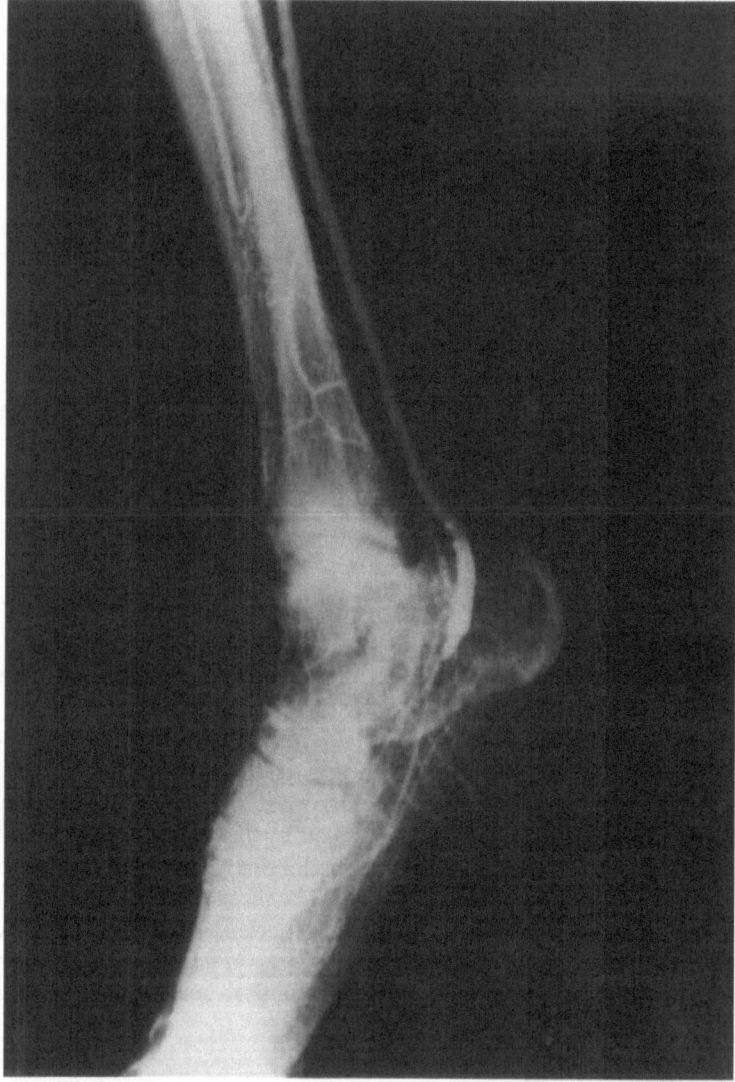

FIGURE 1.9. Postoperative angiogram of a reversed saphenous vein graft to the common plantar artery.

valve is noted. A layer of endothelial cells remains near the valve, although the cells have been deformed (lower picture). Fig. 1.13 shows endothelial cell spreading, starting from the area near the valve 1 week after implantation in a dog. These findings suggest that the residual endothelial cells near the valve may be one of the sources of re-endothelialization, in addition to other sources of endothelial cells such as the ostium of the branch, the site of anastomosis, and the vasa vasorum seen in the vein graft after implantation.[8]

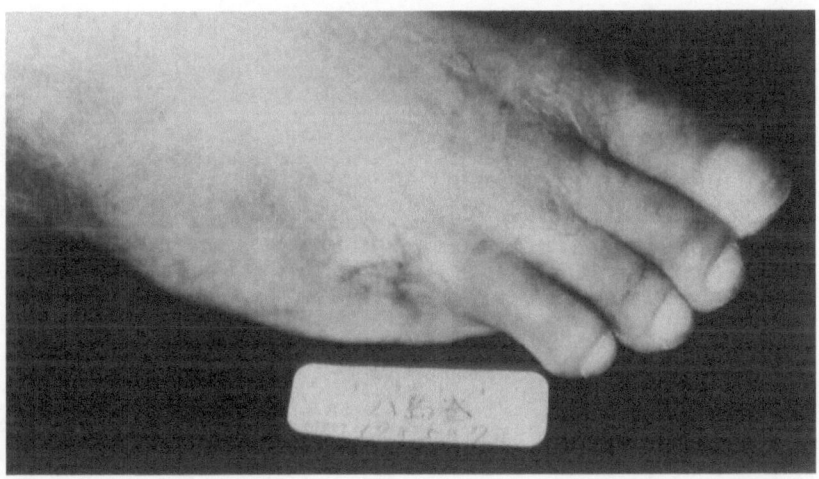

FIGURE 1.10. Foot of the patient in Figure 1.9. The ulcer is completely covered by the skin.

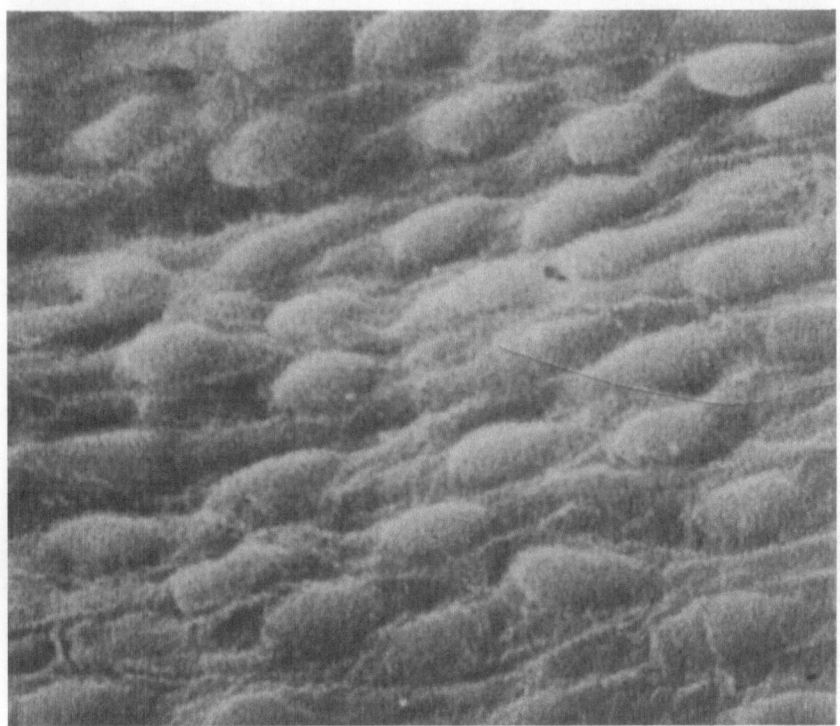

FIGURE 1.11. Scanning electron microscopic finding of the healthy endothelial layer.

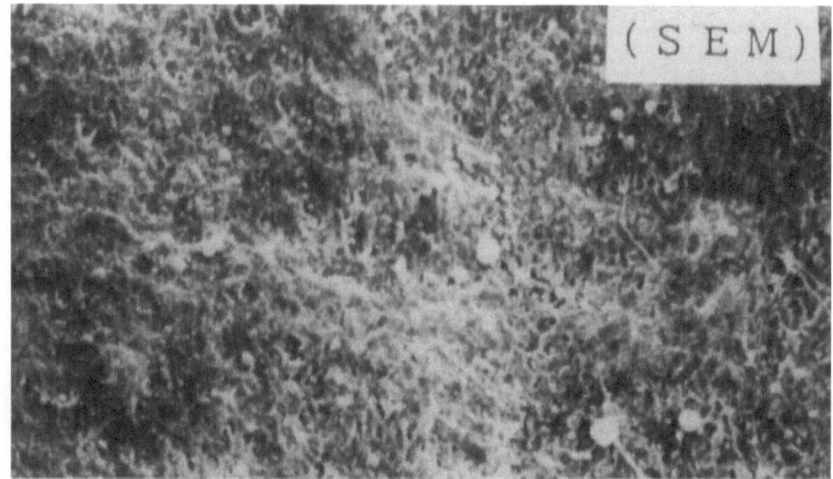

A

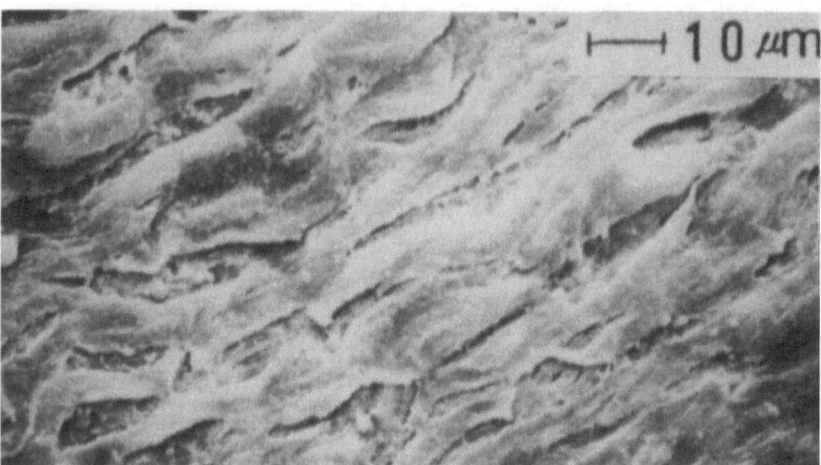

B

FIGURE 1.12. Reversed-vein graft 3 hours after implantation. Upper picture shows the internal surface of the graft away from the valve. Lower picture shows the surface near the valve.

Measurement of prostaglardin I_2 (PGI_2) production of the reversed-vein graft in dogs indicates reduction of PGI_2 production 1 week after implantation, and then favorable recovery at 2 weeks, corresponding with regeneration of the endothelium. On the other hand, measurement of PGI_2 production by a reversed vein during the preservation period after harvesting shows that the inner surface of the graft, which has lost its endothelial lining, does have a relatively high potential to produce PGI_2 under stimulation by arachidonic acid, even after 2 hours of preservation. This result may explain the

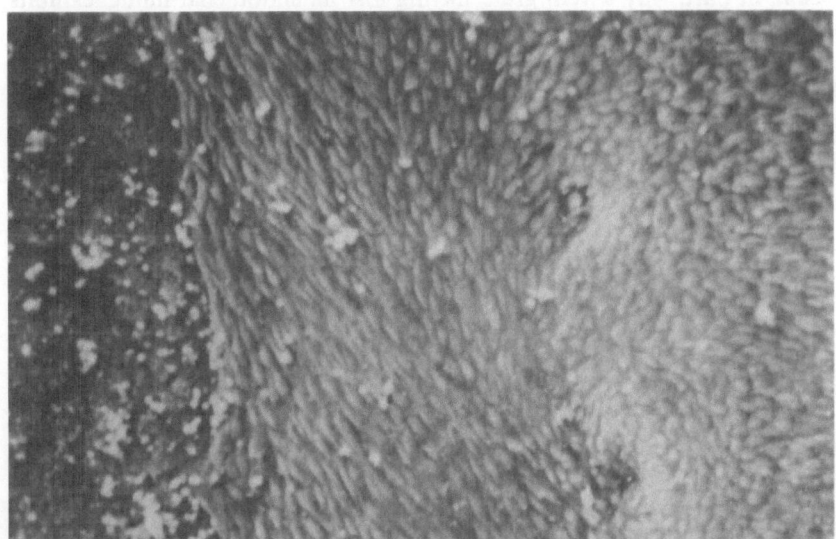

FIGURE 1.13. Endothelial cell spreading near the valve 1 week after implantation.

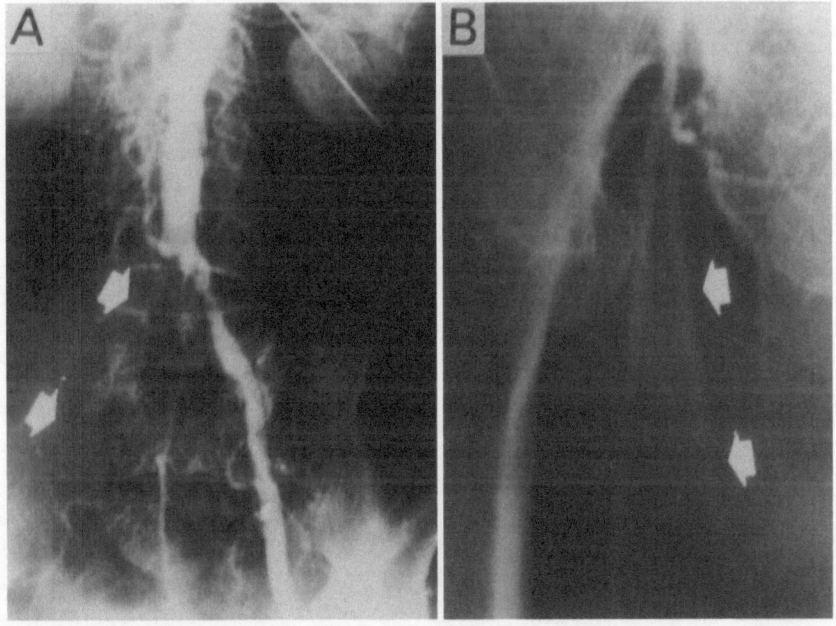

FIGURE 1.14. Angiograms of a patient who has undergone femoropopliteal bypass. (A) The right iliac artery is completely occluded. (B) However, the femoropopliteal graft is still patent.

reason, in part, why a vein graft, having lost its endothelial lining, exhibits relatively good antithrombogenicity during the early postoperative period.[9]

Two to three months after bypass procedure, many of the vein grafts follow the eventual course of definite intimal thickening with complete endothelialization. This is well known as arterialization of the vein graft. Fig. 1.14 shows two angiograms of a patient who underwent right femoropopliteal below-knee bypass with a reversed saphenous vein graft 4 years before. The athero-

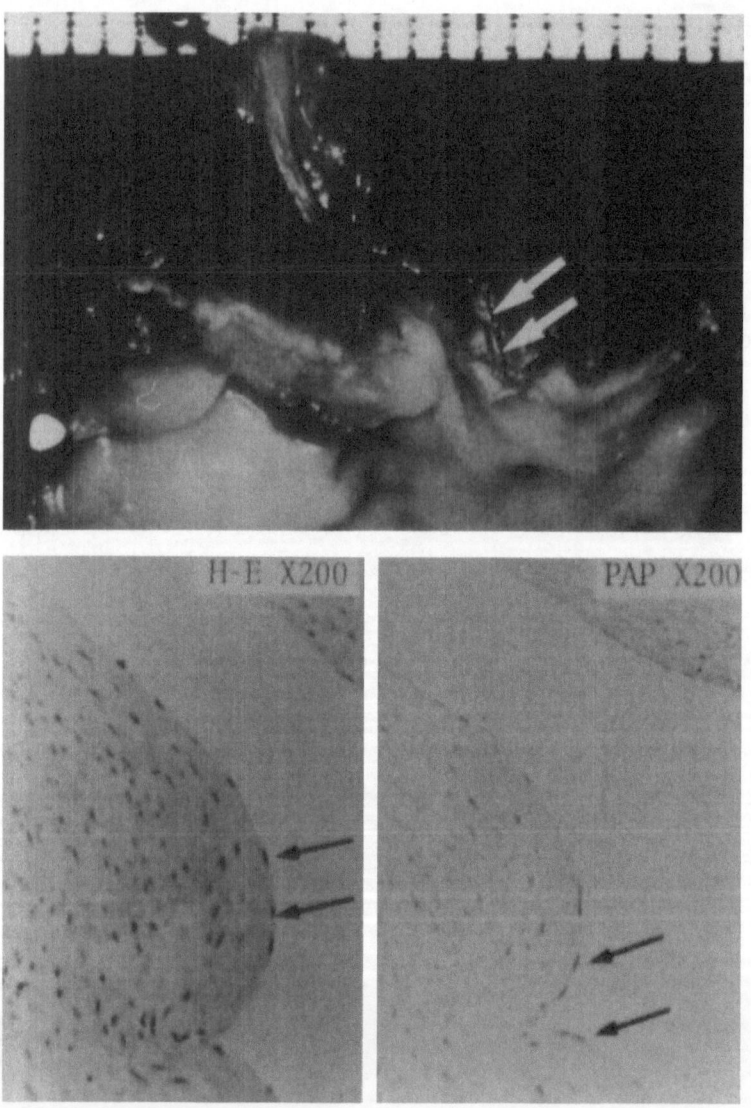

FIGURE 1.15. Proximal anastomotic stenosis. Hematoxylin-eosin (H-E) stain and Peroxidase-antiperoxidase (PAP) stain of the stenotic site in the lower pictures.

sclerotic occlusive lesion had progressed to the iliac region. On the left, the occlusive lesion of the iliac artery can be seen. On the right, the patent femoropopliteal vein graft is fairly well demonstrated despite the proximal occlusion. We call it "pseudo-occlusion." From this observation, we could speculate that there is a very high antithrombogenicity of the vein graft after arterialization.

In the chronic phase beyond 1 month after surgery, very characteristic changes of the vein graft can be observed. One of these is the progressive stenosis due to localized intimal hyperplasia seen preferentially at the site of anastomosis, including that of the veno–venous composite graft, or in the area near the venous valves. When the quality of the vein graft is poor, the stenotic lesion could be diffuse. The other change is the progression of the native disease, resulting in proximal and distal occlusion. The upper picture in Fig. 1.15 shows a typical stenosis at the proximal anastomosis. The lower picture shows that the hyperplastic tissue is made of proliferating smooth muscle cells. It is covered by a monolayer of flattened cells that are not stained by peroxidase-antiperoxidase (PAP), which may immunologically certify the existence of well-functioning endothelial cells. It is questionable if this thin layer is that of the endothelial cells. Scanning electron microscopy of the surface covering the intimal hyperplasia has never found an endothelial cell in good shape (Fig. 1.16). These morphological findings make us speculate

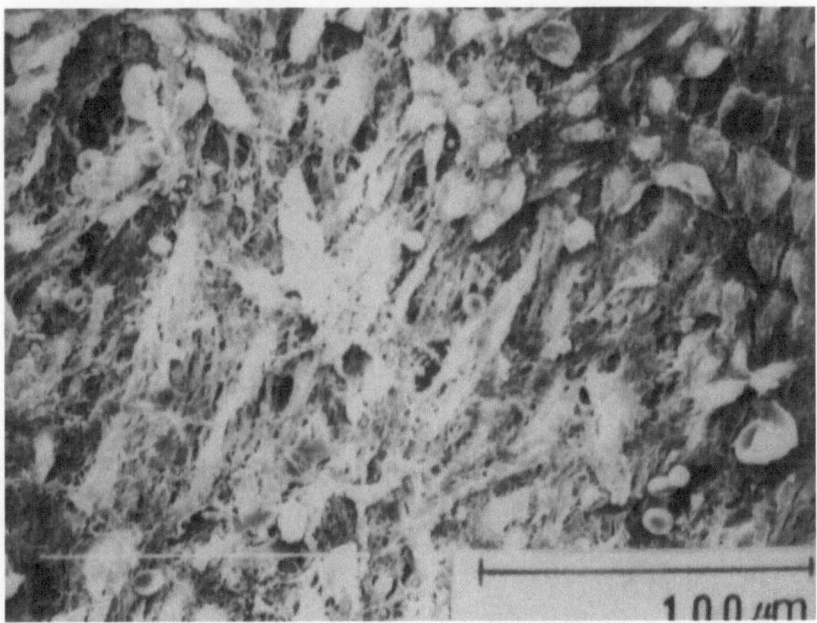

FIGURE 1.16. Scanning electron microscopy of the intimal hyperplasia with deformed endothelial cells.

that the surface of the abnormally hypertrophied intima cannot be covered by healthy endothelial cells.

Another problem of the autogenous vein is atherosclerotic change of the graft itself. This pathological change is observed far less commonly in Japanese than in Caucasians, and we have had only two cases with this condition in our series. Fig 1.17 shows multiple stenosis found in the bilateral femoro-

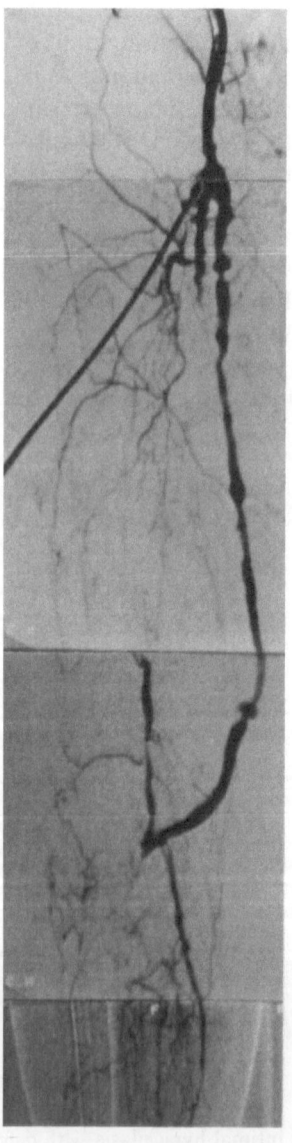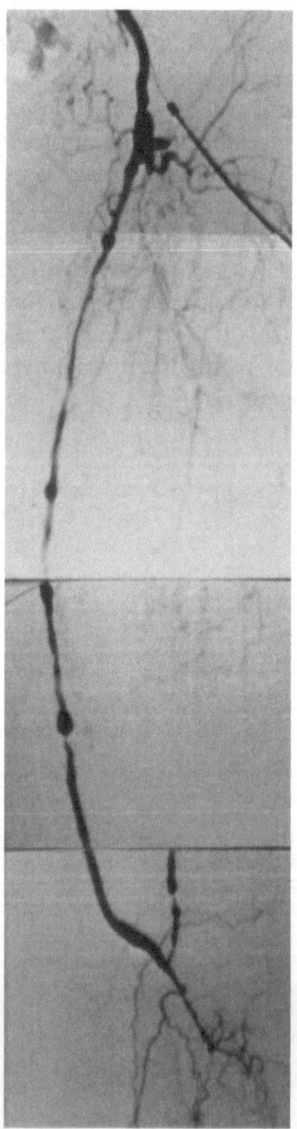

FIGURE 1.17. Multiple-graft stenosis in a patient with hyperlipidemia.

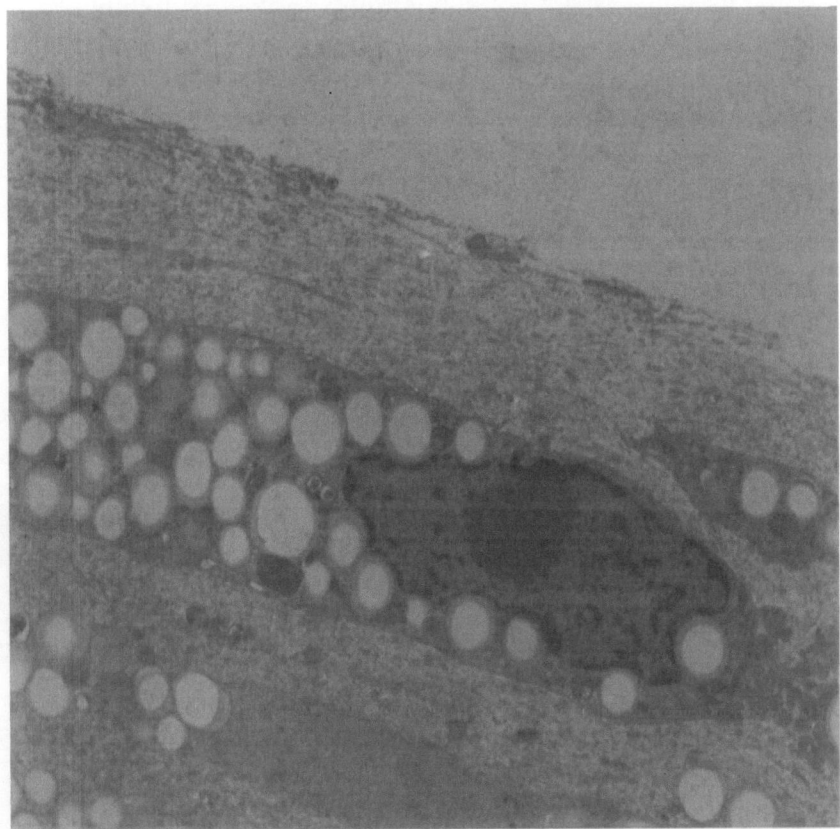

FIGURE 1.18. Graft of the patient with hyperlipidemia contains the macrophage with fatty droplets.

popliteal bypass graft 3 years after operation in a 78-year-old woman with hyperlipidemia. Remarkable atheromatous change with ulceration was seen in the vein graft, and the transmission electron microscopic finding of the graft shows many fatty droplets in the macrophage (Fig. 1.18).

Postoperative Surveillance and Management

Fig 1.19 shows the major modes of primary graft failure of the reversed-vein and in situ saphenous vein. The incidence of vein graft stenosis is almost equal in both grafts. The stenosis of the graft itself appears almost definitely within 2 years.[10] On the other hand, graft failure due to progression of the native disease seems to happen more than 2 years after operation. Therefore we have employed postoperative graft patency surveillance and anticoagulant therapy combined with antiplatelet drugs.[7]

Type of Lesion   Procedures Used to Revise

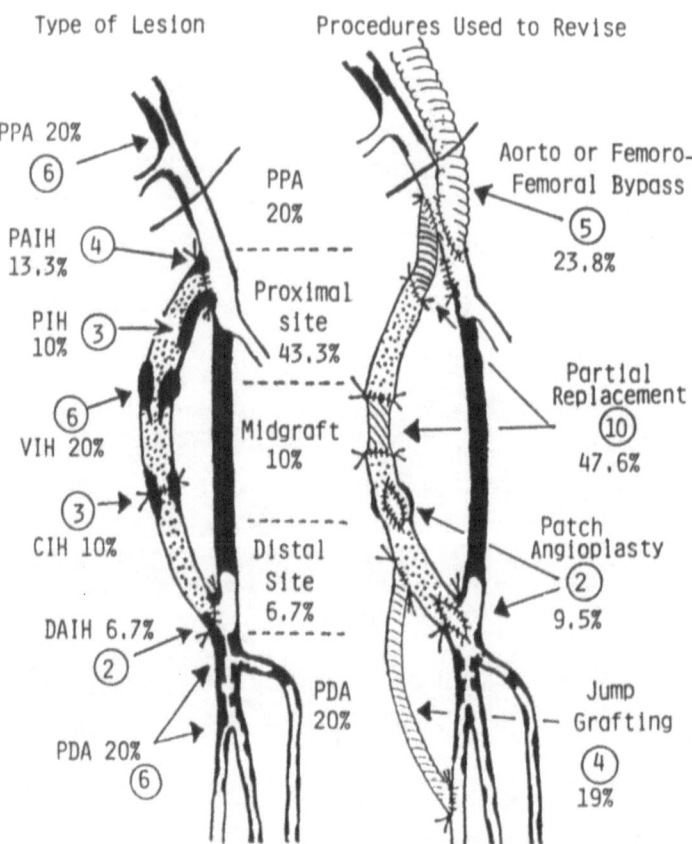

FIGURE 1.19. Modes of failure of vein grafts. IH, Intimal hyperplasia. PIH, Diffuse or localized IH for a 10- to 15-cm segment from the proximal anastomosis. PAIH, Proximal anastomotic IH. CIH, IH at veno–venous anastomosis. VIH, Fused or fibrotic valve. DAIH, Distal anastomotic IH. PPA, Progression of proximal athero-sclerosis. PDA, Progression of distal atherosclerosis.

For patients after arterial reconstruction with autogenous vein grafts, fol-low-up examination is done at 3-month intervals for the first 2 years and then every 6 months thereafter. Special attention is paid to high-pitched bruits on auscultation and to the reduction of the size of the wave in Doppler analysis. Whenever one of these signs develops, the follow-up interval is shortened to 2 to 4 weeks. If the ankle-brachial pressure index then decreases definitely by more than 0.1 during this period, angiography is indicated. If a graft-threatening lesion is then recognized, a corrective operation is per-formed even if the patient is still asymptomatic.

Localized stenosis at proximal and distal anastomosis as well as in the graft is corrected by partial replacement or patch angioplasty. Progression of proximal and distal atherosclerosis is treated by bypass with a new graft

TABLE 1.3. Effect of PEG$_1$ administration to suppress intimal hyperplasia in patients with femoro-crural bypass.

	Intimal hyperplasia (+)	Intimal hyperplasia (−)	Total
PGE$_1$(+)	3* (5.5%)	52	55
PGE$_1$(−)	6* (25.0%)	18	24
Total	9 (11.4%)	70	79

* $p < 0.05$

connecting the patent old graft and the native artery beyond the site of stenosis.

We routinely give antiplatelet agents to patients with grafts in the aortoiliac regions. We add an anticoagulant for patients with infrainguinal grafts. When an autogenous saphenous vein is used, anticoagulant therapy is continued for 2 years and antiplatelet agents for longer. For prosthetic materials in this region, this combination therapy is kept forever. The regimen is considered to help avoid early graft thrombosis and to delay the occurrence of thrombosis in cases with threatened grafts.

In our recent clinical study, we found that prostaglandin E$_1$ (PGE$_1$) administration for 2 weeks following arterial reconstruction has a possibility to suppress intimal hyperplasia. Table 1.3 shows the result of intermediate follow-up of 55 patients with 2 weeks PGE$_1$ administration and 24 patients without it. Significantly fewer patients with the treatment showed intimal hyperplasia.

Concluding Comments

During the past 15 years we have performed arterial reconstruction in the lower extremities of 1,200 patients (1,500 limbs) with occlusive lesions due to ASO or thromboangiitis obliterans.

In the postoperative observation of ASO patients, who were the majority of these patients, the following findings were recognized:

1. Aortoiliac occlusive lesions have been routinely bypassed with Dacron prostheses, and the secondary patency rate at 10 years reached 96.5%. These favorable results seem to be due mainly to our aggressive policy of pursuing as complete revascularization as possible. The operative mortality was 2.7%. The main problems encountered in this region were anastomotic aneurysm in the femoral artery (3.9%), outflow occlusion (2.8%), and graft infection (1.2%).
2. In the infrainguinal region, there are still problems to be solved. First of all, there is no graft material comparable to the autogenous vein. In addition, many of the materials should suffer significant pathological changes

from the environment in the long term following surgery, which we have not understood well enough yet.

3. Biograft could be used at the above-knee level as an alternative graft to autogenous vein, like other small-caliber prostheses. But degradation of a bioprosthesis in human tissue could not be avoided. Animal experiments have made us speculate that the cause of the characteristic anastomotic pannus hyperplasia may be the incapability of the pannus to anchor to the internal surface of the vessel.

4. In our hands, the secondary 5-year patency rates of reversed-vein grafts as well as in situ vein grafts, including femoro-popliteal below-knee and femorocrural bypasses, have exceeded 90%, although their primary patency at 5 years was between 67% and 86%.

5. Postoperative troubles that directly threaten the autogenous vein graft function have mostly been attributed to the intimal hyperplasia and progression of the disease. The former was observed in about 10% of grafts and had a tendency to occur within 2 years after surgery. The intimal hyperplasia of the autogenous vein graft consists of localized and diffuse types. The localized intimal hyperplasia is seen at the sites of anastomosis or the valve sites, and they were corrected relatively easily with minor invasion. On the other hand, the diffuse type of intimal hyperplasia seemed to be due to the poor quality of the autogenous vein graft.

6. As a strategy against postoperative graft occlusion, we have employed anticoagulant therapy combined with antiplatelet drugs mainly for the patients with infrainguinal grafts. Although the effect is difficult to demonstrate at present, it is considered that the regimen should serve to avoid early graft thrombosis and to delay occurrence of thrombosis in cases with threatened grafts.

Acknowledgments. The authors would like to express their appreciation to Dr. John B. Chang for giving us the opportunity to present our paper at the Sixth International Vascular Symposium in Seoul. We also would like to thank Ms. Ann J. Boehme for her help in preparation of the manuscript.

References

1. Rutherford RB, Flanigan DP, Gupta SK, et al. Suggested standards for reports dealing with lower extremity ischemia. J Vasc Surg 1986;4:80–94.
2. Harris PL, Bigley DJC, McSweeney L. Aortofemoral bypass and the role of concomitant femorodistal reconstruction. Br J Surg 1985;72:317–320.
3. Szilagyi DE, Elliott JP Jr, Smith RF, Reddy DJ, McPharlin M. A thiry year survey of the reconstructive surgical treatment of aortoiliac occlusive disease. J Vasc Surg 1986;3:421–436.
4. Kubo Y, Sasajima T, Atsuta T, et al. Early clinical results of the modified human umbilical cord vein homograft (Dardik Biograft). J Cardiovasc Surg 1983;24:101–106.

5. Sasajima T, Kubo Y, Kokubo M, Morimoto N, Yoshida H. The biological compatibility and the fate of chemically modified collagen vascular grafts. Artif Organ Today 1992;2:9–19.
6. Dardik H, Miller N, Dardik A, et al. A decade of experience with the glutaraldehyde-tanned human umbilical cord vein graft for revascularization of the lower limb. J Vasc Surg 1988;7:336–346.
7. Sasajima T, Kubo Y, Kokubo M, Izumi Y, Inaba M. Comparison of reversed and in situ saphenous vein graft for infragenicular bypass: experience of two surgeons. Cardiovasc Surg 1993;1:38–43.
8. Horio M. De-endothelialization and re-endothelialization in autogenous vein grafts—fundamental and clinical study. J Jpn Surg Soc 1991;92:867–873.
9. Nakayama K. Experimental study of the prostacyclin production of autogenous vein graft. J Jpn Surg Soc 1992;93:1341–1346.
10. Whittemore AD, Clowes AW, Couch NP, Mannick JA. Secondary femoropopliteal reconstruction. Ann Surg 1981;193:35–42.

2
Development of Modern Vascular Surgery in Korea

Yong Kak Lee

Introduction

The chronology of modern vascular surgery in Korea is relatively short, as most of the present-day vascular surgical technology was developed during the past 30 years.

Although Carrel in 1905 first developed many of the vascular surgical techniques that are still in use today, progress was greatly hampered by lack of anesthesia and asepsis. According to DeBakey, among thousands of devastating injuries of the extremities during World War II, only one limb was salvaged by direct anastomosis of the severed artery.

Along with Blalock, Gross, and Grafoord, who pioneered in surgical repair of the tetralogy of Fallot, patent ductus arteriosus, and coarctation of aorta in the late 1940s, Dubost in 1952 successsfully resected an abdominal aortic aneurysm and replaced the aorta with a homograft.

Traumatology made great progress during the Korean War from 1950 to 1953, when trauma-related death and sequelae were drastically reduced to the current levels.

The first large series of arterial surgical repairs with or without insertion of homografts on US and Korean soldiers was reported by Frank Spencer, MD, in 1953. It was my good fortune to work with Dr. Spencer during the war and to witness his pioneering work in vascular repair of traumatized limbs at the "E" Medical Company of the First US Marine Division, which was stationed at Munsanni on the Western Front of the Korean War zone near the 38th parallel. Our unit was supporting both the Korean Army and the US Marines. Homografts were harvested from the cadavers of allied soldiers and preserved in Ringer's lactate solution with penicillin and streptomycin added and stored in refrigerators.

When I moved to the United States for surgical training at the Baylor Affiliated Surgical Training Program in Houston, Texas, from 1953 to 1958, the goddess of fortune placed me under the wings of the great pioneers in modern cardiovascular surgery, Michael DeBakey, MD, and Denton A. Cooley, MD. They invented the Dacron vascular prosthesis, which is still in wide use today. Dr. DeBakey and Dr. Cooley developed new surgical techniques for the repair of occlusive diseases of the aortoiliac and popliteal arteries, aneurysms of the abdominal and thoracic aorta, renovascular hypertension, and cerebral ischemia due to extracranial artery stenosis, etc. With dizzying pace, many conditions that were untouchable up to that time became surgically correctable, one by one, by their amazing work.

Vascular Surgery in Korea

When I returned home from the United States in 1958, modern vascular surgery was begging to be born here as well. At Ewha University from 1958 to 1961, I introduced femoral arteriography and abdominal aortography with Urokon contrast solution. I had to manufacture a manual three-film cassette changer made of plywood and lead sheet.

DeBakey's Dacron prostheses were implanted to correct iliofemoral arterial occlusive diseases, and Y-grafts for replacement of abdominal aortic aneurysms. Endarterectomy was also carried out on some occlusive arterial diseases. Homemade wire loops were used for endarterectomy, and similarly handmade vein strippers with components of guitar G-string wire and silver stripper head were used for stripping varicose veins. The vintage contraptions may still be found in the depths of drawers in some operating rooms in Korea.

After I moved to the Catholic University Medical College, my vascular work continued. In 1963 I reported the first surgical series of arterial diseases in Korea: 20 cases of occlusive disease of the lower extremities, 3 cases of aortoiliac thrombosis, 3 cases of abdominal aortic aneurysm 3 cases of aortoiliac occlusion 4 cases of renovascular hypertension, and 5 cases of arterial injuries. By the end of the 1980s when I left the Catholic University, our surgical department had accumulated over 2,000 vascular surgery cases of various categories.

Among these, Buerger's disease, affecting mostly the popliteal artery and its branches, comprised nearly half of the cases. Lumbar sympathectomy had been the only surgical means available for this lesion up to that time, and this was only partially rewarding or totally ineffective. I started to tackle it by direct vascular recanalization or saphenous vein bypass graft. By combining aggressive femoral arteriographic study in all affected limbs, noninvasive diagnostic instruments, and application of microvascular techniques, we succeeded in restoring distal arterial flow and salvaged limbs in one-third of all Buerger's conditions and drastically reduced amputation rates.

Organ Transplantation

As renal transplantation has become a common practice since 1964, this unique therapeutic model has set up an ideal experimental situation in humans regarding the human rejection process, which differs quite a bit from that described from animal experimentation by P. B. Medawar. The impact of new knowledge on cell-mediated immunity affected almost all of the medical specialties, and it altered classification of etiologies and created new therapeutic approaches. Korean medicine was at a standstill in the late 1960s when everybody was waiting anxiously for the introduction of new technology from abroad. The expectation was great.

The first Korean renal transplantation performed by our Catholic University transplantation team on March 25, 1969, sparked a new vitality in Korean medicine. Although not published, we performed a parathyroid transplantation on December 28, 1968, by anastomosing the carotid artery and the jugular vein of a composite thyroid–parathyroid gland obtained from a cadaver of a newborn baby to the femoral vessels of a recipient whose parathyroids had been completely destroyed by repeated thyroid surgery.

The reason for the success for our team, which had little specific training at an overseas transplantation center, was that we had accumulated sufficient vascular surgical techniques and some of us had enough knowledge for preparation of patients and postoperative management.

Since I organized and launched the Korean Transplantation Society in 1972 with vascular surgical colleagues from all over the nation, the number of renal transplants has risen to nearly 800 cases per annum. With the current national mood to accept the concept of brain death, multiorgan transplantation and liver transplantation are taking place more frequently.

Microvascular Surgery

I briefly mentioned microvascular surgery in Buerger's disease. In 1972 Sun Lee, MD, Scripps Clinic, La Jolla, California, was invited here to hold a workshop on microvascular surgery in rats at our department. He was regarded as the father of modern microvascular surgery. It so happens that he was a classmate of mine in medical school. Surgeons from several medical schools throughout the country were invited to attend the session, which lasted for 8 days. Using magnifying glasses and microsurgical instruments, we learned to anastomose arteries and veins in rats for transplant of kidney, liver, heart, and testicles. This workshop produced many brilliant microvascular surgeons, several of whom are now practicing replantation of severed limbs and digits. This experimental model has contributed to numerous research papers as well.

Korean Vascular Surgery Society

The new surgical subspecialty of vascular surgery remained in the infantile stage up to the early 1980s, when only a limited number of surgeons practiced in this field. In 1984, vascular surgeons from 10 medical schools met and decided to launch the Korean Vascular Surgery Society to expand the scope of university participation and to promote exchange of information. Today our membership has grown to 150 regular members, and the Scientific Congress is held twice a year. The *Journal of the Korean Vascular Surgery Society* is issued twice a year with recent clinical and research articles.

John B. Chang, MD, Director of the Vascular Surgery Center, Long Island Jewish Medical Center, and Albert Einstein Medical College, New York, was invited to Korea twice to give special lectures at our Congresses in 1989 and 1990. It was he who suggested that we cosponsor the Sixth International Vascular Symposium in Seoul, Korea, in conjunction with the Korean Vascular Surgery Annual Congress in 1992. On this occasion a new scientific body, the Asian Vascular Society, was organized.

Conclusion

Rapid progress has been achieved in vascular surgery in Korea during the past 30 years, and it is now a routine procedure throughout our 32 medical schools and other major hospitals. Refreshing the memories of olden days serves to give us new insights into the present and the future of learning, as an old Korean adage says, "look back to the old days to find new ways."

3
A Novel Approach to Preventing Intimal Hyperplasia: Inhibition of Smooth Muscle Cell Migration with Enalapril

ERIC T. CHOI, NIRAJ SEHGAL, SHAPING SUN, JEFFREY TRACHTENBERG, UNA S. RYAN, AND ALLAN D. CALLOW

Summary

As a leading cause of restenosis, intimal hyperplasia is common to small-caliber grafting, endarterectomy, and balloon angioplasty. Following surgical injury to the artery, smooth muscle cells (SMC) in the media migrate into the intima and then proliferate. Angiotensin II, which is present in the arterial wall after injury, has been demonstrated to cause SMC migration in vitro without affecting proliferation. Therefore, our experiments were performed to determine if inhibition of angiotensin II production by enalapril had an inhibitory effect on SMC migration in an in vivo model and, in turn, reduced intimal lesion formation.

Forty normotensive Sprague-Dawley rats were subjected to left carotid balloon injury. The first group received enalapril (4 mg/kg/day in saline, subcutaneous) and the second group received vehicle (saline, subcutaneous). Four to five animals were sacrificed at 2, 4, 7, and 14 days postinjury. The blood pressure measurements at the time of sacrifice were consistent with the therapeutic effects of enalapril [83 $\pm$ 7 mm Hg vs. 101 $\pm$ 11 mm Hg (vehicle)]. The carotid arteries were sectioned and immunohistochemically stained for proliferating cell nuclear antigen expressed in replicating SMCs and SMC-specific α actin expressed only in SMCs. Administration of enalapril did not affect the proliferative rate of SMCs in the media or in the intima after balloon injury at any time points. Enalapril, however, signficantly reduced the number of SMCs migrating into the intima at 7 and 14 days (reduction of 60% ($p < 0.01$) and 63% ($p < 0.01$), respectively). Furthermore, there was a reduction in the intimal lesion area on the 7th and 14th postinjury days [reduction of 78% ($p < 0.01$) and 55% ($p < 0.05$), respectively]. These results suggest that enalapril inhibited SMC migration after balloon injury and, in turn, reduced intimal lesion formation. Hence, SMC migration should be targeted as a therapeutic option in the prevention of intimal hyperplasia.

Introduction

Intimal hyperplasia is the leading cause of restenosis following small-caliber grafting, endarterectomy, and balloon angioplasty.[1-3] This disease process is the natural healing response to arterial injury and is characterized by neointimal SMC proliferation and extracellular matrix deposition leading to luminal narrowing and eventual reocclusion.[3,4] Hence, researchers have targeted the proliferating SMC as an approach to control neointimal lesion formation in various experimental models of intimal hyperplasia and atherosclerosis. For instance, antimitotic agents such as steroids, methotrexate, and colchicine have been used to prevent SMC proliferation after balloon angioplasty in animal models.[5-7] Antibodies to various SMC growth factors have been infused into animals to reduce lesion formation after arterial injury.[8,9] However, many of these modalities targeting proliferation alone have been unsuccessful in significantly reducing restenosis after balloon angioplasty in clinical trials.[10]

The migratory activity of the SMC in the development of the neointimal lesion has recently been a research focus. Dilley and coworkers[11] demonstrated the role of SMC migration from host artery to vascular graft in the development of the anastomotic intimal hyperplastic lesion (see Fig. 3.1). At the time of anastomosis, there is perianastomotic endothelial cell and SMC disruption and platelet adherence. This initial event is followed by medial SMC proliferation. Subsequently, proliferating and nonproliferating medial SMCs migrate to the intima of the graft and further divide there. Proliferation does not appear to be a prerequisite for migration.[11]

Similarly, arteries undergoing angioplasty respond to the trauma of the catheter by a series of thrombotic and cellular events seen with vascular grafting, including early platelet accumulation, proliferation of medial SMCs, migration of proliferating and nonproliferating medial SMCs into the intima, and chronic replication of intimal SMCs (see Fig. 3.2).[12-14] In the rat carotid angioplasty model, from which most of this information has been gathered, migration appears to be a critical cellular event in the development of the neointimal lesion, for the media is the only source of SMCs; no SMCs are present in the intima of normal, untraumatized vessels. Clinically, the critical role of SMC migration is also evident. SMCs derived from stenotic post-angioplastied intimal lesions have increased migratory activity compared to those derived from stenotic unangioplastied atherosclerotic lesions.[15] Furthermore, Clowes and colleagues[12] first reported that in the balloon angioplasty model, proliferation is not a prerequisite for the SMC to migrate from the media into the intima. In fact, 50% of all the migrating intimal SMCs do not undergo proliferation according to their results.

Many mitotic and chemotactic agents are present in the artery following injury. Elevation of mRNA expression of platelet-derived growth factor (PDGF) and angiotensinogen, potent chemotactic cytokines, has been reported following balloon injury.[16,17] Recently, Jawien and coworkers[18]

artery   anastomosis   graft

lumen   lumen

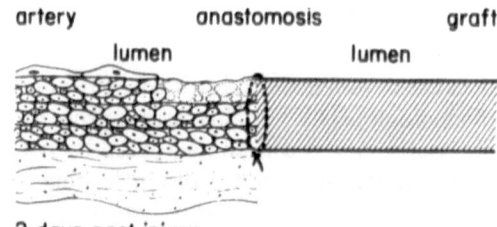

2 days post-injury

FIGURE 3.1. Schematic representation of smooth muscle cell migration from the host artery to vascular graft leading to the development of the anastomotic intimal hyperplastic lesion.

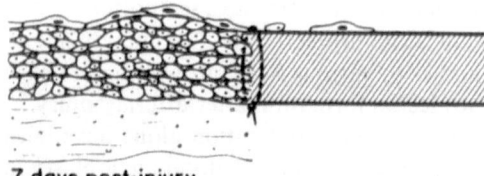

7 days post-injury

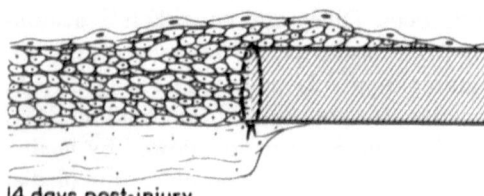

14 days post-injury

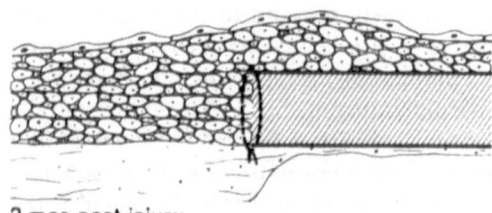

2 mos post-injury

reported that PDGF infused to rats following balloon injury caused significant worsening of the neointimal lesion. The increased lesion size was attributed to both increased SMC migration and proliferation. Conversely, when antibody to PDGF was infused following balloon injury, the neointimal lesion was reduced with attenuation of all cellular activities.[11] Therefore, the role of migration in neointimal lesion formation remains unknown. Recently, an angiotensin-converting enzyme (ACE) inhibitor, cilazipril, was demonstrated to decrease intimal lesion formation following balloon injury in the rat model.[19] Since then, other ACE inhibitors have also been shown to reduce intimal lesion formation in angioplastied arteries and in vein

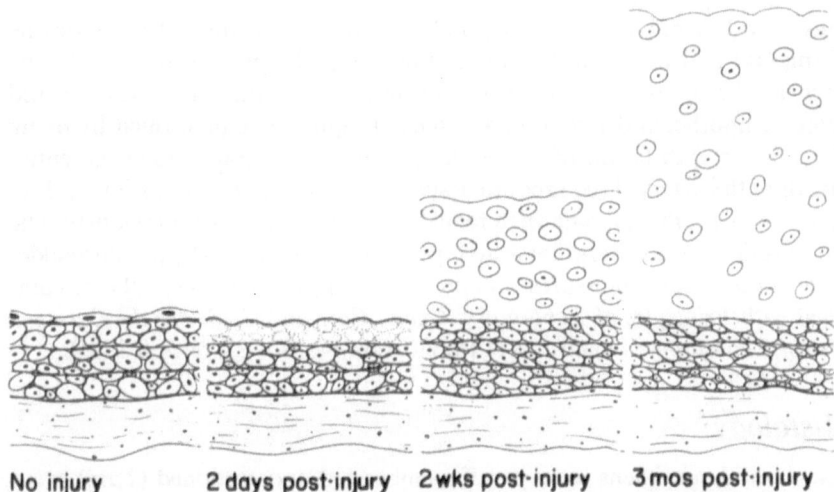

No injury   2 days post-injury   2 wks post-injury   3 mos post-injury

FIGURE 3.2. Schematic representation of smooth muscle cell accumulation in the new intima following balloon angioplasty.

grafts.[20-23] These authors speculated that ACE inhibitors had antiproliferative and antimigratory effects. However, angiotensin II, a product of ACE, has recently been demonstrated to be a migration-inducing agent and not an SMC mitogen.[21,23]

Hence, in this work, we inhibited angiotensin II formation following arterial injury with enalapril in order to determine its effect on intimal hyperplasia. We demonstrated that enalapril blocked angiotensin II-induced SMC migration and in turn reduced the neointimal lesion.

Methods

Arterial Injury Model

Ten male Sprague-Dawley rats (400 g) (Harlan Labs, Indianapolis, IN) were used at 2, 4, 7, 14 days postinjury for a total of 40 animals. The daily subcutaneous enalapril (Sigma, St. Louis, MO) (4 mg/kg in 2 mL of saline) ($n = 5$ per time point) or vehicle (saline) ($n = 5$ per time point) injections were started 3 days before the arterial injury and continued for the course of the study. The arterial pressure of all animals was measured through a cannula placed in the femoral artery using a pressure transducer (Millar Instruments Inc, Houston, TX). Measurements were performed at the time of balloon injury and at the time of harvest.

The procedure for carotid arterial injury is well documented by this laboratory and others.[12-14,24] Briefly, animals were anesthetized with an intramuscular dose of ketamine (40 mg/kg), acepromazine (1 mg/kg), and xylazine (20 mg/kg) and aseptically prepped. Following the midline incision to the neck, a 2 Fr embolectomy catheter was inserted into the left external carotid artery. Endothelial denudation and medial injury were performed by filling the balloon with 0.1 ml of saline and pulling it antegrade along the entire length of the artery three times to assure uniform injury. On postinjury days 2, 4, 7, and 14, the animals were reanesthetized as described previously. The left carotid arteries were harvested, perfusion-fixed with 4% paraformaldehyde at physiologic pressures, and processed for histology. Animal care complied with *Principles of Laboratory Animal Care* and *Guide for the Care and Use of Laboratory Animals* (NIH Publication No. 80–23, revised 1985).

Histology

The carotid specimens were paraffin-embedded and sectioned (2 μm) every 5 mm. The sections were deparaffinized and dehydrated through xylene and graded ethanol series. Following preincubation with 2% normal nonimmune serum and levamisole, an endogenous alkaline phosphatase blocker, the sections were incubated with antiproliferating cell nuclear antigen (anti-PCNA, Coulter Diagnostics, Hialeah, FL) (1:1000 dilution) or anti-SMC-specific α actin (1:10000, Sigma, St.Louis, MO). The sections were rinsed with phos-

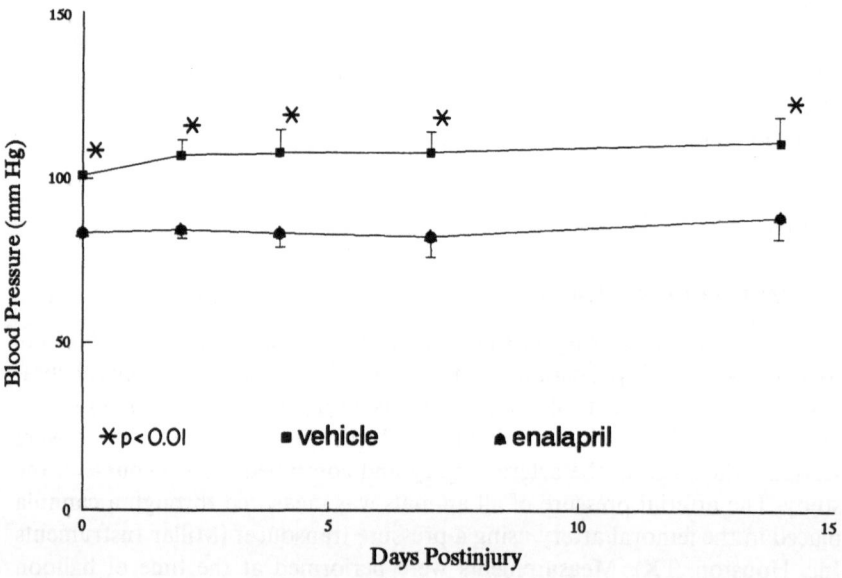

FIGURE 3.3. Mean systemic blood pressure measured following enalapril or vehicle treatment.

phate-buffered saline (PBS), incubated with a biotin-labeled antibody, and treated with an avidin–biotin–alkaline phosphatase complex (10 μg/mL of avidin with 2.5 μg/mL biotin–alkaline phosphatase in Tris buffer) followed by Fast Red substrate (BioGenex, San Ramon, CA) for detection. Finally, the sections were counterstained with hematoxylin for nuclear identification.

Statistics

All data are expressed as the mean ± standard deviation of the mean. Differences in means were tested for significance using two-tailed Student's t test for unpaired data, with p values less than 0.05 regarded as significant.

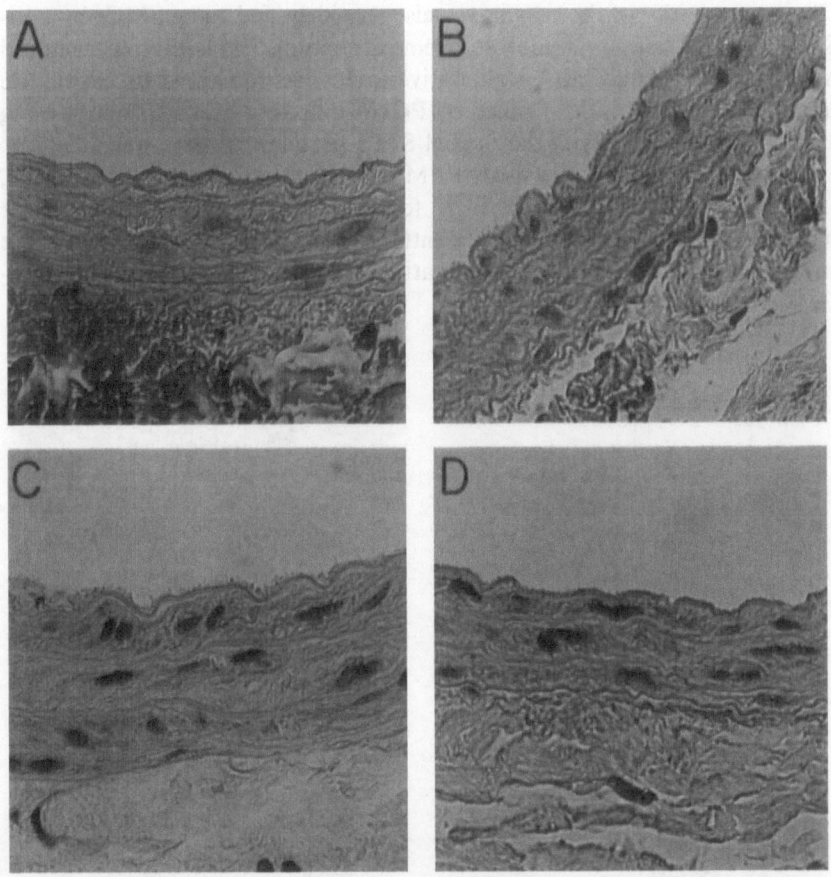

FIGURE 3.4. Immunohistochemical staining with anti-PCNA at 2 days (**A,B**) and 4 days (**C,D**). Panels **A** and **C** are vehicle-treated and panels **B** and **D** are enalapril-treated.

Results

Blood Pressure

Enalapril and vehicle treatments were begun 3 days before the time of balloon injury. Preliminary studies have shown that the antihypertensive effect of enalapril is achieved after 3 days. At the enalapril dose of 4 mg/kg/day, blood pressure reduction was achieved at the time of surgery and maintained throughout the course of the treatment [83 $\pm$ 7 mm Hg (enalapril) vs. 101 $\pm$ 11 mm Hg (vehicle) at the time injury; $p < 0.01$)] (see Fig. 3.3).

SMC Proliferation and Migration

Greater than 95% of the cells in vessels were identified to be SMCs by anti-SMC specific α actin immunohistochemical staining. Enalapril treatment did not affect the medial SMC proliferative rate when compared to the vehicle treatment (control) as determined by PCNA immunohistochemistry (see Fig 3.4). On postinjury day 2, the medial SMC proliferative rate was 25 $\pm$ 7%. On days 4, 7, and 14, the medial SMC proliferative rates were 15 $\pm$ 8%, 11 $\pm$ 4%, and 3 $\pm$ 1.3%, respectively, for the enalapril-treated group. These proliferative rates were not significantly different from the controls on the same days (see Fig. 3.5). Our proliferative rates determined by PCNA stain-

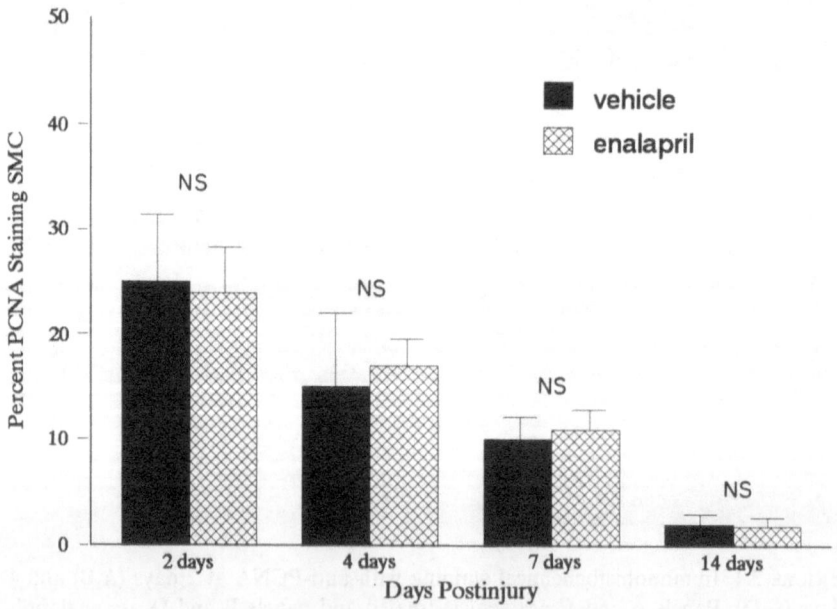

FIGURE 3.5. Proliferative rates in the media as determined by anti-PCNA at 2, 4, 7, and 14 days postinjury.

ing were similar to the reported proliferative rates by tritiated thymidine.[12-14] However, by postinjury day 4, the control arteries had SMCs present in the intima (22 ± 9 SMCs per section). SMCs were not seen in the intima of the vehicle-treated arteries on postinjury day 4, despite having the same medial SMC proliferation. Consequently, on postinjury days 7 and 14, a significantly smaller number of intimal SMCs were seen in the enalapril-treated arteries (142 ± 45 vs. 56 ± 40 SMCs per section on day 7 and 805 ± 198 vs. 297 ± 185 SMCs per section on day 14) (see Fig 3.6 and 3.7). Reduction in intimal SMCs was achieved with enalapril while the intimal SMC proliferation rates remained unchanged (see Fig. 3.8). Since intimal SMC accumulation can only be achieved by SMC migration from the media or intimal

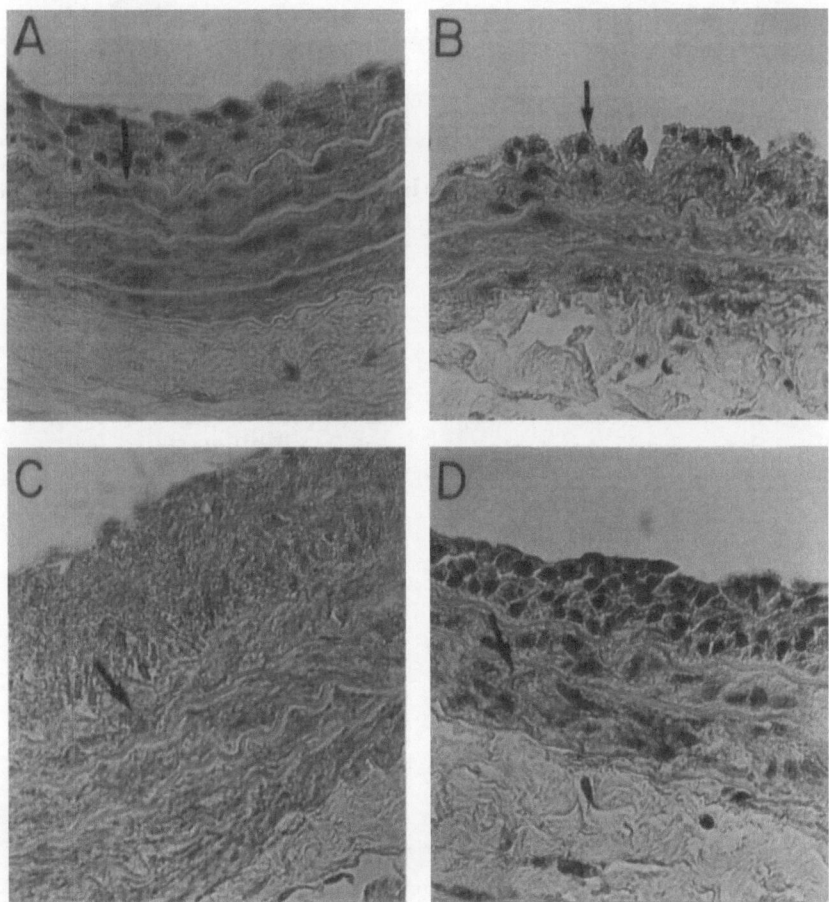

FIGURE 3.6. Immunohistochemical staining with anti-SMC specific α actin at 7 days (**A,B**) and 14 days (**C,D**). Panels **A** and **C** are vehicle-treated and panels **B** and **D** are enalapril-treated. Arrows indicate representative staining of smooth muscle cells.

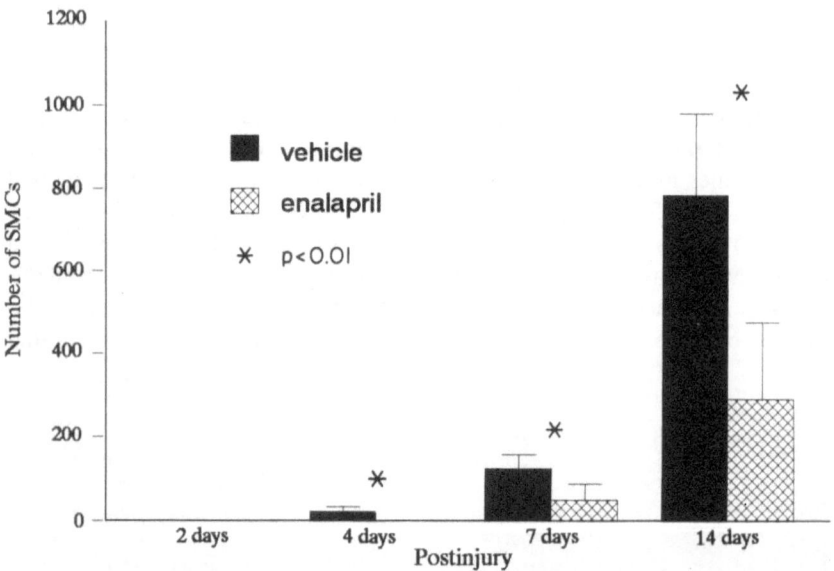

FIGURE 3.7. Total number of SMCs in the intima as determined by anti-SMC specific α actin at 2, 4, 7, and 14 days postinjury.

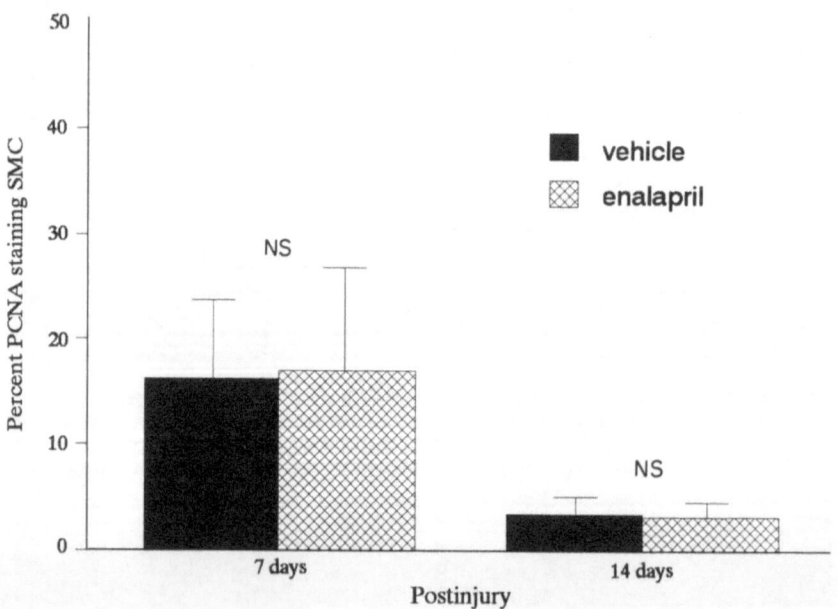

FIGURE 3.8. Proliferative rates in the intima as determined by anti-PCNA at 7 and 14 days postinjury.

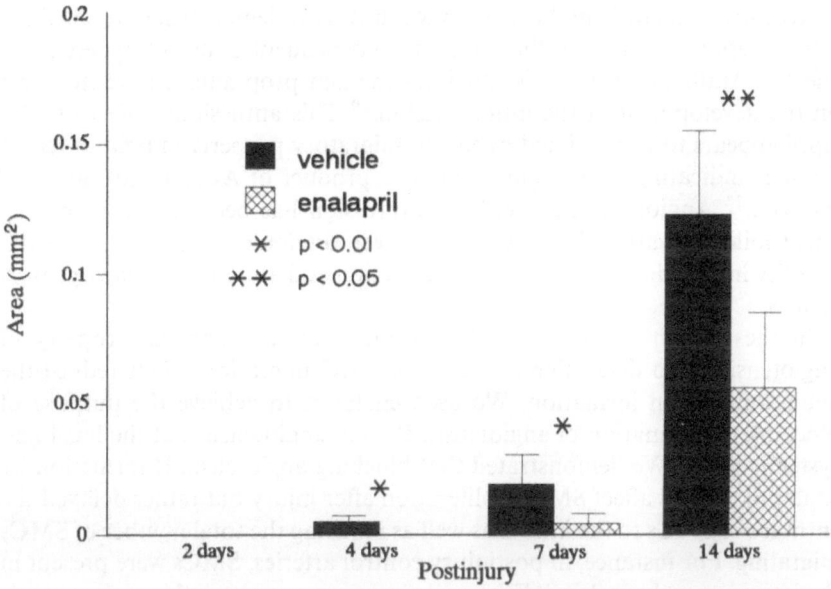

FIGURE 3.9. Intimal lesion area at 2, 4, 7, and 14 days postinjury.

proliferation, it is apparent that enalapril treatment decreased the intimal SMC accumulation by reducing the number of SMCs migrating from the media.

Reduction in Intimal Lesion

Enalapril treatment decreased SMC migration from media to intima without affecting SMC proliferation, which was evident by the reduction in the intimal lesion area on postinjury day 7. Also evident is the significant reduction in the intimal area on postinjury day 14 (see Fig. 3.9).

Discussion

Smooth muscle cell proliferation is pathognomonic for vascular diseases such as intimal hyperplasia and atherosclerosis.[1-3] However, there is increasing evidence that SMC migration may also play a critical role in the development of the neointimal lesion.[5] In the case of the anastomotic intimal hyperplastic lesion, it is intuitive that SMCs from the host artery must migrate to the anastomotic site before further proliferating and creating the restenotic lesion. Hence, it is conceivable that a simple modality of antiproliferative agents may be ineffective.

Recently, cilazipril, an ACE inhibitor, has been demonstrated to decrease intimal lesion thickness in the rat model independent of its antihypertensive effect.[19] Antihypertensives like hydralazine and propranolol have no effect on the development of the intimal lesion.[19] This antilesional effect of cilazipril appears to be mediated by its antimigratory property in light of recent findings indicating that angiotensin II, a product of ACE, is not an SMC mitogen.[22] Angiotensinogen mRNA expression has been shown to be elevated following arterial injury.[16] Moreover, angiotensin II increases SMC motility in addition to stimulating production and secretion of many growth factors.

In the present study, we took advantage of this singular property of angiotensin II to determine if inhibiting SMC migration might reduce the neointimal lesion formation. We used enalapril to achieve the purpose of blocking the formation of angiotensin II from angiotensin I at the local and systemic levels. We demonstrated that blocking angiotensin II formation by enalapril did not affect SMC proliferation after injury but rather delayed the entrance of SMCs to the intima as well as reducing the total number of SMCs migrating. For instance, in postinjury control arteries, SMCs were present in the intima as early as day 4. Enalapril treatment prevented this early appearance/migration of the medial SMCs to the intima. On the 7th day, SMCs were present in the intima in both groups. However, there was a significantly smaller number of SMCs (605 reduction) with enalapril treatment. This reduction in the number of SMCs is in light of equal proliferative rates among the intimal SMCs.

Most importantly, inhibition of migration reduced the neointimal lesion formation. It is uncertain whether, at the termination of enalapril therapy, SMC migration might be restored. To the best of our knowledge, this is the first time reduction in neointimal lesion formation was achieved solely by decreasing SMC migration without affecting cellular proliferation. We believe that inhibiting SMC migration is a strong therapeutic option effective either alone or with an antiproliferative agent.

References

1. McBride W, Lange RA, Hillis LD. Restenosis after successful angioplasty. Pathophysiology and prevention. N Engl J Med 1988;318:1734–1737.
2. Cohen JR, Mannick JA, Couch NP, Whittemore AD. Recognition and management of impending vein graft failure: importance for long-term patency. Arch Surg 1986;121:758–759.
3. Sottiurai VS, Yao JS, Batson RC, et al. Distal anastomotic intimal hyperplasia: histopathologic character and biogenesis. Ann Vasc Surg 1989;3:26–33.
4. Dartsch PC, Voisard R, Bauriedel G, Hofling B, Betz E. Growth characteristics and cytoskeletal organization of cultured smooth muscle cells from human primary stenosis and restenosis lesions. Arteriosclerosis 1990;10:62–75.
5. Colburn MD, Moore WS, Gelabert HA, Quinones-Baldrich WJ. Dose responsive

suppression of myointimal hyperplasia by dexamethasone. J Vasc Surg 1992; 15:510–518.

6. Currier JW, Pow TK, Minihan AC, et al. Colchicine inhibits restenosis after iliac angioplasty in the atherosclerosis in the rabbit (abstr). Circulation 1989;80 (suppl II): II–66.

7. Muller DWM, Topol EJ, Abrams G, et al. Intraluminal methotrexate therapy for the prevention of intimal proliferation after endothelial injury (abstr). Circulation 1990;82 (suppl III): III–429.

8. Lindner V, Reidy MA. Proliferation of smooth muscle cells after vascular injury is inhibited by an antibody against basic fibroblast growth factor. Proc Natl Acad Sci USA 1991;88:3739–3743.

9. Ferns GA, Raines E, Sprugel KM, Motani AS, Reidy MA, Ross R. Inhibition of neointimal smooth muscle accumulation after angioplastry by an antibody to PDGF. Science 1991;253:1129–1132.

10. O'Keefe JH, McCallister BD, Bateman TM, et al. Ineffectiveness of colchicine for the prevention of restenosis after coronary angioplasty. J Am Coll Cardiol 1992; 19:1597–1600.

11. Dilley RJ, McGeachie JK, Tennant M. The role of cell proliferation and migration in the development of a neointimal layer in veins grafted into arteries in rats. Cell Tissue Res 1992;269:281–287.

12. Clowes AW, Schwartz SM. Significance of quiescent smooth muscle migration in the injured carotid artery. Circ Res 1985;56:139–145.

13. Clowes AW, Clowes MM, Reidy MA. Kinetics of cellular proliferation after arterial injury III. Endothelial and smooth muscle growth in chronically denuded vessels. Lab Invest 1986;54:295–303.

14. Clowes AW, Reidy MA, Clowes MM. Kinetics of cellular proliferation after arterial injury. I. Smooth muscle growth in the absence of endothelium. Lab Invest 1983;49:327–333.

15. Bauriedel G, Windstetter U, Demaiosj UR, Kandolf R, Hofling B. Migratory activity of human smooth muscle cells cultivated from coronary and peripheral primary and restenotic lesions removed by percutaneous atherectomy. Circulation 1992;85:554–564.

16. Rakugi H, Jacob JH, Ingelfinger JR, Krieger JE, Dzau VJ, Pratt RE. Angiotensin gene expression in the myointima after vascular injury. Hypertension 1990;16: 345–352.

17. Majesky MW, Reidy MA, Bowen-Pope DF, Hart CE, Wilcox JN, Schwartz SM. PDGF ligand and receptor gene expression during repair of arterial injury. J Cell Biol 1990;111:2149–2158.

18. Jawien A, Bowen-Pope DF, Lindner V, Schwartz SM, Clowes AW. Platelet-derived growth factor promotes smooth muscle migration and intimal thickening in a rat model of balloon angioplasty. J Clin Invest 1992;89:507–511.

19. Powell JS, Clozel JP, Muller RKM, et al. Inhibitors of angiotensin converting enzyme prevent myointimal hyperplasia after vascular injury. Science 1989;245: 186–188.

20. O'Donohoe MK, Schwartz LB, Radic ZS, Mikat EM, McCann RL, Hagen P. Chronic ACE inhibition reduces intimal hyperplasia in experimental vein grafts. Ann Surg 1991;214:727–731.

21. Bell L, Madri JA. Influence of the angiotensin system on endothelial and smooth muscle cell migration. Am J Pathol 1990;137:7–12.

22. Geisterfer AA, Peach MJ, Owens GK. Angiotensin II induces hypertrophy, not hyperplasia, of cultured rat aortic smooth muscle cells. Circ Res 1988;62:749–756.
23. Prescott MF, Webb RL, Reidy MA. Angiotensin-converting enzyme inhibitor versus angiotensin II, AT1 receptor antagonist: effects in smooth muscle cell migration and proliferation after balloon injury. Am J Pathol 1991;139:1291–1296.
24. Hilgarth K, Trachtenberg J, Choi ET, Stevens S, Callow AD. The inhibitory effect of FK506 on intimal hyperplasia. FASEB J 1992;6:A1029.

4
Involvement of Calpain in the Development of Myonephropathic Metabolic Syndrome (MNMS)

Yoshifumi Tsuji, Ei-ichi Shiba, and Jun-ichi Kambayashi

Introduction

Acute obstruction of blood flow to the lower extremities is associated with high morbidity and mortality rates even after successful revascularization.[1] The mechanism behind skeletal muscle injury after ischemia has not been completely elucidated, although data support the concept that cell damage occurs during ischemia as well as during subsequent reperfusion.[2] In 1960 Haimovici et al.[3] reported acute renal failure associated with revascularization of acute arterial occlusion and defined this condition as MNMS (myonephropathic metabolic syndrome). It is well known that the main phenomena of MNMS are marked hypermyoglobinemia, myoglobinuric nephrosis with precipitation of myoglobin in the renal tubules, and metabolic alterations such as metabolic acidosis probably due to acute renal failure, azotemia, and hyperkalemia.[4,5] Several studies suggest that the reperfusion after an acute arterial occlusion of the extremities further enhances the muscle injury as a cause of MNMS.[6-8] The pathogenesis of ischemia reperfusion injury (IRI), which is complicated and involves a number of factors, has not been clearly elucidated, although an increase in intracellular calcium ($[Ca^{2+}]i$) in various organs has been thought to be responsible for the organ failure.[9,10] We presumed the ischemia and/or reperfusion-associated activation of calpain (calcium-activated neutral protease) in muscle is a significant etiologic factor, since the elevation of $[Ca^{2+}]i$ activates calpain and then activated calpain hydrolyzes α-actinin in skeletal muscle.

The purpose of this study was (1) to establish an animal model for the evaluation of myoglobinuria and skeletal muscle injury during ischemia and reperfusion, and (2) to determine whether such injury could be reduced by the administration of calpeptin, a cell-permeable synthetic peptide calpain inhibitor.[11]

Materials and Methods

Animal Model

Ten male Japanese albino rabbits weighing 2.2–2.7 kg were used after overnight fasting. The animals were anesthetized with intravenous sodium pentobarbital (30 mg/kg), and an additional dose was given if necessary to ensure that the animals did not suffer any discomfort. After laparotomy by a median incision, small-caliber plastic catheters were placed in the inferior mesenteric artery (IMA), inferior vena cava (IVC), and bladder for systemic blood pressure monitoring, venous blood collection, and urine collection, respectively. Ischemia of the hind legs was induced experimentally by ligations of the distal collateral branches (Fig. 4.1), and then by cross-clamping of the infrarenal abdominal aorta with a small atraumatic clamp (holding force 65 g). The ischemic state was maintained for 5 hours and then the clamp was released. The subsequent 3 hours of reperfusion state was observed. An intravenous bolus dose of sodium heparin (50 U/kg IV) was administered just before clamping the aorta. Throughout the experiment, saline was continuously infused (5 mL/kg/hr) via IMA and marginal ear vein. Two milliliters of blood was collected from IVC, which was immediately anticoagulated with one-tenth volume of 3.8% trisodium citrate at the following times; before clamping, 300 minutes after clamping; 30, 90, and 180 minutes after reperfusion. The volume of blood removed was replaced with an equal amount of saline. An aliquot of the anticoagulated blood was delivered to an automated blood cell counter for the determination of white blood cell (WBC) count, red blood cell (RBC) count, platelet (PLT) count, hematocrit (Ht), and hemoglo-

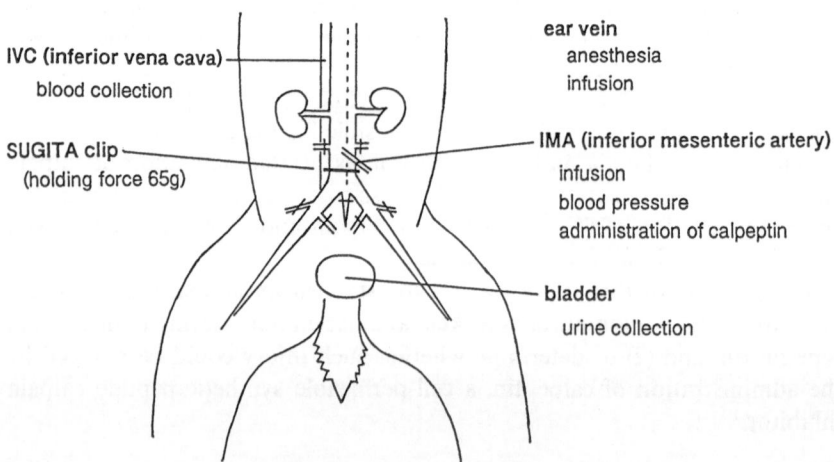

FIGURE 4.1. Animal model.

bin (Hb) value. Then, plasma was prepared from the remaining whole blood, which was kept frozen until the assay of N-acetyl-β-D-glucosaminidase (NAG) by a chromogenic substrate method using MCP-NAG[12] (NAG Test Shionogi, Shionogi Pharmaceuticals, Osaka, Japan). At the end of the 3 hours reperfusion period, the gracilis muscle was harvested fixed in 10% formalin, and stained with hematoxylin–eosin for light microscopic (LM) examination. The animals were sacrificed by an overdose of sodium pentobarbital. Myoglobinuria was detected by the 65% salting-out method.[13]

Experimental Group

Ten rabbits were divided into two groups of five animals each. Group 1 (untreated) received IRI only. group 2 (treated) received IRI + calpeptin. A bolus intraaortic administration of calpeptin (12 mg/kg) was given through IMA just prior to aorta clamping.

Statistical Analysis

Data were presented as the mean ± SD. Statistical differences were analyzed by the unpaired Student's t test.

Results

Blood Pressure

Systemic blood pressure (BP) in both groups was not significantly altered by the aortic clamping and during the subsequent ischemic state (I-300), as shown in Table 4.1. However, BP in group 1 (IRI) markedly dropped from $97 \pm 2.4\%$ (I-300) to $80 \pm 8.9\%$ (R-30) and to $65 \pm 4.9\%$ (R-180). Adminis-

TABLE 4.1. Changes in parameters during ischemia and reperfusion

	Group	pre	I-300	R-30	R-90	R-180
Blood pressure	1	100 ± 0	97 ± 2.4	80 ± 8.9	68 ± 6.8**	65 ± 4.9*
(%)	2	100 ± 0	101 ± 17.3	95 ± 13.5	91 ± 11.1**	87 ± 12.4*
Platelet (%)	1	100 ± 0	89 ± 5.9	82 ± 10.8	78 ± 6.7	69 ± 14.4
	2	100 ± 0	96 ± 7.5	78 ± 16.7	70 ± 16.6	79 ± 6.7
WBC (%)	1	100 ± 0	118 ± 40.0	113 ± 40.9	126 ± 67.8	127 ± 65.7
	2	100 ± 0	112 ± 31.1	102 ± 26.0	105 ± 25.6	106 ± 27.3
Plasma NAG	1	17.2 ± 5.4	40.5 ± 10.0	97.4 ± 19.6**	94.2 ± 13.9**	85.6 ± 25.0*
(U/l)	2	15.1 ± 3.0	40.5 ± 6.3	52.7 ± 11.5**	54.9 ± 9.6**	49.2 ± 15.8*

Group 1, IRI; group 2, IRI + calpeptin
* $p < 0.05$; ** $p < 0.01$; mean ± SD

tration of calpeptin (group 2) significantly attenuated this reperfusion-associated hypotension, 101 ± 17.3% (I-300), 95 ± 13.5% (R-30), and 87 ± 12.4% (R-180).

Blood Cell Counts

No significant change was observed in WBC count, RBC count, Ht, and Hb in both groups. There was no change in platelet count during ischemia. However, platelet count in both groups was gradually decreased and significantly dropped from 89 ± 5.9% (I-300) to 69 ± 14.4% (R-180) in group 1, and from 96 ± 7.5% (I-300) to 79 ± 6.7% (R-180) in group 2, respectively.

Plasma NAG

The plasma level of NAG in group 1 slightly increased during ischemia (40.5 ± 10.0 U/L at I-300) and it was significantly elevated to 97.4 ± 19.4 U/L immediately after reperfusion. Although the plasma level of NAG in group 2 was similarly elevated during ischemia (40.5 ± 6.3 U/L at I-300), the elevation was minimal after reperfusion (52.7 ± 11.5 U/L at R-30). The administration of calpeptin (group 2) significantly prevented the elevation of plasma NAG after reperfusion (Table 4.1).

Myoglobinuria

Myoglobinuria was detected (± − + +) in all group 1 animals after reperfusion. Myoglobinuria was detected in only one animal in group 2. Thus, the administration of calpeptin prevented this reperfusion-associated myoglobinuria (Fig. 4.2).

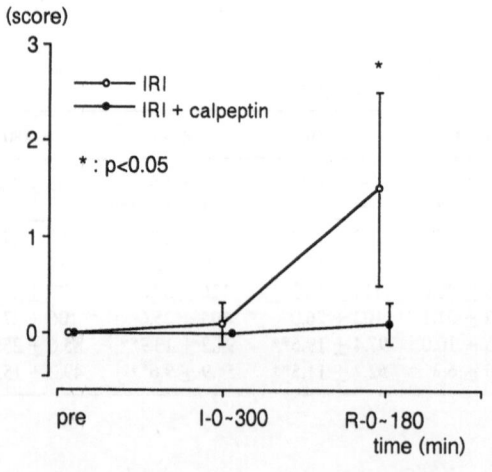

FIGURE 4.2. Changes in myoglobinuria. pre, before ischemia; I-0 ~ 300, 300 min after ischemia; R-0 ~ 180, 0 ~ 180 min after reperfusion.

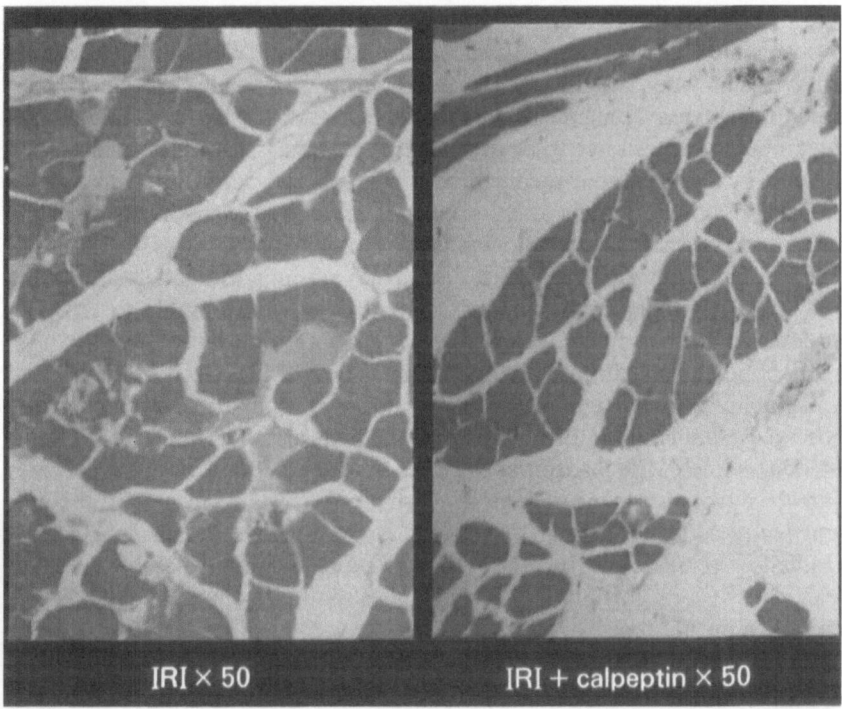

FIGURE 4.3. Histological findings of skeletal muscle in R-180 under light microscopy (x50).

Histological Findings (LM) (Fig. 4.3)

The affected muscle fibers in group 1 (IRI) demonstrated several characteristic histological features, namely, degeneration of the sarcoplasm and marked edema in the interstitial tissues and intramuscular region. However, the muscles in group 2 exhibited minimal histological changes, such as interstitial edema. The administration of calpeptin apparently prevented damage of the gracilis muscle histologically. The kidneys of group 1 animals showed acute tubular necrosis with hemorrhage and dissolution in the renal epithelium of the proximal convoluted tubule. These changes in kidney were not observed in group 2 (data not shown).

Discussion

Calpain (calcium-activated neutral protease) is a cytosolic cysteine protease regulated by Ca^{2+} that shows maximal activity at neutral pH. It exists in different tissues of various species. Although the physiological function of this enzyme has not been fully clarified yet, it has been considered to play important roles in various cell functions through proteolytic processes. Calpain has two isozymes, calpain I and calpain II, according to Ca^{2+} sensitivity. Muscle proteins, enzyme proteins, cytoskeletal proteins, coagulation factor, and other have been recognized as calpain substrates.[14] In skeletal muscle, α-actinin has been shown to be degraded by calpain.[15,16] We have developed a peptide calpain inhibitor, calpeptin,[11] which is cell-permeable and may be applied to animal models as a useful tool to probe the involvement of the enzyme under various physiological or pathological conditions.

First, attempts were made to establish an animal model simulating MNMS. After repeated preliminary experiments, we were able to establish the present animal model, which manifested, with high reproducibility, systemic hypotension, thrombocytopenia, elevation of plasma NAG level, and myoglobinuria after reperfusion, which may be compatible with clinically observed manifestation of MNMS. NAG, with a molecular weight of 13–14 kDa, is one of the lysozomal enzymes that degrade mucopolysaccharides and glycoproteins. Measurement of plasma NAG was performed in the present study as an indicator of skeletal muscle damage. Plasma NAG level gradually increased during the ischemic state and immediately increased after reperfusion. This observation indicates that severe muscle damage was provoked during reperfusion.

A cell-permeable calpain inhibitor, calpeptin, clearly inhibited the increase of NAG after reperfusion. There was no effect on NAG level during ischemia. Concomitant with this observation, calpeptin prevented the degradation of skeletal muscle determined by light microscopy. These data indicate that calpain is supposed to be active during reperfusion via elevation of $[Ca^{2+}]i$, and that activated calpain causes degradation of skeletal muscle and release of NAG from muscle cells. It is also conceivable that calpain was involved in the development of myoglobinuria as well and calpeptin prevented it. The preventive effect of calpeptin on the decrease of blood pressure during reperfusion has not been clarified yet. One can assume that various substances released from muscle cells might induce hypotension directly or indirectly via various cytokines,[17,18] oxygen free radicals,[19,20], complement factors, and so on.[21,22] When calpeptin was administered, calpain would not be activated in the damaged tissues by ischemia and reperfusion. Therefore, the amount of various substances released from the skeletal muscle cells should be diminished, resulting in improvement in the various parameters of MNMS. These observations ensure the possible clinical application of calpain inhibitors for the treatment of MNMS.

References

1. Blaisdell FW, Steele M, Allen RE. Management of acute lower extremity arterial ischemia due to embolism and thrombosis. Surgery 1978;84:822–834.
2. Haimovici H. Metabolic complications of acute arterial occlusions. J Cardiovasc Surg 1979;20:349–357.

3. Haimovici H. Arterial embolism with acute massive ischemic myopathy and myoglobinuria. Surgery 1960;47:739–747.
4. Haimovici H. Muscular, renal, and metabolic complications of acute arterial occlusions. Myonephropathic metabolic syndrome. Surgery 1979;85:461–468.
5. Fisher RE, Fogarty TJ, Morrow AG. Clinical and biochemical observations of the effect of transient femoral artery occlusion in man. Surgery 1970;68:323–328.
6. Perry MD, Fantini G. Ischemia profile of an enemy. Reperfusion injury of skeletal muscle. J Vasc Surg 1987;6:231–238.
7. McCord JM. oxygen-derived free radicals in post-ischemic tissue injury. N Engl J Med 1985;312:159–164.
8. Feller AM, Roth AC, Russell RC, Eagleton B, Suchy H, Debs N. Experimental evaluation of oxygen free radical scavengers in the prevention of reperfusion injury to skeletal muscle. Ann Plast Surg 1989;22:321-329.
9. Pridijian A, Levitsky S, Krukenkamp I, Silverman N, Feinberg H. Intracellular sodium and calcium in the post ischemic myocardium. Ann Thorac Surg 1987; 43:416–421.
10. Smith A, Hayes G, Frcsc AR, Paul W. The role of extracellular calcium in ischemia/reperfusion injury in skeletal muscle. J Surg Res 1990;49:153–156.
11. Tsujinaka T, Kajiwara Y, Kambayashi J, et al. Synthesis of a new cell penetrating calpain inhibitor (calpeptin). Biochem Biophys Res Commun 1988;153:1201–1208.
12. Noto A, Ogawa Y, Mori S. Simple, rapid spectrophotometry of urinary N-acetyl-β-D-glucosaminidase, with use of a new chromogenic substrate. Clin Chem 1983; 29:567–572.
13. Solomon HB, Emanuel M, Elazar S. A simple set of myohemoglobinuria (myoglobinuria). JAMA 1958;167:453–454.
14. Kambayashi J, Sakon M. Calcium dependent proteases and their inhibitors in human platelets. Methods Enzymol 1989;169:442–455.
15. Bullard B, Sainsbury G, Miller N. Digestion of proteins associated with the Z-disc by calpain. J Muscle Res Cell Motility 1990;11:271–279.
16. Goll DE, Dayton WR, Singh I, Robson RM. Studies of the α-actinin/actin interaction in Z-disk by using calpain. J Biol Chem 1991;266:8501–8510.
17. Ascer E, Mohan C, Gennaro M, Cupo S. Interleukin-1 and thromboxane release after skeletal muscle ischemia and reperfusion. Ann Vasc Surg 1992;6:69–73.
18. Walker PM. Ischemia/reperfusion injury in skeletal muscle. Ann Vasc Surg 1991; 5:399–402.
19. Korthuis RJ, Granger DN, Townsly MI, Taylor AE. The role of oxygen-derived free radicals in ischemia-induced increases in canine skeletal muscle vascular permeability. Circ Res 1985; 57:599–609.
20. Rubin B, Tittly J, Chang G, et al. A clinically applicable method for long term salvage of post ischemic skeletal muscle. J Vasc Surg 1991;13:58–68.
21. Cambria RA, Anderson RJ, Dinkdan G, Lysz TW, Hobson RW II. The influence of arachidonic acid metabolites on leukocyte activation and skeletal muscle injury after ischemia and reperfusion. J Vasc Surg 1991;14:549–556.
22. Anderson RJ, Cambria RA, Dikdan G, Lysz TW, Hobson RW II. Role of eicosanoids and white blood cells. The beneficial effects of limited reperfusion after ischemia-reperfusion injury in skeletal muscle. Am J Surg 1990;160:151–155.

II
Anesthesia in Vascular Surgery

5
Anesthesia and Perioperative Cardiac Risk in Vascular Surgery Patients

Thomas R. Eide

Coronary Artery Disease in the Vascular Surgical Patient

Coronary artery disease in the vascular surgical patient continues to represent one of the largest and most clinically significant factors contributing to perioperative morbidity and anesthetic management decisions.

A highly significant relationship exists between the presence of coronary artery disease and patients evaluated for and undergoing vascular surgical procedures. in a series of 1,000 vascular surgical patients beginning in 1978 at the Cleveland Clinic, 25% were found to have severe, correctable coronary disease.[1] Within this group, only 34% of patients were suspected by history and clinical findings of having coronary disease. Severe correctable coronary disease was found in 31% of patients whose primary vascular diagnosis was abdominal aortic aneurysm, in 26% of patients with cerebral vascular disease, and in 21% of patients with lower extremity disease.[2]

Perioperative Myocardial Ischemia

Performing coronary arteriography on all vascular surgical patients is currently not recommended on the basis of both intrinsic procedural risk and increased economic cost. Identifying patients at risk for perioperative cardiac events by means other than coronary arteriography and understanding the nature of perioperative myocardial ischemia is important in order to take steps to reduce morbidity.

Many studies now indicate that the majority of perioperative cardiac ischemic episodes occur postoperatively and that patients with postoperative ischemic episodes are at risk for postoperative cardiac events and have poorer outcomes. Mangano and colleagues[3] prospectively studied 474 men with coronary artery disease undergoing elective noncardiac surgery and found that 41% had electrocardiographic (ECG) findings of myocardial ischemia during the postoperative period, as compared with 20% before surgery and 25% during surgery. They also found that postoperative myocardial ischemia within 48 hours after surgery conferred a ninefold increase in the odds of cardiac death, nonfatal myocardial infarction, or developing unstable angina. Long-term follow-up of this group found that the occurrence of a postoperative ischemic episode and a postoperative adverse cardiac event conferred a greatly increased risk for a subsequent cardiac complication over a 2-year period.[4]

Myocardial Infarction

Perioperative myocardial infarction continues to have a major impact on vascular surgical patients. the rate of perioperative myocardial infarction in studies of vascular surgical patients that included peripheral, carotid, and aortic disease, including emergency procedures,[5,6] has been found to range from 0.7% to 3.9%, with an overall rate of 2%–3% most consistently found.

It has been shown that myocardial infarction has a significant impact on overall outcome in postsurgical follow-up studies. In a group of 273 patients who underwent lower extremity revascularization, fatal postoperative myocardial infarction occurred in 3.3% and accounted for 52% of deaths within 30 days of surgery.[7] In 335 patients undergoing carotid endarterectomy, fatal myocardial infarction occurred postoperatively in 1.8% of patients and accounted for 60% of early postoperative deaths,[8] and in 343 patients who had a repair of an abdominal aortic aneurysm, fatal myocardial infarction accounted for 37% of all postoperative deaths and occurred in 6% of patients.[9]

These studies have shown that the rate of perioperative myocardial infarction is significant in vascular surgical patients and represents a major cause of perioperative and long-term morbidity.

Clinical Risk Factors of Perioperative Myocardial Ischemia

Many clinical characteristics have been identified as predictors of perioperative myocardial ischemia. The presence of left ventricular hypertrophy on ECG, hypertension, diabetes mellitus, the known presence of coronary artery disease (angina, heart failure, previous myocardial infarction), and the use of digoxin have been shown to be significant predictors of perioperative cardiac morbidity.[10]

Clinical conditions common in vascular surgical patients that are of concern to the anesthesiologist are recent myocardial infarction, heart failure, dysrhythmias, and hypertension.

Prior Myocardial Infarction

Patients with a history of prior myocardial infarction have a higher rate of perioperative reinfarction when compared to patients without prior myocardial infarction (5%–7% compared to 0.1%–0.5% for general surgical patients). Rao[11] studied two groups of patients who were undergoing noncardiac surgery who had a previous myocardial infarction. His first group was a retrospective review of 364 patients from 1973 to 1976. This group had a reinfarction rate of 7.7%. A second group of 733 patients followed prospectively from 1977 to 1982 had a reinfarction rate of 1.9%. This second group of patients was managed with arterial lines, pulmonary artery catheters, and a 3- to 4-day stay in a postoperative intensive care unit, and had aggressive intraoperative control of blood pressure and heart rate. It is implied by this study that optimization of cardiovascular status, invasive monitoring, and aggressive intervention and control of intraoperative hemodynamic parameters served to dramatically reduce the rate of reinfarction in these patients.

Rao's study[11] also addressed the length of time it would be prudent to delay elective surgery after a recent myocardial infarction. In his prospectively followed group, the rate of reinfarction after surgery was 5.7% in patients with an infarct less than 3 months old, and 2.3% in patients with an infarction 4–6 months old. Steen[12] found reinfarction rates of 27% for a myocardial infarction less than 3 months old and 11% for a myocardial infarction 4–6 months old. Rao's percentages are much lower than those in many other studies that address the rate of reinfarction relative to the length of time between a myocardial infarction and elective surgery. Despite the large differences in rates found in Rao's study as compared to other studies, nearly all studies have found that waiting 3 months after a myocardial infarction before proceeding with elective surgery significantly reduces the risk of reinfarction. Waiting 6 months further decreases the risk of reinfarction, but to a lesser degree.

Heart Failure

The presence of impaired cardiac function determined clinically by evidence of pulmonary congestion, as S_3, juvenile vascular disease (JVD), or measured as an election fraction by an imaging technique, is widely recognized as a significant and large factor associated with perioperative morbidity. Goldman's [13] multifactorial index of cardiac risk in noncardiac surgery ascribed the highest number of risk points to the presence of JVD or an S_3. In Mangano's[4] study of long-term cardiac events following noncardiac surgery, the presence of preexisting congestive failure was found to correlate with adverse cardiac events for the in-hospital period and for up to 2 years after discharge. In a large study[14] of preoperative predictors of perioperative adverse outcomes on 17,201 patients, a history of congestive heart failure carried a 7.3% risk of a severe outcome event (myocardial ischemia, myocardial infarction, cardiac failure, respiratory failure, or bronchospasm).

Cardiac failure in a surgical patient should be treated aggressively and well in advance of the surgical procedure with every reasonable effort made to optimize cardiac performance.

Ventricular Arrhythmias

In a patient population considered at risk for coronary artery disease, the presence of asymptomatic ventricular arrhythmias (frequent paroxysmal ventricular complex (PVC) or ventricular tachycardia) is regarded as a manifestation of underlying cardiac pathology. The vascular surgical patient population is, however, already presumed to have significant risk for cardiac disease, and the presence of a perioperative ventricular arrhythmia may not be by itself an independent marker for a further increased risk of an adverse cardiac outcome. Shah and colleagues[15] prospectively studied 688 patients with coronary artery disease undergoing noncardiac surgery and found no correlation of arrhythmias with perioperative myocardial infarction. This study, as with most previous studies addressing the significance of arrhythmias, did not continuously record the ECG on patients throughout surgery. In a more recent study using continuous Holter monitoring beginning 24 hours preoperatively, O'Kelly and coinvestigators[16] prospectively followed 230 major noncardiac surgical patients with known or presumed cardiac disease. He found that ventricular arrhythmias were common, occurring in 44% of patients, and that there was no relationship between ventricular arrhythmias and perioperative myocardial infarction or inhospital cardiac death. Increased intraoperative arrhythmias were associated with preoperative arrhythmias and preoperative congestive failure, and were found during new episodes of myocardial ischemia.

There is a need to make reasonable recommendations for patients with asymptomatic ventricular arrhythmias and patients receiving chronic antiarrhythmic therapy. Asymptomatic patients found to have ventricular arrhythmias not thought secondary to ongoing ischemia are not considered to be at increased risk for an adverse cardiac outcome.

The physiologic changes intrinsic to the induction of general anesthesia and the perioperative period, such as alterations in blood pCO_2, pH, electrolytes, and sympathetic activity, can increase arrhythmia activity, which may require intraoperative treatment with an antiarrhythmic agent. These patients should have their ECG monitored continuously for a least 3 days postoperatively to demonstrate a return to baseline arrhythmic activity, but need not be committed to chronic antiarrhythmic therapy.

Patients currently on chronic antiarrhythmic therapy should continue their medications up to surgery and may require intravenous supplementation of their medications during the procedure, depending upon the length of surgery and the half-life of the agents, in order to maintain therapeutic blood levels.

Hypertension

The adequate preoperative control of chronic hypertensive disease as a necessary step to minimize anesthetic risk and postoperative outcome remains controversial and unresolved. The presence of hypertension was found to be an independent predictor of in-hospital mortality among patients undergoing noncardiac surgery,[17] yet it was not found to be a predictor of perioperative myocardial ischemia in vascular surgical patients.[18] Prys-Roberts[19] found that hypertension was associated with intraoperative lability of blood pressure; however, Goldman[20] in a large prospective study of both treated and untreated hypertensive patients found that they did not develop more perioperative cardiac complications and postoperative renal failure, and they did not require more intraoperative fluid challenges or adrenergic agents to control blood pressure decreases than normotensive patients.

The preoperative withdrawal of beta antagonists and clonidine has been studied and found to result in intraoperative blood pressure lability and to exacerbate anginal symptoms.[21,22] This is the basis for the general recommendation that antihypertensive medications should be continued and given on the morning of surgery.

Interpreting studies of hypertensive disease is inherently difficult. The definition of controlled blood pressure varies from study to study and includes subsets of patients whose antihypertensive medications consist of antiischemic agents (beta antagonists and nitrates), antiarrhythmic agents (calcium channel blockers), in addition to agents with only antihypertensive effects (diuretics). When weighing the many conflicting results of studies on hypertension and perioperative complications, no clear determination can be made that the presence of hypertension, whether adequately treated or not, exposes the patient to more risk.

From these nonconclusive finding only seemingly common-sense recommendations can emerge that patients on chronic antihypertensive medications should continue their medication up to surgery, that hypertensive patients may have a more labile intraoperative course and require intraoperative antihypertensive agents, and that there will most likely be no difference in the overall anesthetic outcome of these patients.

It is clear that some cardiovascular conditions are more strongly associated with worse outcomes than others (congestive heart failure, ischemic heart disease, as compared to hypertension or arrhythmias). The optimization of a patient's cardiovascular status before surgery remains imperative and includes the establishment of appropriate and stable drug regimens for cardiac failure, ischemic heart disease, arrhythmias, and hypertension.

Identifying Patients at Risk for Perioperative Myocardial Ischemia

The Holter Monitor

The ability to accurately predict which patients are at high risk for perioperative ischemic events would be valuable. These patients could be evaluated more extensively and treated more aggressively to reduce their cardiac risk before proceeding with vascular surgery. Two potentially useful means of stratifying cardiac risk preoperatively are Holter monitoring and dipyridamole–thallium scintigraphy.

Raby[23] studied 176 elective vascular surgical patients who were not preselected on the basis of risk factors of coronary disease and followed them through their operative course with Holter monitoring beginning 24 hours prior to surgery. They found that 18% of these patients had preoperative ischemic events, nearly all of which were asymptomatic. Of patients who had preoperative ischemic events, 38% had postoperative cardiac events (fatal and nonfatal myocardial infarction and unstable angina), as compared to less than 1% of patients without preoperative ischemic events. In a similar study of 115 patients, Raby[18] was able to show that preoperative Holter screening for ischemic events could identify a group of patients particularly at risk for postoperative cardiac events. In this study, 18% of patients had preoperative ischemia and 30% had postoperative ischemia. Preoperative ischemia was present in 57% of patients with postoperative ischemia, as compared with 4% without postoperative ischemia.

The use of Holter monitoring as simple, risk-free, and cost-effective means of identifying patients at risk for perioperative cardiac events is promising. More investigation is required, however, before the routine use of preoperative Holter monitoring can be recommended for all vascular surgical patients.

Dipyridamole–Thallium Scintigraphy

Dipyridamole–thallium scintigraphy involves the intravenous injection of dipyridamole, an agent that maximally dilates nonstenosed coronary circulation at the expense of stenosed coronary circulation. This "coronary steal phenomenon" is identified by injecting thallium-201, which distributes to regions of the myocardium in proportion to blood flow. The defects seen can represent old scarring or infarcts. These defects are reexamined 4 hours later for evidence of increased thallium uptake. If uptake has occurred in these areas, they are considered to represent regions of viable myocardium placed at risk due to the presence of an arterial stenosis. It is this "redistribution phenomenon" which indicates the presence of a significant coronary lesion.

The results of many studies on the usefulness of dipyridamole–thallium scintigraphy to predict adverse perioperative cardiac events have ranged from findings of a highly sensitive and specific predictor of perioperative myocardial ischemia in a study by Boucher[24] to no predictive value in a study by Mangano.[25] Most of these studies, however, consistently point to the usefulness of dipyridamole–thallium scintigraphy in its high negative predictive accuracy. That is, if no redistribution is found, the chances for an uneventful operative course are very high. The use of dipyridamole–thallium scintigraphy in patients without clinical indications of cardiac disease has not yet been established.

Intraoperative Monitoring for Myocardial Ischemia

The history of the introduction of virtually all intraoperative monitoring equipment has shown that factors of availability, ease of use, and expense, not necessarily those of intrinsic usefulness or predictive value for overall outcome, determine whether or not a monitor is accepted in the operating room.

There are three clinically feasible and commonly accepted ways of monitoring for the detection of intraoperative myocardial ischemia: the electrocardiogram (ECG), the pulmonary artery (PA) catheter, and transesophageal echocardiography (TEE).

Electrocardiogram

Electrocardiography is considered a standard and acceptable method for detecting intraoperative myocardial ischemia. Certain recommendations should be adhered to for optimal use of the ECG as an ischemia detection monitor. Most monitoring manufacturers now make available a computerized and continuous S-T segment evaluation with trending of multiple ECG leads. These monitors should have a frequency response of 0.05–100 Hz and provide for continuous display and trending of the S-T segment 60 msec after the J point. They should also provide a means for adjusting which part of the S-T segment the monitor will follow, since shortening of the S-T segment with tachycardia will result in a sampling of part of the T wave. Also, a digoxin effect, left ventricular hypertrophy, and left bundle branch block can interfere with S-T segment monitoring.

An S-T segment depression of at least 1 mm, lasting at least 1 minute and deviating from a previously normal baseline, should be suspected of being an ischemic episode. Since it is not practicable to continuously monitor all 12 leads on a surgical patient, the sensitivity of using only two or three leads has been investigated. It was found that the continuous trending of at least two leads, II and V_5, will detect 80% or ischemic episodes and that the use of three leads, II, V_4, and V_5, will detect 96% of ischemic episodes relative to the 12-lead ECG.[26]

Pulmonary Artery Catheter

The PA catheter was for many years considered a reliable method for detecting intraoperative myocardial ischemia.[27] Many follow-up studies have found, however, that myocardial ischemia can be present without an elevation in pulmonary capillary wedge pressure (PCWP) or the appearance of a V wave. Haggmark's[28] study of cardiac ischemia in 53 vascular surgical patients compared wall motion changes seen with cardiokymography to ECG changes, coronary lactate production, and PA catheter measurements. They found that the PA catheter was unreliable in detecting ischemic episodes. Leung's[29] study of regional wall motion abnormalities as seen by transesophageal echocardiography found that changes in PA catheter indices were not present during most ECG and TEE ischemic episodes. They concluded that the PA catheter was a very insensitive monitor for detecting intraoperative myocardial ischemia.

Continuous S-T segment trending with multilead ECG and the appearance of new regional wall motion abnormalities with TEE are much more sensitive than the PA catheter for diagnosing intraoperative myocardial ischemia.

Transesophageal Echocardiography

TEE is a relatively new operating room monitoring technique (Fig. 5.1) that has been used in surgical patients since 1985. It has been found that inserting an echo probe in the esophagus produces clear and detailed images of all four cardiac chambers and allows for examination of the left ventricle and the mitral and aortic valves (Fig. 5.2). Changes in wall motion, ventricular size, and valve motion and blood flow are readily determined with a TEE examination (Fig. 5.3).

The benefits of using TEE in all patients undergoing vascular surgical procedures, however, have not yet been demonstrated. In a series[30] of 49 patients undergoing vascular surgical procedures, new wall motion abnormalities were found in 14 patients. In 10 of those 14, resolution of wall motion abnormalities occurred after treatment for ischemia. These patients did not develop myocardial infarction. In the other 4 whose wall motion did not return to normal, 1 sustained a myocardial infarction and 1 had an intraoperative cardiac arrest. In a more recent study, Eisenberg[31] looked at TEE and the 12-lead ECG and compared these to the use of a 2-lead ECG and preoperative clinical data for the ability to identify patients at high risk for perioperative ischemic outcomes (cardiac death, myocardial infarction, unstable angina). He found that TEE yielded little incremental value beyond preoperative clinical indicators to predict perioperative ischemic outcomes.

Proficient use of TEE requires many hours of training for consistent and accurate interpretation of images and changes in wall motion. Manipulating the esophageal probe and viewing the TEE monitor does require a large

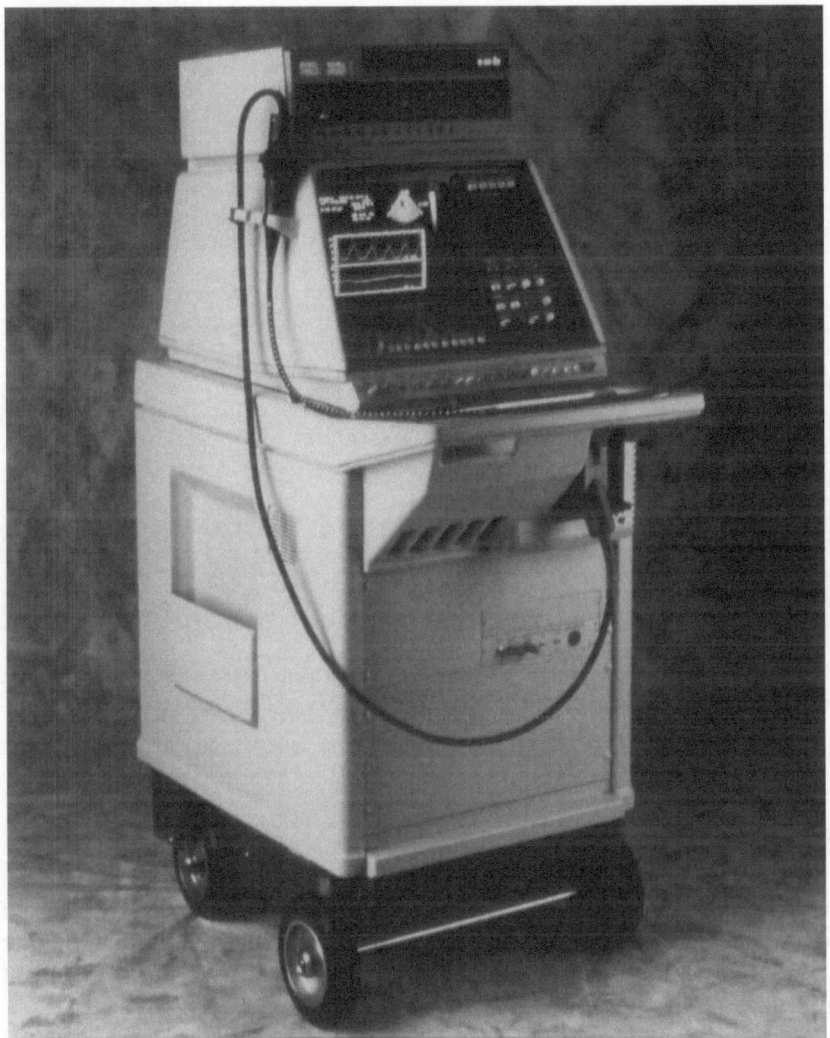

FIGURE 5.1. The Transesophageal Ultrasound Monitoring System consisting of the control panel, monitor, VCR, and attached transesophageal echo probe. Courtesy of The Hewlett-Packard Company, Andover, Massachusetts.

attentional demand from the anesthesiologist and can distract from other areas of patient care. These aspects of TEE use will become more apparent as it is more extensively studied in the operating room.

Apart from these problems, TEE provides the most comprehensive evaluation of cardiac function available for routine clinical use, but more investigation is necessary to determine if the routine use of TEE will improve patient outcome in the vascular surgical patient population.

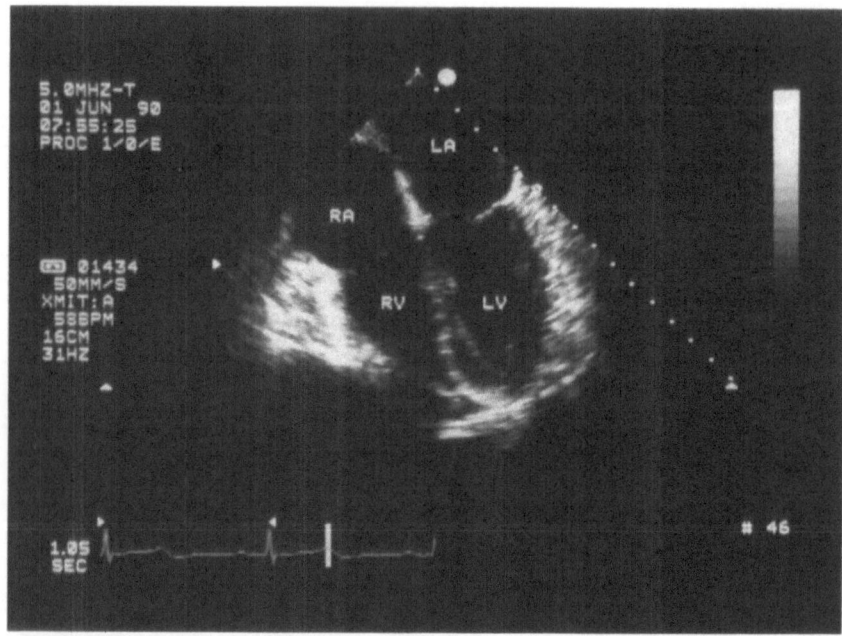

FIGURE 5.2. The four-chamber view allows detailed examination of the mitral valve, left ventricular outflow tract, and left atrium. Courtesy of The Hewlett-Packard Company, Andover, Massachusetts.

Choice of General or Epidural Anesthesia

In recent years the use of an epidural catheter to provide anesthesia and postoperative pain control has gained in popularity. The question of whether epidural anesthesia and postoperative epidural analgesia improves patient outcome is an important topic of ongoing research.

There are many theoretical advantages to regional anesthesia. The gradual delivery of a local anesthetic agent into the epidural space is the only absolute drug requirement. This eliminates the need for intravenous induction and maintenance anesthetics, some of which possess significant cardiac depressant effect. Also, the need for endotracheal intubation and mechanical ventilation with their secondary hemodynamic effects can be avoided. Studies in vascular, urologic, and orthopedic patient populations have demonstrated a decreased intraoperative blood loss,[32] a reduced rate of perioperative deep venous thrombosis and pulmonary embolism,[33] and a reduced postoperative pulmonary complication rate[34] in patients receiving epidural anesthesia either with or without general anesthesia.

Another theoretical advantage of epidural anesthesia is an improvement in myocardial oxygen balance. Myocardial oxygen consumption should be

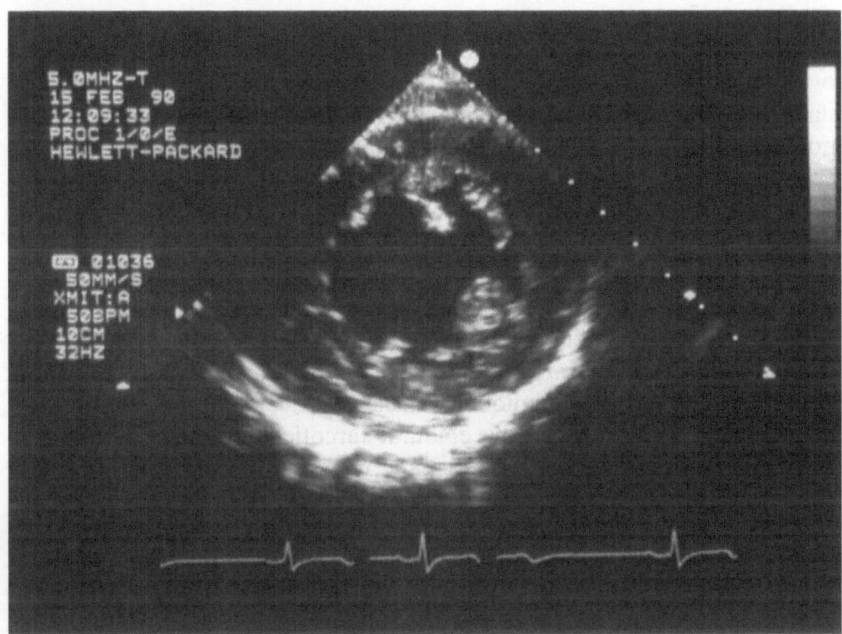

FIGURE 5.3. The short axis view of the left ventricle at the midpapillary muscle level is the standard location for trending wall motion abnormalities. All three coronary arteries contribute blood flow to this level of the left ventricle. Courtesy of The Hewlett-Packard Company, Andover, Massachusetts.

TABLE 5.1. Epidural anesthesia

Complications	Contraindications
Epidural hematoma	Prolonged bleeding time/coagulopathy
Nerve damage	Preexisting neuropathy
Hypotension	Hypovolemia
CNS depression/seizure	Uncooperative/noncommunicative patient
Dural puncture and headache	
Incomplete motor or sensory blockade	

reduced from a decreased preload and afterload and from sympathetic blockade. One study of lumbar epidural anesthesia[35] and a recent study[36] of thoracic epidural anesthesia in vascular surgical patients have shown that epidural anesthetic levels have resolved ischemic symptoms and wall motion abnormalities viewed with TEE.

There are risks associated with epidural anesthesia (Table 5.1), and the benefits of an epidural catheter to reduce intraoperative or postoperative complications in vascular surgical patients have only been inferred and not completely answered.

One study[37] of general anesthesia combined with epidural anesthesia compared to general anesthesia alone in 173 patients undergoing abdominal aortic reconstruction showed no improvement in the rate of myocardial infarction, postoperative cardiac failure, or respiratory complications. Yet in another study[38] of 53 high-risk surgical patients assigned to receive either general anesthesia plus intraoperative epidural anesthesia followed by postoperative epidural analgesia, as general anesthesia with standard intravenous pain control postoperatively, the first group developed fewer cardiac complications (myocardial infarction, congestive heart failure, ventricular arrhythmias) than the second. They also had fewer respiratory complications and a shorter intensive care unit course.

The benefits of epidural anesthesia may be in its use postoperatively. Tuman[39] compared the technique of intraoperative epidural/general anesthesia together with postoperative epidural narcotic infusion for pain control versus general anesthesia with on demand intravenous pain control for patients undergoing lower extremity vascular surgery. He found a decrease in early postoperative thrombotic events, pulmonary infections, and fewer days spent in the intensive care unit. There were no differences in postoperative cardiac ischemia or mortality.

Larger studies comparing outcomes and complications between groups of patients receiving epidural and general anesthesia need to be carried out before definitive conclusions can be stated. However, the current body of evidence indicates that when not contraindicated and when practical, the placement of an epidural catheter for use intraoperatively and, probably more importantly, for pain control postoperatively will be of benefit to patients and reduce major complications.

References

1. Hertzer NR. Clinical experience with preoperative coronary angiography. J Vasc Surg 1985;2:510–514.
2. Hertzer NR, Beven EG, Young JR, et al. Coronary artery disease in peripheral vascular patients. A classification of 1000 coronary angiograms and results of surgical management. Ann Surg 1984;199:223–233.
3. Mangano DT, Browner WS, Hollenberg M, London MJ, Tubau JF, Tateo IM. Association of perioperative myocardial ischemia with cardiac morbidity and mortality in men undergoing noncardiac surgery. N Engl J Med 1990;323:1781–1788.
4. Mangano DT, Browner WS, Hollenberg M, Li J, Tubau JF, Tateo IM. Long term cardiac prognosis following noncardiac surgery. JAMA 1992;268:233–239.
5. Bunt TJ. The role of a defined protocol for cardiac risk assessment in decreasing perioperative myocardial infarction on vascular surgery. J Vasc Surg 1992;15: 626–634.
6. Taylor LM, Yeager RA, Moneta GL, McConnell DB, Porter JM. The incidence of perioperative myocardial infarction in general vascular surgery. J Vasc Surg 1992;15:52–61.

7. Hertzer NR. Fatal myocardial infarction following lower extremity revascularization. Two hundred seventy three patients followed six to eleven postoperative years. Ann Surg 1981;193:492–498.

8. Hertzer NR. Fatal myocardial infarction following abdominal aortic aneurysm resection. Three hundred forty three patients followed six to eleven years postoperatively. Ann Surg 1980;192:667–673.

9. Hertzer NR. Fatal myocardial infarction following carotid endarterectomy. Three hundred thirty five patients followed six to eleven years after operation. Ann Surg 1981;194:212–218.

10. Hollenberg M, Mangano DT, Browner WS, London MJ, Tubau JF, Tateo IM. Predictors of postoperative myocardial ischemia in patients undergoing noncardiac surgery. JAMA 1992;268:205–209.

11. Rao TL, Jacobs KH, El-Etr AA. Reinfarction following anesthesia in patients with myocardial infarction. Anesthesiology 1983;59:499–505.

12. Steen PA, Tinker JH, Tarhan R: Myocardial reinfarction after anesthesia and surgery. JAMA 1978;239:2566–2570.

13. Goldman L, Caldera DL, Nussbaum SR, et al. Multifactorial index of cardiac risk in noncardiac surgical procedures. N Engl J Med 1977;297:845–850.

14. Forrest JB, Rehder K, Cahalan MK, Goldsmith CH. Multicenter study of general anesthesia: III. Predictors of severe perioperative adverse outcomes. Anesthesiology 1992;76:3–15.

15. Shah KB, Kleinman BS, Rao TLK, Jacobs HK, Mestan K, Schaafsma M. Angina and other risk factors in patients with cardiac diseases undergoing noncardiac operations. Anesth Analg 1990;70:240–247.

16. O'Kelly B, Browner WS, Massie B, Tubau J, Ngo L, Mangano DT. Ventricular arrhythmias in patients undergoing noncardiac surgery. JAMA 1992;268:217–221.

17. Browner WS, Li J, Mangano DT. In-hospital and long-term mortality in male veterans following noncardiac surgery. JAMA 1992;268:228–232.

18. Raby KE, Barry J, Creager MA, Cook EF, Weisberg MC, Goldman I. Detection and significance of intraoperative and postoperative myocardial ischemia in peripheral vascular surgery. JAMA 1992;268:222–227.

19. Prys-Roberts C, Meloche R, Foex P. Studies of anaesthesia in relation to hypertension 1: Cardiovascular responses of treated and untreated patients. Br J Anaesth 1971;43:122–137.

20. Goldman L, Caldera DL. risks of general anesthesia and elective operation in the hypertensive patient. Anesthesiology 1979;50:285–292.

21. Miller RR, Olson HG, Amsterdam EA, Mason ST. Propranolol-withdrawal rebound phenomenon. Exacerbation of coronary events after abrupt cessation of anti-anginal therapy. N Engl J Med 1975;293:416–418.

22. Bruce DL, Croley TF, Lee JS. Preoperative clonidine withdrawal syndrome. Anesthesiology 1979;51:90–92.

23. Raby KE, Goldman L, Creager MA, et al. Correlation between preoperative ischemia and major cardiac events after peripheral vascular surgery. N Engl J Med 1989;321:1296–1300.

24. Boucher CA, Brewster DC, Darling RC, et al. Determinations of cardiac risk by dipyridamole-thallium imaging before peripheral vascular surgery. N Engl J Med 1985;321:389–394.

25. Mangano DT, London J, Tubau F, et al. Dipyridamole thallium-201 scintigraphy

as a preoperative screening test—a reexamination of its predictive potential. Circulation 1991;84:493–502.

26. London MJ, Hollenberg M, Wong MG, et al. Intraoperative myocardial ischemia: localization by continuous 12 lead electrocardiography. Anesthesiology 1988;69:232–241.

27. Kaplan JA, Wells PH. Early diagnosis of myocardial ischemia using the pulmonary-artery catheter. Anesth Analg 1981;60:789–793.

28. Haggmark S, Hohner P, Ostman M, et al. Comparison of hemodynamic, electrocardiographic, mechanical and metabolic indicators of intraoperative myocardial ischemia in vascular surgical patients with coronary artery disease. Anesthesiology 1989;70:19–25.

29. Leung JM, O'Kelly BF, Mangano DT. Relationship of regional wall motion abnormalities to hemodynamic indices of left ventricular function. Anesthesiology 1990;73:802–814.

30. Gewertz BL, Kremser PC, Zarins CK, et al. Transesophageal echocardiographic monitoring of myocardial ischemia during vascular surgery. J Vasc Surg 1987; 5:607–613.

31. Eisenberg MJ, London MJ, Leung JM, et al. Monitoring for myocardial ischemia during noncardiac surgery. JAMA 1992;268:210–216.

32. Hendolin H, Alhava E. Effect of epidural versus general anesthesia on perioperative blood loss during retropubic prostatectomy. Int Urol Nephrol 1982;14:399–405.

33. Modig J, Hjelmstedt A, Sahlstedt B, Maripuu E. Comparative influences of epidural and general anaesthesia on deep venous thrombosis and pulmonary embolism after total hip replacement. Acta Chir Scand 1981;147:125–130.

34. Mason RA, Newton GB, Cassel W, Maneksha F, Giron F. Combined epidural and general anesthesia in aortic surgery. J Cardiovasc Surg 1990;31:442–447.

35. Baron JF, Coriat P, Mundler O. Left ventricular global and regional function during lumbar epidural anesthesia in patients with and without angina pectoris: influence of volume loading. Anesthesiology 1987;66:621–627.

36. Saada M, Catoire P, Bonnet F, et al. Effect of thoracic epidural anesthesia combined with general anesthesia on segmental wall motion assessed by transesophageal echocardiography. Anesth Analg 1992;75:329–335.

37. Baron JF, Bertrand M, Barre E, et al. Combined epidural and general anesthesia versus general anesthesia for abdominal aortic surgery. Anesthesiology 1991;75:611–618.

38. Yeager MP, Glass DD, Neff RK, Brinck JT. Epidural anesthesia and analgesia in high-risk surgical patients. Anesthesiology 1987;66:729–736.

39. Tuman KJ, McCarthy RJ, March RJ, DeLaria GA, Patel-Rajesh V, Ivankovich AD. Effects of epidural anestheisa and analgesia on coagulation and outcome after major vascular surgery. Anesth Analg 1991;73:696–704.

III
Angiography

6
Brachial Approach for Lower Limb Arteriography

Seok Kil Zeon, Soo Jhi Suh, Won Hyun Cho, Ki Yong Chung, and You-Sah Kim

Introduction

Traditionally, lumbar puncture has been performed for abdominal aortogram or bilateral lower limb arteriogram in case of occlusion or stenosis of those vessels. In addition to the fact that the needles tend to be improperly placed, many complications have been noted, such as pneumothorax, hemothorax, and chylothorax; puncturing of the left ventricle; selective placement of the needle into the renal artery, the celiac artery, or the superior mesenteric artery; incidental placement of the needle into the occluded aorta; and retroperitoneal hematoma. There has also been injury to the spinal canal or peripheral nerve.[1]

In the axillary approach, the axillary fold should be opened for a prolonged period of time during the procedure. This causes much discomfort for patients. The brachial approach has been used as an alternative route for coronary arteriogram and brain four vessels angiogram in patients in whom the femoral route was not feasible, in primary vascular diseases of the upper extremities, for evaluation of the arteriovenous shunting in renal dialysis patients,[1,2] and as a routine puncture site for outpatient arterial digital subtraction angiogram.[3] We studied the usefulness of the brachial approach in abdominal aortography, pelvic arteriography, or simultaneous opacification of bilateral lower limbs. Furthermore, the specially designed catheters were evaluated to negotiate the anatomic structure of the thoracic aorta.

Materials and Methods

The brachial approach was utilized on 51 patients (2 females and 49 males) who were clinically diagnosed as having peripheral lower limb arterial occlusive disease or abdominal aortic occlusion. The ages of the patients were between 23 and 87 years with the average age 55.

Although a weak pulsation could be felt in one or both groins, the brachial approach was undertaken for the simultaneous opacification of both lower limbs and of the recanalized vessels distal to the completely occluded or stenosed lower adominal aorta or pelvic arteries.

The right arm was placed on a flat wooden board keeping the hand supinated. The skin was prepared and a wide area around the puncture site was draped as usual, and a small amount of a local anesthetic was used for the puncture site. The maximum pulsation point of the distal brachial artery at or just above the elbow (proximal to the bifurcation of the brachial artery) was selected (Fig. 6.1), and was punctured with the Seldinger technique. An introducer sheath (6 Fr) was placed to enable easy manipulation of the catheter or to exchange it with the other type.

Just before the catheterization, 5,000 IU heparin mixed with 5 mL of normal saline was slowly infused into the side port of the introducer sheath to prevent distal arterial thrombosis.

At times the axillary fold was opened for a short period of time in elderly patients in order to advance the catheter beyond the axillary region. The guide wire was helpful during that time.

Two types of specially designed catheters (Zeon-1 and Zeon-2, Cook Co., Australia) (Fig. 6.2) were manufactured, taking into consideration the ana-

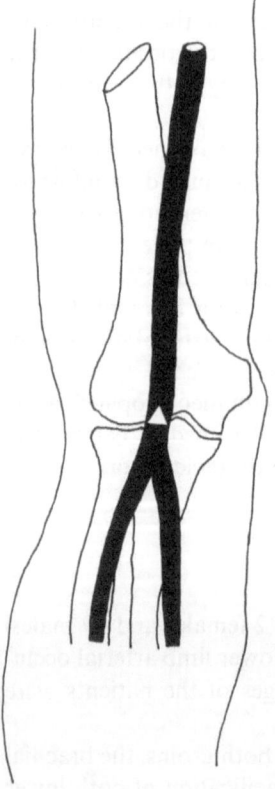

FIGURE 6.1. Puncture site of the forearm.

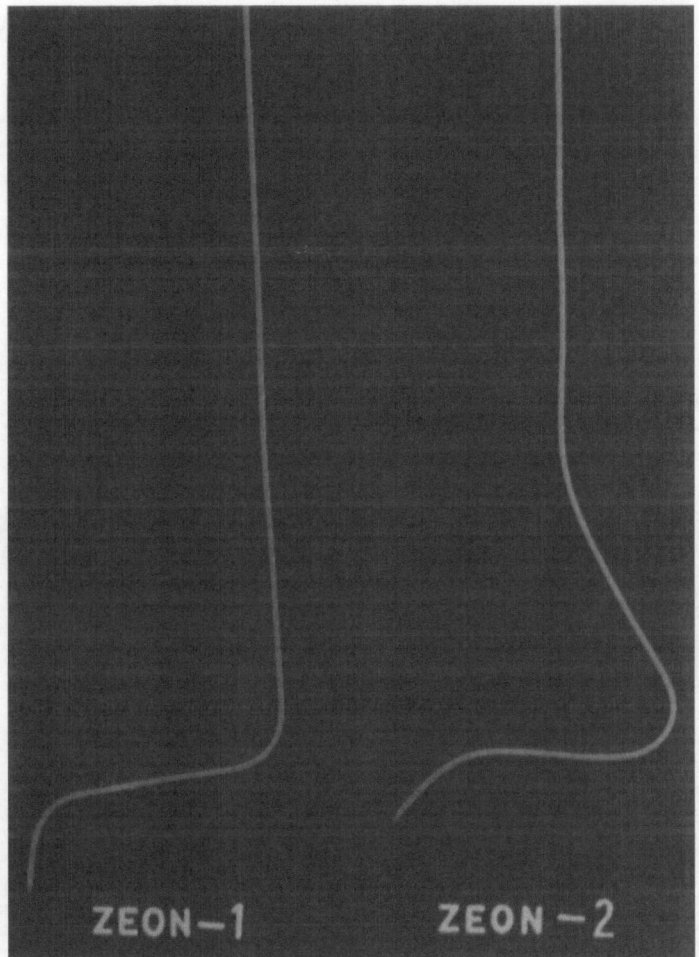

FIGURE 6.2. Radiography of two types of catheters for brachial approach (Cook Co., Australia)

tomic structure of the thoracic aorta and especially the aortic arch (Fig. 6.3). The catheters are 6 Fr in size. They are thin-walled and highly radiopaque. A stainless steel mesh is embedded in the catheter wall, to ensure high torque control for superselection and easy manipulation. However, a 10-cm curved area is left without mesh. There are four side holes within 1 cm of the end of the catheter with an open end (end hole). This allows the large bolus delivery of the contrast medium (up to 10 to 15 mL or more per second) to visualize the abdominal aorta and bilateral iliofemoral arteries simultaneously. The catheter is long enough (120 cm) to be selectively inserted into the common femoral artery or the superficial femoral artery for the selective opacification

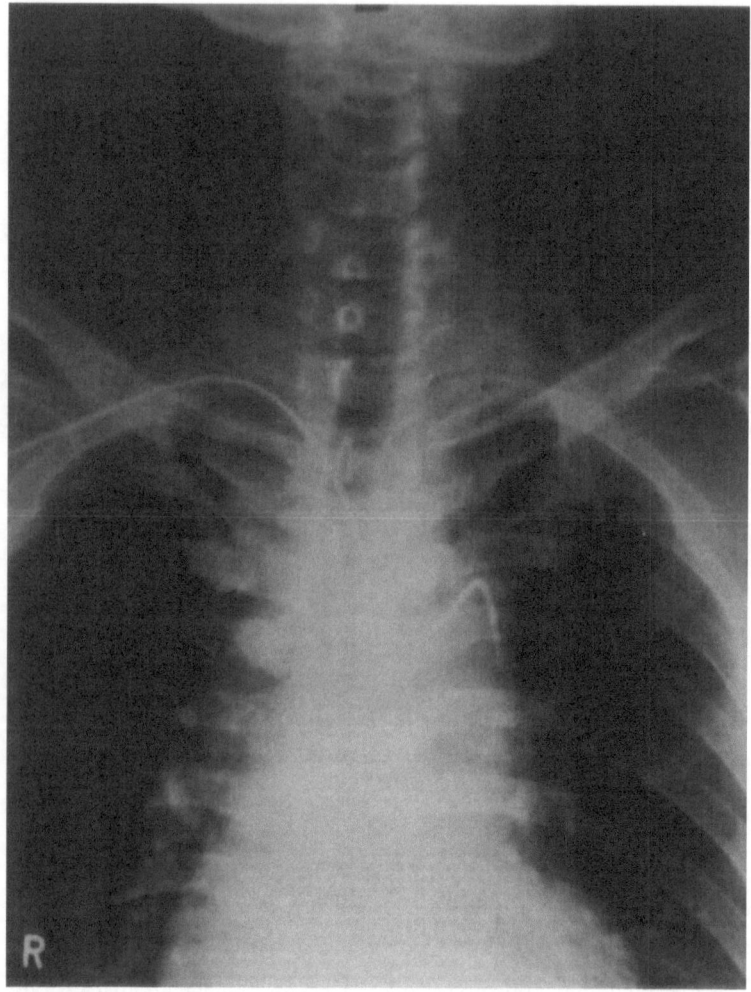

FIGURE 6.3. Catheter in aortic arch.

of one limb, which is another reason that high torque control with the stainless steel mesh in the catheter wall is needed.

The Zeon-2 catheter has a longer curved tip length, and a more complicated curve than Zeon-1.

Results

The insertion of the catheter beyond the aortic arch, down to the descending thoracic and abdominal aorta, further into the iliac and femoral arteries was successful in all 51 cases. The indications included arteriosclerotic

TABLE 6.1. Indications for brachial approach.

Arteriosclerotic occlusion or stenosis	33
Buerger's disease*	7
Thromboembolism**	7
Trauma	4
Total	51

* Including two postsurgical cases of a left hip disarticulation
and a left B-K amputation.
** Including one case of postsurgical thromboembolism.

occlusion or stenosis, Buerger's disease, trauma, and thromoboembolism (Table 6.1).

Abdominal aortograms were obtained in three cases, and they revealed the occlusion of the mid or lower abdominal aorta. The pelvic arteries distal to the occlusion were also examined to evaluate the collateral circulation (Fig 6.4).

Pelvic arteriograms were obtained in 48 patients (Figs. 6.5 and 6.6) with simultaneous bilateral lower limb arteriograms. They were done according to the step-by-step movements of the table in order to evaluate the distal run-offs. In six patients, one or both lower limb arteriograms were obtained separately after the pelvic arteriogram (Fig. 6.7).

Three patients (6%) developed transient cardiac arrhythmias upon unintentional passage of the catheter into the left ventricle, but the arrhythmias spontaneously disappeared within 5 to 6 seconds as the catheter was removed from the left ventricle. The postprocedural absence of the right radial arterial pulse was noted in two patients (4%). Vigorous physical exercise and local application of heat pack was recommended for these patients. In one patient the pulse returned within 2 days and in the other within 3 days, without anticoagulant therapy. The absence of the pulse was probably due to the longstanding compression of the puncture site for hemostasis after the procedure, rather than to thrombus formation during the procedure. There was no obvious large hematoma at the puncture site in any of the patients.

The Zeon-2 catheter negotiated the severely tortuous and dilated thoracic aorta in the aged persons better.

All the examinations in this study were satisfactory in evaluating the diseases, the collaterals, and the distal runoffs.

Discussion

When the femoral pulse is absent, lumbar puncture has been the procedure of choice in the angiographic diagnosis of occlusion or stenosis of the lower abdominal aorta. It has been used for the bilateral pelvic arteries and bilateral lower limb arteries.[1] However, several complications have been noted

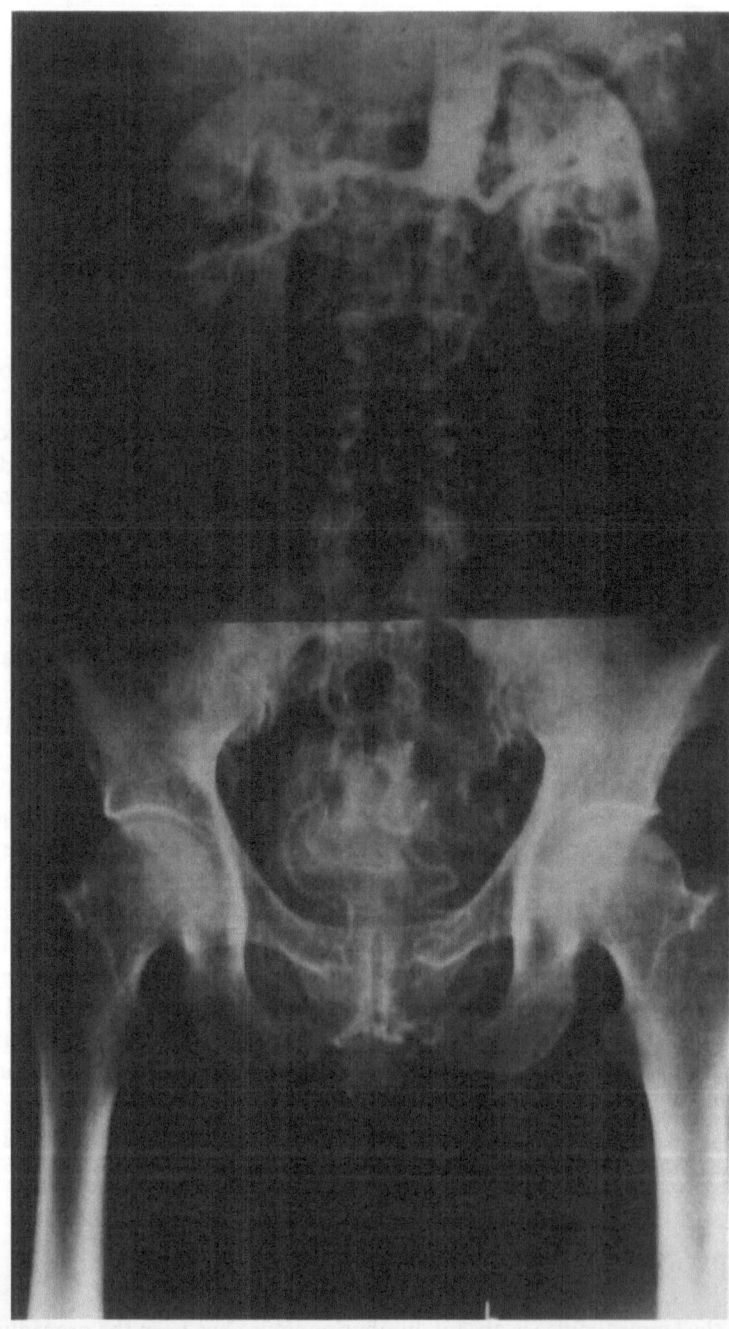

FIGURE 6.4. Arteriosclerotic occlusion of the abdominal aorta, just distal to renal arterial origins in 48-year-old male patient.

FIGURE 6.5. Pelvic arteriogram of the occluded bilateral external iliac arteries, with well-visualized recanalized left common femoral artery and its major branches, and right deep femoral artery. Good opacifications of bilateral popliteal arteries, but poor distal runoffs.

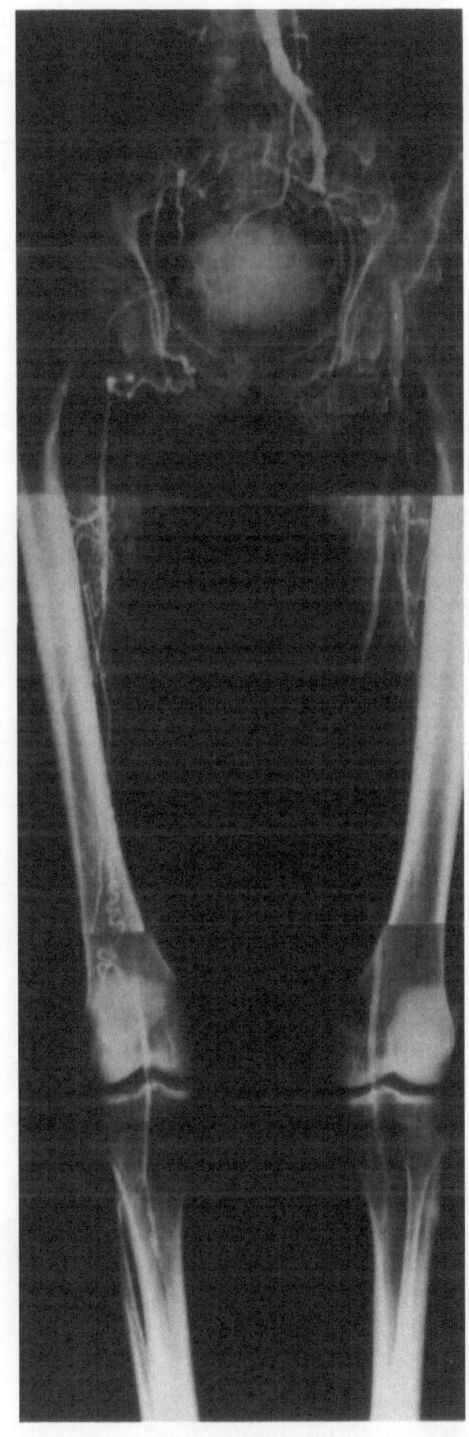

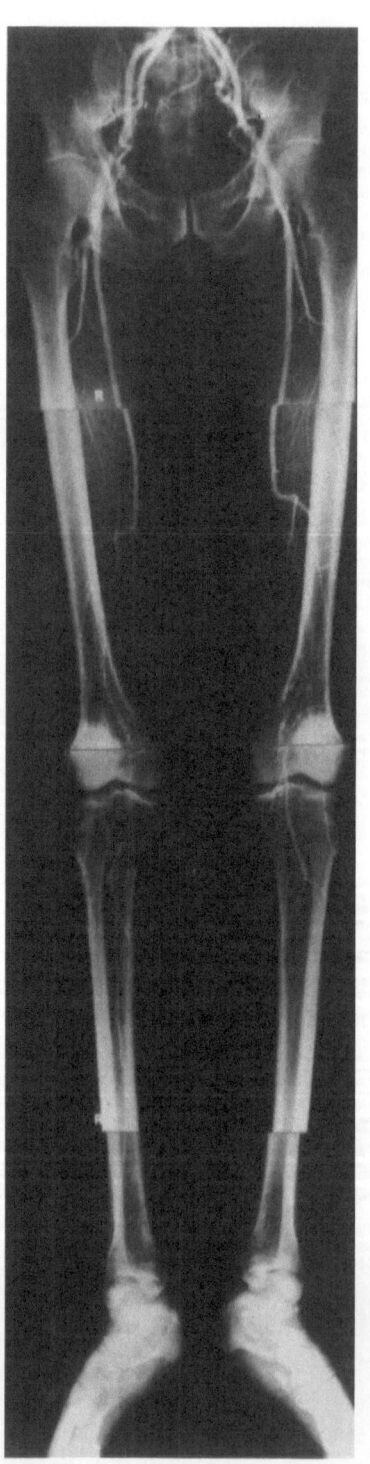

FIGURE 6.6. Simultaneous bilateral lower limb arteriogram of completely occluded bilateral superficial femoral arteries with good visualization of both recanalized popliteal arteries but poor distal runoffs down to both feet.

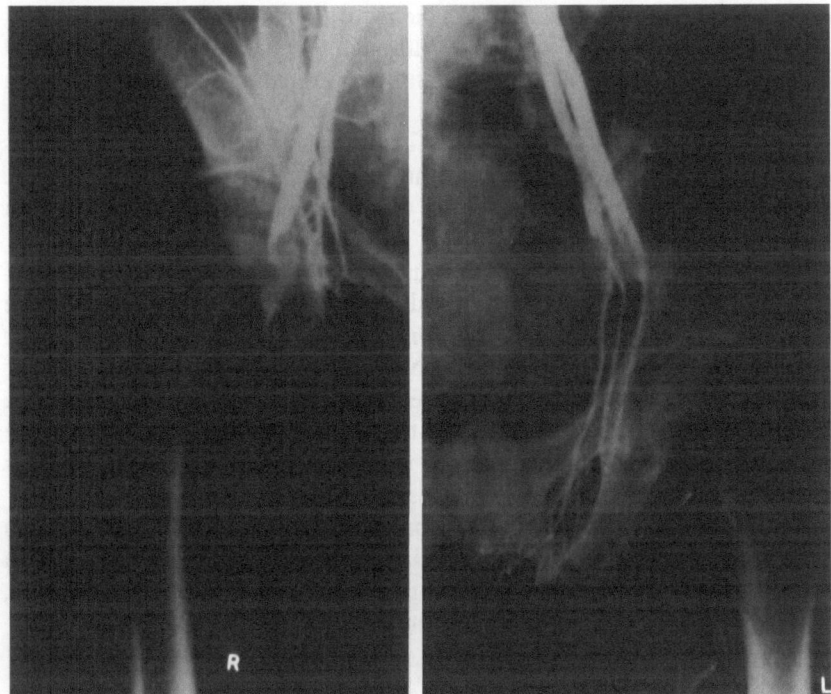

FIGURE 6.7. Separately bilateral lower limb arteriograms of thrombotic occlusions of right common femoral artery and left distal external iliac artery.

upon the improper placement of the puncture needle into the thoracic cavity and left ventricle. Accidental placement of the needle into the visceral arteries may also cause complications. Furthermore, other complications, such as retroperitoneal hematoma and injury to the spinal canal or peripheral nerve, have been noted.[1] The patients have been kept in the prone position during the whole procedure, and this also causes much discomfort. The brachial approach avoids the complications mentioned above and the distress caused by the necessary prone position.

The axillary approach is an alternative method for aortography, and for visceral and lower limb arteriography, in patients with access problems from the femoral approach.[2] However, there is severe distress during the whole procedure because the axillary fold must be kept open with the arm in 90 degree abduction. The brachial approach, which avoids the necessity of keeping the axillary fold open, eliminates the discomfort and pain. Possible complications of axillary hematoma and plexus lesions can also be avoided.[4]

Earlier studies reported that thrombosis occurred two to nine times more often in the brachial than in the femoral arterial approach.[5,6] In this series, 5,000 IU heparin was infused into the artery to prevent thrombus formation.[7]

As a result, there has been no permanent thrombus formation in the distal arteries down to the wrist joint area. Although two patients (4%) experienced transient loss of the radial pulse, spontaneous recovery was observed within 3 days.

Although three cases (6%) of cardiac arrhythmia were noted upon unintentional insertion of the catheter into the left ventricle while overcoming the tortuous aortic arch, it spontaneously disappeared as the catheter was with drawn from the left ventricle.

Two previous studies reported an incidence of surgical complications of 0.3%[3] and 4%.[8] There were no surgical complications in this series. The use of the introducer sheath[4] and heparin infusion[7] probably reduced major complications in this series. The brachial approach eliminates the need for the prone position, which is used in the lumbar approach, and the 90 degree abduction of the arm, which is used in the axillary approach. Although there are some possibilities of complications with the brachial approach, there has no mortality or severe morbidity in this series.

We propose that the brachial approach with specially designed catheters could be used as a routine method of diagnostic angiography in examination of occluded or stenotic abdominal aorta, pelvic artery and femoral artery, and bilateral lower limb arteries, enabling better diagnosis and therapy plan.

References

1. Johnsrude IS, Jackson DC, Dunnick NR. *A Practical Approach to Angiography.* 2nd ed. Boston: Little, Brown and Company, 1988, pp. 44–47.
2. Kadir S. *Diagnostic Angiography.* Philadelphia: WB Saunders, 1986, pp. 40–41.
3. Gritter KJ, Laidlaw WW, Peterson NT. Complications of outpatient transbrachial intraarterial digital subtraction angiography. Radiology 1987;162:125–127.
4. Anderson PE. Brachialis Seldinger puncture with use of introducer sheath. Br J Radiol 1985;58:777–778.
5. Campion BC, Frye RL, Pluth JR, Fairbairn JF, Davis GD. Arterial complications of retrograde brachial artery catheterization: A prospective study. Mayo Clin Proc 1971;46:589–592.
6. Chahine RA, Herman MV, Gorlin R. Complications of coronary arteriography: comparison of the brachial to the femoral approach. Ann Intern Med 1972;76:862.
7. Watkinson AF, Hartnell GG. Complications of direct brachial artery puncture for arteriography: A comparison of techniques. Clin Radiol 1991;44:189–191.
8. Grollman JH, Marcus R. Transbrachial arteriography: Technique and complications. Cardiovasc Interven Radiol 1988;11:32–35.

7
Angiographic and Doppler Evaluation of Profunda Femoris Artery Runoff

HIROSHI YASUHARA, HIROSHI SHIGEMATSU, TOSHIYUKI KUBO, TAKASHI KOMIYAMA, and TETSUICHIRO MUTO

Introduction

The deep femoral artery provides a major collateral channel to the calf and foot. It also plays an important role as an outflow artery in inflow reconstruction grafting to the common femoral artery, especially in the presence of superficial femoral artery occlusion.[1]

Many surgeons have advocated the use of the profunda femoris artery as an outflow tract because of its relative sparing in the atherosclerotic process.[2,3] The blood flow induced by papaverine vasodilatation is twice that measured through femoropopliteal vein grafts and is frequently equal to the flow through the external iliac artery when both superficial and deep femoral vessels are patent.[4] There is also evidence that the graft patency of suprainguinal proximal reconstruction is affected by occlusion in the superficial femoral artery. No report, however, has demonstrated any effect of profunda femoris runoff on the result of a proximal bypass. Therefore, it is of prognostic importance to estimate the profunda femoris artery runoff.

The purpose of this study is to evaluate the efficacy of a combination of preoperative angiography and segmental Doppler measurement to assess profunda femoris runoff. In this paper we retrospectively review our experience of inflow arterial reconstruction to the profunda femoris arteries associated with superficial femoral artery occlusion. The influence of profunda femoris runoff on graft patency is also determined.

Materials and Methods

From January 1980 to June 1991, 208 suprainguinal arterial reconstructions including profundaplasty were performed in 194 patients at the First Department of Surgery in the University of Tokyo and its affiliated hospitals. The series consisted of 78 limbs in 76 patients with superficial femoral artery occlusion and 118 patients with patent superficial femoral arteries. There were 68 male and 8 female patients. The mean age of those patients was 62 years, ranging from 55 to 87 years. Indications for the operation included rest pain in 20 limbs (20%) and severe claudication in 58 limbs (75%).

The procedures were classified as suprainguinal reconstructions to the patent superficial femoral arteries (PSFA) in 130 limbs, to the occluded superficial femoral arteries without any associated distal bypass [OSFA(−)] in 45 limbs, and to the occluded superficial femoral arteries combined with distal bypass [OSFA(+)] in 33 limbs. In the patients with an occlusion of the superficial femoral artery, the proximal arterial reconstructions were always done with the associated profundaplasty (Fig. 7.1.).

Inflow profundaplasty was performed in 66 limbs with an associated proximal procedure: aortofemoral bypass in 41 limbs (62%), iliofemoral bypass in 22 limbs (33%), aortoiliac bypass in one limb (1.5%), axillofemoral bypass in one limb (1.5%), and femorofemoral crossover bypass in one limb (1.5%). Primary profundaplasty was done in 12 limbs without any other additional procedures. The OSFA(+) group consisted of 30 patients who underwent profundaplasties in conjunction with femoropopliteal bypass in 32 limbs and one patient with femorotibial bypass.

All the patients underwent preoperative angiography. Runoff resistance values (RRV) were determined by the preoperative angiographic findings according to the reporting standard of the ad hoc committee in 1986.[5] Segmental Doppler pressures were obtained preoperatively in the patients without distal reconstructions. Profunda-popliteal collateral index (PPCI) was calculated as described by Boren et al.[6] The runoff of the profunda femoris was evaluated from the findings of both preoperative angiography and the segmental Doppler pressure measurements using RRV and PPCI values.

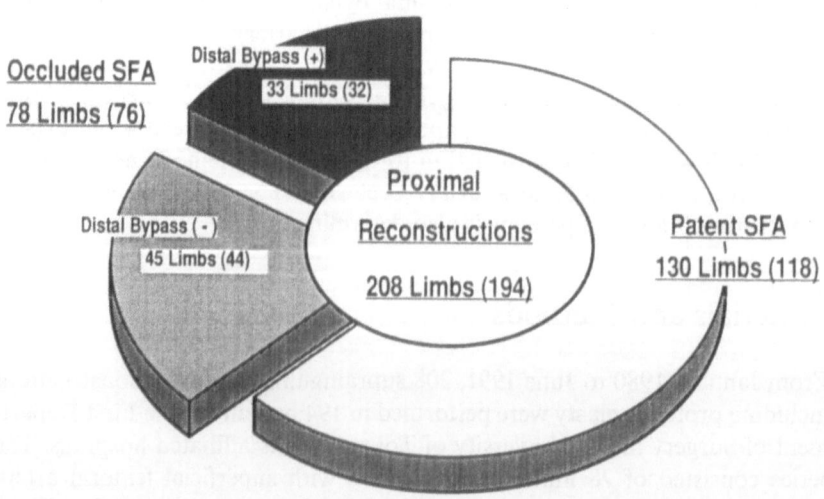

FIGURE 7.1. Patient group. SFA, Superficial femoral artery.

Their influences in predicting success and failure of the arterial reconstructions were determined.

The results of the OSFA(−) group were assessed in relation to the values of PPCI and RRV. The graft patency rate was calculated by the life table method.

Results

A graft failure was defined as the deterioration of Doppler signs and symptoms or as angiographic findings of graft occlusion. Overall clinical success was achieved in 61 limbs over the period of clinical follow-up.

The operative mortality rate was 1.0%. One patient died from postoperative myocardial infarction and the other from postoperative bleeding. Postoperative morbidity occurred in 11 extremities, including 5 wound hematomas and 2 lymphatic fistulas that responded to local wound care.

The life table analysis demonstrated that the outcome of the suprainguinal bypass was affected by the existence of the patent superficial femoral artery: the graft patency of the PSFA patient group was significantly higher than that of the OSFA(−) group (Fig. 7.2.). The patency rate of the suprainguinal graft appeared to be improved by the associated distal bypass, although the difference in the cumulative patency between the OSFA(+) and OSFA(−), groups was not significant.

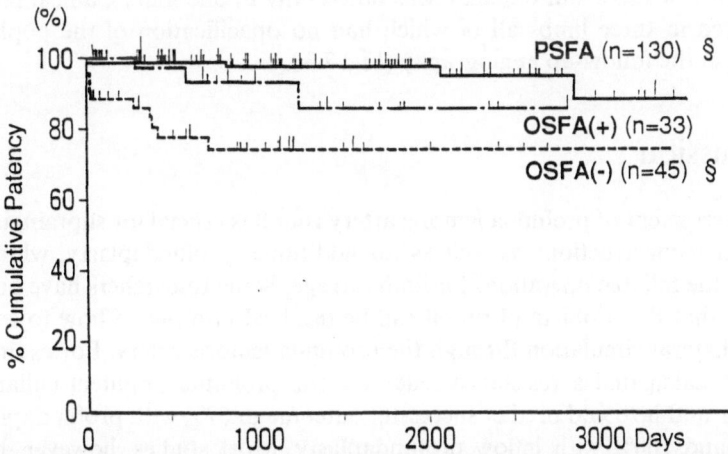

FIGURE 7.2. Cumulative patency by the life-table analysis. The horizontal bars on each graph represent the numbers of patients whose grafts were occluded during the follow-up. PSFA, patients with patent superficial femoral artery; OSFA(+), patients with occluded superficial femoral artery who underwent distal bypass; OSFA(−) patients with occluded superficial femoral artery who underwent distal bypass. § $p <$ 0.05 (PSFA vs. OSFA(+)).

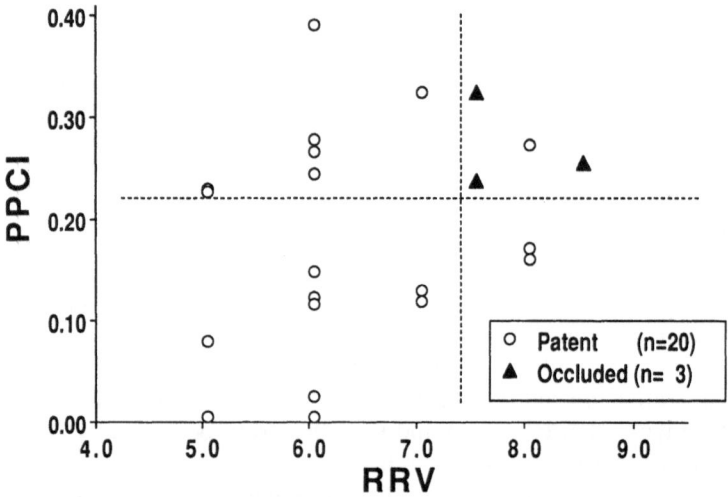

FIGURE 7.3. PPCI and RRV values were plotted in the OSFA(−) group, presenting high incidence of graft failures among the patients of high PPCI and RRV values.

During a follow-up period, there was a high incidence of graft failure in the patients with high preoperative RRV and PPCI values, although each value alone could not predict graft patency. In the patient with good PPCI and/or RRV, success was achieved in 42 extremities. In the group with poor PPCI and RRV, a successful outcome was noted only in one limb. Clinical failure occurred in three limbs all of which had no opacification of the popliteal artery in the follow-up angiography (Fig. 7.3.).

Discussion

The assessment of profunda femoris artery runoff is crucial for suprainguinal arterial reconstructions as well as for additional profundaplasty, which is one of the reliable operations for limb salvage. Some researchers have pointed out that the problem of runoff can be resolved into one of how to assess the collateral circulation through the profunda femoris artery. For example, Boren[6] calculated a resistance index for the profunda popliteal collateral system, and he could predict successful outcome in 67% with profundaplasty alone and 100% with inflow profundaplasty. Most studies, however, have failed to show a correlation between any single predictive value and graft patency.

Bernhard[7] reported a guide for selection of the operation when profunda femoris obstruction is demonstrated in patients with superficial femoral occlusion but unimpaired aortoiliac inflow. He classified distal runoff into six categories using three criteria: profunda femoral stenosis, PPCI, and popliteal-

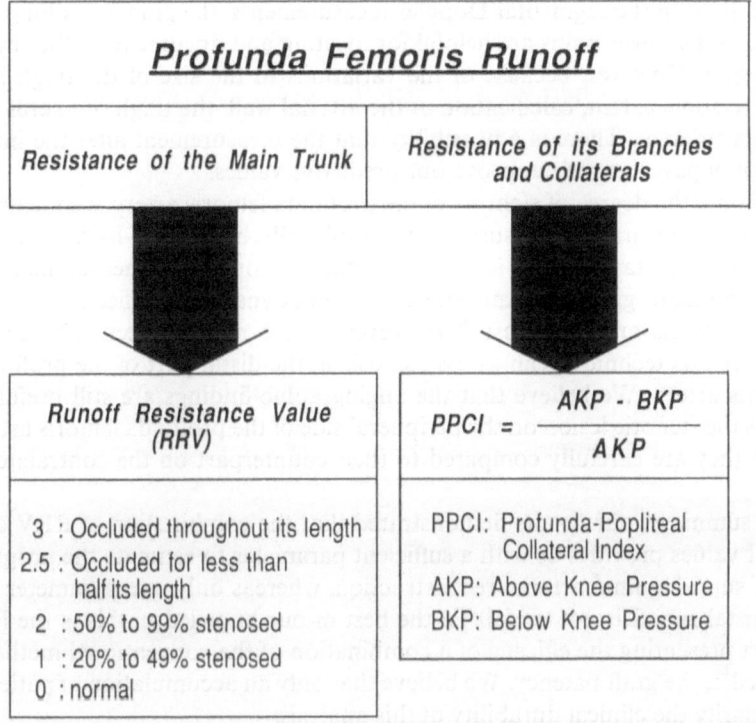

FIGURE 7.4. The profunda femoris runoff was mainly determined by two factors: (1) the resistance of the main trunk of the profunda femoris artery assessed by preoperative angiography, (2) the resistance of the small branches evaluated by segmental Doppler pressure measurements.

tibial runoff. The reliability of the evaluation for popliteal-tibial runoff still remains questionable.

Our results suggested that the profunda femoris runoff was determined by two factors (Fig. 7.4). One is its hemodynamically significant lesion in the main trunk of the profunda femoris artery, in other words, the extension of the atherosclerotic lesion in the deep femoral artery. The other is the resistance produced by the branches of the bypass arteries. Therefore, the development of the collateral communication between profunda femoris and popliteal arteries is also supposed to be measured by the PPCI values.

Our major hypothesis is that the PPCI value provides the popliteal-tibial runoff indirectly, since in the chronic stage of the disease the development of the collateral channels appeared to reflect the popliteal runoff. In fact, many of our cases with low PPCI values are associated with occluded or isolated popliteal arteries Although a combination of the angiographic findings and Doppler measurements provides useful information, there are still several problems to be discussed. The first is the accuracy of the Doppler measurement itself. In the segmental Doppler measurements, the gradients along the levels in the lower limbs are helpful for locating and documenting the site of occlusion. However, because of the variations in the size of the thigh and also, to some extent, calcification of the arterial wall, the thigh pressures are subject to error. There is a possibility that the measurement after the injection of papaverine may improve our predictive values.

Second, the degree of stenosis of the profunda femoris artery is sometimes difficult to accurately measure arteriographically because of its anatomical variation and tapering. It is reported that intraoperative measurement of mean pressure gradients can detect the hemodynamic significance of profunda femoris artery stenosis.[8] However, it has not yet been determined whether this technique can assess stenosis in the distal part of the profunda femoris artery. We believe that the angiographic findings are still useful to assess the stenotic lesion on the peripheral side of the profunda femoris artery when they are carefully compared to their counterpart on the contralateral side.

In summary, our results demonstrated that the combination of RRV and PPCI values provides us with a sufficient parameter to estimate the prognosis of suprainguinal arterial reconstruction, whereas only one parameter for the distal runoff is not useful. To the best of our knowledge, this is the first report presenting the efficacy of a combination of the conventional methods to predict the graft patency. We believe that only an accumulation of patients will clarify the clinical durability of this analysis.

References

1. Leeds FG, Gillfillan RS. Importance of the profunda femoris artery in revascularization of the ischemic limb. Arch Surg 1961;82:25–31.
2. Malone JM, Goldstone J, Moore WS. Autogenous profundaplasty the key to long-term patency in secondary repair of aorto-femoral graft occlusion. Ann Surg 1978; 188:817–823.
3. Jamil Z, Hobson RW, Lynch TG, et al. Revascularization of the profunda femoris artery for limb salvage. Am Surg 1984;50:109–111.
4. Bernhard VM, Ray LI, Militello JM. The role of angioplasty of the profunda femoris artery in revascularization of the ischemic limb. Surg Gynecol Obstet 1976; 142:840–844.
5. Rutherford RB, Flanigan DP, Gupta SK, et al. Suggested standards for reports dealing with lower extremity ischemia. J Vasc Surg 1986;4:80–94.
6. Boren CH, Towne JB, Bernhard VM, et al. Profundapopliteal collateral index. A guide to successful profundaplasty. Arch Surg 1980;115:1366–1372.
7. Bernhard VM. Limitations of profunda femoris revascularization. In: Veith FJ (ed.) Critical Problems in Vascular Surgery. New York: Appleton-Century-Crofts, 1982, p.260.
8. Archie JP, Feldtman RW. Intraoperative assessment of the hemodynamic significance of iliac and profunda femoris artery stenosis. Surgery 1981;90:876–880.

IV
Carotid Artery Surgery

8
Endarterectomy and Reimplantation for Carotid Stenosis

RUDOLPH G. VANMAELE, PAUL E. VAN SCHIL,
MARIANNE G. DE MAESENEER, PHILIPPE LEHERT, AND
ROBIN F. VAN LOOK

Introduction

Since its introduction by DeBakey in 1953,[1] carotid endarterectomy through a longitudinal arteriotomy followed by direct suture has become the most widely used technique for this surgical procedure.

Based on hemodynamic considerations, patch angioplasty, as had been proposed by Carrel,[2] was soon introduced [3,4] and enjoyed an increasing popularity. During the last decade a number of papers (see Table 8.1) have reported the superiority of patch angioplasty over direct suture in the prevention of recurrent stenosis.[5-14] The results with the saphenous vein patch seemed better than those with synthetic material.[15]

The saphenous vein, however is a precious graft material, and its value has been increasing with the development of coronary revascularization and distant infrapopliteal bypass surgery. The vein segment is generally harvested at ankle level, a part that is most appropriate for coronary surgery, although some authors recommend the use of the proximal part at groin level for its superior wall quality.[16] The harvesting of a saphenous vein segment might jeopardize the future of a significant part of this vessel and preclude its further use as graft material. Furthermore, the saphenous vein patch has its intrinsic disadvantages and complications: prolonged operating time, dilatation, rupture, and embolism.

For these reasons, it could be of interest to develop a surgical technique for carotid endarterectomy which could avoid the risk of depleting the precious vein graft resources of the patient, provided the results were comparable with regard to morbidity, mortality, and recurrence rate.

Since a longitudinal arteriotomy is not the only way to gain access to the arterial lumen for endarterectomy, some authors have used a division of the carotid bifurcation.[3,17-24] This was based on the techniques currently used for the treatment of kinking, loop, or coil formation,[18,25] combined with eversion endarterectomy as described at aortoiliac level.[26]

We describe here this technique, division–endarterectomy–anastomosis (DEA) as it is routinely performed in this department and discuss its value based on our results.

TABLE 8.1. Recurrent stenosis rate after patch angioplasty compared to direct suture in 10 recent studies

Author	Year	n	Method	Mean follow-up	Patch	Direct suture
Hamman	1985	798	Duplex + angio	4.6 y	1.0%	5.5%
Van Berge-Henegouwen	1985	87	Doppler	<1 y	2.1%	15%
Archie	1986	200	Doppler + OPG	<1 y	0%	4%
Curley	1987	66	Doppler	1–3 y	12.5%	16.6%
De Vleeschauwer	1987	94	Doppler + angio	1 y	26%	35.5%
Hertzer	1987	332	Doppler + angio	3 y	9%	31%
Katz	1987	89	Duplex + angio	2 y	2.4%	18.1%
Ouriel	1987	102	Duplex	1.5 y	5.7%	28.6%
Eikelboom	1988	129	Duplex	1 y	3.5%	21%
Clagett	1989	152	Duplex + OPG	22 mo	12.9%	1.7%

Description of the DEA Technique

General Management

The patient is positioned supine on the table with the shoulders elevated on a roll to obtain maximal extension of the neck, the head turned as much as possible to the contralateral side. Preparation of the skin and draping leaves access to the lateral neck region, from the earlobe to the clavicle, and to the ankle region of one leg. This routine is a wise precaution, but in our experience the saphenous vein has never had to be harvested unless planned for a patch procedure.

A general anesthesia is preferred, aiming at "fine-tuning" of the patient's vital parameters, cerebral monitoring with electroencephalographic (EEG) spectral analysis, and quick arousal allowing clinical assessment of the neurologic status.

Exposure of the Carotid Bifurcation and Assessment of the Tolerance to Cross-Clamping

The carotid bifurcation is exposed through a standard incision that parallels the anterior border of the sternocleidomastoid muscle. If the incision has to be extended cephalad, as in very high bifurcations, care is taken to proceed behind the earlobe, in order to avoid injury to the marginal mandibular branch of the facial nerve.

The carotid sheath is entered at the lowest level, and the common carotid artery (CCA) is encircled with a tape. Great caution is taken to respect the vagus nerve and the hypoglossal nerve.

In order to reduce the risk of atheroma embolism, further control of the carotid arteries is obtained, avoiding manipulation of the atheromatous area as much as possible until clamping is completed.

The internal carotid artery (ICA) is encircled with a tape, preferably above the level of the plaque. Gently pulling down will allow further mobilization of the ICA, which is important in the DEA technique. This mobilization requires gentle, strictly blunt dissection, in order to avoid injury to the vagus and glossopharyngeal nerves and to respect the innervation of the pharynx.

The external carotid artery (ECA) is controlled, together with the superior thyroid artery on one tape. The sinus nerve is carefully dissociated from both ICA and ECA to its endings.

Five thousand units heparin are administered intravenously. Atraumatic clamps are applied to the ECA and CCA. Cross-clamping is maintained for 5 minutes and the EEG is observed. If signs of ischemia appear, the clamps are removed promptly and arrangements are made for shunt insertion. If the EEG shows no alterations after 5 minutes, no shunt is used, the ICA is clamped with an angulated Kartchner vascular clamp, and the DEA is started without delay. Once the risk of embolism is excluded by cross-clamping, the atheromatous bifurcation is completely mobilized, which is important in the DEA technique.

Division–Endarterectomy–Anastomosis: Standard Technique

To start the endarterectomy, the ICA is divided at its origin. As the section runs through the plaque, this has to be performed with heavy scissors, a sharp surgical blade, or both.

It is very important to start the section about 5 mm above the true bifurcation and extend it downward, almost parallel to the axis ECA–CCA, in order to obtain an opening of not less than 25 mm in its longitudinal diameter (Fig. 8.1A). In doing so, a 5-mm ridge of ICA is left on the bifurcation.

If the ICA is properly mobilized, it can be straightened and pulled downward on average 1.5 cm. The incision on the ICA is extended cephalad in regard to the ECA to the level of the ridge on the bifurcation. The incision on the CCA is extended in the caudal direction over the same distance, in order to make both circumferences match and to have a good view inside the CCA and on the origin of the ECA (Fig 8.1B).

The endarterectomy is performed with a fine curved mosquito forceps. It is started on the ICA. With the mobilization and incision of the ICA, it is most frequently possible to get the top of the plaque under direct visual control and to start a retrograde endarterectomy at this point. In some cases the plaque comes loose at the caudal edge of the incision, without interfering with the visual control of the top of the endarterectomy.

On the CCA the endarterectomy usually starts in the thickest part of the atheroma. It is extended caudally as far as the plaque. The sequester is divided with fine scissors, or crushed with the forceps, always taking care to leave a smooth edge on the CCA. The endarterectomy is continued circumferentially on the CCA and also on the ridge of the ICA which was left on the

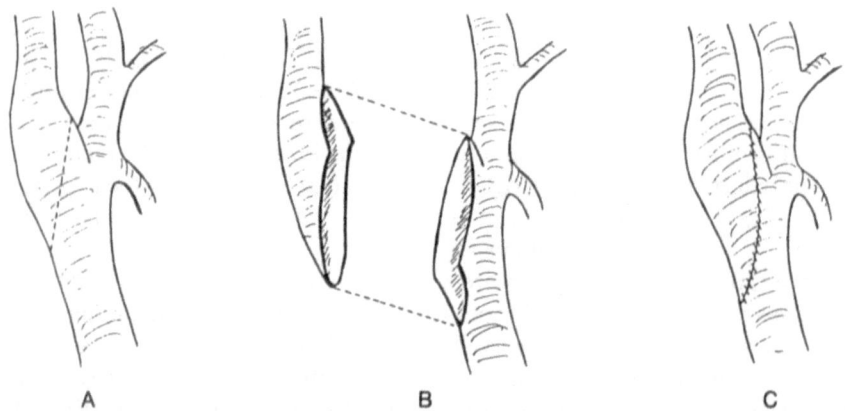

FIGURE 8.1. DEA standard technique. Right carotid bifurcation. (Reprinted with permission, from Vanmaele et al., Acta Chir Belg 1990;90:255–261)

bifurcation. The point is reached where the atheroma extends into the ECA. The endarterectomy is continued blindly into the ECA, until the plaque comes out entirely, or at least over 1 cm, to make sure that the blood supply to the carotid body is restored and that no residual atheroma can protrude into the CCA–ICA lumen.

The edges and the whole site of the endarterectomy are carefully inspected under copious diluted heparin saline irrigation in order to detect and remove any loose debris or smooth muscle flaps. The ICA is then anastomosed with a running 6/0 Prolene twin-needled suture, starting at the top of the incision. Prior to completion of the closure, clamps are released separately so that air and clots are extruded, the diameters of the CCA, ECA, and ICA are measured with DeBakey calibrators, and the lumen is again flushed with saline by introducing a blunt needle in the three arteries until it reaches the clamps. The suture is then completed and tied. The clamp on the ECA is released first.

Back-pressure is usually sufficient to identify bleeding points on the suture and insert additional stitches. When the suture line is dry, the clamp on the CCA is released and the endarterectomy site is twisted between thumb and forefinger. This "massage" is meant to encourage dislodgement of any residual clots or debris into the ECA. Finally, the ICA clamp is removed and blood flow to the brain is restored (Fig. 8.1C).

Some technical details are of paramount importance for the quality of reconstruction with the DEA technique. The preservation of a 5-mm ICA ridge on the bifurcation has a triple function. First, it will protect the carotid body and the sinus nerve from being tacked in the suture. Second, it will provide a solid grip for the first stitches of the anastomosis. Finally and essentially, it will prevent narrowing of the "heel" of the anastomosis due to

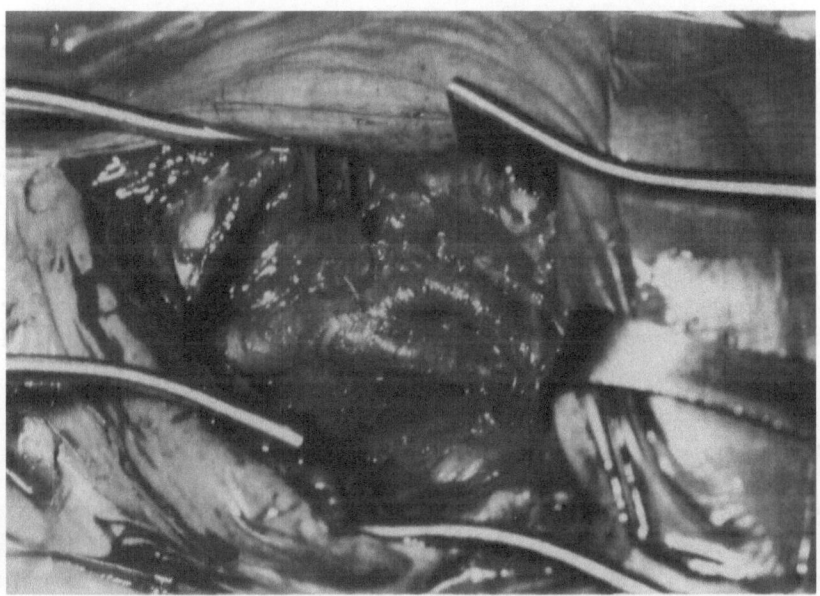

FIGURE 8.2. Operative view of a completed DEA procedure.

its elliptic form. This is especially important in cases where the ICA has been pulled down and longitudinally incised.

Also of utmost importance is that the incision line has to be almost parallel to the axis CCA–ECA in order to be very oblique on the ICA and to create a wide lid that can be removed from the CCA, allowing a good view inside the artery and giving enough space to manipulate the atheroma and remove it entirely.

The anatomic result after completion of the anastomosis is excellent (Fig. 8.2).

After hemostasis has been assured, a Redon suction drain is inserted and the platysma is closed with a running suture Vicryl 2/0. The skin is closed with a running intradermal suture fast-resorbing Vicryl 3/0, as is the ankle wound, if present.

Division–Endarterectomy–Anastomosis: Special Problems

Two problems may interfere with the standard execution of the DEA technique: difficulty in mobilizing the ICA enough to have visual control on the end of the plaque, and intolerance to cross-clamping, thus requiring the use of a temporary indwelling shunt.

If the ICA cannot be mobilized and brought down enough to allow a cephalad incision and retrograde endarterectomy, two solutions can be proposed.

The first is to extend the incision cephalad on both the ICA and the ECA. In this option, it is important to make the incision on the ECA behind the carotid body in order to preserve its innervation. The ECA should then be carefully endarterectomized. This solution may jeopardize the benefits of the ICA ridge on the bifurcation. The difficulty of the anastomosis is considerably increased because it starts almost on the deep aspect of the bifurcation (Fig. 8.3).

The other solution is the eversion endarterectomy. The plaque is held with a pick-up forceps and the endarterectomy is started at the most caudal part of the divided ICA. The plaque is freed with the mosquito forceps and the arterial wall is progressively everted over the plaque. The atheroma will

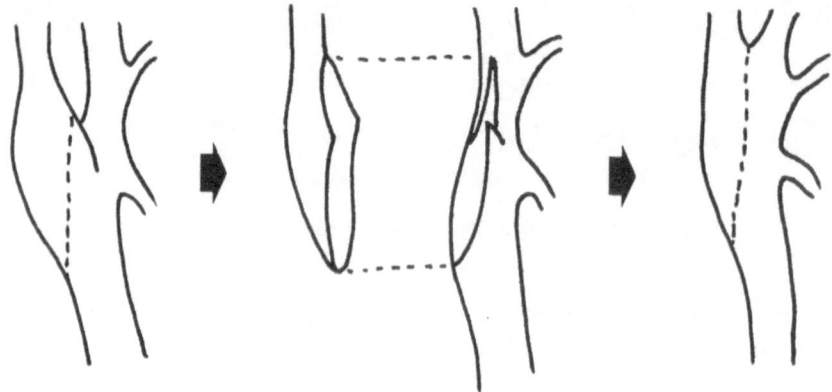

FIGURE 8.3. DEA technique with incision on the ECA. Right carotid bifurcation. See text.

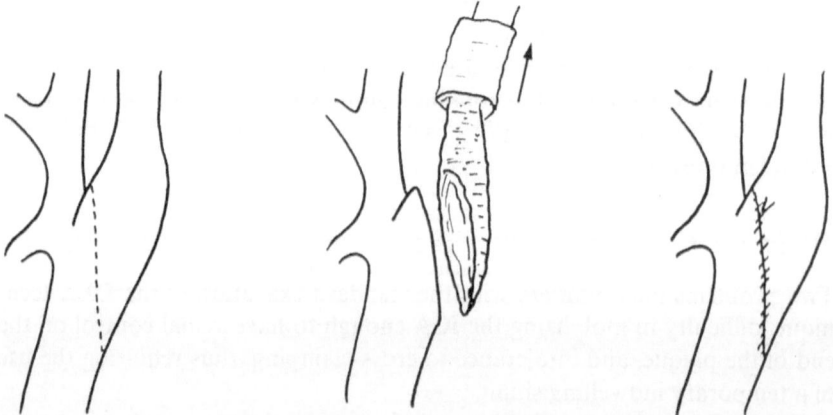

FIGURE 8.4. DEA technique with eversion endarterectomy of the ICA. Left carotid bifurcation. See text.

break spontaneously at its end (Fig. 8.4). It is very important to keep the artery everted until it is absolutely sure that no loose flaps are left.

The whole wound is flooded and profusely irrigated with diluted heparin saline, as in the underwater technique used in microsurgery. Loose intima will be floating in the fluid and can easily be grasped.

When the distal end of the endarterectomy is absolutely clean, the artery is inverted again, and the operation is continued in the standard way.

Once the artery is inverted, it is very difficult to evert it again! In case of any doubt, a control by angiography, angioscopy, or ultrasound is strongly recommended.

The use of an indwelling shunt is possible but difficult in the DEA. In our experience we have used the Javid shunt with its clamps. When a shunt has to be inserted, it is important to have access to at least 4–5 cm of CCA. The three carotids are clamped as in the standard technique, with the CCA clamp placed as far caudally as possible. The ICA is divided in the standard way and endarterectomized properly. A small transverse incision is made in the CCA, and the proximal end of the shunt is inserted and secured with its clamp. The CCA cross clamp is removed and placed on the shunt after copious flushing to expel air and eventually clots and debris.

The distal end of the shunt is inserted in the ICA, which is profusely

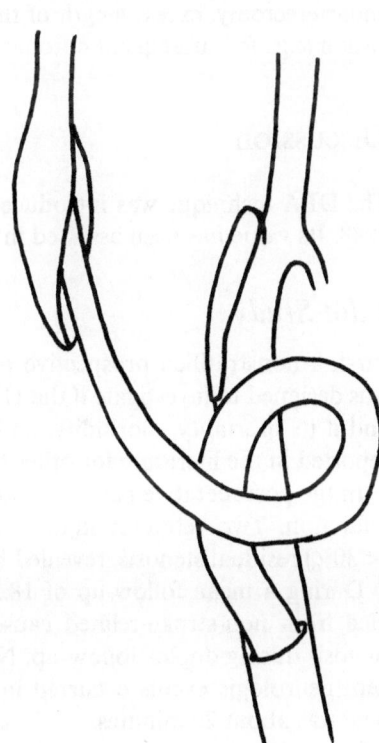

FIGURE 8.5. Position of the Javid shunt during a DEA procedure. Right carotid bifurcation. See text.

backbled to remove any air bubbles or debris. It is also secured with its corresponding clamp.

The cross clamps on the ICA and on the shunt are removed and the blood supply to the brain is restored. This procedure can be performed well within the limit of 5 minutes cross-clamping time (Fig. 8.5).

Ischemic signs on the EEG should resolve immediately if the shunt is functioning properly. Thus use of a shunt without any monitoring is unwise, since the flow through the shunt is out of visual control.

The endarterectomy of the CCA and ECA is performed in the standard way. The anastomosis is very difficult, since the elastic recoil of the shunt pushes both sides away. When the anastomosis is almost finished, the transverse incision on the CCA is loosely sutured around the shunt with 6/0 Prolene. The shunt is quickly removed and the ICA and CCA are cross-clamped. The running suture on the transverse incision is completed, and after the procedures described in the standard technique, the anastomosis is completed as well. Blood flow to the brain is restored within 5 minutes cross-clamping time. Ischemic signs on the EEG, if any, resolve immediately.

The difficulty of the DEA technique with a shunt is very great. For this reason, the use of the DEA technique with a shunt requires extensive experience with the standard technique. It can only be justified under strict indications, such as very high lesions on the ICA requiring eversion endarterectomy, excess length of the ICA, or absence or mandatory preservation (e.g., for subsequent coronary surgery) of the saphenous vein.

Discussion

The DEA technique was introduced in this department at the beginning of 1988. Its value has been assessed in two consecutive studies.

Pilot Study

First, a nonstratified prospective pilot study in 25 patients (26 operations) was designed to investigate if the DEA technique was routinely reproducible and if its mortality, morbidity, and recurrence rates were within the range reported in the literature for other techniques.[27]

In the postoperative period (< 30 days), one patient died from myocardial infarction. Two retractor injuries to the hypoglossal nerve and one mild (< 30%) residual stenosis, revealed by control angiogram, were reported.[28]

During a mean follow-up of 18.5 ± 7.0 months (range 1–27), 7 patients died from non-stroke-related causes and one developed < 50% recurrent stenosis during duplex follow-up. No postoperative late transient or permanent neurologic events occurred in this study. The average cross-clamping time was about 20 minutes.

There were no complications intrinsically related to the technique. It never had to be abandoned during the procedure in favor of another technique. It can easily be performed by a vascular surgeon familiar with carotid procedures. The results proved to be comparable to those obtained with other techniques, including saphenous vein patch angioplasty.

Prospective Randomized Comparative Study

Encouraged by these results, we performed a prospective randomized nonstratified comparative study in 200 consecutive operations (170 patients) to assess the value of the DEA technique compared to vein patch angioplasty in the same hands.[29]

Patients were assigned at random by sequential selection to either of two groups (102 DEA and 98 patch) with most characteristics and risk factors equally distributed. The DEA technique was performed as described here. The patch angioplasty technique was similar to the classic techniques described by other authors.[30-32] During a mean follow-up of 365 ± 276 days, patients were seen for clinical and color duplex evaluation at regular intervals.

The main features are compared for both groups in Table 8.2. The overall perioperative mortality was 2.5% (5 patients). One death was due to acute myocardial infarction, the other four to stroke. Thus, the cumulative mortality-morbidity rate (CMMR), including death, disabling stroke, or any other stroke producing symptoms for more than 7 days, was 4% in the DEA group and 8% in the patch group. Significant differences were observed in cross-clamping time ($p < 0.001$) and cranial nerve dysfunction ($p = 0.002$) in favor of the reimplantation technique.

Late neurologic events were exceptional and transient. No late stroke-related deaths were reported. There were no significant differences between the groups in survival or in events. There was no significant difference between the groups in recurrent stenosis ($p = 0.524$), and all recurrences were apparent within 9 months. Although the small number of events makes this

TABLE 8.2. Comparative study ($n = 200$)—main features

	DEA	PATCH	p
Perioperative Mortality	2%	3%	n.s.
CMMR	4%	8%	n.s.
Residual stenosis >60%	0	2	n.s.
Early occlusion	3	5	n.s.
Cranial nerve injury	1	11	0.002
Cross-clamping time (min. sec.)	24.11 ± 5.40	29.85 ± 5.86	0.001
False aneurysm	0	1	n.s.
Late mortality	5%	6%	n.s.
Recurrent stenosis >60%	1	2	n.s.
Turbulence	5%	24%	0.005

difference nonsignificant, it should be mentioned that the recurrence rate in the DEA group was only 2.7% in cases with retrograde endarterectomy versus 7% after eversion endarterectomy. There was significantly more turbulence after patch angioplasty ($p = 0.005$), and dilatation is definitely more pronounced after patch angioplasty.

Conclusions

In a total of 128 operations, it has been shown that the DEA technique is routinely reproducible as an alternative to the widely used techniques for endarterectomy as reported in the literature. In our hands, the results with this technique were equivalent to those with saphenous vein patch angioplasty in terms of mortality, morbidity, and recurrence rates. These results were obtained without breaking into the patient's precious venous graft capital. In addition, the DEA technique offers attractive solutions for combined problems, such as high carotid bifurcations, high ICA plaque, ICA kinking, etc.

The DEA technique can therefore be considered a valuable alternative technique for the surgical treatment of carotid stenosis, provided these results are confirmed in a long-term study.

"It usually requires a considerable time to determine with certainty the virtues of a new method of treatment and still longer to ascertain the harmful effects..." Alfred Blalock (1899–1964)

Acknowledgment. The authors are gratefully indebted to Miss Carine Aerts for preparing the manuscript with great accuracy and expediency.

References

1. DeBakey ME. Successful carotid endarterectomy for cerebrovascular insufficiency. Nineteen-year follow-up. JAMA 1975;233:1083–1085.
2. Carrel A, Guthrie CC. Uniterminal and biterminal venous transplantation. Surg Gynecol Obstet 1906;2:266–286.
3. DeBakey ME, Crawford ES, Cooley DA, Morris GC Jr. Surgical considerations of occlusive disease of innominate, carotid, subclavian and vertebral arteries. Ann Surg 1959;149:690–710.
4. Imparato AM. The role of patch angioplasty after carotid endarterectomy. J Vasc Surg 1988; 7:715–716.
5. Hamman H, Badmann A, Vollmar JF. Residustenosen nach carotis TEA. Langenbecks Arch Clin 1985;366:323–326.
6. Van Berge Henegouwen DP, Reimer F. Early restenosis after carotid endarterectomy. Vasa 1985;14:55–58.
7. Archie JP. Prevention of early restenosis and thrombosis occlusion after carotid endarterectomy by saphenous vein patch angioplasty. Stroke 1986;17:901–905.

8. Curley S, Edwards WS, Jacob TP. Recurrent carotid stenosis after autologous tissue patching. J Vasc Surg 1987;6:350–354.

9. De Vleeschauwer PH, Wirthle W, Holler L, Krause E, Horsh S. Is venous patch grafting after carotid endarterectomy able to reduce the rate of restenosis? Prospective randomized pilot study with stratification. Acta Chir Belg 1987;87:242–246.

10. Hertzer NR, Bevend EG, O'Hara PJ, Krajewski LP. A prospective study of vein patch angioplasty during carotid endarterectomy: three-year result for 801 patients and 917 operations. Ann Surg 1987;206:628–635.

11. Katz MM, Jones GT, Degenhardt J, Gunn B, Wilson J, Katz S. The use of patch angioplasty to alter the incidence of carotid restenosis following thromboendarterectomy. J Cardiovasc Surg 1987;28:2–8.

12. Ouriel K, Green RM. Clinical and technical factors influencing recurrent carotid stenosis and occlusion after endarterectomy. J Vasc Surg 1987;5:702–706.

13. Eikelboom BC, Ackerstaff RGA, Hoeneveld M, et al. Benefits of carotid patching: a randomized study. J Vasc Surg 1988;7:240–247.

14. Clagett GP, Patterson CB, Fisher DF J, et al. Vein patch versus primary closure for carotid endarterectomy. A randomized prospective study in a selected group of patients. J Vasc Surg 1989;9:213–223.

15. Fode NC, Sundt TM Jr, Robertson JT. Multicenter retrospective review of results and complications of carotid endarterectomy in 1981. Stroke 1986;17:370–376.

16. Petitjean C, Richard T, Ruotolo C, Kieffer E. Les reinterventions tardives apres chirurgie carotidienne. In: Kieffer E, Natali J (eds.) Aspects techniques de la chirurgie carotidienne. Paris: AERCV, 1987, pp. 299–315.

17. Najafi M, Javid M, Due WS, Hunter JA, Julian OL. Kinked internal carotid artery: clinical evaluation and surgical correction. Arch Surg 1964;89:134–143.

18. Etheredge SN. A simple technique for carotid endarterectomy. Am J Surg 1970; 120:275–278.

19. Chino ES. A simple method for combined carotid endarterectomy and correction of internal carotid artery kinking. J Vasc Surg 1987;6:197–199.

20. Kasprzak PM, Raithel D. Eversionsendarteriektomie der A. Carotis Interna (EEA). Angio 1990; 12:1.

21. Dall' Antonia F, Germani B, Danieli D, et al. The advantages of eversion endarterectomy and local anesthesia in carotid surgery. In: Strano A, Novo S (eds.) Advances in Vascular Pathology. Amsterdam: Excerpta Medica, 1989, pp. 439–444.

22. Jones CE. Carotid eversion endarterectomy revisited. Am J Surg 1989;157:323–328.

23. Vanmaele RG, Van Schil PE, De Maeseneer MG. Closure of the internal carotid artery after endarterectomy: the advantages of patch angioplasty without its disadvantages. Ann Vasc Surg 1990;4:81–84.

24. Reigner B. L'endarteriectomie par retournement de la carotide interne (Dissertation). Angers, France: Universite d'Angers, 1991.

25. Quattlebaum JK Jr, Upson ET, Neville RL. Stroke associated with elongation and kinking of the internal carotid artery: report of 3 cases treated by segmental resection of common carotid artery. Ann Surg 1959;150:824–832.

26. Connolly JE, Stemmer EA. Simplified technique of eversion endarterectomy for aortoiliofemoral occlusive disease. Arch Surg 1972;105:520–523.

27. Vanmaele RG, Van Schil PE, De Maeseneer MG, Meese G, Lammens GP,

Schoofs EL. Division and reanastomosis of the internal carotid artery for endarterectomy. Acta Chir Belg 1990;90:255–261.

28. Baker JD, Rutherford RB, Bernstein EF, et al. Suggested standards for reports
dealing with cerebrovascular disease. Prepared by the subcommittee on reporting
standards for cerebrovascular disease, ad hoc committee on reporting standards,
Society for Vascular Surgery/North American chapter, International Society for
Cardiovascular Surgery. J Vasc Surg 1988;8:721–729.

29. Vanmaele RG. The technqiue of Division-Endarterectomy-Anastomosis for the
surgical treatment of extracranial carotid artery atheromatosis. (Thesis). Antwerp,
Belgium: Antwerp University UIA, 1992, 175 pp.

30. Moore WS. Technique of carotid endarterectomy. In: Moore WS (ed.) *Surgery for
Cerebrovascular Disease*. New York: Churchill-Livingstone, 1987, pp. 491–502.

31. Sundt TM Jr. Techniques of carotid endarterectomy. In: Sundt TM Jr (ed.) *Occlusive Cerebrovascular Disease. Diagnosis and Surgical Management*. Philadelphia:
W.R. Saunders Company, 1987, pp. 191–225.

32. Baker WH. Personal method of carotid endarterectomy. In: Chang JB (ed.) *Modern Vascular Surgery. Volume 4*. California: PMA Publishing Company, 1991,
pp. 79–86.

V
Cardiac Hemodynamics

9
Effect of Acute Normovolemic Hemodilution on Blood Coagulation

ZSOLT A. VARGA, JILL C. LOCKE-EDMUNDS, PETER M. LAMONT, ROGER N. BAIRD, AND JOHN F. THOMPSON

Summary

Acute normovolemic hemodilution (ANH) is one of the autotransfusion options currently in use to minimize homologous blood exposure to the patient. Fresh autologous blood reinfused at the end of surgery can help to establish surgical hemostasis, as ANH blood contains functioning platelets and clotting factors. ANH was used in 47 patients undergoing abdominal aortic aneurysm (AAA) repair or major general surgical procedures (GS). Direct arterial blood pressure, electrocardiogram (ECG), pulse oximetry, and bedside packed cell volume (PCV) measurements were used to safeguard the procedure. The target PCV was 0.30 in the AAA and 0.28 in the GS groups and was calculated using a nomogram. Gelatin solution was used for volume replacement. There were no adverse events related to ANH. After hemodilution the international normalized ratio (INR) and the activated partial thromboplastin ratio (APTR) were prolonged but platelet numbers remained within the normal range, and the overall coagulability of the blood (activated clotting time ACT) was unaffected. ANH is a straightforward and safe autotransfusion method and can be used even in high-risk arteriopathic patients. The alteration in coagulation studies may become more significant if higher blood volumes are removed and underlines the need for a preoperative clotting screen.

Background

Autologous blood transfusion is gaining popularity because of current concerns regarding transfusion-transmitted diseases and the immunosuppressive effect of homologous blood. Autotransfusion is now backed by the law in Germany and some states in the United States. Preoperative donation, preoperative plasma or plateletpheresis, acute normovolemic hemodilution (ANH), intraoperative salvage autotransfusion, and postoperative wound drainage autotransfusion are the options available. The most effective method to reduce transfusion is to withold it until absolutely necessary by enforcing strict transfusion policy.[1] Drugs such as aprotinin may also reduce bleeding during surgery.[2] A combination of different autotransfusion methods can usually eliminate the need for homologous transfusion in elective surgery and can significantly decrease it in emergency and trauma surgery.

Acute normovolemic hemodilution is one of the easiest blood-saving methods and probably the cheapest. It involves withdrawal of calculated volume of blood immediately before surgery—preferably in the anesthetized patient—and isovolemic replacement with cell-free fluids. For dilution, colloid or crystalloid infusions can be used. Crystalloids are cheap but have the disadvantage of a short intravascular half-life and a tendency to extravasate, thus producing interstitial edema. Three times the venesected blood volume of crystalloid should be administered to maintain intravascular normovolemia, and this is not recommended.[3] Hydroxyethyl starches are also in use, and some authors prefer them as they have been shown to decrease perioperative thromboembolic complications. The highest recommended dose is 20 mL/kg. Hydroxyethyl starch has a specific effect on hemostasis, namely a decrease of factor VIII.[4] Albumin solutions are physiological, but their use is limited by cost. Only pasteurized plasma products do not carry transfusion-transmitted viruses. Short- (2–3 hours) half-life gelatin solutions are ideal for volume replacement during ANH. They are inexpensive, do not have a direct effect on platelets and blood coagulation, do not have a maximum dose, and the danger of circulatory overload is minimal if the venous pressure is monitored as an excess is excreted by the kidneys.[5]

ANH is useful for surgery when the expected blood loss is 1,500–2,000 mL. When combined with other blood-saving methods, its role can be extended to surgical procedures with a higher anticipated blood loss. It can also be used in cancer surgery when intraoperative salvage autotransfusion is contraindicated because of the danger of salvaging and reinfusing cancer cells. Tumor cells are present in the reinfusate after centrifuging and washing the shed blood.[6] Although intraoperative salvage autotransfusion has been used in cancer surgery,[7] salvage and reinfusion of blood from wounds containing malignant cells remains a contraindication.[8]

It is mandatory to test predonated blood for transmissible disease in the same way as bank blood in case of clerical error leading to inadvertent transfusion to the wrong recipient. As ANH blood is stored in the operating theatre, it does not need to be tested for hepatitis C, human immunodeficency virus, or other diseases.[9]

Pooled platelet concentrates are produced by centrifuging fresh homologous blood within 8 hours of collection. It has been shown that platelets stored in whole blood for 3 days retained better aggregability responses to adenosine diphosphate (ADP) and collagen than platelets stored as platelet concentrates (PC) for the same period.[10] Coagulation factor deterioration proceeds more slowly than assumed. Factor V and VIII concentration decreases the fastest but activity is still 30%–50% for factor VIII and 80% for factor V after 5 days storage.[11] Therefore it is not surprising that ANH blood stored for up to 6 hours retains its hemostatic ability.

Storage of red blood cells for 2 weeks at 4°C leads to severe depletion of 2,3-diphosphoglycerate.[12] ANH blood has a high level of this compound, which improves oxygen handling. ANH provides a superior oxygen supply to the tissues compared to bank blood because of increased capillary blood flow,[13] an increased cardiac output,[14] and a right shift of the hemoglobin dissociation curve.[15]

Bacterial growth was not observed in a study where homologous blood was repeatedly refrigerated and exposed to room temperatures.[16] There are no studies that describe bacterial contamination of ANH blood which should remain sterile if collected under strict aseptic conditions.

Two thousand milliliters of blood loss from a patient with a PCV of 0.45 represents 900 ml of red cell loss. The same volume of blood loss represents only 600 ml of red cell loss if the PCV is 0.30. Provided normovolemia is maintained during the operation, the PCV at the end of surgery would be 0.27 in the case of concentrated but 0.33 in the diluted patient if the ANH blood was reinfused after the surgical bleeding had stopped. In the literature an 18%–100% reduction in homologous blood transfusion requirement has been reported using ANH.[17–19]

The effect of hemodilution on general circulation, regional blood flow (especially coronary and cerebral blood flow), and blood oxygenation has been investigated in both experimental and clinical studies. Blood pressure, central venous pressure, and heart rate remain stable provided normovolemia is maintained. Blood viscosity decreases, and venous return and therefore stroke volume increases, so tissue oxygenation is maintained by increased cardiac output. Venous blood oxygen content decreases only under a PCV of 0.20. With accumulating clinical experience in this field, contraindications have been relaxed, and ANH has been shown to be a safe method in elderly,[20] cardiovascular[21], vascular,[22] and pediatric[23] patients undergoing surgery.

In this study the effect of ANH on blood coagulation was addressed in both general and vascular surgical patients.

Patients and Methods

After ethical committee approval, 47 patients underwent acute preoperative normovolemic hemodilution before elective surgery. The indication for surgery was abdominal aortic aneurysm (AAA) in 30 cases (group 1) and major general surgery (GS) in 17 cases (group 2). In group 2,4 patients had subtotal colectomy: 3 for ulcerative colitis and 1 for chronic constipation. Seven had an anterior resection for rectal cancer, 3 had thoracoscopic-assisted transhiatal esophagectomy, and there was an abdominoperineal resection, a rectal stump excision, and iliac pouch formation after a previous subtotal colectomy for ulcerative colitis and a choledochoduodenostomy for irresectable chronic pancreatitis.

Informed written consent was obtained. Full blood count and coagulation studies (international normalized ratio INR; activated partial thromboplastin ratio APTR; and fibrinogen, FBNG were performed on the day before surgery. The patients were anesthetized and monitored using radial arterial pressure, precordial electrocardiogram (ECG), and pulse oximetry. Initially a dose of 500 mL gelatin solution [20 g of succinylated gelatin, average molecular weight 30,000, in each 500 mL (Gelofusine, Hausmann Laboratories Ltd, St. Gallen, Switzerland/Vifor, UK, Ltd)] was administered into a peripheral vein. A sample was then taken from the arterial line; deadspace plus 8 mL was discarded; and from a 5-mL aliquot, packed cell volume (PCV) and activated clotting time (ACT) were determined immediately, using a microcentrifuge (Hematastat Model-70, Separation Technology Inc., Altamonte Springs, FL, USA) and ACT tubes containing 12 mg of diatomaceous earth as a contact activator and a dual-channel automated clotting time device using a magnetic clot detection system (Hemochron 801, International Technidyne Corp, Edison, NJ, USA). The volume of blood to be withdrawn for ANH was calculated using a nomogram based on weight, height, gender, and initial PCV, measured after the "preload" Gelofusine.[24] Autologous blood was taken from a peripheral vein via a 14-gauge (2 mm OD) Venflon cannula (Viggo-Spectramed, Helsingborg, Sweden), and an equal volume of colloid solution (Gelofusine) was administered into a vein in the opposite arm. The blood was collected into plastic bags containing 63 mL citrate, phosphate, dextrose (CPD) solution. Two bags were connected with a Y-shaped coupling equipped with clips and a luer lock connector (autologous blood collection kit, Baxter-Fenwal, Deerfield, IL, USA). Venipuncture was performed under strict aseptic conditions and the cannula was connected to the collection kit immediately. The blood collection bags were weighed continously on a spring balance to measure the volume withdrawn. The replacement fluid was administered under pressure if the blood withdrawal was rapid, to maintain normovolemia. When the calculated blood volume had been collected, the lines of the bags were sealed using hand sealing clips and the bags were disconnected. The intravenous cannula was flushed with normal saline, connected to an infusion set, and used for volume replacement during surgery. The blood was numbered, labeled with the patient's details, and kept on the anesthetic machine at room temperature until reinfusion. During the procedure, blood pressure, heart rate, and blood oxygen saturation were closely monitored. After hemodilution an arterial sample was taken for coagulation studies (APTR, INR, FBNG, ACT, and PCV).

Four and one-half milliliters of blood was collected into a glass tube containing 0.5 mL 0.105 M sodium citrate (Vacutainer, Becton-Dickinson, Rutherford, NJ, USA). The sample was analyzed using an automated coagulation system (ACL 300 Instrumentation Laboratory UK, Ltd) and rabbit brain calcium thromboplastin for INR and FBNG (Instrumentation Laboratory UK, Ltd) and Diagen kaolin-platelet substitute for APTR (Diagnostic Reagent Ltd, UK) within an hour after sampling. PCV was measured using the microcentrifuge, and ACT was measured on a Hemochron system. In the general surgical group, 4.5 mL of blood was collected into ethylenediamine tetraacetate (EDTA) K_3 for a full blood count using an automated cell counter (Technicon H*1 Technicon Division, Bayer Diagnostic, Basingstoke, UK).

During surgery, blood loss was replaced with Gelofusine and Hartman's solution to maintain normovolemia. The PCV was measured every half hour, or whenever the patient's condition indicated (for example, if the blood pressure dropped) or before blood transfusion was started. Bank blood was administered when the blood loss was thought to be clinically significant or when the PCV fell below 23–27, depending on the patient's cardiovascular status. The autologous blood was reinfused in a reverse order (the second collected unit first) after "surgical" bleeding had been controlled. In vascular cases this was when the anastamoses had been completed and heparin had been reversed with a half dose of protamine sulfate. Correct reversal of heparin was checked using ACT, to return it to the postdilution level. Postoperatively, blood coagulation and full blood count samples were taken either in the recovery or in the intensive care unit after reinfusion of all the autologous blood.

The results were recorded on record sheets, transferred to a database, and analyzed using the C-Stat (Oxtech Ltd, UK) statistical package. Means and 95% confidence intervals were calculated and the Mann-Whitney U test was used. A p value of 0.05 was accepted as the limit of significance.

Results

There were 24 males and 6 females in the arteriopath group with a median age (range) of 70 (51–85 years) and 8 males and 9 females in the GS group with a median age of 65 (19–81). Among the patients with AAA, 8 had a history of myocardial infarction (MI), 5 had angina pectoris, and 9 were hypertensive. Twenty-six had clinical, radiographic, or respiratory functional evidence of chronic obstructive airway disease (COAD), and 16 admitted smoking. In the GS group, no patient had a previous history of MI but 3 had angina pectoris. Five patients were hypertensive, 4 were diabetics, and 6 had evidence of COAD.

The calculated mean blood volume was 4,282 mL (3,921–4,644) in the general surgical and 4,700 mL (4,411–4,989) in AAA patients. This difference reached statistical significance ($p = 0.035$). The mean volume of blood withdrawn in the AAA group was 832 mL (726–939) or 17.7% and 951 mL (866–1,037) or 22.2% in the GS group, but the difference was not statistically significant ($p = 0.258$). The mean preoperative hemoglobin (Hb) was 13.6 g/L (13.2–14.1) in the AAA group and 13.2 g/L (12.6–13.7) in the GS group; the difference was nonsignificant. Changes in PCV and clotting studies in the two groups are summarized in Table 9.1. The decrease in PCV in each group after preload Gelofusine infusion was 0.4 and 0.7, but this was not significant. The PCV after dilution was significantly lower in the GS group, in which the blood volume was lower and the volume of withdrawn blood higher: 0.28 (0.27–0.29) versus 0.31 (0.29–32) ($p = 0.017$). Blood loss during AAA surgery was significantly higher than during other surgical procedures, 1,694 mL (1,218–2,169) versus 1,035 mL (667–1,402) ($p = 0.018$). Intraoperative bank blood replacement was also significantly higher during aneurysm repair (0.18 versus 1.97 units), so the mean postoperative PCV did not differ significantly between the two groups: 0.30 (29–32) versus 0.28 (26–30) ($p = 0.053$). Only 13 patients of the 30 needed postoperative transfusion of a mean of 1.03 units after aneurysm repair, and 6 of 17 in the GS group required a mean of 0.76 unit. Nine patients out of 30 AAA patients did not receive any blood product transfusions during their hospital stay, and 11 out of 17 were not exposed to bank blood after general surgery (Table 9.2).

Preoperative coagulation studies were normal in both groups (Tables 9.3 and 9.4). There was no statistical difference between the two groups' preoper-

TABLE 9.1. Changes in PCV and clotting studies in the two groups. Values are means and 95% CI except age (median and range).

	Group 1 AAA repair	p value	Group 2 GS
Age (range)	70 yrs (51–85)	NS	65 yrs (19–81)
Blood volume	4,700 mL (4411–4989)	0.035	4,282 mL (3921–4644)
ANH volume	832 mL (726–939)	NS	951 mL (866–1037)
PCV preop	0.40 (0.39–0.42)	NS	0.40 (0.39–0.41)
PCV predil	0.39 (0.38–0.41)	NS	0.39 (0.37–0.40)
PCV postdil	0.31 (0.29–0.32)	0.017	28 (0.27–0.29)
PCV postop	0.30 (0.29–0.32)	NS	0.28 (0.26–0.30)
INR preop	1.04 (1.01–1.08)	NS	1.06 (1.02–1.11)
INR postdil	1.33 (1.28–1.38)	0.013	1.37 (1.27–1.47)
APTR preop	0.97 (0.93–1.01)	NS	1.02 (1.04–1.31)
APTR postdil	1.04 (0.99–1.1)	NS	1.18 (1.04–1.31)
FBNG preop	3.8 (3.43–4.16)	NS	4.4 (3.61–5.19)
FBNG postdil	2.58 (2.32–2.84)	NS	2.71 (2.3–3.12)
FBNG postop	2.13 (1.9–2.36)	0.037	2.56 (2.16–2.97)
ACT predil	130 sec (123–137)	NS	124 sec (115–133)
ACT postdil	131 sec (122–139)	NS	123 sec (114–132)

TABLE 9.2. Homologous transfusion data. Values are means and 95% CI.

	Group 1 AAA repair	p value	Group 2 GS
Blood loss	1,694 mL (1218–2169)	0.018	1,035 mL (667–1402)
No transfusion	9/30 patients		11/17 patients
Transfusion volume	3 units (2.1–3.9)	0.003	0.88 unit (0.7–1.7)

TABLE 9.3. Changes in coagulation studies and PCV after hemodilution in AAA patients.

	Predilution	p value	Postdilution
PCV	0.39 (0.38–0.41)	<0.001	0.31 (0.29–0.32)
INR	1.04 (1.01–1.08)	<0.001	1.33 (1.28–1.38)
APTR	0.97 (0.93–1.01)	NS	1.04 (0.97–1.1)
FBNG	3.8 (3.43–4.16)	<0.001	2.58 (2.32–2.84)
ACT	130 s (123–137)	NS	131 (122–139)

TABLE 9.4. Changes in coagulation studies and PCV after hemodilution in GS cases.

	Predilution	p value	Postdilution
PCV	0.39 (0.37–0.40)	<0.002	0.28 (0.27–0.29)
PLT count	275 g/l (236–315)	<0.002	189 g/l (157–220)
INR	1.06 (1.02–1.11)	<0.002	1.37 (1.27–1.47)
APTR	1.02 (0.93–1.11)	NS	1.18 (1.04–1.31)
FBNG	4.40 (3.61–5.19)	<0.002	2.71 (2.3–3.12)
ACT	124 (115–133)	<0.005	123 (114–132)

ative coagulation results. Due to hemodilution, FBNG concentration decreased in each group to 2.71 (2.3–3.12) and 2.58 (2.32–2.84), respectively, but there was no statistically significant difference between the two groups after dilution. However, after vascular surgery, fibrinogen concentration decreased further, and the difference between the postdilution and postoperative FBNG levels was statistically significant: 2.13 (1.9–2–36) ($p = 0.007$). This did not occur after general surgery, when the postoperative FBNG was 2.56 (2.16–2.97) ($p > 0.05$).

The INR was prolonged in both groups after dilution: 1.33 (1.28–1.38) in AAA patients and 1.37 (1.27–1.47) in the GS group. Both changes were statistically significant ($p < 0.02$ and $p < 0.001$) compared to preoperative values.

The postdilution INR results were not different between the two groups, but the APTR results were. In the GS cases, where PCV after dilution was significantly lower than in the AAA group, the APTR was significantly raised (Tables 9.3 and 9.4).

The ACT was not affected by dilution in either group.

If the patients are divided into two groups with regard to the volume of hemodilution, in 25 patients the withdrawn blood volume was under 1,000 mL because of the lower blood volume [mean 4,288 mL (3,168–4,608)] (Table 9.5 and 9.6). In the other 22 patients, when the blood volume was higher [4,846 mL (4553–5,138)], over 1,000 mL could be withdrawn. The mean volume of blood withdrawn was 703 mL (613–791) versus 1,072 mL (1,025–1,119). Analysis of clotting studies dependent on the volume of blood

TABLE 9.5. Preoperative data in patients having venesection of $>1,000$ mL and $<1,000$ mL.

	ANH $<$ 1,000 mL $N = 25$	p value	ANH $>$ 1,000 mL $N = 22$
Blood volume	4,288 mL (3,968–4,608)	$p = 0.038$	4,845 mL (4,553–5,138)
ANH volume	703 mL (613–792)	$p < 0.001$	1,072 mL (1,025–1,119)
INR predil	1.05 (1.01–1.08)	NS	1.06 (1.02–1.11)
APTR predil	0.98 (0.91–1.04)	NS	0.995 (0.951–1.101)

TABLE 9.6. Changes in coagulation studies predilution and postdilution in patients having $<1,000$ mL and $>1,000$ mL of hemodilution.

	Predilution	p value	Postdilution
ANH $<$ 1000			
INR	1.05 (1.01–1.08)	<0.001	1.31 (1.24–1.37)
APTR	0.98 (0.91–1.04)	$=0.144$	1.04 (0.97–1.12)
ANH $>$ 1000			
INR	1.06 (1.02–1.11)	<0.001	1.42 (1.35–1.49)
APTR	0.99 (0.95–1.01)	$=0.003$	1.15 (1.04–1.25)

withdrawn revealed a more marked prolongation of the APTR in the more diluted patients: 1.15 (1.04–1.25) ($p = 0.003$).

The pulse oximetry recordings were constant before, during, and after the dilution and reflected adequate blood oxygenation throughout the entire process.

Discussion

The ANH procedure was easy to perform and took an average of 23.5 minutes to remove a mean of 875 mL (801–950) of blood. Draining the blood from a peripheral arm vein appears to be adequate for hemodilution. A triple-lumen central venous line does not provide an adequate channel for rapid venesection, but some authors have used Swan-Ganz catheter sheaths. Central venous pressure monitoring is not mandatory during hemodilution and was not used in this study. When a central venous line is indicated for intraoperative monitoring and rapid fluid replacement, hemodilution can be performed from a peripheral vein during venous line insertion. Use of the arterial line is not as speedy as one may think and precludes simultaneous arterial blood pressure monitorings.

There was one intraoperative complication during aortic aneurysm repair. During the procedure the patient's airway pressure increased and his blood oxygen saturation fell below 90. Intraoperative bronchoscopy revealed a mucous plug which was removed. Approximately 30 minutes later the ECG showed ST segment elevation and the blood pressure fell. At the same time the autologous blood was being reinfused. Postoperative ECG and enzyme changes were consistent with an MI. The patient did not have a previous history of coronary artery disease and did not have ischemic changes on his preoperative ECG. His postoperative course otherwise was uneventful. There were no other perioperative complications related to the procedure. Despite the fact that 13 of 47 patients had either a previous MI or angina, all underwent hemodilution without cardiac complication.

Normovolemia during hemodilution is essential, and therefore the accepted ANH method was modified by using a preload colloid infusion before blood withdrawal. This is because general surgical and vascular surgical patients are often dehydrated and may be hypovolemic at the time of anesthetic induction, and this prehydration may compensate for vasodilatation caused by anesthetic drugs. This preload did not alter the PCV significantly.

The direct blood-saving effect of the method was not calculated in this study using prospective controls. However, 20 of 47 patients (42.5%) did not receive bank blood transfusion. It has been reported that hemodiluted patients bleed more during surgery,[25] but this was not observed in this study. Surgical bleeding shows a close relation to platelet counts and function. The platelet count decreased significantly as the result of dilution in general surgical patients. The difference of the means of preoperative and postdilution platelet count was 32%; the postdilution platelet count was still within the normal range and so did not present any danger of impaired hemostasis. There were significant differences between the predilution and postdilution coagulation studies in the general surgical cases, where the final mean PCV was 0.28. The APTR showed significant prolongation only in the general surgical group but remained normal in the vascular surgical patients. Therefore there were statistically significant changes in coagulation studies reflecting both the extrinsic and intrinsic coagulation pathways. However, the intrinsic pathway seemed to be less sensitive to dilution.

The ACT is a functional measure of the intrinsic clotting pathway and reflects the overall coagulability of blood.[26] It has been reported that during cardiopulmonary bypass surgery the ACT is prolonged by other factors than heparin.[27] Although hemodilution contributes toward this prolongation, in extracorporeal circulation other factors, such as enhanced fibrinolysis and a marked drop in platelet counts, also contribute to this effect.

In conclusion, blood coagulation appears to be altered by moderate hemodilution, but from this clinical experience the maximum INR of 1.5 or APTR of 1.3 did not represent clinically significant coagulopathy. Blood coagulation factors are normally present in excess amounts, and surgical hemostasis can be achieved when their level is approximately 20–30% of the normal. However, in view of the mild dilutional coagulopathy seen in this study, it is recommended that a normal preoperative coagulation screen be mandatory for patients undergoing ANH.

Reinfusion of functioning platelets at the end of a procedure has a beneficial effect in achieving hemostasis. This is supported by the clinical observation of decreased oozing after reinfusion of the patient's own blood. This effect is very beneficial in vascular surgery when platelets have been exposed to heparin and protamine.[28,29]

In summary, ANH appears to be a practical, safe method for blood conservation, even in high-risk patients. The minor degree of dilutional coagulopathy that occurs following the technique is not associated with clinically important bleeding, and the method deserves widespread application, especially in cancer surgery, where other methods of intraoperative autotransfusion may be contraindicated.

Acknowlegments. The authors are grateful for the generous support of Haemocell Bellhouse Bio-Sciences PLC, Abingdon, Oxfordshire, UK, who provided financial support for Dr. Varga, and to Baxter Fenwal UK Ltd, Compton Newbury, Berkshire, UK, who provided the Autologous Blood Collection Kits.

References

1. National Institutes of Health, Bethesda, Md: Perioperative red blood cell transfusion JAMA 1988;260:2700–2703.
2. Bidstrup BP, Royston D, Sapsford N, Taylor KN. Reduction in blood loss and blood used after cardiopulmonary bypass with high dose aprotinin (Trasylol). J Thorac Cardiovasc Surg 1989;97:364–372.
3. Messmer K, Kreimer U, Intaglietta M. Present state of intentional haemodilution. Eur Surg Res 1986;18:254–263.
4. Halonen P, Linko K, Myllyla G. A study of haemostasis following the use of high doses of hydroxyethyl starch 120 and dextran in major laparotomies. Acta Anaesthesiol Scand 1987;31:320–324.
5. Testas P. Clinical experience with polygeline in the surgical field. Arch Emerg Med 1989;1(Suppl):39–45.
6. Dale RF, Kipling RM, Smith MF, Collier DStJ, Smith PG. Separation of malignant cells during autotransfusion. Br J Surg 1988;75:581.
7. Hart OJ III, Klimberg IW, Wajsman Z, Baker G. Intraoperative autotransfusion in radical cystectomy for carcinoma of the bladder. Surg Gynec Obstet 1989;168: 302–306.
8. Guidelines for blood salvage and reinfusion in surgery and trauma. American Association of Blood Banks, 1990.
9. BCSH Blood Transfusion Task Force: Guidelines for autologous transfusion. Clin Lab Haemat 1988;10:193–201.
10. Rodgers SE, Lloyd JV, Russel WJ. Platelet function in platelet concentrates and in whole blood. Anaesth Intensive Care 1985;13:355–361.
11. Nilsson L, Hedner U, Nilsson IM, et al. Shelf-life of bank blood and stored plasma with special reference to coagulation factors. Transfusion 1983;23:377–381.

12. Duhm J, Meul A, Wood L. Depletion and regeneration of 2,3-diphosphoglyceric acid in stored red blood cells. Transfusion 1969;9:109.
13. Briden KL, Telster M, Weiss HR. The effect of mild normovolaemic haemodilution on regional blood flow, oxygenization and small vessel blood content in the rabbit heart subjected to acute coronary occlusion. Circ Shock 1979;6:223–233.
14. Shah DM, Prichard MN, Newell JC, et al. Increased cardiac output and oxygen transport after intraoperative isovolaemic haemodilution. Arch Surg 1980;115:597–600.
15. Parris WCW, Kambam JR, Blanks S, Dean R. The effect of intentional haemodilution on P_{50}. J Cardiovasc Surg 1988;29:560–562.
16. Saxena S, Adono V, Uba J, Nelson JM, Lewis WL, Shulman IA. The risk of bacterial growth in units of blood that have warmed to more than 10°C. Am J Clin Pathol 1990;94:80–83.
17. Hallowell P, Bland JHL, Buckley MJ, et al. Transfusion of fresh autologous blood in open heart surgery: A method for reducing bank blood requirements. J Thorac Cardiovasc Surg 1972;64:941.
18. Davies MJ, Cronin KD, Domaingue C. Haemodilution for major vascular surgery—using 3.5% polygeline (Haemaccel). Anaesth Intens Care 1982;10:265–270.
19. Rose D, Coutsoftides T. Intraoperative normovolaemic haemodilution. J Surg Res 1981;31:375–381.
20. Vara-Thorbeck R, Guerrero-Fernandez Marcote JA. Haemodynamic response of elderly patients undergoing major surgery under moderate normovolemic haemodilution. Eur Surg Res 1985;17:372–376.
21. Hardesty RL, Bayer WL, Bahnson HT. A technique for the use of autologous fresh blood during open heart surgery. J Thorac Cardiovasc Surg 1968;56:683.
22. Krämer AH, Hertzer NR, Bevan EJ. Intraoperative haemodilution during elective vascular reconstruction. Surg Gynec Obstet 1979;149:831–836.
23. Haberken M, Dangel P. Normovolaemic haemodilution and intraoperative autotransfusion in children: Experience with 30 cases of spinal fusion. Eur J Pediatr Surg 1991;1:30–35.
24. Zetterström H, Wiklund L. A new nomogram facilitating adequate haemodilution. Acta Anaesthesiol Scand 1986;30:300–304.
25. Parker MC. Pre-operative normovolaemic haemodilution in major general surgery. Surg Res Comm 1987;1:181–194.
26. Hattersley PG. Activated clotting time of whole blood. JAMA 1966;196:436–440.
27. Kesteven PJ, Pasaoglu I, Williams BT, Savidge GF. Significance of the whole blood activated clotting time in cardiopulmonary bypass. J Cardiovasc Surg 1986;27:85–89.
28. Brace LD, Fareed J. An objective assesment of the interaction of heparin and its fractions with human platelets. Semin Thromb Hemost 1985;11:190–198.
29. Horrow JC: Protamine: A review of its toxicity. Anaesth Analg 1985;64:348–361.

10
Percutaneous Bidirectional Femoral Artery Cannulation for Extended Extracorporeal Circulatory Support

HIROSHI MATSUURA, XI MING YANG, JAMES D. FONGER, GABRIEL S. ALDEA, and RICHARD J. SHEMIN

Summary

Femoral artery cannulation for the return of blood from an extracorporeal perfusion circuit to the systemic circulation causes near or complete occlusion of distal blood flow to the cannulated limb. Although intraoperative limb ischemia is generally tolerated, extended circulatory support with femoral artery cannulation can result in severe ischemic limb complications. A percutaneous bidirectional femoral artery cannula has been developed which maintains distal perfusion and thus prevents ischemia in the cannulated limb.

To evaluate the benefits of bidirectional cannulation, seven adult pigs were cannulated with a 17 Fr unidirectional cannula in one groin and a 17 Fr bidirectional cannula in the opposite groin. Venous drainage was established by cannulating the right atrium. On full cardiopulmonary bypass, distal arterial flows, pressures, and femoral venous oxygen saturation values were measured over a range of flows from the extracorporeal circuit.

At circuit flows of 4 L/min, the distal mean flow was 206.6 mL/min in the bidirectional limbs and unmeasurable in the unidirectional limbs ($p < 0.01$). The distal mean pressure was 76.3 mm Hg in the bidirectional limbs and 18.8 mm Hg in the unidirectional limbs ($p < 0.01$). Femoral venous oxygen saturation was 71.6% in the bidirectional limbs and 27.8% in the unidirectional limbs ($p < 0.01$).

These results demonstrate that this fenestrated percutaneous bidirectional femoral artery cannula significantly improved distal perfusion in the cannulated limb.

Introduction

Recent developments in cannula materials and design have allowed the establishment of full cardiopulmonary bypass via percutaneous femoral cannulation.[1-3] Extracorporeal membrane oxygenation and left ventricular assist can also be established using femoral artery cannulation.[4,5] However, current femoral artery cannulation for the return of blood from the perfusion circuit to the systemic circulation causes near or complete occlusion of flow distally in the cannulated limb. Although intraoperative limb ischemia is usually tolerated, extended circulatory support with femoral artery cannulation can result in severe ischemic limb complications. Therefore, we have evaluated a percutaneous fenestrated bidirectional femoral artery cannula that maintains distal perfusion to prevent ischemia in the cannulated limb.

Methods

Cannula Design

This percutaneous bidirectional cannula (DLP Inc., Grand Rapids, MI, USA) (Fig. 10.1) has two distinctive features. The body is standard 17 Fr polyurethane femoral artery cannula. However, one new feature is a proximal side hole or fenestration with a neighboring ridge to hold the fenestration away from the arterial wall and direct a portion of the femoral flow distally (Fig. 10.2). Also, the obturator is fashioned with a reduced proximal diameter so that when the proximal side hole enters the vessel this is signaled by a burst of blood in a "flash chamber" in the cannula hub.

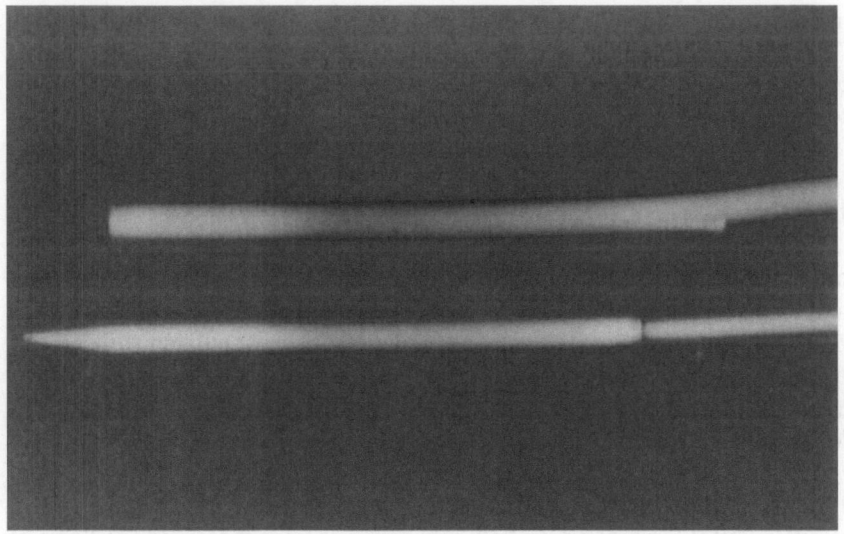

FIGURE 10.1. Percutaneous bidirectional femoral artery cannula.

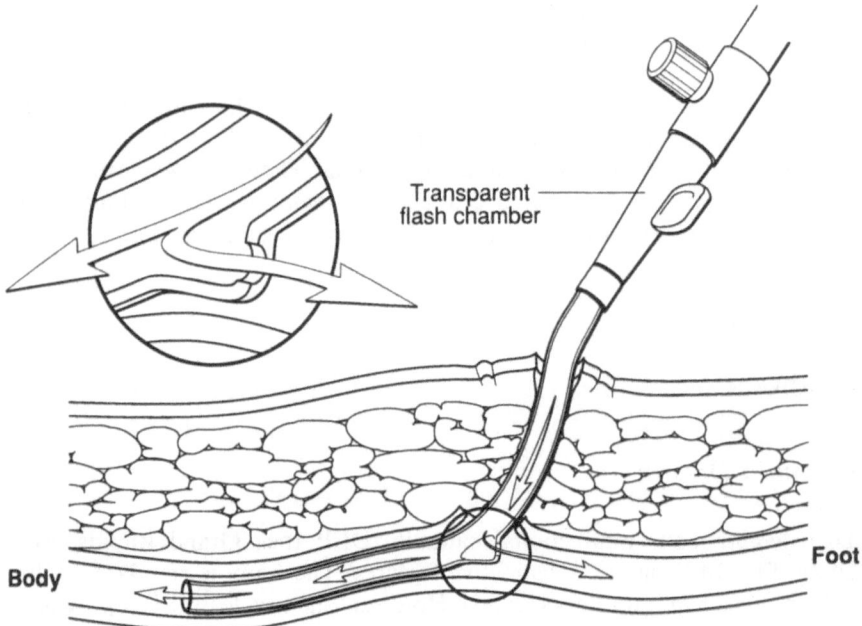

Transparent flash chamber

Body

Foot

FIGURE 10.2. Schematic view of percutaneous bidirectional femoral artery cannulation.

Experimental Study

Seven adult pigs (78–92 kg) were premedicated with intramuscular ketamine hydrochloride (20 mg/kg), anesthetized with intravenous α-chloralose (75 mg/kg), and placed on positive-pressure endotracheal ventilation. Catheters were placed into the left carotid artery and left jugular vein for monitoring systemic pressure and administering fluids. Distal portions of both femoral arteries were exposed and electromagnetic flow probes (Carolina Medical Electronics, Inc.) and pressure monitoring lines were placed (Fig. 10.3).

Following control measurements of flow, pressure, and femoral venous oxygen saturation (SVO_2), a median sternotomy was performed. After systemic heparinization, a 42 Fr venous drainage cannula was placed in the right atrium. One femoral artery was percutaneously cannulated with a 17 Fr bidirectional cannula by means of the Seldinger needle technique, and then cardiopulmonary bypass (Sarns delphin 2 centrifugal pump and Sarns SMO Membrane Oxygenator, Sarns 3M, Ann Arbor, MI) was initiated.

Flow in the bypass circuit was increased in increments of 0.5 L/min from 1.5 to 4.5 L/min. After each additional 0.5 L/min of flow had stabilized for 5 minutes, distal femoral artery flow and pressure were measured. At flows of 2, 3, and 4 L/min, ipsilateral SVO_2 was also obtained. Then the opposite femoral artery was percutaneously cannulated with a conventional 17 Fr

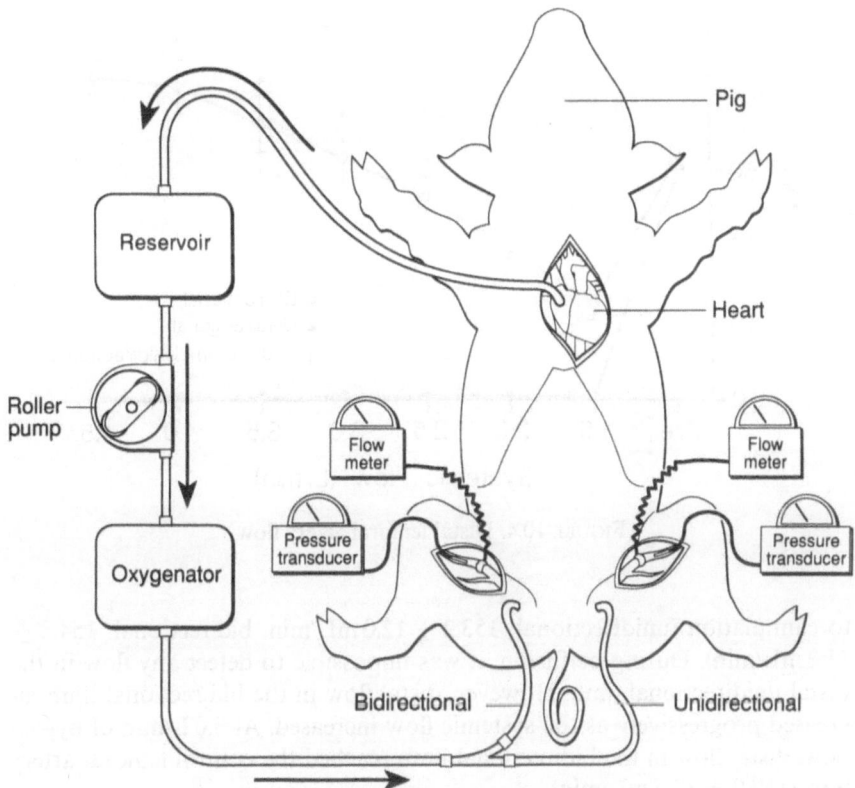

FIGURE 10.3. Schematic of experimental model.

unidirectional cannula and connected to the circuit. After clamping the bi-directional cannula, another series of similar measurements was made. During cardiopulmonary bypass the arterial Po_2 was maintained at 300 mm Hg.

All data were expressed as the mean $\pm$ standard error of the mean. Paired t-tests between the bidirectional and unidirectional limb in the same animal were used for statistical analysis using each animal as its own control. Data were considered significant at the $p < 0.05$ level.

All animals received humane care in compliance with *Principles of Laboratory Animal Care* formulated by the National Academy of Sciences and published by the National Institutes of Health (NIH Publication No. 80–23, revised, 1978).

Results

Distal Femoral Artery Flow

The changes in distal femoral artery flow are shown in Fig. 10.4. There was no difference between control femoral artery flows in either limb prior

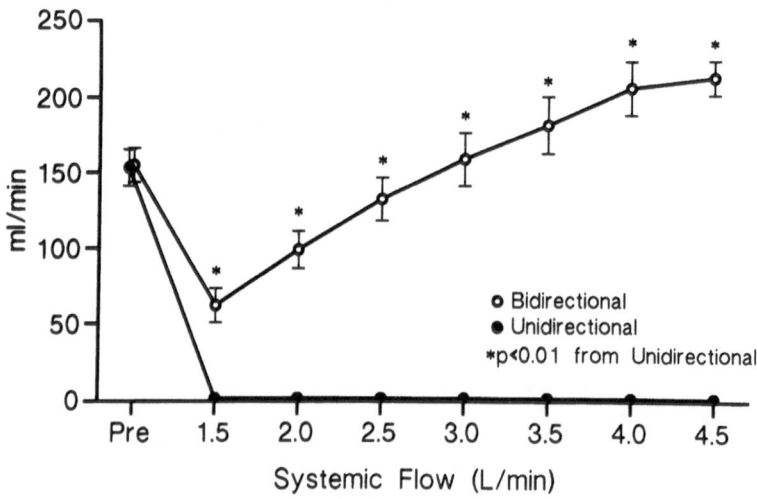

FIGURE 10.4. Distal femoral artery flow.

to cannulation (unidirectional: 153.2 ± 12.0 mL/min, bidirectional: 154.8 ± 11.2 mL/min). During perfusion, it was impossible to detect any flow in the distal unidirectional limb. However, distal flow in the bidirectional limb increased progressively as the systemic flow increased. At 3.0 L/min of bypass flow, distal flow in the bidirectional limb reached the control femoral artery flow (159.0 ± 17.7 mL/min).

Distal Femoral Artery Pressure

The changes in distal femoral artery pressure are illustrated in Fig. 10.5. Both femoral arteries had equal mean pressures prior to cannulation (unidirectional: 84.7 ± 6.2 mm Hg; bidirectiona: 81.3 ± 3.3 mm Hg). During bypass, pressures in the unidirectional limb remained low despite increases in bypass flow (15.0 ± 5.2 mm Hg at 1.5 L/min; 17.1 ± 5.7 mm Hg at 3.0 L/min; 19.9 ± 5.1 mm Hg at 4.5 L/min). However, pressure in the bidirectional limb rose with increases in bypass flow (35.8 ± 4.1 *mm Hg at 1.5 L/min; 67.3 ± 6.1 +mm Hg at 3.0 L/min; 74.7 ± 9.1 +mm Hg at 4.5 L/min).

Femoral Venous Oxygen Saturation (SVO_2)

The changes in SVO_2 in the ipsilateral femoral vein are summarized in Fig. 10.6. The control femoral vein SVO_2 before cannulation was similar in both limbs (77.6 ± 3.2% unidirectional; 75.4 ± 3.5% bidirectional; not significant). After cannulation, at 2.0 L/min of bypass flow, SVO_2 decreased in both limbs

*$p < 0.05$, +$p < 0.01$ from unidirectional.

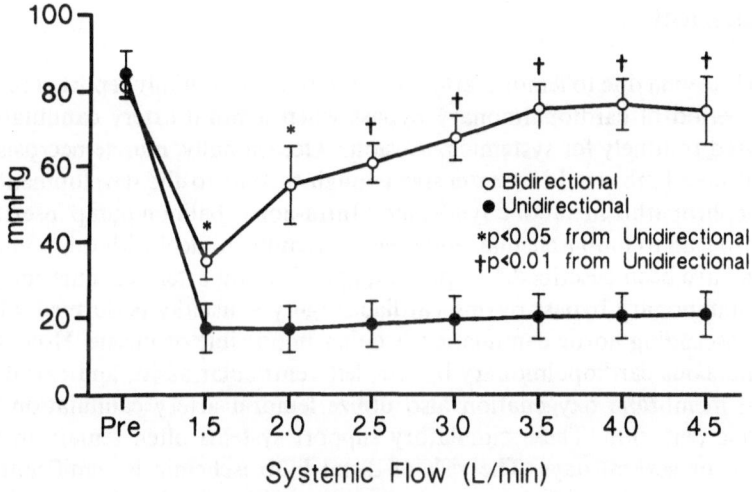

FIGURE 10.5. Distal femoral artery pressure.

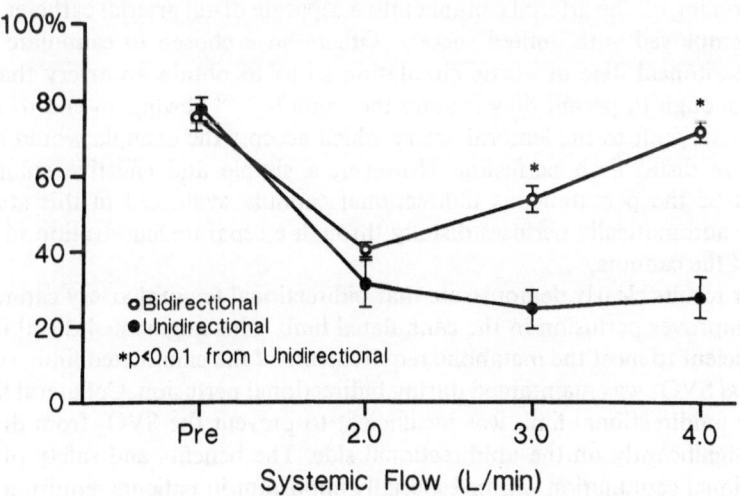

FIGURE 10.6. Femoral venous oxygen saturation (SVO_2).

($31.2 \pm 6.3\%$ unidirectional; $40.2 \pm 2.1\%$ bidirectional, not significant). In the unidirectional limbs, SVO_2 remained low ($24.5 \pm 5.3\%$ at 3.0 L/min; $27.8 \pm 5.6\%$ at 4.0 L/min). However, SVO_2 in the bidirectional limbs improved significantly ($53.8 \pm 3.5\%$* at 3.0 L/min; $71.6 \pm 2.8\%$* at 4.0 L/min). At 4.0 L/min of bypass flow, the SVO_2 in the bidirectional limbs almost returned to the control level.

*$p < 0.01$ from unidirectional.

Discussion

Limb ischemia due to femoral artery cannulation was initially reported in the early period of cardiopulmonary bypass when femoral artery cannulation was used routinely for systemic perfusion.[6] Occasionally, muscle necrosis in the affected limb would be extensive enough to lead to the development of myonephropathic metabolic syndrome.[7] Intra-aortic balloon pump insertion can also lead to limb ischemia, and several attempts to deal with this complication have been described.[8] At present, open femoral artery cannulation for cardiopulmonary bypass during cardiac surgery is usually performed when direct ascending aortic cannulation is either impossible or unsafe. However, percutaneous cardiopulmonary bypass, left ventricular assist, and extracorporeal membrane oxygenation also utilize femoral artery cannulation for systemic perfusion. These circulatory support systems often remain in the patient for several days. The risk of distal limb ischemia is significant in this setting, yet it is often too soon to remove the cannula when problems develop.

In an attempt to augment distal perfusion to the cannulated limb, a side-arm coming off the arterial cannula into a separate distal arterial catheter has been employed with limited success. Others have chosen to cannulate the retroperitoneal iliac or aortic circulation so as to obtain an artery that is large enough to permit flow around the cannula.[9,10] Sewing an end-to-side prosthetic graft to the femoral artery which accepts the cannula would also preserve distal limb perfusion. However, a simple and effective solution would be the percutaneous bidirectional cannula evaluated in this study, which automatically perfuses distally through a separate fenestration in the heel of the cannula.

Our results clearly demonstrate that bidirectional femoral artery cannulation improves perfusion in the cannulated limb. This augmented distal flow is sufficient to meet the metabolic requirements of the cannulated limb, since femoral SVO_2 was maintained during bidirectional perfusion. Collateral flow to the unidirectional limb was insufficient to prevent the SVO_2 from dropping significantly on the unidirectional side. The benefits and safety of bidirectional cannulation will be especially important in patients requiring extended periods of femoral artery perfusion.

References

1. Phillips SJ, Ballentine B, Slonine D, Hall J. Percutaneous initiation of cardiopulmonary bypass. Ann Thorac Surg 1983;36:223–225.
2. Phillips SJ, Zeff RH, Kongtaworn C, Skinner JR. Percutaneous cardiopulmonary bypass: Application and indication for use. Ann Thorac Surg 1989;47:121–123.
3. Mooney MR, Arom KV, Joyce LD, Mooney JF. Emergency cardiopulmonary bypass support in patients with cardiac arrest. J Thorac Cardiovasc Surg 1991; 101:450–454.

4. Glassman E, Engelman RE, Boyd AD, Lipson D. A method of closed-chest cannulation of the left atrium for left atrial-femoral artery bypass. J Thorac Cardiovasc Surg 1975;69:283–290.
5. Sasaki E, Nakatani T, Taenaka Y, Noda H. Easy access for left ventricular assist system without thoracotomy. ASAIO Transactions 1991;37:M280–M281.
6. Fisher RD, Fogarty TJ, Morrow AG. Clinical and biochemical observations of the effect of transient femoral artery occlusion in man. Surgery 1970;68:323–328.
7. Kugimiya T, Shirabe J, Kusaba E, Hadama T. Myonephropathic-metabolic syndrome as a complication of cardiopulmonary bypass. Jpn J Surg 1983;13:431–437.
8. Gold JP, Cohen J, Shemin RJ, DiSesa VJ. Femorofemoral bypass to relieve acute leg ischemia during intra-aortic balloon pump cardiac support. J Vasc Surg 1986; 3:351–354.
9. Read R, St Cyr J, Tornabene S, Whitman, G. Improved cannulation method for extracorporeal membrane oxygenation. Ann Thorac Surg 1990;50:670–671.
10. Duncan JM, Burnett CM, Vega JD, et al. Rapid placement of the hemopump and hemofiltration cannula. Ann Thorac Surg 1990;50:667–669.

11
Plain Chest Radiographic Assessment of Cardiac Tamponade in Patients with Penetrating Chest Injury Using Vascular Pedicle Width Measurements

FELISBERTO M. SORIANO, JR., AND ROMULO G. VEA

Introduction

Recent increases in injuries resulting from civilian violence have been noticeable in the past several years in the Philippines. The most dramatic of these is the injured heart in its entire spectrum, from cardiac rupture to penetrating wounds with cardiac tamponade.[13] Cardiac penetration in civilian trauma is most often caused by stab wounds from knives or ice picks or missile injuries from gunshot wounds.[13,32,33]

Hippocrates noted the fatal outcome of cardiac injury, but it is no longer true that all wounds of the heart are mortal, as initially thought by Boerhaave.

The importance of prompt diagnosis and treatment of these injuries is underscored by the possibility of achieveing a significant survival rate.[13] Plain chest radiographs have commonly been employed in patients with chest injuries. However, many prominent surgeons and clinicians think of chest radiographs as having little or no value in diagnosing cardiac tamponade.[13,32,33]

The chest radiograph is commonly employed and has become an established part of chest interpretation. Systemic vessels are visible on chest radiographs, i.e., the superior vena cava can be traced on the right, while the aorta and takeoff of the left subclavian artery can be traced on the left. These vessels, which form the border of the superior mediastinum, have been termed the vascular pedicle.[24,25,29,36] Pistolesi proposed a method of measuring this (vascular pedicle width, VPW) and found good positive linear correlation of this measurement with the total blood volume (TBV), systemic blood volume (SBV), and mean right atrial pressure. Local studies done by Vea et al. showed a good correlations in acute myocardial infarction patients with cardiac output, stroke volume plus ejection fraction in mitral stenosis, and cardiac output in normal subjects.[8,24,27,36]

To our knowledge, there have been no systematic attempts to make use of the chest radiograph in an objective assessment of cardiac tamponade in penetrating chest injury. This study was undertaken to evaluate the detection of cardiac tamponade in patients with penetrating chest injury via chest radiography. Our specific objectives were (1) to assess the ability of the chest radiograph to diagnose cardiac tamponade using vascular pedicle width measurements in chest trauma, (2) to determine the diagnostic accuracy of these measurements, and (3) assess the applicability of other radiographic findings (pneumothorax, hemothorax, pneumomediastinum, pulmonary contusion) and clinical findings (hypotension, tachycardia, normal blood pressure, hypotension with tachcycardia, nature and site of injury) in determining the presence of cardiac tamponade, independent of VPW.

Methods

Study Population

The subjects were 94 patients seen at the emergency room of San Juan de Dios Hospital from September 1986 to September 1990 who had chest trauma and whose injuries could result in cardiac tamponade based on the guidelines proposed by Evans and Murdock.[13] The basis of patient selection is illustrated in Fig. 11.1. The initial chest films (prior to fluid resuscitation) of all chest trauma patients seen in this period were assessed by one radiologist. The films were assessed as to the adequacy of techniques using the following criteria: (1) no obliquity, (2) good inspiratory film, (3) good penetration, adequate for accurate measurement of VPW, and (4) taken before volume replacement. All subjects satisfied all criteria. The subjects were divided into two populations. Population 1 consisted of 33 patients who had cardiac tamponade, verified by surgery, and population 2 consisted of patients who had injury without cardiac tamponade (assessed clinically during admission, during stay in the hospital, and in subsequent follow-up). Excluded from the study were patients with clinical signs of cardiac tamponade who were not admitted, patients who died on arrival at the emergency room, and those who were transferred to other hospitals.

Radiologic Evaluation

Qualitative Parameter

The presence in the initial chest radiograph of any of the following was assessed and recorded for each patient: (a) pneumothorax, (b) pneumomediastinum, (c) hemothorax, (d) pulmonary contusion, (e) subcutaneous emphysema.

Quantitative Parameter

VPW measurement is proposed in this study as a quantitative parameter for cardiac tamponade. Fig. 11.2 shows how VPW is measured. The right border

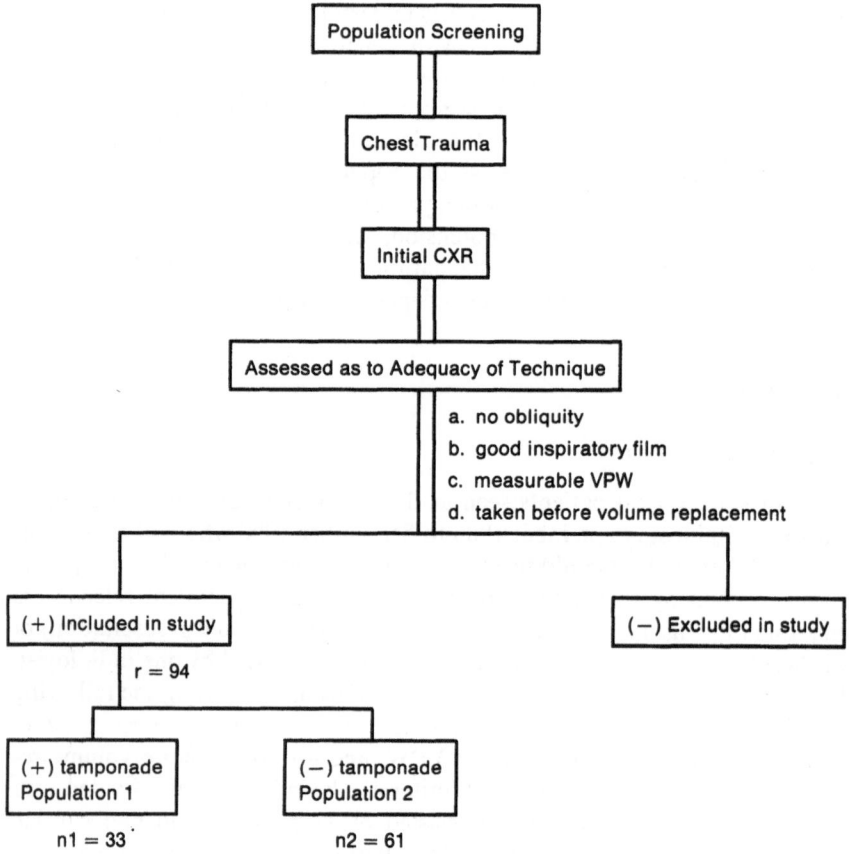

FIGURE 11.1. Algorhythm for the selection of population.

(dark area) is all venous and the left border (light area) is all arterial. The measuring points for VPW are R the point at which the superior vena cava (SVC) crosses the superior border of the right main stem bronchus and L the point of the takeoff of the subclavian artery from the aorta. The right VPW (RVPW) is measured from point R to the midline and the left VPW (LVPW) is measured from point L to the midline. The total VPW (TVPW) is determined by adding the RVPW and LVPW. Since these measurements are affected by magnification, all the chest films taken in the supine position were corrected by subtracting 20% of the value to make them uniform with those taken posteroanteriorly (the magnification factor of 20% is based on the studies of Pistolesi and locally by Vea[24,25,27,36]). All measurements were done in millimeters using the same ruler in all subjects.

The following arguments underlie the fundamental assumption and the physiologic basis of this proposed method:

FIGURE 11.2. Method of measurement of vascular pedicle width (VPW) in millimeters.

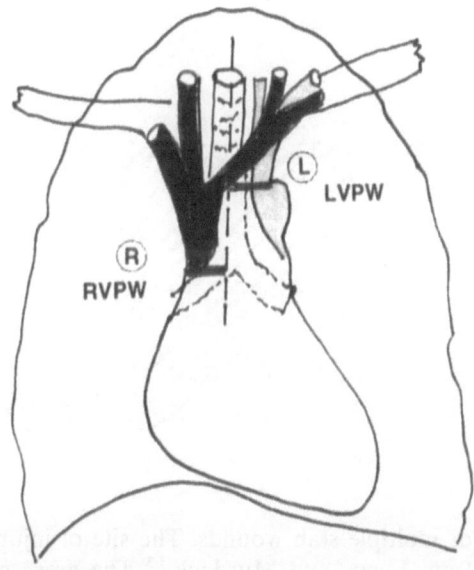

(1) In the presence of cardiac injury, blood accumulates in the pericardium and produces tamponade, which raises the central venous pressure (CVP) and significantly impairs cardiac contractililty and cardiac output, subsequently causing profound hypotension.[30,32,33]

(2) RVPW is affected by CVP. The measurement increases with increasing CVP. (This assumption has been validated by the published work of Pistolesi.[24,25,29])

(3) LVPW is affected by cardiac output. The measurement decreases with decreasing cardiac output. (This assumption has been validated by the studies of Vea et al. on normal subjects, patients with acute myocardial infarction, and patients with mitral stenosis.[24,25,29])

Based on the above arguments, we hypothesize that in the presence of cardiac tamponade, the RVPW increases while LVPW decreases. The following were therefore measured: (1) TVPW, (2) RVPW, (3) LVPW, (4) RVPW/ TVPW, (5) LVPW/TVPW, and (6) LVPW/RVPW. Measurements 4 and 5 are indices to correct the effect of magnification. All measurements were done to the nearest hundredth of a millimeter. All radiographs were assessed without knowledge of the patient's clinical condition.

Clinical Evaluation

In the clinical evaluation, the following parameters were reviewed in the chart: (1) nature of injury, (2) site of injury, and (3) presence of peripheral signs of decreasing cardiac output, namely, hypotension and tachycardia. The cause of the injury was classified as single stab wound, gunshot wound,

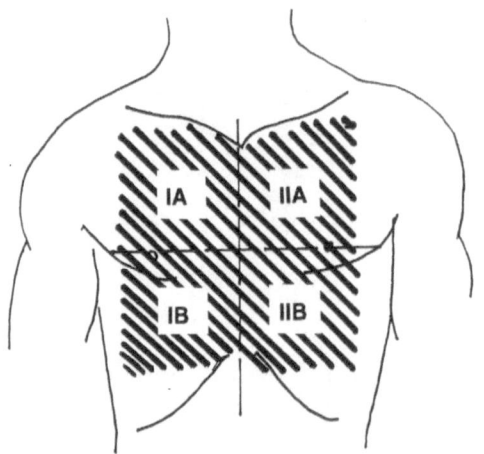

FIGURE 11.3. Penetrations in the shaded area are frequently associated with cardiac injuries. Cardiac injuries must be ruled out if mediastinal penetration has occurred.

or multiple stab wounds. The site of injury was then classified as modified from Evans and Murdock.[13] The areas of the chest that frequently affect cardiac injury are the precordium, epigastrium, and left upper chest. An imaginary line in the midsternal area divided the chest from the suprasternal notch down to the xiphoid area, and another horizontal line was made on the nipple area to the posterior axillary line. The right half of the chest was called region I and it was then subdivided on the nipple line into IA (above the nipple line, right side) and IB (below the nipple line, right side). The left side was similarly divided into IIA and IIb. Region III contained injuries incurred outside the study area (regions I and II) (Fig. 11.3)

The presence or absence of hypotension and tachycardia was recorded. The other peripheral signs known to be associated with cardiac tamponade, such as increased jugular venous pressure, pulsus paradoxicus, and Kussmaul's breathing, were not assessed because these data were not recorded in the available charts.

Statistical Evaluation

All VPW measurements were individually tested by ANOVA and covariance through stepwise linear regression to see if the two populations had significant differences in their mean values.

To assess the validity (diagnostic accuracy), of the different VPW measurements, namely, RVPW/TVPW, LVPW/TVPW, and LVPW/RVPW, in predicting the presence of cardiac tamponade, the following were computed for each measurement: (a) sensitivity, (b) specificity, (c) positive predictive value, and (d) negative predictive value.

To test if the radiographic finding of pneumothorax, pneumomediastinum, hemothorax, pulmonary contusion, or subcutaneous emphysema can separate chest trauma patients with cardiac tamponade from those without, the percentage accuracy of these parameters in population 1 and population 2 were compared using the one-way ANOVA test.

To assess if the clinical findings of hypotension, tachycardia, hypotension with tachycardia, and normal BP and pulse rate can be used to segregated patients with chest trauma with cardiac tamponade from those without tamponade, the percentage accuracy in population 1 and population 2 was compared using the one-way ANOVA test. The one-way ANOVA test was also used to test if the site and nature of injury influenced the occurrence of cardiac tamponade.

Results

There were 94 chest trauma patients included in the study, 3 females and 91 males. The youngest patient was 12 years old and the oldest was 57. The most frequent age group affected was between 20 and 30. The majority of the patients were from the vicinity of Pasay. One patient had an industrial accident in which a fan blade of a car flew off hitting his precordial area and resulting in cardiac tamponade. Thirty percent of the total study population had alcoholic breath, and the majority of the incidents occurred between 10 PM and 1 AM. The population in the study consisted of 33 patients diagnosed by operation to have cardiac tamponade and 61 patients without tamponade.

Using VPW measurements on population 1 diagnosed to have cardiac tamponade and population 2 without tamponade, each measurement was individually tested by one-way ANOVA and covariance through stepwise linear regression to see if a significant correlation existed. The results are shown in Tables 11.1 and 11.2. There is a significant positive linear correlation between the two populations in TVPW ($r = .233, t = 2.31, p = .021$) and RVPW ($r = .233, t = 2.31, p = .000$), and a negative linear correlation in LVPW ($r = .442, t = 4.75, p = .000$). The last three variables, RVPW/TVPW

TABLE 11.1. Quantitative radiographic parameter (vascular pedicle width (VPW) measurement results using analysis of variance and covariance through stepwise regression).

Variable	Pop. 1 mean (mm)	Pop. 2 mean (mm)	r	t	p	Conclusion
TVPW	52.41	49.59	.233	2.31	.021	*
RVPW	31.59	25.47	.233	2.31	.000	*
LVPW	20.85	24.11	−.442	−4.75	.000	*
RVPW/TVPW	0.60	0.51	.714	9.84	.000	***
LVPW/TVPW	0.39	0.49	−.583	−6.92	.000	***
LVPW/RVPW	0.67	0.94	−.637	−7.96	.000	***

* Significant; *** highly significant.

TABLE 11.2. Validity of vascular pedicle width (VPW) measurements as predictors of cardiac tamponade in penetrating chest injury.

VPW (mm)	Value (mm)	Sensitivity (%)	Specificity (%)	(+) Pred. value (%)	(−) Pred. value (%)
LVPW/TVPW	0.40	62%	98%	95%	82%
RVPW/TVPW	0.60	65%	98%	96%	83%
LVPW/RVPW	0.67	80%	93%	87%	89%

($r = .7144$, $t = 9.874$, $p = .000$), LVPW/TVPW ($r = .583$, $t = 6.92$, $p = .000$) and LVPW/RVPW ($r = .637$, $t = 7.96$, $p = .000$), showed the greatest correlation, as shown by the high r values and .000 probability values. To determine the diagnostic accuracy of these three variables, the sensitivity, specificity, positive predictive value, and negative predictive value were computed in each using the mean value in population 1 rounded to the nearest hundredth of a millimeter. The following criteria were used:

(1) RVPW/TVPW of 0.6 and above is considered positive for cardiac tamponade.
(2) LVPW/TVPW of 0.4 and below is considered positive for cardiac tamponade.
(3) LVPW/RVPW of 0.67 and below is considered positive for cardiac tamponade.

Of the three variables, LVPW/RVPW showed the highest sensitivity, 80%, compared to 62% and 65% for LVPW/TVPW and RVPW/TVPW, respectively. All values are highly specific (LVPW/RVPW, 93%; RVPW/TVPW and LVPW/TVPW, both 98%) meaning that they are valid radiographic indices for excluding the possibility of having cardiac tamponade in chest trauma. The positive predictive values are likewise high: 95%, 96%, and 87% for LVPW/TVPW, RVPW/TVPW, and LVPW/RVPW, respectively. Although the two variables LVPW/TVPW and RVPW/TVPW showed lower sensitivity, they had very high specificity (98%), making them a good diagnostic tool for excluding cardiac tamponade, because a negative test will be expected to be truly negative.

Table 11.3 compares the percentage occurrence of pneumothorax, hemothorax, pulmonary contusion, and subcutaneous emphysema. Hemothorax and pulmonary contusion occurred in 27% and 39%, respectively, of population 1; these values are significantly different from the 4% value shown by population 2 ($t = 3.237$, $p = .0020$; $t = 4.671$, $p = .0000$). The rest of the variables showed no significant correlation with the presence or absence of cardiac tamponade. Pneumomediastinum, which is highly indicative of cardiac injury, was not tested because of the small sample size.

Table 11.4 summarizes the clinical hemodynamic parameters. The one-way ANOVA test showed a significant difference between population 1 and

TABLE 11.3A. Qualitative radiographic parameters. Percentage occurrence in pop. 1 and pop. 2

	Pop. 1		Pop. 2	
Variables	n	(%)	n	(%)
Pneumothorax	6/33	18%	9/61	14%
Pneumomediastinum	1/33	3%	1/61	1%
Hemothorax	9/33	27%	3/61	4%
Pulmon. contusion	13/33	39%	3/61	4%
Subcut. emphysema	2/33	6%	3/61	4%

TABLE 11.3B. Radiographic parameters. Results of one-way ANOVA test.

Variables	Pop. 1	Pop. 2	t	p	Conclusion
Pneumothorax	.1818	0.1479	0.429	.6722	ns
Hemothorax	.2727	4.9800	3.237	.0020	*
Pul. contusion	.3939	4.9100	4.671	.0000	*

ns, Not significant; * significant.

population 2 in terms of the presence of hypotension and hypotension plus tachycardia ($t = 3.237$, $p = .0020$; $t = 2.238$, $p = .0259$). Tachycardia alone or normal BP showed no significant correlation with the test.

Table 11.5 compares the nature of injury in population 1 and population 2. The nature of injury does not influence the occurrence of cardiac tamponade except in cases of gunshot wounds, where there is a significant difference between population 1 and population 2 ($t = 2.833$, $p = .0058$).

The site of injury does not influence the occurrence of cardiac tamponade, as summarized in Table 11.6a&b. The one-way ANOVA test showed no significant difference in all variables. This means that the classification of chest injury adapted in the study is not a good method of determining the chance of having cardiac tamponade.

Discussion

The fundamental pathological alteration underlying cardiac tamponade in penetrating chest wounds is the accumulation of blood and clots in the pericardium causing hemodynamic instability.[13] The degree of pericardial tamponade is determined by the size of the rent in the pericardium, the rate of bleeding from the cardiac wound, and the chamber of the heart involved. With knife wounds, the pericardial laceration may be sealed rapidly by clot or adjacent fat. Consequently 80%–90% of patients with stab wounds present

TABLE 11.4A. Clinical-hemodynamic parameters. Percentage occurrence in pop. 1 and pop. 2.

Variables	Pop. 1		Pop. 2	
	n	(%)	n	(%)
Hypotension	9/12	75%	3/12	25%
Tachycardia	6/17	35%	11/17	65%
Hypotension and tachycardia	9/15	60%	6/15	40%
Normal BP, PR	15/43	35%	28/43	65%

TABLE 11.4B. Results of one-way ANOVA.

Variables	Pop. 1	Pop. 2	t	p	Conclusion
Hypotension	0.2727	0.1276	3.237	0.0020	*
Tachycardia	0.1818	0.1803	0.018	0.9340	ns
Hypotension and tachycardia	0.2727	9.8360	2.238	0.0259	*
Normal BP, PR	0.4545	0.4590	0.041	0.9188	ns

ns, Not significant; * significant.

TABLE 11.5A. Site of injury. Percentage occurrence in pop. 1 and pop. 2.

Variables	Pop. 1		Pop. 2	
	n	(%)	n	(%)
Stab wounds	24/62	38%	38/62	61%
Gunshot wounds	8/12	66%	4/12	33%
Multiple stab wounds	1/8	12%	7/8	87%

TABLE 11.5B. Result of one-way ANOVA test.

Variables	Pop. 1	Pop. 2	t	p	Conclusion
Stab wounds	0.7272	0.6229	1.014	.3144	ns
Gunshot wounds	0.2750	6.5570	2.833	.0058	*
Multiple stab wounds	3.0300	0.1147	1.400	.1612	ns

ns, Not significant; * significant.

with tamponade. On occasion, a small cardiac wound, especially of the left ventricle, seals promptly and the hemorrhage ceases with a resultant absence of signs of tamponade.[32,33]

When the pericardial laceration seals, continued rapid hemorrhage favors clotting rather than defibrination of the blood. As little as 60 to 100 mL of blood and clots in the pericardium may produce the clinical symptoms of

TABLE 11.6A. Site of injury. Percentage occurrence in pop. 1 and pop. 2.

Variables	Pop. 1		Pop. 2	
	n	(%)	n	(%)
IA	6/22	27%	16/22	73%
IB	4/11	36%	7/11	63%
IIA	5/14	35%	9/14	64%
IIB	12/30	40%	18/30	60%
IA, IIAB	3/6	50%	3/6	50%
IIA, IIB	2/6	33%	4/6	66%
IIA, III	0		1/1	

TABLE 11.6B. Results of one-way ANOVA test.

Variables	Pop. 1	Pop. 2	t	p	Conclusion
IA	0.1818	0.2626	.874	.6114	ns
IB	0.1212	0.1147	.092	.8882	ns
IIA	0.1162	0.1475	.456	.6538	ns
IIB	0.3636	0.2950	.675	.5084	ns
IA, IIAB	9.0900	4.9180	.784	.5590	ns
IIA, IIB	6.0606	6.5570	.093	.8876	ns
IIA, III	0	1.6390	.734	.5280	ns

cardiac tamponade. At this stage, however, raising the cardiac filling pressure by rapid volume infusion may overcome the tamponade and maintain cardiac output and systemic blood pressure, the stage of compensated tamponade. When the limits of distensibility of the pericardium are reached, however, accumulation of even a small amount of additional blood significantly impairs cardiac contractility and cardiac output. A sudden and profound systemic hypotension ensues. If unrelieved, the tamponade causes a progressive decrease in coronary and cerebral perfusion and the rapid demise of the patient.

In contrast to stab wounds, gunshot wounds of the pericardium and cardiac chambers often are large. The ensuing hemorrhage, in the presence of an open pericardial sac, will dominate the clinical presentation. Major associated injuries in the thorax and abdomen contribute to the blood loss and hypovolemia. Pericardial tamponade often is not present.[13]

The classic clinical description of tamponade, Beck's triad, is useful but not entirely reliable as a diagnostic criterion of tamponade, according to several studies.[13] Agitation, lack of cooperation, air hunger, cool and clammy skin, neck vein distention, Kussmaul's sign, paradoxical pulse, muffled heart sounds, and elevated central venous pressure in patients with penetrating wounds of the precordium, neck, chest, and upper abdomen strongly suggest

penetrating injury to the heart with tamponade. Although cardiac tamponade is relatively easy to diagnose with those clinical findings, it may not be so
easy in certain clinical settings. Ethanol intoxication, for example, many produce many of the signs of tamponade, particularly the neurological manifestations. Such patients should be thoroughly examined and pericardial tamponade excluded the agitation and lack of cooperation are attributed to
intoxication. In patients with hemothorax and pericardial tamponade, the
clinical picture may be attributed to intoxication. In patients with hemothorax and pericardial tamponade, the clinical picture may be attributed to
just blood loss when volume expansion markedly improves the hemodynamic parameters. In such patients, however, cardiac tamponade should be
strongly suspected and searched for, since volume expansion, which increase
the filling pressure, will result in clinical improvement of patients with hemothorax and tamponade or with tamponade alone. Neck vein distention and/
or a CVP of 12 cm saline or greater in such instances strongly suggests pericardial tamponade rather than hypotension due to blood loss. These signs
may be misleading, however, particularly when other conditions that may
produce elevation of the CVP are present.

According to Symbas et al.,[33] when signs of cardiac tamponade are present
in a patient with an external wound that might result in cardiac perforation,
pericardiocentesis should be performed at once. If nonclotting blood is
obtained, the diagnosis is established and the decompression of the pericardial
sac provides the initial effective treatment of the injury. Other diagnostic
parameters are the pericardial window with local anesthesia. Fluoroscopy,
when done, will show decreased cardiac motion and is of slight value in
diagnosing cardiac tamponade. According to several investigators, chest
radiographs have almost no value in the diagnosis of cardiac injury[13,32,33]
and should only be used to diagnose injury to other organs.

Systemic vessels are seen on chest radiographs; e.g., the superior vena cava
can be traced on the right side of the chest radiograph while the aorta and the
takeoff of the left subclavian artery can be traced on the left side. These
vessels, which form the border of the superior mediastinum, are now termed
the vascular pedicle, as proposed by Pistolesi who also developed a method
of measuring it. His studies found good positive linear correlation for his
measurement, as seen in Figure 11.2, related to the total blood volume, systemic circulation, blood volume, and mean right atrial pressure. Studies done
at the Philippine Heart Center for Asia by Vea et al. verified his findings, and
aside from the previous findings, the VPW showed good correlation with
measurement of the cardiac index in acute myocardial infarction patients,
stroke volume plus ejection fraction in mitral stenosis, and also cardiac output in normal patients.[27] The VPW measurement has therefore been validated as a measure of systemic circulation.[8,24,25,27,29] We believe this is the
first systematic attempt to use the chest radiograph in objective assessment
of cardiac tamponade in penetrating chest injury using VPW measurement.
The assumption proposed in this study has been validated. In cardiac injury,

blood accumulates in the pericardium, producing tamponade which raises the CVP and significantly impairs cardiac contractility and cardiac output; subsequently, profound hypotension ensues. The RVPW is affected by the CVP, and, as shown by Pistolesi, with increasing CVP the RVPW is widened. The LVPW, on the other hand, is affected by cardiac output such that the measurement decreases with decreasing cardiac output (CO) (Vea et al.)[36] as in a cardiac tamponade. The study therefore showed that in the presence of cardiac tamponade, the RVPW will increase and the LVPW will decrease.

The presence of hemothorax and pulmonary contusion on chest radiograph is suggestive of cardiac tamponade, but because of their low percentage occurrence (27% and 29%, respectively), they are nonreliable screening parameters in the diagnosis of cardiac tamponade, and their presence or absence will not rule out the possibility. Likewise, the clinico-hemodynamic findings of hypotension with tachycardia and hypotension alone showed good correlation with the presence of cardiac tamponade but had low percentage occurrence (75% and 60%, respectively). The site of injury based on a modification from Evans and Murdocks showed no significant relationship between the two populations. For these reasons, these variables are not recommended as screening parameters; they only become significant when they are present, but their absence does not rule out the possibility of cardiac tamponade.

Contrary to what has been claimed by several investigators about the limited usefulness of radiography in diagnosing cardiac tamponade, the study of VPW has clinical applications with traumatic cardiac tamponade and is practical, economical, and highly diagnostic.

Conclusion and Recommendations

1. The proposed VPW measurement correlates significantly with the presence or absence of cardiac tamponade in patients with penetrating chest injury. Contrary to what has been claimed earlier, the present study shows the usefulness of the chest radiograph as a simple, economical, and noninvasive diagnostic tool for the determination of cardiac tamponade.

2. The quantitative parameters (1) LVPW/TVPW, (2) RVPW/TVPW, and (3) RVPW/LVPW have been shown to be valid diagnostic tests. Using 0.67 mm as a cutoff, LVPW/RVPW values of 0.67 and below are associated with cardiac tamponade with a subsequent sensitivity of 80%, a specificity of 93%, a positive predictive value of 87%, and a negative predictive value of 89%. RVPW/TVPW value of 0.6 mm and above, on the other hand, are strongly associated with cardiac tamponade with a sensitivity of 65%, a specificity of 98%, a positive predictive value of 96%, and a negative predictive value of 83%. LVPW/TVPW values of 0.4 and below are associated with cardiac tamponade with a sensitivity of 62%, a specificity of 98%, a positive predictive value of 96%, and a negative predictive value of 82%.

3. Although the two variables LVPW/TVPW and RVPW/TVPW showed lower sensitivity, they have very high specificity (98%), making them a very good diagnostic tool for excluding cardiac tamponade, because a negative test will be expected to be truly negative.

4. The presence of hemothorax and pulmonary contusion is highly suggestive of cardiac tamponade; however, their percentage occurrence is low (27% and 29%, respectively), making them nonreliable as screening parameters. Likewise, the clinico-hemodynamic findings of hypotension with tachycardia show good correlation with the presence of cardiac tamponade but have likewise low percentage occurrence (75% and 60%, respectively). For these reasons these variables are not recommended as screening parameters: they only become significant when they are present, but their absence does not rule out the presence of cardiac tamponade.

5. Based on these findings, it is valid to assume that the quantitative radiographic parameters are superior to the qualitative radiographic and clinico-hemodynamic parameters. For this reason, a routine evaluation of the three VPW measurements is recommended for every patient with chest injury: first for assessment of the presence of tamponade, and second as a screening test to decide whether the patient needs further investigation, such as a 2-day echocardiogram or pericardiocentesis or pericardial window. This study has disproved the claim of other authors that the plain radiograph has limited usefulness in the evaluation of traumatic cardiac tamponade.

Bibliography

1. Beall AC Jr., Patrick TA, Okies JE, et al. Penetrating wounds of the heart: Changing patterns of surgical management. J Trauma 1972;12:468.
2. Beall AC, et al. Gunshot wounds of the heart: Changing patterns of surgical management. Ann Thorac Surg 1972;11:523.
3. Blalock A, Ravitch MM. A consideration of the non operative treatment of cardiac tamponade resulting from wounds of the heart. Surgery 1943;14:157.
4. Blalock A, et al. A consideration of the non operative treatment of cardiac tamponade. Surgery 1962;52:330.
5. Bland EF, Beebe GW. Missiles in the heart: A twenty years follow up report of WWII cases. N Engl J Med 1966;274:1039.
6. Decristofaro D, Liu CK. The hemodynamics of cardiac tamponade and blood volume overload in dogs. Cardiovasc Res. 1969;3:392.
7. Drilon C, Vea RG. The Vascular Pedicle Width in Mitral Stenosis. Unpublished. Philippine Heart Center for Asia Library. 1989.
8. Ebert PA. The pericardium. In: Gibbon (ed.) Surgery of the Chest. Philadelphia: WB. Saunders, 1969, pp. 552–572.
9. Eiseman, B. Prognosis of Surgical Disease. Chest Injuries. 1st ed. Philadephia: WB Saunders, 1979.
10. Elkin DC. The diagnosis and treatment of cardiac trauma. Ann Surg 1941;114: 169.

11. Evans J. et al. Principles for the management of penetrating cardiac wounds. Ann Surg 1980;191:228.
12. Fallahnejad M, Kutty ACK, Wallace H. Secondary lesions from cardiac injuries: A frequent complications Ann Surg 1980;191:228.
13. Fillmore SJ, Scheidt S, Killip T. Objective assessment of cardiac tamponade, right heart catheterization at bedside. Chest 1971;59:312.
14. Griswold RA, Maquire C. Penetrating wounds of the heart and pericardium. Ann Surg 1954;139:783.
15. Griswold RA. Cardiac wounds. Ann Surg 1970;101:683.
16. Hardy JD. *Rhoads Textbook of Surgery. Principles and Practice.* 5th ed. Philadelphia: JB Lippincott, 1977, pp. 1508–1517.
17. Hewitt RL, et al. Penetrating cardiac injuries: Current trends in management. Arch Surg 1970;101:683.
18. Lemos PC, Okumura M, Azevedo A, Cardiac wounds; Based on 121 operated cases. J Cardiovasc Surg 1976;17:1.
19. Levitsky S. New insights in cardiac trauma. Surg Clin North Am 1975;55:43.
20. Maquire CH, Griswold R. Further observations on penetrating wounds of the heart. Am J Surg 1947;74:721.
21. Milne ENC. The vascular pedicle of the heart and the veno azygous. Part I. Normal subjects. Radiology 1984;152:1.
22. Milne ENC. Correlation of physiologic findings with chest roentgenology. Radial Clin North Am 1973;11:17–47.
23. Mattox KL, et al. Logistic and technical consideration in the treatment of the wounded heart. Circulation 51&52 (suppl 1): 1975;1210.
24. Obusan J, Vea RG. Normal plain chest radiographic measurement of cardiovascular structures among normal Filipinos. Unpublished. Philippine Heart Center for Asia. 1988.
25. Oparah S, Mandal A. Penetrating stabwounds of the chest: Experience with 200 consecutive cases. J Trauma 1976;16:868.
26. Pistolessi M. The vascular pedicle of the heart and the veno azygous: Part II. Acquired diseases of the heart. Radiology 1984;152:9.
27. Shabetai R, Fowler N, Guntherof, WG. The hemodynamics of cardiac tamponade and constrictive pericarditis. Am J Cardio 1970;26:480.
28. Sugg WL, et al. Penetrating wounds of the heart. An analysis of 459 cases. J Thorac Cardiovasc Surg 1968;56:531.
29. Symbas PN. Cardiac trauma. Am Heart J 1976;92:387.
30. Symbas PN, Harlaftis, Waldo W. Penetrating cardiac wounds: A comparison of different therapeutic methods. Ann Surg 1976;183:377.
31. Szentpetery S. Changing concepts in the treatment of penetrating cardiac injuries. J Trauma 1977;17:457.
32. Trinkle J, et al. Affairs of the wounded: Penetrating cardiac wounds. J Trauma. 1979;19:467.
33. Vea RG, et al. A radiologic hemodynamic subset classification of acute myocardial infarction. Phil J Cardiol 1988;17(2):77–87.
34. Von Berg A. et al. Ten years experience with penetrating injuries of the heart. J Trauma. 1961;1:186.
35. Wilkinson A, et al. Cardiac injuries: An evaluation of the immediate and long range results of treatment. Ann Surg 1958;147:347.
36. Yao ST, et al. Penetrating wounds of the heart. Ann Surg 1968;168:67.

12
Incidence and Anatomy of the Posterior Gastric Artery and Its Surgical Importance

You-Sah Kim, Seok Kil Zeon, Wansik Yu, and Il Woo Whang

Introduction

The posterior gastric artery is a branch of the splenic artery. This artery was described by many authors under various names, including ramus gastricus,[1] arteria gastrolienalis,[2] and ascending posterior esophagogastric branch, cardioesophageal branch, or accessory left gastric artery.[3,4] Walther[5] described this artery in 1729 for the first time, and Haller[6] in 1745 named it for the first time.

Ischemic necrosis of the gastric remnant is a serious complication of high subtotal gastrectomy. Rutter[7] reported the first case of ischemia of the remaining stomach after gastric resection, and Thompson[8] in 1963 reported four cases and stated that up to that time only 12 other cases had been recorded in the world literature. Strode[9] in 1970 reported a single case of perforation of an ischemic proximal gastric remnant in approximately 1,500 gastric resections.

When performing a high gastric resection, the left gastric artery is usually ligated at its origin, and if the spleen is not removed, there should be enough blood supply to the remaining stomach through the short gastric branches of the splenic artery, the esophageal artery, and the inferior phrenic artery. If the spleen is removed, the blood supply is then dependent upon the esophageal and the phrenic arteries, and the risk of complications of ischemia increases. Operations on older patients with arteriosclerosis may further increase the incidence of these complications.

The blood supply to the remaining stomach after high subtotal gastrectomy is of some interest, especially in view of the rarity of ischemic necrosis of the gastric remnant. Damage to the posterior gastric artery may cause operative complications such as bleeding and ischemic necrosis.

The incidence, anatomy, and surgical importance of the posterior gastric artery were investigated through careful dissections during subtotal gastrectomies in patients with distal gastric cancer.

Materials and Methods

A total of 59 consecutive patients with preoperative diagnosis of operable distal gastric cancer, between March 1988 and February 1990, were included in this study. They consisted of 39 males and 20 females and their ages ranged from 30 to 72 years (Table 12.1).

During distal subtotal gastrectomy, the celiac trunk and the origin of the splenic artery were first identified, and branches of the splenic artery were carefully searched from the origin of the splenic artery to the splenic hilum. Special attention was paid to the branches running behind the posterior parietal peritoneum of the lesser omental bursa.

The number, diameter, location, course, and distributing areas of the posterior gastric artery were carefully observed and recorded. After the search had been accomplished, the gastrectomy was completed after ligation of the left gastric artery at its origin from the celiac trunk.

In order to determine the areas supplied by the posterior gastric artery, the splenic artery just distal to the origin of the posterior gastric artery was temporarily clamped with a vascular clamp, and 0.5 mL of 1% methylene blue solution was injected into the splenic artery just proximal to the posterior gastric artery.

Results

The posterior gastric artery was identified in 49 of 59 patients (83.1%). In 2 female patients, two posterior gastric arteries were found originating independently from the splenic artery; thus the total number of posterior gastric arteries identified was 51. The frequency of the posterior gastric artery identified during gastrectomies is summarized in Table 12.2.

The majority of the posterior gastric arteries originated from the middle third of the splenic artery (40); and 6 originated from the proximal third and 5 from the distal third (Table 12.3).

The size of the posterior gastric artery measured by its external diameter

TABLE 12.1. Age and sex distributions of 59 patients.

Age	Male	Female	Total
30–39	—	3	3
40–49	4	2	6
50–59	22	8	30
60–69	13	6	19
70–79	—	1	1
Total	39	20	59

TABLE 12.2. Frequency of posterior gastric arteries identified during gastrectomies.

Sex	No. of patients	No. pts with PGA	Percent
Male	39	33	84.6%
Female	20	16	80.0%
Total	59	49	83.1%

TABLE 12.3. Location of the origin of the posterior gastric artery on the splenic artery.

Location	No. identified	Percent
Proximal 1/3	6	11.8%
Middle 1/3	40	78.8%
Distal 1/3	5	9.8%
Total	51	100.0%

TABLE 12.4. External diameter of the posterior gastric artery

Size	No. of PGAs	Percent
0.5–0.9 mm	1	2.0%
1.0–1.4 mm	40	78.4%
1.5–1.9 mm	2	3.9%
2.0–2.5 mm	8	5.9%

was between 1.0 and 1.4 mm in 40 arteries and between 2.0 and 2.5 mm in 8 arteries (Table 12.4).

The posterior gastric artery usually coursed upward behind the posterior parietal peritoneum of the lesser omental bursa and reached the upper part of the posterior gastic wall. The anterior wall as well as the posterior wall of the gastric remnant were stained blue immediately after the injection of methylene blue solution, after which the bluish color gradually disappeared.

Discussion

The posterior gastric artery was recognized as early as 1729 by Walther[5] but had been ignored or neglected by surgeons and anatomists alike until its rediscovery and description by Suzuki et al.[10] in 1978. The posterior gastric artery was named in the *Nomina Anatomica* for the first time in 1980,[11] from the contributions of Suzuki et al.[10] and DiDio et al.[12]

The incidence of the posterior gastric artery has been reported in extremes of figures. Angiographic studies have reported incidences between 36.8%[13] and 46%,[12] and studies using anatomical dissections have reported incidences between 62.3%[10] and 66%.[2] The discrepancy of incidence rates between radiographic and anatomic studies was explained by DiDio et al.[12] who stated that there is a natural source of error in the interpretation of radiograms, in which the superimposition of images may influence the identification of an inconstant vessel, and failure of penetration of the contrast medium, because of pathologic obliteration of the posterior gastric artery, may also lead to a negative diagnosis from the radiograms. Our result of 83.1% is better than the reports from anatomical studies using cadavers, and the reason probably is that we identified the artery through careful dissection during gastrectomy in living patients and verified it by injecting methylene blue, staining the gastric remnants.

It is interesting that Tanigawa[2] found the posterior gastric artery in 67.8% of 121 fetuses and only 36% of 100 adult cadavers. Whether or not this artery may undergo atrophic changes in adult life will require further investigation. Most of our patients were more than 50 years old, and our results do not agree with Tanigawa's.

The location of the origin of the posterior gastric artery from the splenic artery has been described by many authors. We found that the origin was in the middle third of the splenic artery in 78.8% of patients, and this agrees with the findings of Suzuki et al.,[10] Haller,[6] and Tanigawa.[2]

According to Suzuki et al.,[10] the posterior gastric artery runs obliquely upward and toward the left, usually raising a fold of the posterior parietal peritioneum, then reaching the gastric posterior wall through the gastrophrenic ligament; it supplies the superior portion of the posterior wall of the gastric body, near the cardiac area, and the fundus. Some authors[1,14] have reported distribution limited to the posterior wall of the fundus, while others[6] have reported distribution to the superior and left portion of the stomach as well as to the area near the lesser curvature. These findings are probably based on the distribution of the terminal branches of the vessel itself to the stomach. In this study, areas of the stomach supplied by the posterior gastric artery were investigated by injecting a small amount of methylene blue solution into the splenic artery just proximal to the posterior gastric artery after the splenic artery distal to the posterior gastric artery was temporarily clamped with a vascular clamp. The posterior wall as well as the anterior wall of the remaining stomach after gastrectomy was stained blue. This suggests that blood supplied through the posterior gastric artery can fill the entire intramural arterial network of the remaining stomach. Methylene blue is sometimes used in the treatment of methemoglobinemia by intravenous injection of 1–2 mg/kg, and severe untoward reactions can occur with injection of a very large dose.[15] However, in this study, 0.5 mL of 1% solution was used per patient and no side effects were noted.

A few authors[2,16] mentioned the relationship between the posterior gastric artery and the superior polar artery supplying the superior pole of the spleen in cadaveric studies, but we could not examine this relationship due to technical limitations of surgical dissection in living patients.

The surgical importance of the posterior gastric artery comes from its high incidence, from being another source of blood supply to the stomach, and from having a deep and almost hidden origin from the splenic artery and its course in the retroperitoneum. Inadvertent transection of this vessel during gastrectomy, especially in high subtotal gastrectomy with associated splenectomy, pancreatoduodenectomy, or distal pancreatectomy, may cause serious bleeding or necrosis of the gastric remnant,[12] and special attention to this artery is also needed during the operation for reflux esophagitis.[17]

During radical gastrectomy for gastric cancer, it is essential to clear lymphatics around the celiac trunk and to divide the left gastric artery at its origin.[18] In this kind of situation, Jackson[19] even thought that the risk of ischemic necrosis of the remaining stomach was a chance surgeons might have to take, especially in patients with severe generalized arteriosclerosis; this complication can be prevented, however, if the posterior gastric artery is preserved, since this artery can supply the remaining stomach independently, as shown in this study.

Since the lymphatics around the posterior gastric artery constitute one of the primary routes draining the posterior wall of the gastric fundus,[2] complete dissection should be performed around this vessel during the operation for proximal stomach cancer.

References

1. Michels NA. The variational anatomy of the spleen and splenic artery. Am J Anat 1942;70:21.
2. Michels NA. Blood supply and anatomy of the upper abdominal organs with a descriptive atlas. London: Pitman, 1955.
3. Walther A. De arteriae coeliacae tabula. Lipsiae Titius, 1729.
4. Haller A. Tabulae arteriae coeliacae. In: Icones anatomicae partes corporis humani, fasc. II. Vandenhoeck, Gottingae, 1745.
5. Adachi B. Das Arteriensystem der Japaner. Vol 2. Universitätsverlad, Kyoto, 1928, p. 65.
6. Rutter AG. Ischemic necrosis of the stomach following subtotal gastrectomy. Lancet 1953;2:1021–1022.
7. Thompson NW. Ischemic necrosis of proximal gastric remnant following subtotal gastrectomy. Surgery 1962;54:434–440.
8. Strode JE. Perforation of an ischemic proximal gastric remnant following gastric resection. Surg Cl N Am 1970;50:301–307.
9. Suzuki K, Prates JC, DiDio LJA. Incidence and surgical importance of the posterior gastric artery. Ann Surg 1978;187:134–136.
10. DiDio LJ, Christoforidis AJ, Chandnani PC. Posterior gastric artery and its significance as seen in angiograms. Am J Surg 1980;139:333–337.

11. International Anatomical Nomenclature Committee. *Nomina Anatomica*. 5th ed. Amsterdam: Excerpta Medica Foundation, 1980.
12. Kupic EA, Marshall WH, Abrams HL. Splenic arterial patterns. Angiographic analysis and review. Invest Radiol 1967;2:70–98.
13. Tanigawa K. On the arteria gastrolienalis branching from lienal artery. Fukuoka Acta Med 1963;54:592–600.
14. Barbin JY, Guntz M. La Circulation Arterielle Viscerale. Essai de Systematisation. Bull Assoc Anat 1972;153:817.
15. Gilman AG, Goodman LS, Gilman A. *The Pharmacological Basis of Therapeutics*. 6th ed. New York: Macmillan Publishing Co, 1980, pp. 964–987.
16. Trubel W, Rokitansky A, Turkof E, Firbas W. Correlation between posterior gastric artery and superior polar artery in human anatomy. Anat Anz 1988;167:219–223.
17. Wald H, Polk HC. Anatomical variations in hiatal and upper gastric areas and their relationship to difficulties experienced in operations for reflux esophagitis. Ann Surg 1983;197:389–392.
18. Yu, W, Whang I. Surgical treatment of gastric cancer. J Korean Med Assoc 1988;31:1153–1160.
19. Jackson PP. Ischemic necrosis of the proximal gastric remnant following subtotal gastrectomy. Ann Surg 1959;150:1070–1074.

13
Coronary Artery Bypass Surgery with Right Gastroepiploic Artery

Thay-Hsiung Chen

Introduction

Ever since the first myocardial revascularization surgery by Vineberg in 1946, scientists have been seeking ideal bypass conduits that last forever with very little success. The greater saphenous vein has been routinely used for coronary artery bypass graft (CABG) operation for more than 20 years, and left internal mammary artery (LIMA) has become popularized in the last 10 to 15 years to its better long-term patency. Yet, the limitations of LIMA, such as the limited flow, the length, the location, and the difficulties in harvesting without inducing spasm, led to use of other graft conduits such as the right internal mammary artery, the inferior epigastric artery, and the right gastroepiploic artery (Rt GEAR)[1-5] in recent years.

Materials and methods

Between February 1991 and January 1992, 130 patients underwent CABG surgery in our hospital. Among them, 115 patients received the saphenous vein and/or LIMA as the graft material; the rest, 15 patients, received Rt GEAR with the LIMA and/or the saphenous vein as the graft conduit. The latter constituted the patient population of this study. The patients with Rt GEAR in CABG operations (Table 13.1) included 5 patients who had previous CABG surgery and marked wound adhesion prohibiting LIMA harvesting, 3 patients who had their LIMA jeopardized during operation, 4 patients who had received optimal arterial revascularization using Rt GEAR + LIMA, and 3 patients who had received suboptimal arterial revascularization using Rt GEAR + LIMA + SV. In all 15 patients, either Rt GEAR was utilized to achieve arterial revascularization, or the ideal conduit LIMA was not available.

All the patients were in supine position and were anesthetized with endotracheal general anesthesia. The radial arterial line, Swan-Ganz catheter, EKG monitoring, Foley catheter, etc. were routinely placed. After antiseptic

TABLE 13.1. Reasons for using right gastroepiploic artery for CABG.

Reasons	No. of patients
2nd operation (LIMA not attempted)	5
LIMA injured	3 (1 redo)
Total arterial CABG (LIMA + GEAR)	4 (1 redo)
Subtotal arterial CABG (LIMA + GEAR + GSV)	3
Total	15

CABG, Coronary artery bypass graft; GEAR, gastroepiploic artery; LIMA, left internal mammary artery; GSV, greater saphenous vein.

FIGURE 13.1. Skin incision for CABG with Rt GEAR.

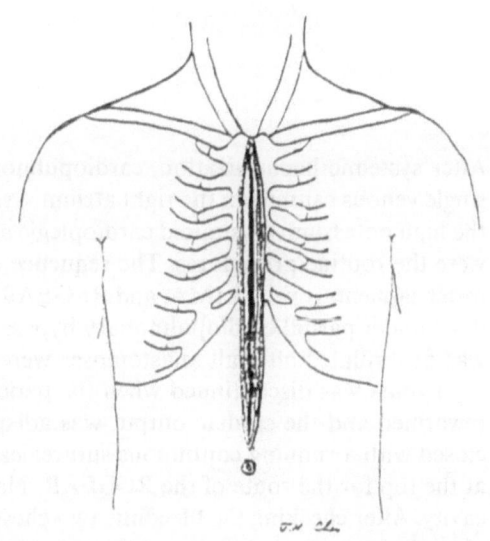

painting and draping, the greater saphenous vein was harvested starting from the groin to just above the knee level. In the meantime, a midline incision from 1 inch below the sternal notch to 1 inch above the umbilicus was performed (Fig. 13.1) The LIMA was isolated using a Favaloro sternal retractor. The peritoneal cavity was opened, the stomach and the greater omentum were identified, and the Rt GEAR was checked for its pulsation, length, and feasibility as the anticipated anastomosis. Then, by dividing its communicating branches with the greater curvature of the stomach and the greater omentum on either side, the Rt GEAR was isolated from its connection with the left GEAR to its origin from the gastroduodenal trunk in order to obtain an optimal redundancy of the vessel (Fig. 13.2). If the patient was a reoperation case, the sequence of LIMA and Rt GEAR harvesting was reversed to avoid the possibility of sternotomy bleeding, which sometimes brought about an urgent cardiopulmonary bypass, and the operation proceeded quickly.

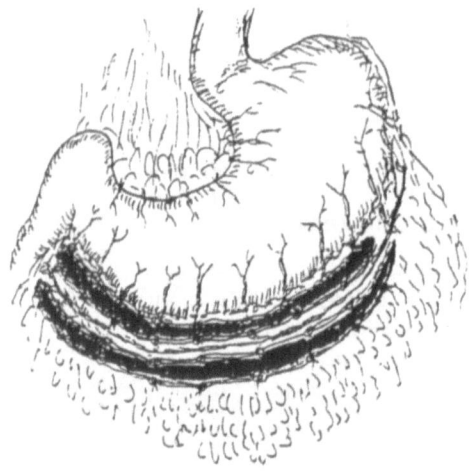

FIGURE 13.2. Rt GEAR isolated from its origin near the gastro-duodenal trunk to its communication with Lt GEAR.

After systemic heparinization, cardiopulmonary bypass was started with a single venous cannula in the right atrium. Systemic hypothermia to 25°C and the high potassium crystalloid cardioplegic arrest for myocardium protection were the routine procedures. The sequence of distal anastomosis was in the order saphenous vein, LIMA, and Rt GEAR. The proximal anastomosis was done under partial cardiopulmonary bypass with aortic de-clamp. The heart was defibrillated after all anastomoses were completed. The cardiopulmonary bypass was discontinued when the patient's body temperature was fully rewarmed and the cardiac output was adequate. The peritoneal cavity was closed with a running continuous suture, leaving a window about $3 \times 3 \, cm^2$ at the top for the route of the Rt GEAR. No drain was left in the peritoneal cavity. After checking the bleeding, two chest tubes in the pericardial and the pleural spaces were placed, and the wound was closed in the usual fashion.

After moving the patient to the intensive care unit, the postoperative measures were the same as those of other CABG operations except that the patients with Rt GEAR did not start food intake until flatus passage and a good bowel movement began, which was usually on the second or third postoperative day. The patients were transferred to general wards when their general conditions were stabilized and the drain tubes removed. They were usually discharged on the seventh or eighth postoperative day.

Results

Among the 15 patients with Rt GEAR for the CABG operation, a total of 40 coronary arteries were revascularized (Table 13.2). The Rt GEAR was connected to the left anterior descending (LAD) in 11 patients, the right coronary artery (RCA) in 3 patients, and the left circumflexartery (LCx) in 1 patient;

TABLE 13.2. CABG operations with Rt GEAR, LIMA, and saphenous vein.

Patient's name	Sex	Age (yr)	Rt GEAR to	LIMA to	Saphenous vein to	CABG No.
Huang	M	59	LCx	LAD	—	II
Leu	M	51	LAD	X	—PG—OMB—PDA	III
Lee	M	63	RCA	LAD	—	II
Hao	M	64	RCA	LAD	Intermediate	III
Tsaur	M	66	LAD	X	—RCA—OMB	III
Chen	M	67	LAD	Diagonal	—	II
Tzeng	F	61	LAD	X	LCx	II
Nieh	M	62	LAD	Diagonal	LCx	III
Kao	M	57	LAD	Injured	—PDA—OMB	III
Leu	F	55	RCA	LAD	Diagonal	III
Shieh	M	56	LAD	X	—OMB—PDA	III
Tsai	F	62	LAD	Injured	—OMB—PDA	III
Hsu	F	62	LAD	X	—PDA—OMB	III
Liang	M	57	LAD	Injured	—Diagonal—PDA	III
Chen	M	65	LAD	Diagonal	—	II
Total						40

GEAR, Gastroepiploic artery; LAD, left anterior descending; OMB, obtuse marginal branch; PDA, posterior descending artery; RCA, right coronary artery; PG, previous graft.

LIMA was connected to LAD in 4 patients and to the diagonal artery in 3 patients. The saphenous vein was used to bypass Lcx in 8 patients, the diagonal artery in 3 patients, and RCA in 7 patients. There was no perioperative hospital mortality in comparison with 2 deaths in the other 115 patients who received the CABG operation without GEAR during the same period (no significant difference by chi-square test). During the follow-up period (3 to 15 months; average 7.4 months), all 15 GEAR patients returned to their angina-free daily life. Postoperative recatheterization was done in 3 patients 2 weeks to 6 months after the operation. Eight grafts were studied, and all of them were patent.

Comments

Coronary artery disease has been the major cause of death in most developed countries. In the past 40 years, it has been dealt with by various maneuvers. In 1946 Vineberg implanted the first LIMA to the ischemic myocardium.[6] Later the saphenous vein became the popular routine bypass graft material in the 1960s. The inevitable graft failure of the saphenous vein beyond 10 years has made the LIMA a better choice of graft due to its long-term patency.[7-10] However, the LIMA has limitations,[11] such as difficulties in harvesting, length limited to a certain location of the anastomotic site, limited flow in the early postoperative period, and capability of bypassing only one vessel. Therefore, surgeons have been seeking other arterial graft substitutes such as radial artery, splenic artery, right IMA, free LIMA, free right IMA, epigastric artery, etc.[12-17] Yet, the clinical results suggest that those graft substitutes are not compatible with the performance of the LIMA, and may even not be superior to the results with the saphenous vein. In 1987 Pym et al.[3] pointed out the possibility of Rt GEAR for coronary bypass. In the same year, Suma et al.[4] also reported their clinical observation that the results with Rt GEAR were very similar to those with LIMA. In 1989, Lytle et al.[5] began the clinical application of Rt GEAR for CABG operations. In 1992, during the 41st American College of Cardiology meeting in Dallas Texas, Ishimura et al.[18] presented the midterm follow-up and the clinical results of Rt GEAR. They reported that the midterm patency of Rt GEAR was excellent, and the physiological response of Rt GEAR was very similar to that of LIMA. They further suggested that the long-term results would be equally promising. From our clinical experience with those 15 cases, we confirmed the findings of these earlier investigations. The long-term patency of the Rt GEAR, however, was not confirmed in the present studies. There remain many uncertainties. For instance, does it have postprandial or diurnal flow variation? Does the operation make future abdominal surgery complicated or even contraindicated? From our observations and those of others, we suggest that Rt GEAR is an ideal graft substitute in the case that LIMA is not sufficient or unavailable and the saphenous vein is diseased or has prominent varicosity. In the CABG reoperations, there usually are marked wound adhesions, making the isolation of LIMA and RIMA extremely difficult, and the patients commonly have diffuse diseases with distal lesions beyond the reaching range of LIMA or RIMA. Also, the saphenous vein may have already been taken for the first operation. These situations make the Rt GEAR an ideal graft of choice. Thus, our current indications are:

1. The Rt GEAR is usually utilized for CABG reoperations.
2. When the greater saphenous vein and/or the LIMA are either not suitable or unavailable, the Rt GEAR is the second-best choice.
3. If the long-term results of the Rt GEAR are proven to be compatible with LIMA, then the Rt GEAR can be used routinely in all CABG operations.

Finally, the last question is, Is the routine preoperative celiac arteriogram necessary when using Rt GEAR for coronary artery bypass surgery? According to Suma et al.,[10] the Rt GEAR was found too small to use intraoperatively in only 5% of patients. Also, celiac arteriogram can preduce iatrogenically induced spasm both in free GEAR graft, as reported by Mills and Everson,[19] and in in situ GEAR graft as reported by Suma.[20] For the above reasons, currently we do not routinely perform the preoperative celiac arteriogram. Instead, we accept the strategy proposed by Suma et al.[21] When the Rt GEAR was found too small or spastic, first vasodilators such as papaverine or nitroglycerine were tried to increase flow, and if the initial resuscitative maneuver failed, then the next option was to turn the in situ graft into the free graft. This usually can be accomplished without much difficulty.

References

1. Bailey CP, Hirose T, Aventura A. Revascularization of the ischemic posterior myocardium. Chest 1967;52:273–285.
2. Bailey CP, Hirose T, Aventura A, Yamamoto N. Revascularization of the posterior portion of the heart. Ann Thorac Surg 1966;2:791–805.
3. Pym J, Brown PM, Charrette EJP, Parker JO, West RO. Gastroepiploic-coronary anastomosis. J Thorac Cardiovsc Surg 1987;94:256–259.
4. Suma H, Fukumoto H, Takeuchi A. Coronary artery bypass grafting by utilizing in situ right gastroepiploic artery: Basic study and clinical application. Ann Thorac Surg 1987;44:394–397.
5. Lytle BW, Cosgrove DM, Ratriff NB, Loop FD. Coronary artery bypass grafting with the right gastroepiploic artery. J Thorac Cardiovasc Surg 1989;96:826–831.
6. Vineberg AM. Development of the anastomosis between coronary vessel and the transplanted internal mammary artery. Can Med J 1946;55:117–119.
7. Galbut DL, Traad EA, Dorman MH, et al. Twelve-year experience with bilateral internal mammary artery grafts. Ann Thorac Surg 1985;40:264–270.
8. Loop FD, Lytle BW, Cosgrove DM, et al. Influence of the internal mammary artery graft on the 10 year survival and other cardiac events. N Engl J Med 1986;314:1–6.
9. Spencer FC. The internal mammary artery: The ideal coronary artery bypass graft? N Engl J Med 1986;314:50–51.
10. Tector AJ, Schmachl TM, Canino VR. Expanding the use of the internal mammary artery to improve patency in the coronary artery bypass grafting. J Thorac Cardiovasc Surg 1986;91:9–16.
11. Loop FD, Lytle BW, Cosgrove DM, Golding LAR, Taylor PC, Stewart RW. Free internal mammary artery grafts. J Thorac Cardiovasc Surg 1986;92:827–831.
12. Mueller CF, Lewis CE, Edward WS. The angiographic appearance of splenic to coronary anastomosis. Radiology 1973;106:513–516.
13. Fisk RL, Brooks CH, Callaghan JC, Dvorkin J. Experience with the radial artery graft for coronary artery bypass. Ann Thorac Surg 1976;21:513.
14. Stoney WS, Alfold WC Jr, Burrus GA, Glassford DM, Petracek MR, Thomas CS. The fate of arm veins used for aorto-coronary bypass grafts. J Thorac Cardiovasc Surg 1980;30:550–557.
15. Sansford RN, Oakley GD, Talbot S. Early and late patency of expanded polytetrafluoroethylene vascular grafts in aorto-coronary bypass. J Thorac Cardiovasc Surg 1981;81:860–864.
16. Prieto I, Basilo F, Abdulncur E. Upper extremity vein graft for aorto-coronary bypas. Ann Thorac Surg 1984;37:218–221.
17. Puig LB, Neto LF, Rati M, Ramires JAF, Lui PLD, Jatene AD. A technique of anastomosis of the right internal mammary to the circumflex artery and its branches. Ann Thorac Surg 1984;38:533–534.
18. Ishimura T, Funauchi T, Umezawa T, Wakabayashi A, Suma H. Mid-term results of right gastroepiploic artery grafts: Sequential angiographic follow-up. JACC 1992;19:160A;755–766.

19. Mills NL, Everson CT. Right gastroepiploic artery: A third arterial conduit for coronary artery bypass. Ann Thorac Surg 1989;47:706–711.
20. Suma H. Spasm of the gastroepiploic artery graft. Ann Thorac Surg 1990;49: 168–169.
21. Suma H, Takeuchi A, Hirota Y. Myocardial Revascularization with combined arterial grafts utilizing the internal mammary and the gastroepiploic arteries. Ann Thorac Surg 1989;47:712–715.

14
Inferior Epigastric Artery for Coronary Bypass

Hendrick B. Barner

The recognized effectiveness of the left internal thoracic artery (ITA) with regard to enhanced survival and freedom from ischemic events when grafted to the left anterior descending coronary artery is well known.[1] This success has resulted in widespread use of this configuration for coronary bypass grafting and increasing use of the right ITA. It has not been possible to demonstrate enhanced survival when the right ITA is added to use of the left, but freedom from ischemic events has been positively influenced at 8 years in patients under the age of 60[2] and at 15 years in all treated patients.[3] These positive clinical results, combined with freedom of the ITA from atherosclerosis to 21 years after coronary grafting,[3] has resulted in the use of alternative arterial conduits in an effort to improve results achieved with saphenous vein grafts. These have included the gastroepiploic artery (GEA), the radial artery, and the inferior epigastric artery (IEA). It is this latter conduit which is the subject of this report and which was first utilized by Puig and associates in 1987 and reported in 1990.[4]

Preparation

The IEA can be harvested with a midline or paramedian incision from symphysis pubis to umbilicus. The midline approach allows harvesting of one or both IEAs using lateral retraction of the rectus muscle. The paramedian incision allows medial rectus retraction or splitting of the muscle, which provides better exposure and is our incision of choice. In 20% to 30% of patients, the IEAs bifurcate or enter the rectus muscle before reaching the level of the umbilicus so that length is thereby limited, but a bifurcation graft is occasionally useful. Mobilization begins in the middle third of the IEA and is continued proximally, including the venae comitantes and a small amount of areolar fatty tissue, to within 1 cm of the external iliac artery. Branches are controlled with small clips and the proximal IEA with medium clips or a silk ligature. Distal dissection continues until the desired length is attained, but this may be limited by branching or by the artery entering the rectus muscle, beyond which dissection is extremely difficult. The mean length of the IEA was 11.9 cm (range 8–16 cm),[5] which is significantly less than 16.5 cm for the ITA and 20–22 cm for the GEA.

The harvested IEA is placed in room temperature normal saline containing papaverine, 0.5 mg/mL. Prior to use, it is flushed with 10 mL of heparinized blood containing papaverine, 0.5 mg/mL, using a plastic needle with a 2-mm olive and without distal occlusion. Axial orientation is marked with a silk suture or methylene blue.

Usage

Because of limited length, the IEA is usually anastomosed to a site close to the aorta, such as the left anterior descending coronary, a diagonal artery, the ramus marginalis, or the first obtuse marginal artery, although most distal sites can be reached if the proximal anastomosis is made to another arterial conduit.

The distal anastomosis is accomplished with a 3–4 mm arteriotomy, spatulation of the IEA, and continuous 7–0 or 8–0 polypropylene. The associated areolar tissue may be tacked to the epicardium with a fine suture to reduce tension and prevent angulation. The proximal anastomosis is directly to the aorta using a 4-mm punch and 7–0 polypropylene or to the aortic hood of an associated saphenous vein graft using a 4–5 mm incision. If the aorta is thickened and there is no vein graft, then a patch of spahenous vein or pericardium would be placed in the aorta and the conduit attached to it as with a vein graft hood.

Results

In general, the IEA has been used in patients having multiple arterial grafts, including both ITAs and, in some instances, the GEA as well. Patients are frequently under the age of 65 with good left ventricular function,[5] but in the case of reoperative coronary bypass, there has been no age limit because of the desire to utilize arterial conduits to replace failed atherosclerotic saphenous vein grafts.[5-8]

Operative mortality has been in the acceptable range.[5-8] The incidence of perioperative complications, including reoperation for bleeding, perioperative myocardial infarction, and mediastinal wound infection, has not been increased.[5-8] Major abdominal wound infection occurred in 1/108,[6] superficial infection in 5/38,[8] and hematoma requiring surgical drainage in 4/69.[7] In 2/17 patients having bilateral ITA and IEA harvesting, there was abdominal wall necrosis including skin, subcutaneous tissue, and the rectus muscle (unilateral only) but sparing the tissue posterior to the muscle.[6] Both wounds healed after debridement and delayed skin closure without other intervention. One of these two patients had Raynaud's phenomenon.

Follow-up of patients having IEA grafting is limited. Postoperative angiography has demonstrated graft patency of 88% at 10 days[4] and 84% at 6 months,[7] which is less than that for ITA and GEA grafts.

Likewise, clinical follow-up is brief and numerically small. In 69 patients followed 1–28 months (mean = 9), there was one extracardiac death, no myocardial infarction, and no recurrence of angina with all patients free of symptoms.[7]

Discussion

At this time, the IEA is known to have a short-term patency which is not as good as that of the ITA or GEA and is more comparable to that of saphenous vein. It is not clear whether this represents a learning curve or whether patency with the IEA is inferior to that of the other arterial conduits. Abdominal wound complications have been in the acceptable range for a clean wound in the heparinized patient except when both IEAs and ITAs were utilized, with 2/17 having abdominal wall necrosis. Other complications specific to IEA harvest have not been recognized, but the potential for them exists and includes isolated rectus muscle necrosis. The ductus deferens approaches the IEA from a posteromedial position and is joined by the spermatic artery (a branch of the IEA) before entering the internal spermatic ring and could be injured. It is unlikely that dividing the external spermatic artery would cause testicular necrosis because of collateral flow. The genitofemoral nerve passes close to the IEA and could be damaged if dissection strays. A major branch of the IEA can be the anomalous obturator artery, which arises within 1.0–1.5 cm of the origin of the IEA and courses posteriorly to the obturator canal. Because this branch is large, it can be confused as the main trunk of the IEA and not a branch. The two venae comitantes of the IEA join to form a single trunk before entering the external iliac vein, where care must be taken to avoid injuring the latter. Some surgeons have advocated taking a wedge of the external iliac artery about the orifice of the IEA to facilitate the aortic anastomosis.[9] We have not practiced this approach, which would entail clamping of the iliac artery and perhaps reconstruction with a pericardial or venous patch, which would carry some risk in the unheparinized patient. The external iliac artery is frequently atherosclerotic, which may compromise its reconstruction and also the appropriateness of incorporating the diseased tissue into the aortic anastomosis, with the potential for atherosclerotic stenosis of the orifice of the IEA.

All arterial conduits have the potential problems of limited graft flow due to a small-sized conduit, disproportion between conduit size and the mass of myocardium to be supplied, the potential for conduit injury, technical anastomotic errors, and conduit spasm. The GEA and IEA develop spasm more readily than the ITA during harvesting, but this spasm resolves quickly when flow is restored. Persistent spasm is usually a result of injury, but vigorous treatment with topical papavarine, nifedipine, glyceral trinitrate, or sodium nitropusside (in order of increasing effectiveness) is indicated.[10] In my experience, the ITA is more vulnerable to injury (intimal dissection) than the GEA or IEA, which do not manifest the tendency for separation of the intima and media noted for the ITA.

Late postoperative assessment demonstrating adequacy of arterial conduit flow has been obtained for the ITA but not the IEA. These observations of the ITA include measurement of graft flow using radioactive xenon washout with isoproterenol stimulation,[11] exercise stress testing,[12] exercise thallium testing,[13] and coronary flow reserve assessed by contrast-induced vasodilation.[14] Because these conduits closely approximate one another in diameter and because intraoperative conduit flows were identical,[5] it is likely that late graft flow measurements will be similar.

Because the IEA has the least clinical follow-up and late angiographic assessment of all the arterial conduits, it must remain as the last choice among the available arterial conduits. Experience with the radial artery is also limited, but because it was used by a few groups in the mid-seventies, there is some long-term follow-up, which, therefore, places it ahead of the IEA and also the GEA with respect to long-term follow-up. Thus, indications for IEA use are related to the perceived advantage of this arterial conduit versus saphenous vein, the availability of the other arterial conduits, and the experience of the surgeon.

References

1. Loop FD, Lytle BW, Cosgrove DM, et al. Influence of the internal mammary artery graft on 10 year survival and other caridac events. N Engl J Med 1986;314: 1–6.
2. Cosgrove DM, Hill A, Lytle BW, et al. Are two internal mammary arteries better then one? J Thorac Cardiovasc Surg (in press).
3. Fiore AC, Naunheim KS, Dean P, et al. Results of internal thoracic artery grafting over 15 years: Single versus double grafts. Ann Thorac Surg 1980;49:202–209.
4. Puig LZ, Ciongolli W, Cividances GVL, et al. Inferior epigastric artery as a free graft for myocardial revascularization. J Thorac Cardiovasc Surg 1990;99:251–255.
5. Barner HB, Naunheim KS, Fiore AC, Fischer VW, Harris HH. Use of the inferior epigastric artery as a free graft for myocardial revascularization. Ann Thorac Surg 1991;52:429–437.
6. Barner HB, Naunheim KS, Peigh PS, Willman VL, Fiore AC. Inferior epigastric artery for myocardial revascularization. Eur J Cardiovasc Thorac Surg (in press).
7. Buche M, Schoevaerdts J-C, Louagie Y, et al. Use of the inferior epigastric arteries for coronary bypass. J Thorac Cardiovasc Surg 1992;103:665–670.

8. Milgalter E, Pearl JM, Laks H, et al. The inferior epigastric arteries as coronary bypass conduits. J Thorac Cardiovasc Surg 1992;103:463–465.
9. Vincent JG, Vanson JAM, Skotnicki SH. Inferior epigastric artery as a conduit in myocardial revascularization: The alternative free arterial graft. Ann Thorac Surg 1990;49:323–325.
10. Cooper GJ, Wilkinson GAL, Angelini D. Overcoming perioperative spasm of the internal mammary artery: Which is the best vasodilator? J Thorac Cardiovasc Surg 1992;104:465–468.
11. Schmidt DH, Blau F, Hellman C, Grzelak L, Johnson WD. Isoproterenol-induced flow responses in mammary and vein bypass grafts. J Thorac Cardiovasc Surg 1980;80:319–326.
12. Siegal W, Loop FD. Comparison of internal mammary artery and saphenous vein bypass grafts for myocardial revascularization: Exercise test and angiographic correlations. Circulation 1976;54 (Suppl 3): III–1–3.
13. Johnson AM, Kron IL, Watson DD, Gibson RS, Nolan SP. Evaluation of postoperative flow reserve in internal mammary artery bypass grafts. J Thorac Cardiovasc Surg 1986;92:822–826.
14. Hodgson J M, Singh AK, Drew TM, Riley RS, Williams DO. Coronary flow reserve provided by sequential internal mammary artery grafts. J Am Coll Cardiol 1986;7:32–37.

15
Significant Decrease in Mortality in Surgery for Ventricular Septal Defect with Serious Pulmonary Hypertension by Use of Vasodilators

LIU ZONG-GUI, LIU WEI-GONG, JU MING-DA, ZHANG WEI-LIAN, YAN JING-XUE, AND LIANG JI-HE

Summary

We operated on 58 cases of ventricular septal defect (VSD) with serious pulmonary hypertension (SPH) from November 1960 to July 1989. The ratio of pulmonary artery pressure to systemic artery pressure (Pp/Ps) was 0.75 or more in 56 cases and 0.65 and 0.72 in the other two, but the pulmonary vascular resistance (Rp) was 10 and 14 (Wood) in those two. The patients were divided into control and vasodilator groups. In the latter, IV and oral vasodilators were given before and after operation. The average mortality was only 7% overall, but it was 18% in the control group and only 2.4% in the vasodilator group. Therefore the use of vasodilators in surgery for VSD with SPH was effective in decreasing postsurgical mortality.

Introduction

Patients with large ventricular septal defects associated with serious pulmonary hypertension should have their defects closed as soon as possible after diagnosis. Operational mortality is high (from 20% to 54%).[2-5] Mortality in our cases was 18% before 1983 (the control group). Since 1983, we used preoperative and postoperative vasodilators and the mortality was only 2.4% in these cases.[7]

Materials and Methods

Patient Description

There were 58 patients: 36 males and 22 females, with a mean age of 12.4 ± 4.2 years. They all had severe growth failure. A bulging precordium, or so-called pigeon breast deformity, was a common finding. A systolic thrill was felt in the third to fifth intercostal spaces on the left in all but six cases.

Systolic murmurs of third to fourth degree were heard on the left. The second sound at the base of the heart was usually louder and split. Pp/Ps was 0.85 ± 0.08; Rp was 6.71 ± 3.62 and 33% of patients had Rp ≥ 8. The percentage of patients with left-to-right shunt was 63.2 ± 13.5. On ECG, 16% of the patients had left ventricular hypertrophy (LVH), 29% had right ventricular hypertrophy (RVH), and 55% had double ventricular hypertrophy (DVH). We defined Pp/Ps ≥ $0.75^{3,7}$ or Rp ≥ 10 as severe pulmonary hypertension. Pp/Ps was equal to or larger than 0.75 in 56 cases and the other 2 were 0.65 and 0.72 but the Rp in these 2 was 10 and 14 respectively.

Vasodilators Before Surgery

Since 1983 vasodilators, such as captopril, hydralazine, or dihydralazine, were given orally for 3 to 12 months before surgery. Regitine should be given IV for 1 or 2 or more weeks before surgery. Stronger vasodilators such as nitroprusside or regitine should be administered IV after surgery for 3 to 7 days or more, followed by other vasodilators given orally for several months or years, depending on the degree of pulmonary vascular disease. Our 58 patients comprised two groups, according to whether or not vasodilators were used.

Cardiopulmonary Bypass Surgery for Ventricular Septal Defect

All patients had large VSD with a mean diameter of 2.13 ± 0.56 cm. Prosthetic patches were used for all patients. The VSD was repaired by cardiopulmonary bypass with medium hypothermia and with the aorta closed by the insertion of a tube into the aorta at the base. Cold cardioplegia solution at 4°C was injected by pump within 3 to 4 minutes and then once every 20 minutes during the operation. Ice bags and cooled 0.9% sodium chloride solution, which filled the precordium and cooled the surface of the heart, were changed every 30 minutes.

Vasodilators After Surgery

After the operation, IV vasodilators were given immediately when the blood volume was sufficient for circulation; for example, regitine (1.04 ± 0.36 to 1.41 ± 0.73 g/kg/min) or nitroprusside (1.10 ± 0.51 to 1.43 ± 1.35 g/kg/min). The former drug is gentler and the latter one is stronger.

We kept the central venous pressure (CVP) at 11.0 ± 3.5 cm H_2O, the systolic pressure at 106.5 ± 10.8 to 109.4 ± 11.48 or the diastolic pressure at 176.2 ± 11.67 mm Hg. Sometimes this was maintained for 1 or more weeks. Oral vasodilators would usually be used at the third to seventh day after operation, when pulmonary pressure of Rp became lower.

The IV vasodilators should be started slowly by dripping, for example, nitroprusside from 1.104 g/kg/min to 1.429 g/kg/min or more. Increasing or decreasing the dosage was decided according to the pulmonary pressure and whether or not it was lowered. In this way, the breath sounds in the lungs became clearer, the limbs became warmer, and vessels throughout the body dilated, which could be seen in the flushed face, neck, and even trunk. The more red in the skin, the more clear the lungs, the less secretion in the lungs. Redness of the upper trunk after the use of vasodilators was an indication of whether to maintain or decrease dosage of nitroprusside, depending, of course, on whether the lungs were clear or not.

While using vasodilators, the volume of circulation must be kept balanced, because dilatation of vessels has the effect of decreasing the volume of circulation and may increase bleeding at the incision. Careful monitoring is important.

Dosages of vasodilators differ among patients, depending on differential changes in the disease of the pulmonary vessels. For example, the dosage of nitroprusside has been as high as 7.06 µg/kg/min in a 6-year-old child who had an Rp of 12 and whose VSD was 2.0 cm in diameter. We also found that the drugs were not needed several days later when patients felt better. At that time, oral vasodilators such as captopril (22.16 ± 18.72 mg/kg/day) would be given instead for several months or even for a year or more. In this way, tracheotomy has rarely been necessary in our cases since 1983.

When the patients had auriculoventricular block (AVB) II to III degree, or when the heart rate was under 60 or under 80 in children, especially with obvious enlarged heart or irregular ventricular rhythms, a pacemaker would be used or isoprenaline given IV or by mouth. We have not encountered any serious problems of this type. Vasodilators, heart drugs such as digitalis, and diuretics were used for patients who still had left-to-right shunt and those with III degree AVB after surgery. Sometimes continuous mechanical ventilation is needed for these patients for 3 to 7 days or more. This may prevent patients from reaching more dangerous stages requiring a second operation.

Results

In Table 15.1 we see the 18% mortality in the control groups and the 2.4% mortality of the vasodilator group. This difference is quite significant ($p < 0.005$). Table 15.2 shows the 47% incidence of RVH in the control group on ECG and the 15% incidence in the vasodilator group. This difference is

TABLE 15.1. Mortality.

Group	Number	Mortality
Control	17	18%
Vasodilator	41	2.4%
Results		$p < 0.005$

TABLE 15.2. ECG.

Group	Number	RVH	% (in the group)
Control	17	8	47%
Vasodilator	41	6	15%
Results			$p < 0.001$

RVH = right ventricular hypertrophy

TABLE 15.3. Other factors.

Group	Number	TCA	Pp/Ps	Rp	Shunt (%)	Age (mean)
Control	17	50.71	0.84	6.79	58.73	13.2
Vasodilator	41	50.28	0.85	6.67	65.85	12.2
Results		$p > 0.05$	$p > 0.05$	$p > 0.05$	$p > 0.05$	$p > 0.05$

TCA = time of closed aorta
Rp = pulmonary vascular resistance
Pp/Ps = pulmonary artery pressure/systemic artery pressure

TABLE 15.4. Hospital death after operation.

Name	Sex	Age	Pp/Ps	Rp	Shunt	ECG
Yang	m	6	0.83	10.9	70%	DVH
Chang	f	11	0.88	10.2	45%	RBBB
Dung	m	15	0.83	2.86	74.6%	DVH
Zai	f	9	0.75	5.29	76%	DVH

Rp = pulmonary vascular resistance
DVH = double ventricular hypertrophy
Pp/Ps = pulmonary artery pressure/systemic artery pressure

also significant ($p < 0.001$). Table 15.3 gives the figures for comparisons of other factors between the two groups. We see that there are no significant differences between the groups for Pp/Ps, Rp, time of closed aorta (TCA), age, or left-to-right shunt ($p > 0.05$ for each of these factors). Table 15.4 details the four patients who died in the hospital after surgery. Three of these (75%) had DVH and one (25%) showed RBBB on ECG. There were no deaths among the patients with RVH.

Discussion

Indications for cardiac surgery are controversial for VSD with SPH. A large ventricular septal defect could develop and progress into pulmonary vessel disease, increasing right outflow tract obstruction and aortic valve functional failure. Without surgery, bacteria-infective endocarditis, congestive heart failure, even Eisenmenger's syndrome might occur. Surgery to close the defect prevents these.[1,4] In short, before pulmonary vessel disease could lead to irreversible changes we operated on patients, for example, 1 to 2 years old.[1,4,5] If children appear with pulmonary hypertension and heart failure before age 1, pulmonary banding is necessary.[4]

Many authors think that patients having VSD with Pp/Ps $\geq$ 0.75 should have surgery as soon as possible,[3] but the mortality in surgery for VSD with SPH is high at 20% to 54%.[2-5] In our experience, overall mortality was only 7%. However, it is 18% among cases in our control group and only 2.4% in our vasodilator group. We found no significant differences between these two groups in Pp/Ps, Rp, age, TCA, or shunt ($p > 0.05$ for each). There is a significant difference between the two groups on RVH ($p < 0.001$, but this factor was not applicable to any of the four postoperative deaths, three of which (75%) had DVH and one RBBB on preoperative ECG. Therefore, the use of vasodilators in surgery for VSD with SPH is a very important factor in lowering postoperative mortality.

Pharmacology Review

Nitroprusside and hydralazine are direct-acting vasodilators. Nitroprusside is used intravenously for acute left ventricle failure and severe hypertension. Hydralazine is used for chronic heart failure and also for hypertension. Nitroprusside acts rapidly and dilates both arterioles and veins. So it decreases the return venous blood volume from dilating veins. In this way, blood volume is decreased preload along with energy consumed in the right ventricle; the ratio of ventilation and blood flow in the lungs is increased with dilatation of pulmonary vessels in the lungs, preventing right ventricular failure. On the other hand, nitroprusside dilates arterioles, so the systemic resistance is decreased which decreases the postload of the left ventricle and improves its function. The right ventricular function is improved further from the improvement on the left. This is why the lungs remain clear without accumulation of secretions and why postoperative tracheotomy is rarely necessary in the vasodilator group.

Dilatation effects on vessels can increase bleeding in the incision so it is necessary to prevent this. Patients need enough blood for circulation. We find the use of vasodilators leads to flushed face, neck, and trunk. Therefore reddened skin and clear lungs are effective signs for maintaining or decreasing dosages. However, hypotension can also limit the therapeutic effect of nitroprusside, so we watch the blood pressure to see that the systolic pressure does not go below 90 mm Hg and that the diastolic pressure does not fall below 60 mm Hg.

We increase vasodilator dosage for the patient with complicated III degree AVB or with left-to-right shunt postoperatively. We also used other therapy for low cardiac output, such as dopamine, digitalis, diuresis, pacemaker, isoproterenol, etc., which enabled the patient to pass safely through a dangerous stage.

Hydralazine acts by arteriolar dilatation and probably has a direct action which would explain why the cardiac output rises so steeply for a small drop in left-side filling pressure. We used it for a long time both before and after surgery to improve heart function and decrease pulmonary hypertension.

Phentolamine has a nonspecific vasodilator effect but it also specifically blocks presynaptic adrenoceptors. It increases cardiac output and decreases systemic vascular resistance with a lesser effect on filling pressure. We used single doses of it before and after surgery as a gentler drug than nitroprusside; we also used it in place of nitroprusside postoperatively when the patient lacked tolerance for nitroprusside.

Captopril is an angiotensin inhibitor which acts on the angiotensin-renin system at two sites: it inhibits the angiotensin converting enzyme and it inhibits angiotensin II at their respective receptor sites. Captopril is given orally in low doses and is increasingly seen as the logical therapy to counter the activation of the renin-angiotensin-aldosterone system. We found that it reduced the resistance of small pulmonary vessels. Two patients with Rp of 12 both took captopril for over 12 months preoperatively and they experienced no difficulties.

We offer the following recommendations, based on our experience with patients with VSD and SPH:

1. CVP can be maintained nearly normal at 9.44 ± 4.06 to 11.0 ± 3.5 cm H_2O and the systemic pressure at $106.0 \pm 10.8/71.83 \pm 7.28$ mm Hg. If there is no bleeding and no low cardiac output, most patients will not need medications such as dopamine or adrenaline.
2. After using vasodilators, the limbs will be warmer, urine output will increase to 52.2 ± 13.3 mL/hr, moist or dry rales in both lungs will be decreased or eliminated, respiratory sounds will be clear, and peripheral circulation will be good. When there is flushed skin on the face, head, and neck, warmed limbs, and clear lungs the effective dosage has been reached. Flushed upper trunk and approximately 60 mm Hg diastolic pressure generally indicate the most effective dose. Higher pulmonary resistance indicates higher dosage is needed. Generally speaking, the turning point for maintaining or decreasing dosage falls on the second to the fourth postoperative days; the condition of the lungs is the determining factor.
3. If low cardiac output with blood loss is recognized, restoration of sufficient blood volume is the first step necessary.
4. Vasodilators, respirator treatment, and cardiac and diuretic drugs were used with the patients. Most of them passed safely through the dangerous stages without need for tracheotomy. However, when Rp is high, postoperative dyspnea is more serious and may continue for 3 to 7 days. Only when both lungs are clear are increases in vasodilator dosage unnecessary.
5. These procedures were successfully used in patients with III degree AVB or left-to-right shunt with low cardiac output postoperatively.

References

1. Hallidie-Smith KA, Wilson RSE, Hart A, et al. Functional status of patients with large ventricle septal defect and pulmonary vascular disease 6 to 16 years after surgical closure of their defect in childhood. British Heart J 1977;39:1093–1101.
2. John S, Korule R, Jaira JP, et al. Results of surgical treatment of ventricular septal defect with pulmonary hypertension. Thorax 1983;38:279–283.
3. Cartmill TB, Dushane JW, Mcgoon DC, et al. Results of repair of ventricular septal defect. J Thorac Cardiovasc Surg 1966;52:486–499.
4. Friedli B, Kidd BSL, Mustard WT, et al. Ventricular septal defect with increased pulmonary vascular resistance. Am J Cardiol 1974;33:403–409.
5. Kirklin JW, Mcgoon DC, Dusbane JW, et al. Surgical treatment of ventricular defect. J Thorac Cardiovasc Surg 1960;40:763–765.
6. Opie LH, Harrison DC. Vasodilating drugs. In: Lionel H, Opie LH, eds. *Drugs for the Heart*. Philadelphia: Grune & Stratton; 1984:129–149.
7. Liu Z-G, Ju M-D, Zhang W-T, Liu W-Y, et al. Operational indications of congenital ventricular septal defect (V.S.D.) with serious pulmonary hypertension (S.P.H.). In: Chang JB, ed. *Modern Vascular Surgery*, Vol. 4. California: PMA Publishing; 1991:125–129.

VI
Aortoiliac Occlusive Disease

16
Early Functional Outcome After Treatment of Chronic Aortoiliac Occlusive Disease

Young Wook Kim, Thomas C. Park, Jae Seok Choi, and
Soo Il Chang

Introduction

Early results after vascular surgery are directly influenced by surgical technique.[1] Assessment of the early postoperative results is often qualitative without measuring the degree of functional improvement. In patients with chronic aortoiliac occlusive disease (AIOD) and multilevel arterial occlusion, various treatment procedure(s) can be used to treat lower extremity (LE) ischemia. By quantitatively analyzing the early functional outcomes after treatment of chronic AIOD, we compared the results among patients with different extent of disease, grades of ischemic symptoms, and treatment procedures.

Materials and Methods

From March 1989 to February 1992, 5,000 or more general surgical procedures were performed at Kyungpook National University Hospital in Taegu, Korea. During the same period, 34 patients with chronic AIOD were admitted, and 28 of them were treated. Inflow procedures included 10 aortobifemoral bypass grafts (ABF), 3 axillounifemoral, 9 femorofemoral, 2 iliofemoral crossover, and 1 iliofemoropopliteal sequential bypasses, and 3 iliac percutaneous transluminal angioplasties (PTA). Adjunctive outflow procedures performed in 25 limbs included 18 profundoplasties performed with an extended graft limb, 5 femoropopliteal bypasses, 1 popliteal artery embolectomy, and 1 femoral PTA. The patients were classified according to the extent of the disease documented by arteriograms (Brewster's classification): type I (disease localized to distal aorta and common iliac arteries), type II (suprainguinal disease), and type III (multilevel disease with associated infrainguinal occlusive disease).[2] Patients were also classified according to the severity of the ischemic symptom as follows: grade I (intermittent claudication), grade II (rest pain), and grade III (gangrene or nonhealing foot ulcer). We examined the symptomatic improvements and changes in the ankle–

brachial index (ABI) of the 39 limbs (30 days after the primary treatment), and categorized the results according to the criteria of "Suggested standards for reports dealing with lower extremity ischemia."[3] Cases of acute aortic occlusion and atheroembolism due to aortic lesions were not included in this report.

Results

There were 32 males and 2 females with ages ranging from 26 to 76 years (mean, 57.6 years). The extent of disease defined by the arteriographic findings revealed 1 patient (3%) with type I, 8 patients (23.5%) with type II, and 25 patients (73.5%) with type III. Patient populations defined by the clinical categories of chronic limb ischemia were 13 patients (38.2%) in grade I, 6 patients (17.6%) in grade II, and 15 patients (44.1%) in grade III. Associated disease in these patients included hypertension ($>150/90$ mm Hg) in 11 (32.4%), including 2 renovascular hypertension; symptomatic coronary artery disease in 6 (17.6%); diabetes mellitus in 5 (14.7%); symptomatic cerebrovascular disease in 4 (11.4%); upper extremity arterial occlusive disease in 5 (14.7%); and chronic obstructive pulmonary disease in 1 (2.9%). Early functional outcomes of 39 treated limbs were 64.1% *markedly improved*, 30.8% *moderately improved*, 2.6% *mildly improved*, and 2.6% *markedly worse*. Early outcomes categorized according to the extent of arteriographic disease, the

TABLE 16.1. Early outcomes of treatment according to the type of aortoiliac occlusive disease (39 limbs)

Type (no. of patients)	No. of limbs	Outcomes[a] (no. of limbs)						
		+3	+2	+1	0	−1	−2	−3
I (1)	1	—	1	—	—	—	—	—
II (8)	12	8	4	—	—	—	—	—
III (19)	26	17	7	1	—	—	—	1
Total (28)	39	25	12	1	0	0	0	1

[a] Outcome criteria (suggested standards for reports dealing with lower extremity ischemia in J Vasc Surg; 1986)[3]

+3 *Markedly improved*: asymptomatic with ABI increased to normal limits ($>.95$).

+2 *Moderately improved*: still symptomatic but as least single category improvement; ABI increase greater than 0.10, but not normalized.

+1 *Minimally improved*: greater than 0.10 increase in ABI, but no categorical improvement or upward categorical shift without an increase of ABI greater than 0.10.

0 *No change*: no categorical shift and less than 0.10 change in ABI.

−1 *Mildly worse*: no categorical worsening, but ABI decreased more than 0.10 or downward categorical shift with ABI decreases less than 0.10.

−2 *Moderately worse*: one category worse or unexpected minor amputation (skin intact, preoperatively).

−3 *Markedly worse*: more than one category worse or unexpected major amputation.

TABLE 16.2. Early outcomes of treatment according to the grade of the lower extremity ischemic symptom

Grade[a] (no. of patients)	No. of limbs	Outcomes (no. of limbs)						
		+3	+2	+1	0	−1	−2	−3
I (10)	12	11	1	—	—	—	—	—
II (6)	10	4	6	—	—	—	—	—
III (12)	17	10	5	1	—	—	—	1
Total (28)	39	25	12	1	0	0	0	1

[a] Grade I, Intermittent claudication; grade II, rest pain; grade III, nonhealing ulcer or gangrene.

TABLE 16.3. Early outcomes of primary treatment according to the procedures

Procedure (no. of patients)	No. of limbs	Outcomes (no. of limbs)						
		+3	+2	+1	0	−1	−2	−3
Aortobifemoral bypass								
With distal bypass (2)	4	4	—	—	—	—	—	—
Without distal bypass (8)	16	12	4	—	—	—	—	—
Extraanatomical bypass								
With femoral PTA (1)	1	1	—	—	—	—	—	—
Without distal bypass (13)	13	6	5	1*	—	—	—	1+
Ilio-fem-pop sequential (1)	1	1	—	—	—	—	—	—
Iliac PTA								
With distal bypass (1)	1	—	1	—	—	—	—	—
Without distal bypass (2)	3	1	2	—	—	—	—	—
Total (28)	39	25	12	1	0	0	0	1

[a] Untreated distal arterial occlusive disease
[b] Immediate postoperative graft thrombosis

severity of the ischemic symptom, and the treatment procedures are outlined in Tables 16.1–16.3.

Discussion

The early outcome after treatment of chronic AIOD can be measured by graft patency or symptomatic improvement. Traditionally, vascular surgeons have used graft patency as the objective parameter of surgical success. However, the patency of the reconstruction does not sufficiently reflect the symptomatic relief in the early postoperative period.[4] Disparity between graft patency and symptomatic relief can occur up to 20% for several reasons: 1) residual or overlooked significant LE arterial occlusive disease in the same leg, 2) irreversible ischemic damage in those patients who present with profound ischemia, and 3) misdiagnosis of chronic AIOD (nonvascular causes of LE symptoms).[4,5]

Since two-thirds of the patients with chronic AIOD have concomitant LE arterial disease, proper selection of treatment procedure and accurate surgical technique are equally important in treating multilevel arterial occlusive disease.[6] To determine the proper procedure, various anatomic [arteriography, computed tomography (CT), magnetic resonance imaging (MRI), duplex ultrasound] and hemodynamic (femoral artery pressure measurement with papaverine, femoral artery Doppler waveform analysis, segmental limb pressure measurement, segmental pulse volume recorder, etc.) assessments are currently available.[7-10]

Although ABF is the standard treatment for chronic AIOD, alternatives including extraanatomical bypasses, endarterectomy, and endovascular procedures have been used as inflow procedures. Reflecting a changing trend in the treatment of chronic AIOD, Davies et al.[11] recently reported increased use of PTA, decreased use of ABF, and no change in extraanatomical bypasses. In the majority of the patients with chronic AIOD, successful inflow procedure can treat LE ischemia, but 9% to 20% of them ultimately require infrainguinal bypass surgery or PTA.[12,13] The adjunctive outflow procedures are usually performed as a staged operation if necessary. However, some authors reported better functional results with the same morbidity and mortality rates after simultaneous inflow and outflow procedures than had been reported after single-level repair for the patients with type III chronic AIOD.[14]

Early functional outcomes after treatment of chronic AIOD were reported by some authors, but their outcome criteria, treatment procedures, and patient groups involved were different in each report (Table 16.4). As these functional outcome data in these reports were not standardized as recommended by the reporting standards published in the *Journal of Vascular Surgery*, it is difficult to compare the results. Brewster et al.[13] reported early functional outcomes 3 months after ABF in patients with chronic AIOD. They reported "good results" (symptomatic relief or improvement) in 74% of patients, "unsatisfactory results" (symptomatically unchanged or worse) in 26% of patients, and full relief of ischemic symptoms in only 24% of patients.[13]

Although most authors claim early patency rates more than 95%, full relief of the ischemic symptoms occur in only 24% to 69% of patients.[12,13,15] In our patients, we experienced *marked* and *moderate improvements* in 64.1% and 30.8% of limbs, respectively. There were no differences in outcome among types of patients classified by the extent of disease. However, 91.6% of the patients with claudication had *markedly improved* limbs as compared to 56% for the limb salvage group. In addition, the limbs treated with ABF and distal bypass grafting had the best functional results, 100% *markedly improved*, as compared to 46% *markedly improved* results in the limbs treated by

TABLE 16.4. Early functional outcome after treatment of chronic aortoiliac occlusive disease

Author	No.	Procedure	Functional outcome		Early patency	Operative mortality
Malone et al. (1975)[15]	342 (limbs)	ABF (100%)	Asymptomatic 38% Improved 53% No change 9%		99.2%	2.8%
Jone and Kempczinski (1981)[12]	100 (pts.)	ABF (100%)	Claud. Excellent 62% Good 24% Poor 14%	Limb salv. 76% 16% 8%	n/a	0%
Brewster et al. (1982)[13]	177 (pts.)	ABF (100%) + LS[a]	Good (74%) Cured 24% Improved 50%	Unsatisfactory (26%) Unchanged 18% Worse 8%	n/a	2.2%
Szilagyi et al. (1986)[16]	1,748 (pts.)	ABF (68%) Endarterectomy (10%) Extraanatomic (7%)	Better 87.6% Same 3.0% Worse 1.8% Amputation 2.6%		87.6–90.6%	5.0%
van den Akker et al. (1992)[4]	747 (pts.)	ABF (45.5%) Endarterectomy (30.7%)	Functional success Functional failure	Claud. 98.2% 1.8% / Limb salv. 95.1% 4.9%	99.4%	2.6%

[a] LS, Lumbar sympathectomy in 72%.

extraanatomical bypass without distal bypass grafting. Our 2 initial treatment failures (1 *minimally improved*, 1 *markedly worse*) occurred in the patients with LE arterial disease and nonhealing foot ulcer and were treated by axillounifemoral bypass without distal bypass grafting.

In summary, our functional results confirm that optimal early surgical outcomes are achieved by careful preoperative evaluation of multilevel occlusive disease and total correction of chronic AIOD in conjunction with LE occlusive disease. In our experience, ABF with outflow procedure yielded the best funtional outcome in the early postoperative period.

References

1. Johnston KW. Prevention and management of common complication of vascular surgery: An overview. In: Rutherford RB (ed.). *Vascular Surgery*. Philadelphia: WB Saunders, 1989, pp. 487–491.
2. Brewster DC, Darling RC. Aortoiliofemoral bypass grafting. In: Kempczinski RF, (ed.). *The Ischemic leg*. Chicago: Year Book, 1985, pp. 305–326.
3. Rutherford RB, Flanigan DP, Gupta SK, et al. Suggested standard for reports dealing with lower extremity ischemia. J Vasc Surg 1986;4:80–94.
4. van den Akker PJ, van Schilfgaarde R, Brand R, et al. Long term success of aortoiliac operation for arteriosclerotic obstructive disease. Surg Gynec Obst 1992;174:485–496.
5. Mozersky MJ, Sumner DS, Strandness DE. Long-term results of reconstructive aortoiliac surgery. Am J Surg 1972;123:503–509.
6. Sawchuk AP, Flanigan DP, Tober JC, et al. A rapid, accurate, noninvasive technique for diagnosing critical and subcritical stenoses in aortoiliac arteries. J Vasc Surg 1990;12;158–167.
7. Langsfeld M, Nepute J, Hershey FB, et al. The use of deep duplex scanning to predict hemodynamically significant aortoiliac stenoses. J Vasc Surg 1988;7:395–399.
8. Flanigan DP, Ryan TJ, Williams LR, et al. Aortofemoral or femoropopliteal revascularization? A prospective evaluation of the papaverine test. J Vasc Surg 1984;1:215–223.
9. Harward TRS, Bernstein EF, Fronek A. The value of power frequency spectrum analysis in the identification of aortoiliac arterial disease. J Vasc Surg 1987;5:803–813.
10. Charlesworth D. Simultaneous proximal and distal reconstruction in aortic surgery. In: Bergan JJ, Yao JST (eds.) *Aortic Surgery*. Philadelphia: WB Saunders, 1989, pp. 373–380.
11. Davies AH, Aamarakha P, Collin J, et al. Recent changes in the treatment of aortoiliac occlusive disease by the Oxford Regional Vascular Service. Br J Surg 1990;77:1129–1131.
12. Jone AF, Kempczinski RF. Aortofemoral bypass grafting: A reappraisal. Arch Surg 1981;116:301–305.
13. Brewster DC, Perier BA, Robinson JG. Aortofemoral graft for multilevel occlusive disease: Predictors of success and need for distal bypass. Arch Surg 1982;117:1593–1600.

14. Dalman RL, Taylor LM, Moneta GL, et al. Simultaneous operative repair of multilevel lower extremity occlusive disease. J Vasc Surg 1991;13:211–221.
15. Malone JM, Moore WS, Goldstone J. The natural history of bilateral aorto-femoral bypass grafts for ischemia or the lower extremities. Arch Surg 1975;110: 1300–1306.
16. Szilagyi DE, Elliot JP, Smith RE, et al. A thirty-year survey of the reconstructive surgical treatment of aortoiliac occlusive disease. J Vasc Surg 1986;3:421–436.

17
Intrapleural and Preperitoneal Route of Axillofemoral and Axilloiliac Bypass for the Treatment of Leg Ischemia or Stenotic/Obstructive Lesion of the Aorta

Nobuyuki Nakajima, Shigeyasu Takeuchi, Masahisa Masuda, Mitsuru Nakaya, and Narutsugu Adachi

Introduction

The aortofemoral bypass procedure has been the standard for the treatment of leg ischemia in a majority of patients. This procedure is the most direct method to restore the blood flow to the lower extremities. However, abdominal exploration is needed to create a bypass, and therefore there is a certain operative risk to a patient. To eliminate these operative risks, extra-anatomical bypass procedures such as axillofemoral bypass have been used to minimize the operative risk to poor-risk patients.

The conventional method of axillofemoral bypass is by the subcutaneous route, with the graft lying in subcutaneous tissue. To maintain patency of the graft, patients have to take constant care not to apply external compression over the graft, such as sleeping on the contralateral side, not wearing a belt, and so on. For these reasons, most surgenons consider the axillofemoral bypass less durable in comparison to the direct type of reconstructive procedure.

Since the externally supported ring graft was introduced, which claims a better patency rate, the inconvenience to the patient is minimized. In this report, we describe our new technique of axillofemoral or iliac bypass, including the surgical results as well as long-term follow-up.

Materials and Methods

During the period from February 1984 to August 1992, a total of 28 patients underwent axillofemoral or axilloiliac bypass by the intrapleural and preperitoneal route. The age ranged from 34 to 81 years with a mean of 62.2 ± 12.4 years; 21 patients were male, and 7 were female. The underlying disorders that prompted these procedures were severe leg ischemia due to

TABLE 17.1. Materials.

Patient no.		Age (mean)	Male/female	Follow-up (mean)
ASO	19	45–81 yr (67.8 ± 7.4)	18:1	4–96 mo (42.5 ± 28.4)
Non-ASO	9	34–70 yr (50.2 ± 12.6)	3:6	0.1–91 mo (25.6 ± 33.8)
Overall	28	34–81 yr (62.2 ± 12.4)	21:7	0.1–96 mo (37.0 ± 30.7)

atherosclerosis obliterans (ASO) in 19 patients and non-ASO in 9 (Table 17.1).

In the ASO group, the age ranged from 45 to 81 years with a mean of 67.8 ± 7.4 years. There were 18 males and 1 female. All the patients in this ASO group received axillofemoral bypass. The follow-up period ranged from 4 to 96 months with a mean of 42.5 ± 28.4 months. The underlying disorders of 9 patients in the non-ASO group were atypical coarctation of the aorta in 4 patients; interruption of the aorta in a 2 patients; and coarctation of the aorta, esophageal perforation with infected graft following graft replacement surgery at the descending aorta, and esophageal perforation of descending thoracic aortic aneurysm in one patient each. The age in this group ranged from 34 to 70 years with a mean of 50.2 ± 12.6 years. There were 3 males and 6 females. The follow-up periods in this group were 0.1 to 91 months with a mean of 25.6 ± 33.8 months. The surgical procedure employed with these patients was axilloiliac bypass by the intrapleural and preperitoneal route.

Surgical Technique (Fig. 17.1)

The details of the surgical technique of our new method of axillofemoral or axilloiliac bypass by the intrapleural and preperitoneal route are as follows. The patients lie in the supine position; preparation and draping are done as usual. Exposure and anastomosis to a graft at the axillary artery are also done using conventional technique. Following completion of proximal graft anastomosis, small skin incisions about 5 cm in length are made below the nipple and below the costal margin. Through these incisions; tunneling in intrapleural space is performed as the next step. The pleural cavities are entered through the first intercostal space from an axillary incision; at the fifth intercostal space from below the nipple incision, the diaphragm is penetrated through a subcostal skin incision and intertunnel connections are created in each segment, eventually a long tunnel is made at the anterior portion of the intrathoracic cavity. Then the graft with the already completed proximal anastomosis is brought inside the thoracic cavity, passed through the intrapleural space, and finally is brought out through a subcostal incision. Occasionally a second rib where the graft emerged into the thoracic cavity is partially or totally resected in the segment to prevent any kinking of the graft.

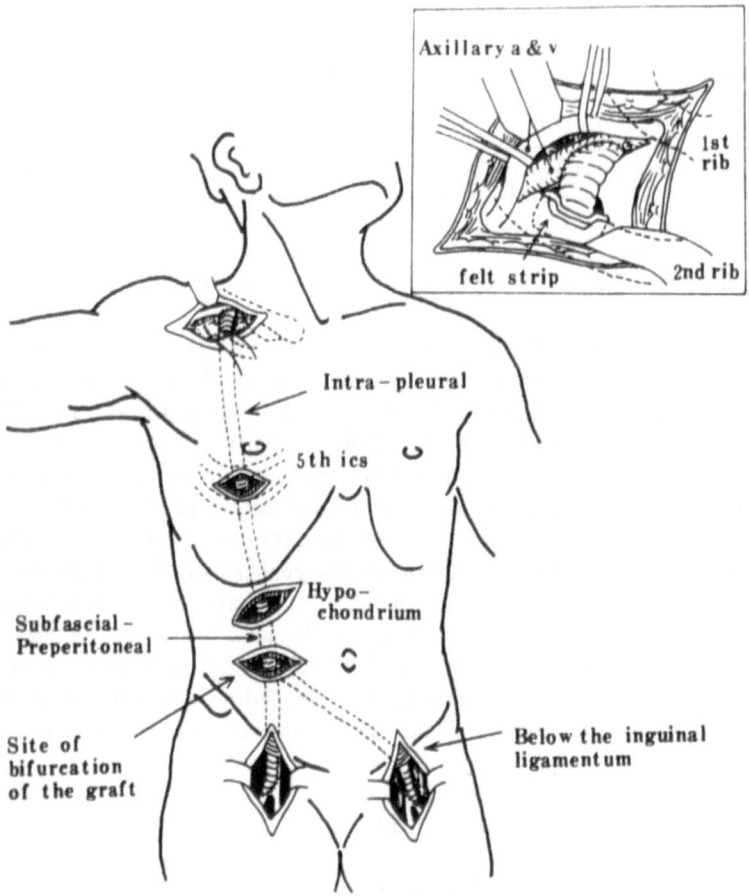

FIGURE 17.1. Schematic drawing of site of skin incisions and the route of the graft.

When axillofemoral bypass for ASO is intended, an additional skin incision is made above the inguinal ligament, a tunnel is created at the space below the muscle layer but over the peritoneum, and the graft is passed through this space between the muscle layer and the peritoneum. Finally, the femoral artery is explored and the tunnel is also created below the inguinal ligament and connected to the previously made supraligament incision. The graft is passed through, below the inguinal ligament, and the distal anastomosis to the femoral artery is done last. In the non-ASO group whose original pathology existed at the descending thoracic aorta, the distal anastomosis was created at the infrarenal abdominal aorta in some patients or at the common iliac artery in the majority. In this situation, the distal abdominal aorta and iliac artery are exposed through a retroperitoneal approach. The graft is brought from the subcostal incision to the retroperitoneal space directly, and distal anastomosis to either the distal aorta or the iliac artery is completed. The vascular prostheses used for the bypass were usually 8 mm in diameter for axillofemoral bypass and 10 to 12 mm for axilloiliac bypass.

Results

In the entire group of patients, two operative deaths and one hospital death were recorded for an overall mortality rate of 16%. Two operative deaths were attributed to postoperative acute myocardial infarction (AMI), and one hospital death was caused by sepsis. Two cases of hemothorax and one case of coronary spasm were encountered as perioperative complications. In the long-term follow-up, 9 patients died; the causes were cerebral hemorrhage in 4 and hepatic cancer, pneumonia, disseminated intravascular coagulation (DIC), traffic accident, and cause unknown in one patient each (Table 17.2). In the ASO group there were no operative or hospital deaths; however, two cases of hemothorax and one coronary spasm were experienced. Hemothorax was treated by inserting a chest drainage tube. In long-term follow-up, 6 deaths were recorded: 4 from cerebral hemorrhage, 1 from hepatic cancer, and 1 from unknown cause. As for the graft patency, only one graft occlusion was experienced. The cumulative patency rate of this procedure for ASO was 100% at 4 years and $80 \pm 8.4\%$ at 8 years (Fig. 17.2). In the non-ASO group, 2 operative deaths and 1 hospital death were encountered, which resulted in a 33% mortality rate. In long-term follow-up, 3 patients were lost (DIC, pneumonia, and traffic accident); therefore, only 3 patients survive at the moment. In the majority of patients in this group, the bypass procedures

TABLE 17.2. Results of the intrapleural and preperitoneal route of axillofemoral bypass, March 1984–August 1992

	ASO ($n = 19$)	Non-ASO ($n = 9$)	Overall
Mortality			
Early death	0	3	3
		(AMI 2, sepsis 1)	
Late death	6	3	9
	(Cerebral hemorrhage 4, liver cancer 1, unknown 1)	(DIC 1, pneumonia 1, traffic accident 1)	
Perioperative complication	3	2	5
	(Hemothorax 2, coronary spasm 1)	(AMI 2)	
Graft occlusion	1	0	1

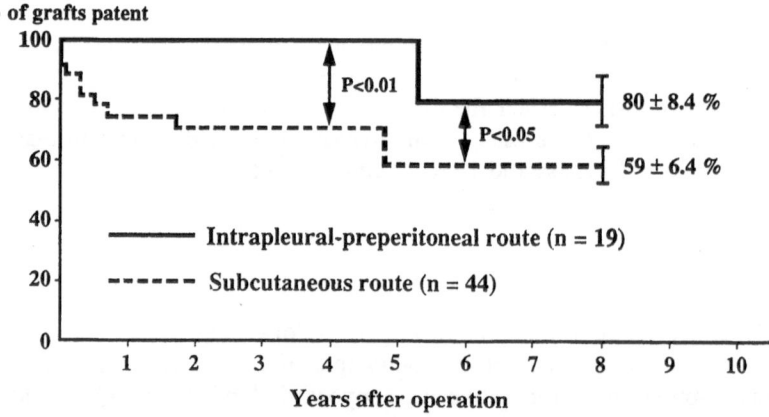

FIGURE 17.2. Patency of axillofemoral bypass for ASO.

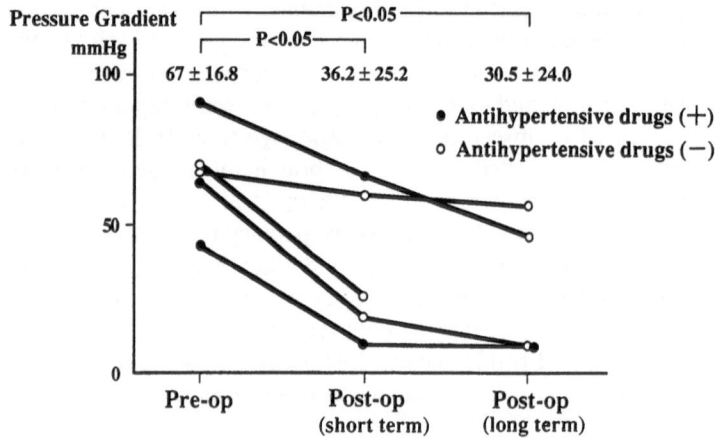

FIGURE 17.3. Pressure gradient between pre- and postoperation of axilloiliac bypass (intrapleural–preperitioneal route).

were employed in combination with other types of operative procedures, such as surgery to the descending aorta, resection of the esophagus, or valve replacement surgery. The pressure study in the long-term follow-up showed significant reduction of the pressure gradient between the upper and lower extremities ($p < 0.05$) (Fig. 17.3).

Discussion

It is important to maintain a good patency rate in bypass grafting. Although patient factors such as distal runoff, aging, and associated risk factors are influential the advantages and disadvantages of surgical procedures that affect patency have to be taken into consideration. In general, it is agreed that a subcutaneous graft is apt to be externally compressed, and that disruption of skin sutures or poor wound healing may influence graft infection. These superficial grafts also have disadvantages to a patient in daily life. For all these reasons, we believe that the subcutaneous route of bypass should be avoided when possible.

With the development of anesthetic management, operative techniques, and so on, direct reconstruction by aortofemoral bypass has become increasingly preferred over the extraanatomical bypass procedure. However, a certain number of patients need extraanatomical bypass. The purpose of this newly designed procedure is to try to eliminate the disadvantages described above, while yielding a better patency rate in long-term follow-up studies. As described in Surgical Technique, the graft lies in the thoracic cage, below the abdominal muscles layer, and when anastomosed to the femoral artery, it lies under the inguinal ligament. Therefore, the entire graft lies deep in the tissues, where it is completely protected from external compression.

The long-term follow-up study showed that ASO patients who received axillofemoral bypass by our procedure were significantly better than those who received axillofemoral bypass by our procedure were significantly better than those who received axillofemoral bypass by the conventional subcutaneous route. The former group had 100% patency at 4 years and $80 \pm 8.4\%$ patency at 8 years, compared to $71 \pm 6.3\%$ at 4 years and $59 \pm 6.4\%$ at 8 years for the subcutaneous route. Our conclusion from the present study is that the intrapleural and preperitoneal route of axillofemoral bypass was superior in regard to graft patency rate in the long-term follow-up compared to the conventional subcutaneous route. There were no complications relating to the procedure itself, and the procedure appeared to impose no disadvantage to a patient.

After we realized that this technique gave definitely better patency rates, we extended the indication to lesions requiring bypass between the upper and lower extremities (obstruction/stenosis of the descending aorta) and to certain types of emergency surgery imposed on the descending aorta. Several procedures have already been introduced to restore the blood flow in the descending aorta, such as direct reconstruction, patch-type angioplasty, graft replacement, and ascending to distal aortic bypass. All these procedures have certain advantages, and the indication for selection is probably based on the individual circumstances. The advantage of our technique of axilloiliac bypass for descending aortic pathology remains the minimum operative risk; however, the primary disadvantage of this procedure is that the bypass does not provide sufficient blood flow to maintain distal perfusion in a certain number of patients. Our study in this group of patients showed that the overall operative results were not satisfactory. The reasons were mainly attributed to the serious condition of the patients and their associated operative procedures. However, for a simple case of descending aortic lesion such as interruption or coarctation of the aorta, this procedure will be indicated. Our long-term follow-up results are not complete but appear to be acceptable.

Summary

1. A significantly higher patency rate was obtained in the long-term follow-up study for the treatment of ASO.
2. It was useful as an alternative bypass procedure for the reduction of pressure gradients caused by aortic stenosis/obstruction.
3. It will be applied in emergency circumstances to restore blood flow from the thoracic to the abdominal aorta in rare types of thoracic aortic complications

Bibliograpy

1. Schneider JR, McDaniel MD, Walsh DB, et al. Axillofemoral bypass: Outcome and hemodynamic results in high-risk patients. J Vasc Surg 1992;15:952–963.
2. Szilagyi DE, Elliott JP, Smith RF, et al. A thirty-year survey of the reconstructive surgical treatment of aortoiliac occlusive disease. J Vasc Surg 1986; 3:421–436.
3. Eugene J, Goldstone J, Moore WS. Fifteen year experience with subcutaneous bypass grafts for lower extremity ischemia. Ann Surg 1977; 186:177–183.
4. Harris EJ, Jr, Taylor LM, McConnell DB, et al. Clinical results of axillobifemoral bypass using externally supported polytetrafluoroethylene. J Vasc Surg 1990;12: 416–421.

VII
Aortic Dissection

18
Follow-up of Aortic Dissection with Thrombosed False Lumen

Nobuhiko Mukohara, Kyoichi Ogawa, Tatsuro Asada, Masami Nishiwaki, Tetsuya Higami, and Takaki Sugimoto

The prevalence of computerized tomography (CT) has revealed a high incidence and good prognosis of aortic dissection with thrombosed false lumen (ADTFL).[1,2] However, if patients have local communication (LC) between the aortic true lumen and the clotted false lumen, they may show various outcomes.[3,4] In this report, we describe the results of follow-up of those patients and discuss clinical problems and operative indications of ADTFL.

Materials and Methods

From August 1981 to April 1992, we treated 153 patients with aortic dissection, consisting of 63 Stanford type A and 90 Stanford type B cases; there were 99 males and 54 females, and the mean age was 67 years. Among them, 73 of 153 patients (48%) had ADTFL, including 17 of the 63 (27%) who had type A dissections, and 56 of the 90 (62%) who had type B dissections. Diagnosis and follow-up of ADTFL were mainly performed by CT. The typical finding of ADTFL in an enhanced CT scan was a crescentic low-density area along the aortic wall and the large opacified true lumen. As a follow-up measure, CT was performed 1 month and 3 months after the onset, and every 6 to 12 months in the follow-up period. LC between the true and false channels was depicted as "ulcerlike projection" on angiography, but on CT, it was shown as either partial opacification of the false lumen or protrusion of the true lumen (Fig. 18.1).

Results

Among the 17 type A ADTFL patients (11 males, 6 females; mean age, 66 years 14 acute phase patients; 3 chronic phase patients), 6 patients had hypertension, 7 had cardiac tamponade, 4 had pleural effusion, 2 had mediastinal bleeding, and 1 had ischemic heart disease (Table 18.1). LCs were found in 4 patients. They were located at the aortic arch in 3 patients and the ascending

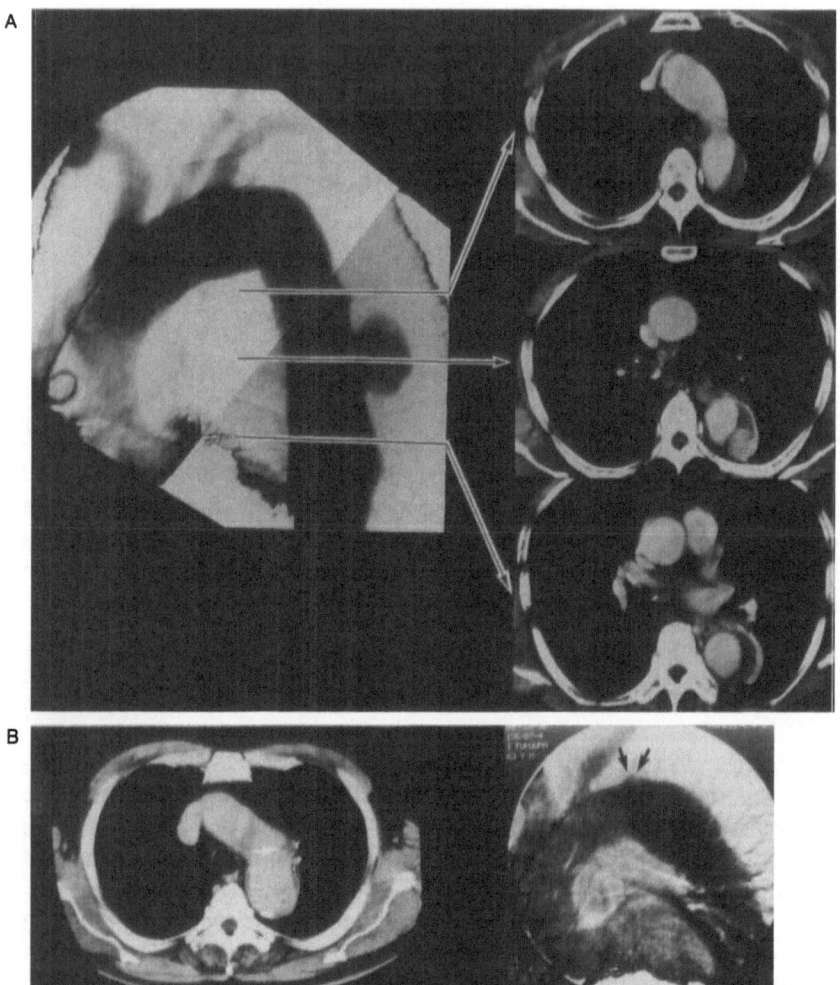

FIGURE 18.1. Findings of local communication (LC) between false and true lumen in angiography and CT. LC was depicted as "ulcerlike projection" in angiography. In CT, it was shown as either partial opacification of the false lumen (A) or protrusion of the true lumen (white arrow) (B).

aorta in 1 patient (Table 18.2). Nine patients underwent operation within 2 weeks after the onset. Indications of surgery were cardiac tamponade (6 patients), enlargement of the aorta (2 patients), and persistent pain (1 patient). Ringed intraluminal graft insertion was carried out in 6 patients; replacement of the total aortic arch, primary anastomosis, and pericardial drainage were performed in 1 patient each. Two patients died of bleeding and pons infarction (hospital mortality, 22%). Among 8 patients who were treated medically

TABLE 18.1. Profiles of patients.

	Type A ($n = 17$)	Type B ($n = 56$)
Male:female	11:6	35:21
Mean age (years)	66	66
Acute:chronic	14:3	46:10
Complications		
Hypertension	6	38
Cardiac tamponade	7	0
Pleural effusion	4	21
Mediastinal bleeding	2	1
AAA	0	11
Renal dysfunction	0	7
IHD	1	6

AAA, Abdominal aortic aneurysm; IHD, ischemic heart disease.

TABLE 18.2. Local communication between the false and true channel.

	Type A	Type B
Incidence	4/12 (33%)	18/39 (46%)
Location		
Ascending aorta	1	
Arch	3	
Descending aorta		18

in the acute phase, 1 died of cardiac tamponade. One patient showed enlargement of the LC with recurrent pain; she underwent replacement of the distal aortic arch and one coronary artery bypass grafting. On operation, 2 entries were found at the site that CT and angiography had revealed (Fig. 18.2). The patient who had been treated by pericardial drainage in the acute stage had recurrence of type A aortic dissection with patent false lumen 58 months after the initial onset. Ringed intraluminal graft insertion was carried out, but he died of renal failure.

Among the type B ADTFL patients (35 males, 21 females; mean age, 66 years; acute phase, 46; chronic phase, 10), 38 patients had hypertension, 21 had pleural effusion, 11 had abdominal aortic aneurysm, 7 had renal dysfunction, 6 had ischemic heart disease, and 1 had mediastinal bleeding (Table 18.1). Three patients underwent pleural drainage without complications. LC was detected in 18 of 39 patients who could be evaluated by CT or angiography (Table 18.2). All but one patient, who died of rupture to the left pleural cavity, recovered from the acute events. Late recurrence was seen in 2 patients: one had a relapse of ADTFL 5 years after the initial onset, another had two recurrences (26 and 82 months) (Fig. 18.3). Eleven patients without

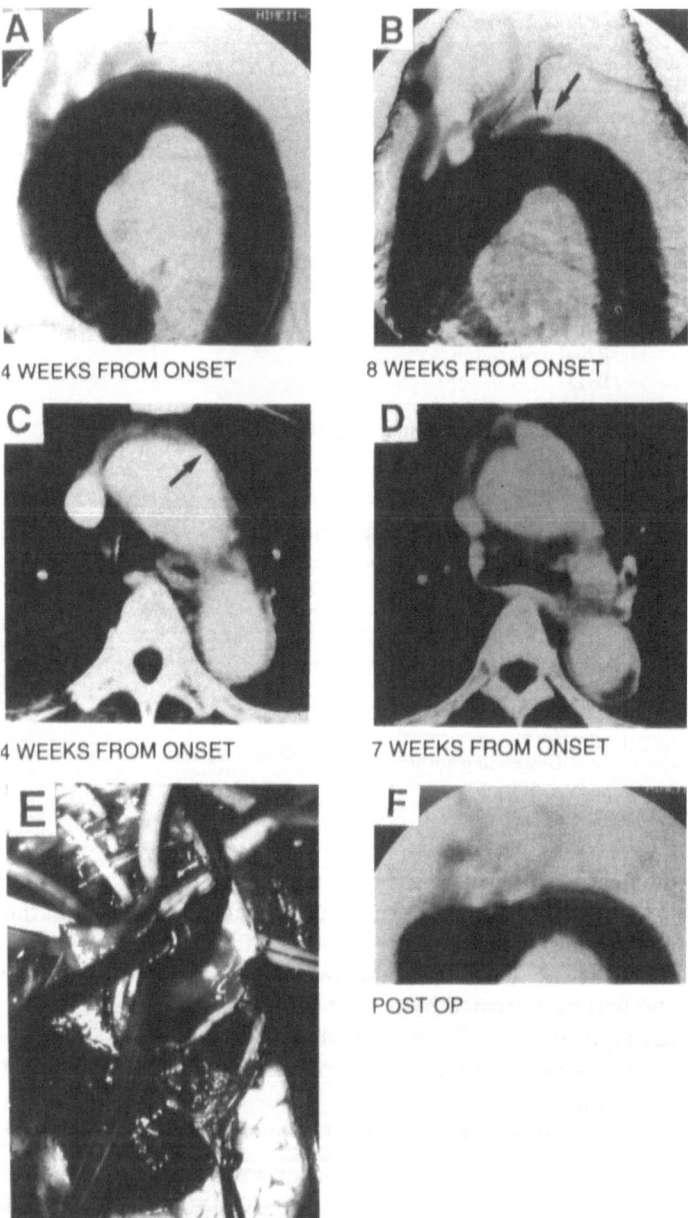

4 WEEKS FROM ONSET

8 WEEKS FROM ONSET

4 WEEKS FROM ONSET

7 WEEKS FROM ONSET

POST OP

FIGURE 18.2. A 67-year-old woman with Stanford type A ADTFL. An angiogram and an enhanced CT scan showed LC at 4 weeks after the onset (A and C) (black arrow). She had recurrent symptoms. The angiogram and CT scan revealed enlargment of LC (B, black arrows, and D). Partial replacement of the aortic arch was performed under selective cerebral perfusion (E). Postoperatively, no residual LC was found (F).

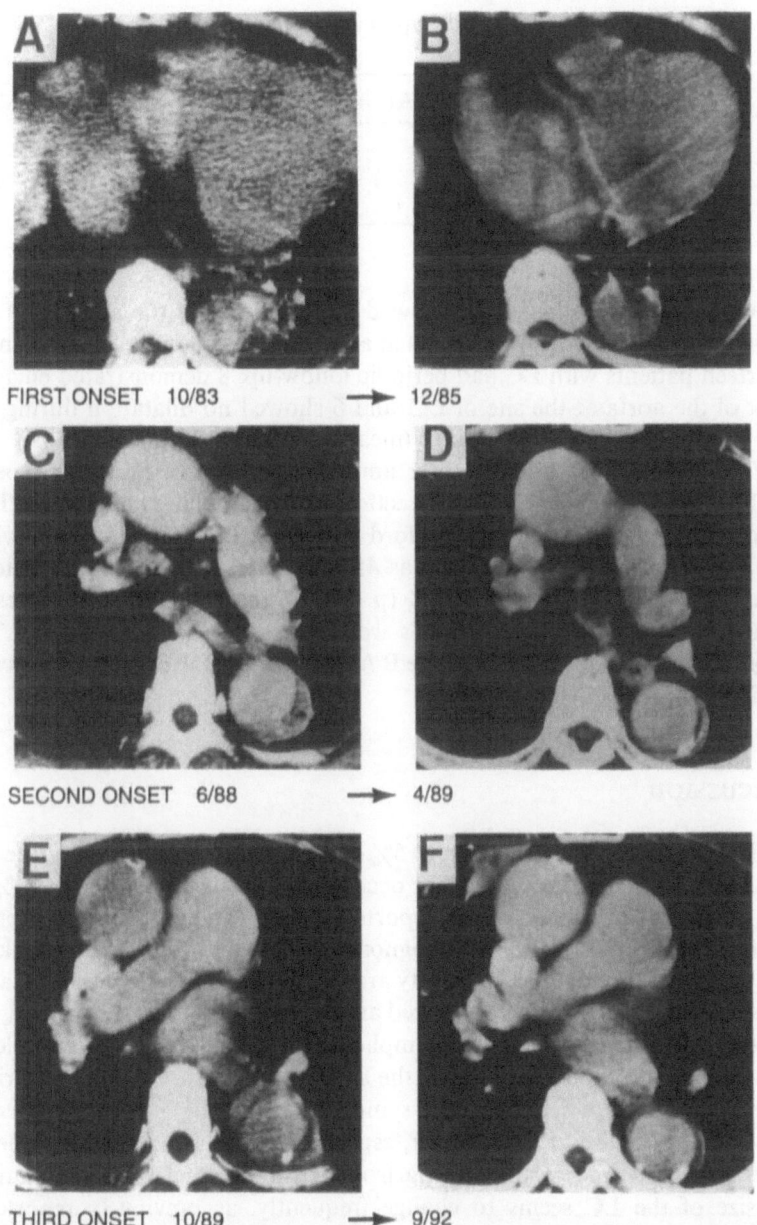

FIGURE 18.3. A 72-year-old woman had two recurrences of ADTFL. Each onset [A (initial), C (second), E (third)] and absorption of low-density area in CT after the onsets (B, D, F).

TABLE 18.3. Follow-up of aortic diameter at the
LC site

	Type A ($n = 1$)	Type B ($n = 14$)
Enlargement		8
> 5 cm		6
No change	1	6

LC who could be followed up showed no dilatation of the aorta, and the
low-density area on CT disappeared in an average 7.3 months after the onset.
Fourteen patients with LC had periodic follow-up; 8 demonstrated enlargement of the aorta at the site of LC, and 6 showed no dilatation during the
follow-up period of 2 to 78 months (mean 35) (Talbe 18.3 and Fig. 18.4).

We compared the survival rate among four groups: Stanford type A
ADTFL, Stanford type A aortic dissection with patent false lumen (ADPFL),
Stanford type B ADTFL, and Stanford type B ADPFL. The 6-year survival
rate of Stanford type A ADTFL was 45%, and the 10-year survival rate of
Stanford type B ADTFL was 88% ($p < 0.01$); the 8-year survival rates of
ADPFL of Stanford type A and B were 34% and 37%, respectively. The
difference between the Stanford type B ADTFL and ADPFL was statistically
significant ($p < 0.001$) (Fig. 18.5).

Discussion

ADTFL has been reported in 3% to 5% of autopsy cases[5,6]; however, the use
of CT has revealed a more frequent occurrence. ADTFL occurred in 20% to
30% of total aortic dissections in reported series[1,2] and in 48% of our series.
Patients without LC had good prognosis. Follow-up CT showed shrinking
and disappearance of the low-density area and normalization of the aorta. In
our series, almost all patients survived an acute event. On the other hand, the
patients with LC showed rather complicated clinical courses. The problems
in managing the patients are that 1) the LC may expand and can be the origin
of redissection with recurrence of symptoms[3,7]; 2) the aorta may present
progressive increase in its diameter, especially at the LC site, and come to
resemble a true aneurysm. Judging from the findings of CT examination,
the size of the LC seems to change frequently, as previously reported,[2]
because of repeated blood coagulation and fibrinolysis in the clotted false
lumen. Although this phenomenon in itself is not considered an operative
indication, if it accompanies relapse of symptoms, careful management is
necessary, as it may present the sign of extension of dissection or expansion
of the false channel. In follow-up, aortic dilatation was seen at the LC site
where there seemed to be a tissue defect. Tissue weakness could induce aortic
expansion against pressure.

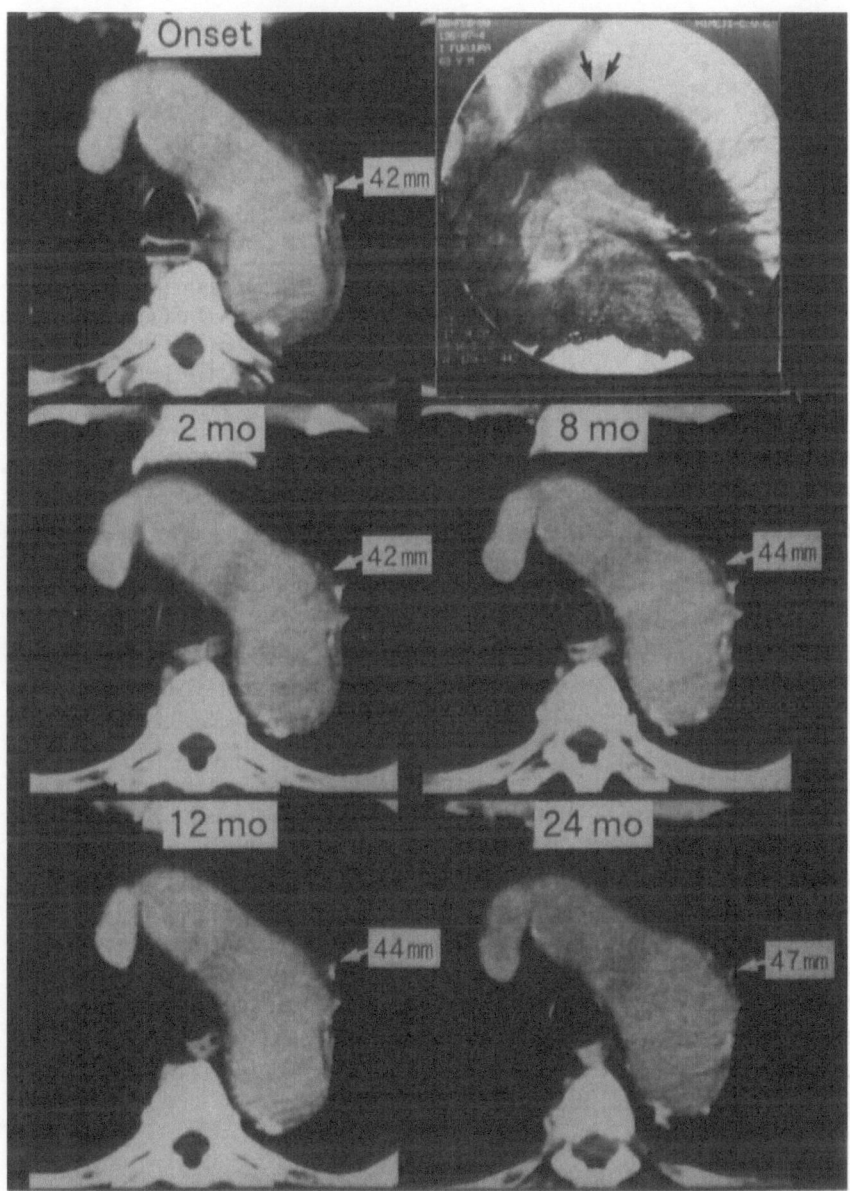

FIGURE 18.4. A 65-year-old man demonstrated enlargement of the aorta at the LC site in follow-up.

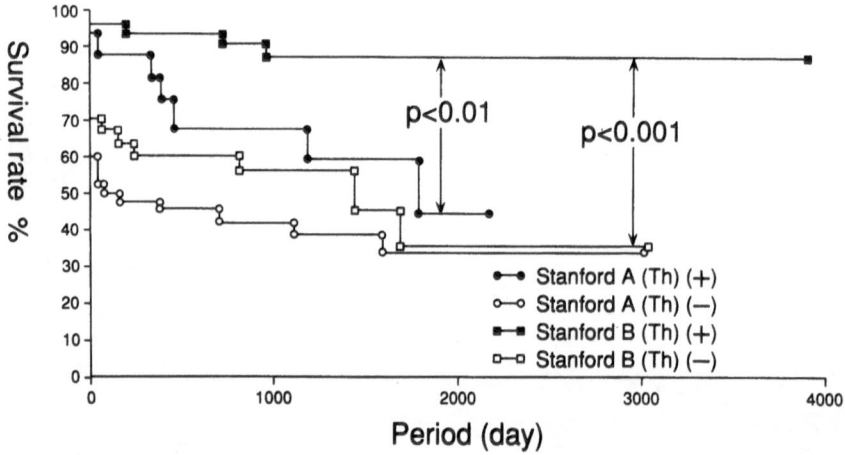

FIGURE 18.5. Survival curves comparing each type of dissection. Th(+), aortic dissection with thrombosed false lumen; Th(−), aortic dissection with patent false lumen.

Basically, acute type B ADTFL should be treated medically. Whether patients with acute type A ADTFL accompanying cardiac tamponade should be operated or not is still controversial. It is said that pericardial effusion of type A ADTFL is due not to open rupture but to extravasation.[1] As massive pleural effusion of type B ADTFL was successfully managed by drainage only in our series, cardiac tamponade might be managed in the same way. But the patients with LC in type A ADTFL should be considered candidates for emergency operation because of the reason previously mentioned. The patients with enlargement of the aorta should be operated, but not always in the acute phase.

In conclusion, 1) ADTFL occupied 48% of total aortic dissections; 2) the patients with LC should be managed and followed up carefully, because they may have recurrence of aortic dissection with patent false lumen or show enlargement of the aorta at the LC site; 3) almost all patients with acute ADTFL can be treated medically; however, surgery should be considered for those with LC in acute type A ADTFL.

References

1. Yamada T, Tada S, Harada J. Aortic dissection without intimal rupture: Diagnosis with MR imaging and CT. Radiology 1988;168:347–352.
2. Nakajima N, Matsuo H, Takamiya M, Hiramori K. "Thrombosed type aortic dissection"—Its clinical features and long term follow up results. In: Strano A, Novo S, (eds.). *Advances in Vascular Pathology 1989*. Amsterdam: Excerpta Medica, 1989, pp. 1325–1330.
3. Tisnado J, Cho S, Beachley MC, Vines FS. Ulcerlike projections: A precursor angiographic sign to thoracic aortic dissection. AJR 1980;135:719–722.

4. Sanderson CJ, Rich S, Beere PA, Anagnostopoulos CE, Levett JM, Lawrence JM. Clotted false lumen: Reappraisal of indications for medical management of acute aortic dissection. Thorax 1981;36:194–199.
5. Hirst AE, Johns VJ, Kime SW. Dissecting aneurysm of the aorta: A review of 505 cases. Medicine 1958;37:217–279.
6. Hayashi K, Meaney TF, Zelch JV, Tarar R. Aortographic analysis of aortic dissection. AJR 1974;122:769–782.
7. Dinsmore RD, Willerson JT, Buckley MJ. Dissecting aneurysm of the aorta. Aortographic features affecting prognosis. Radiology 1972;105:567–572.

VIII
Aortic Aneurysm

19
Evolution of Treatment of Aortic Aneurysms

Denton A. Cooley

The term "aneurysm" probably derives from the Greek "aneurysma," which means "to widen or dilate." The first description of an aneurysm was given by Galen in the second century: "When the arteries are enlarged, the disease is called an aneurysm.... If the aneurysm is injured, the blood gushes forth, and it is difficult to staunch it."[1] Little was known then about abdominal aneurysms; however, in 1555, Vesalius[2] first diagnosed a pulsating tumor near the vertebrae in a patient's back and called it "a dilation of the aorta." In 1670, Elsner said that "since aneurysms are rarely, if ever, found in the larger arteries, it seems strange that they could have occurred in the aorta."[3] Within another century, however, aneurysms would be reported frequently, and in 1728, Lancisi published *De Motu Cordis Et Aneurysmatibus*,[4] which includes the etiology, pathology, and case studies of abdominal aortic aneurysms. In 1847, Crisp[5] published a statistical analysis of the now recognized disease, and much thought began to be directed toward therapy and prevention of rupture. The relevant history began just two centuries ago with the intrepid direct surgical attacks made even before the era of general anesthesia by John Hunter, Astley Cooper, and others.

In 1888, Rudolph Matas[6] reported a historic case in which he successfully repaired a large, painful brachial aneurysm. In that operation, the afferent and efferent branches of the aneurysm were ligated, and the sac was opened. Each of the segmental tributaries was oversewn, thus permanently obliterating pulsation in the lesion. No attempt was made to restore continuity of the brachial artery; however, pain was relieved, and the patient's arm was saved. The name "obliterative aneurysmorrhaphy" was given to this technique. Although the technique of obliterative aneurysmorrhaphy offered advantages over the Hunterian ligature,[7] the disadvantages were apparent. An obliterative aneurysmorrhaphy could not be done satisfactorily if the artery to be sacrificed proved necessary to prevent ischemia or gangrene, nor could the technique be applied to the aorta or major arteries of the extremities without potentially serious consequences.

Subsequently, Matas described a method for internal repair of aneurysms in which continuity of blood flow was restored by creating a tunnel to the efferent branch of the brachial artery from the more normal portion of the lesion after excising the remainder. The name "restorative" or "reconstructive endoaneurysmorrhaphy" was applied to this approach. Although the technique produced more acceptable results when applied to major peripheral vessels, it was limited by the pathologic condition of the aneurysmal sac. Nevertheless, reconstructive aneurysmorrhaphy was revived 30 years ago for excisional therapy of sacciform aneurysms of the thoracic aorta and arch[8] and called tangential excision with lateral aortorrhaphy."

Tangential excision and lateral repair were satisfactory techniques for restoring circulatory continuity for sacciform lesions when less than 50% of the aortic circumference was involved by the aneurysm. Fusiform lesions, however, proved more difficult, since vascular grafts (mostly fresh or preserved homografts) were in limited supply. With the development of fabric grafts made of synthetic fibers, excision with graft replacement became standard.

The current method used to repair aortic aneurysms disregards excision of the aneurysmal wall. Instead, the aneurysm is relined with a sturdy fabric graft, generally a tightly woven, low-porosity Dacron graft. This advance in materials for vascular grafts improved the results of surgical treatment substantially.[9] By limiting the dissection, blood loss at the operating table can be reduced to a minimum.

After having tried many methods to reduce porosity in fabric grafts, we developed a method that proved to be highly satisfactory and that we used until recently. In this method, we made autologous plasma in the operating room from the patient's heparinized blood.[10] After the blood was centrifuged, the plasma was decanted and applied to the woven graft. Placing the moistened graft into the steam autoclave for 5 minutes rendered it almost impervious to interstitial bleeding. Grafts prepared in this manner could withstand not only the full heparinization of the patient's blood but also prolonged perfusion, which was sometimes necessary in patients undergoing deep hypothermic techniques. Because grafts that are already impregnated with bovine collagen or gelatin are now readily available, we no longer use the plasma-autoclave technique.

Surgical Treatment

Surgical treatment depends upon the anatomic location of the aneurysm, which may be anywhere from the aortic annulus and aortic valve to the distal thoracic aorta and the visceral vessels in the abdomen. Aneurysms may be located in the aortic root, as in annuloaortic ectasia; the ascending aorta; the transverse arch; the descending aorta; or the thoracoabdominal aorta.[11]

The type of aneurysm raises additional problems. The aneurysm may be true and of a fusiform or of a sacciform type. From a prognostic standpoint in surgical treatment, the operation may be an elective repair, or it may be an emergency repair of an acute rupture. The other major group of aortic aneurysms are dissecting aneurysms, in which there is an inframural separation in the aortic wall.

Our experience has shown that in most patients without serious associated disease, the presence of an aneurysm is an indication for surgery, since further expansion and rupture of the lesion will most likely result in death. For patients in whom aneurysmal rupture has already occurred or is definitely impending, the decision to operate should be almost unquestioned, since, without surgery, a fatal outcome is inevitable.

After the aorta is rendered bloodless by circulatory arrest during induced hypothermia or by cross-clamping, the internal reconstruction is performed. Pulsatile circulation is restored to the patient's entire body. By leaving the wall of the aneurysm intact, anatomic structures such as the lung, phrenic and vagus nerves, duodenum, and left kidney are not disturbed. The limited dissection also reduces blood loss (Fig. 19.1).

Annuloaortic Ectasia

Surgical repair of lesions resulting from annuloaortic ectasia has been performed since the development of cardiopulmonary bypass, suitable fabric grafts, and artificial valves. Annuloaortic ectasia is usually related to an aortic pathology known as Erdheim's cystic medial necrosis. Often, Erdheim's cystic medial necrosis is associated with Marfan's syndrome, but it may also appear as an isolated lesion of the forme fruste type. Bentall and DeBono's[12] original repair using a composite graft remains the standard of surgical treatment. The technique has been modified, however, especially the manner in which the coronary arteries are implanted. In addition, creating a fistula between the perigraft space and the right atrium may help to control postoperative bleeding.[13]

Ascending and Proximal Arch

In patients with lesions of the ascending aorta and proximal arch, hypothermic circulatory arrest using cardiopulmonary bypass has provided a practical solution to a critical problem. By reducing body temperature to approximately 18° to 20°C, the surgeon gains 30 to 45 minutes of relative safety while the circulation is completely arrested. During this period, the critical central nervous system tissues remain protected against ischemic damage. Special problems arise, however, when a type A acute dissection of the ascending aorta is discovered. The most practical way to diagnose an acute dissection is by transesophageal echocardiography. Because the tissues are friable, however, repair may be difficult. Recently, the use of a simple resorcinol glue[14] has made it possible to seal the layers of the aneurysm together, so that repair can be accomplished.

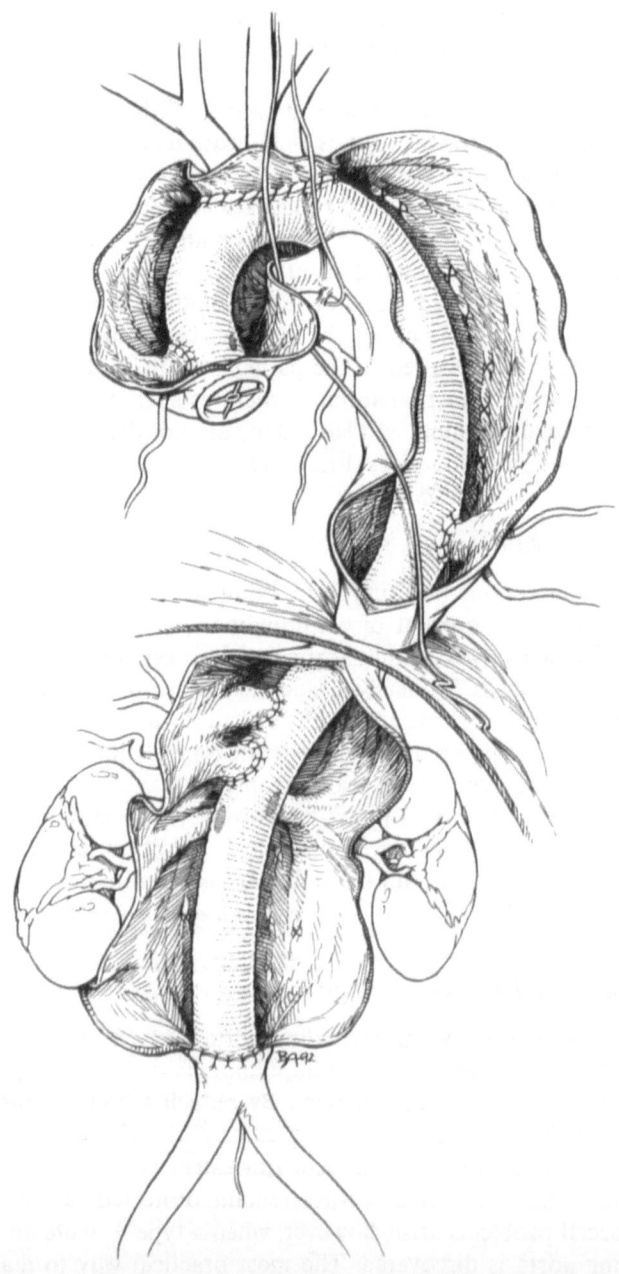

FIGURE 19.1 Repair of aortic aneurysm by reconstructive endoaneurysmorrhaphy.

Transverse Arch

The object in patients with aneurysms of the transverse arch is complete restoration of brachiocephalic circulation. This can usually be accomplished under arrested circulation by implanting the innominate, left common carotid, and left subclavian arteries as a unit. Performing an open distal anastomosis also simplifies repair of transverse arch lesions.

Descending Aorta

In patients with aneurysms of the descending aorta, the threat of paraplegia is the most common and most feared complication. The risk factors for paraplegia include location and extent of the lesion, duration of clamp time, intraoperative hypotension, elevated cerebral-spinal fluid pressure, variability of spinal cord blood supply, and others. Many preventive measures have been tried in the past, mostly to establish and maintain the distal circulation during the period of aortic cross-clamping. These methods have included shunts, pumps, pump oxygenators with femoral vein to femoral artery bypass, and others.

Recently, after extensive experience with all of these modalities, we have begun to employ a technique of exsanguination, or open distal repair.[15] In open distal repair, only a single, proximal aortic clamp is applied. The aneurysm is opened longitudinally, and the distal anastomosis is accomplished (Fig. 19.2). Blood from the distal circulation is aspirated into an autotransfusion unit and slowly replaced into the systemic circulation. During the period of open repair, we have noted that the proximal arterial pressures remain relatively normal, but central venous pressure and, more importantly, cerebral-spinal fluid pressure are reduced. The absence of neurologic complications in our patients may be related only to the brevity of the clamp time; however, the reduced cerebral-spinal fluid pressure may also be a responsible factor. We first reported a relationship between spinal fluid pressure and incidence of paraplegia following temporary aortic occlusion in 1960.[16]

Laboratory and clinical investigations are underway to ascertain the most satisfactory means of preventing paraplegia. These investigations include the use of local hypothermia, systemic calcium channel blockers, and other neuroleptic drugs. A recent report of an experimental investigation revealed that some protection from ischemia may be obtained by intrathecal injection of oxygenated Fluosol.[17]

Conclusion

Aeurysms of the thoracic aorta have long challenged the cardiovascular surgeon. Only during the past several decades has any effective treatment been developed. New techniques, such as hypothermic circulatory arrest with

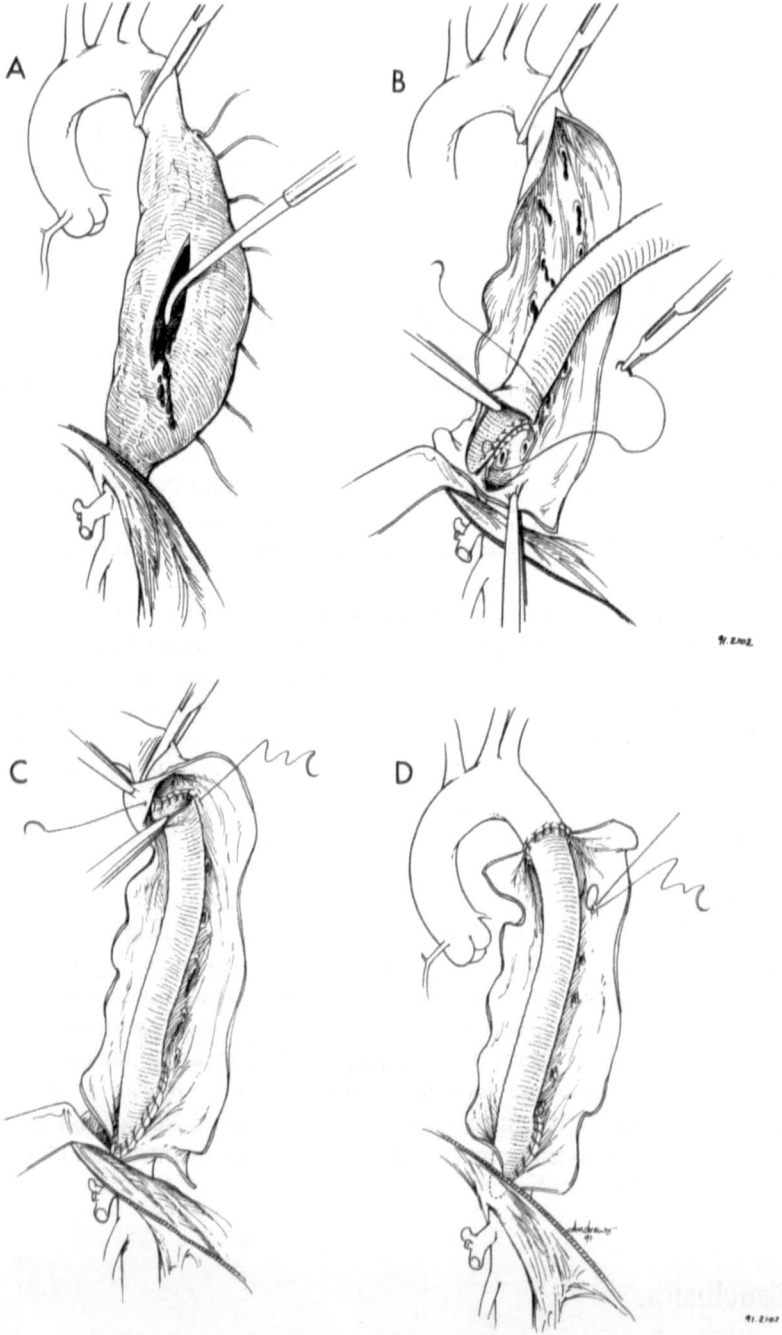

FIGURE 19.2. Open repair of descending thoracic aneurysm. Continuous aspiration of blood to the autotransfusion reservoir maintains a clear operative field. Reprinted with permission from the *Annals of Thoracic Surgery* 1992;54(5):932–936.

open aortic anastomosis and pretreatment of grafts with autologous plasma and autoclaving to prevent interstitial bleeding, have attained a degree of success for thoracic surgeons not possible before. As these techniques are increasingly applied, mortality should decrease significantly.

References

1. Galen J. *Observations on Aneurysm*, translated by JE Erichsen. London: Syndenham Society, 1944, p. 3.
2. *De Aneurysmatibus*, revised and edited by WC Wright. New York: MacMillan, 1952, p. 3.
3. *De Aneurysmatibus*, revised and edited by WC Wright. New York: MacMillan, 1952, p. 333.
4. Lancisi GM: *De Aneurysmatibus*, revised and edited by WC Wright. New York: MacMillan, 1952, p. 24.
5. Crisp E. *Structure, Diseases, and Injuries of Blood Vessels*. London: J Churchill, 1847.
6. Matas R. Traumatic aneurysm of the left brachial artery. Med News 1888;53:462.
7. Hunter J. *Ashhurst Encyclopedia of Surgery*. Vol III, p. 434. Power, Sir D'Arcy. Br J Surg 1929;17:196.
8. Cooley DA, DeBakey ME. Surgical considerations of intrathoracic aneurysms of the aorta and great vessels. Ann Surg 1952;135:660.
9. Cooley DA, Wukasch DC, Bennett JG, Trono R. Double velour knitted Dacron grafts for aortoiliac vascular replacements. In: Sawyer PN, Kaplitt MJ (eds.). *Vascular Grafts*. New York: Appleton-Century-Crofts, 1978, pp. 197–207.
10. Cooley DA, Romagnoli A, Milam JD, Bossart MI. A method of preparing woven Dacron grafts to prevent interstitial hemorrhage. Cardiovascular Diseases Bulletin of the Texas Heart Institute 1981;8:48.
11. Cooley DA. *Surgical Treatment of Aortic Aneurysms*. Philadelphia: WB Saunders, 1986.
12. Bentall H, DeBono A. A technique for complete replacement of the ascending aorta. Thorax 1968;23:338.
13. Lewis CTP, Cooley DA, Murphy MC, Talledo O, Vega D. Surgical repair of aortic root aneurysms in 280 patients. Ann Thorac Surg 1992;53:38.
14. Carpentier A. "Glue aortoplasty" as an alternative to resection and grafting for the treatment of aortic dissection. Semin Thorac Cardiovasc Surg 1991;3:213.
15. Cooley DA, Baldwin RT. Techniques of open distal anastomoses for repair of descending thoracic aortic aneurysms. Ann Thorac Surg 1992;54(5):932–936.
16. Blaisdell FW, Cooley DA. Relationship of spinal fluid pressure and incidence of paraplegia following temporary aortic occlusion: An experimental study. Surg Forum 1960;11:153.
17. Maughan RE, Mohan C, Nathan IM, et al. Intrathecal perfusion of an oxygenated perfluorocarbon emulsion prevents paraplegia after extended normothermic aortic cross-clamping. Abstracts, Society of Thoracic Surgeons 28th Annual Meeting, 1991, p. 104.

20
Abdominal Aortic Aneurysm with Perianeurysmal Fibrosis: An Analysis of 27 Cases in 1,004 AAAs Treated in a Single Vascular Center

MIKAEL BITSCH, JØRGEN E. LORENTZEN, AND TORBEN V. SCHROEDER

Summary

During the twenty-two-year period 1969–1990, 1,004 patients with abdominal aortic aneurysms (AAA) were admitted to the vascular service at Rigshospitalet. In 27 patients (2.7%), the AAA was associated with perianeurysmal fibrosis (PF). The diagnosis was based on preoperative computed tomographic (CT) scan and on macro- and microscopic evaluation. The age and sex distribution of patients with AAA associated with PF did not differ from that of patients with AAA. The male:female ratio was 4:1; the median age was 65 for males and 67 for females. Ureteral obstruction was present in 17 (63%) patients, of whom 5 had bilateral obstruction, all presenting with progressive uremia as the symptom that eventually led to the diagnosis of AAA and PF. None of the patients had overt rupture, but 3 had signs of threatened rupture.

Surgery involved duodenal release and, in 14 instances, ureterolysis. One patient died on the 27th postoperative day due to cardiopulmonary failure, giving a perioperative mortality of 4%. Within this period, renal function was normalized in all cases except in one of the uremic patients. This patient developed progressive renal insufficiency and uncontrollable hypertension, eventually leading to his death 5 years postoperatively. During follow-up, another 6 patients died after a median of 5 years (range 1 to 17 years) of cancer and ischemic heart disease. The cumulative 5- and 10-year survival rates of 82% and 62%, respectively, were not significantly different from that of an age- and sex-matched Danish population. During follow-up, no signs of progression of fibrosis were found, as assessed by renal function. Additionally, postoperative CT scans performed in three instances documented disappearance of PF in all cases.

Introduction

The combined finding of an abdominal aortic aneurysm (AAA) and retroperitoneal fibrosis is more frequent than can be explained by coincidence. It has been suggested that the disease has a background in an allergic reaction,

194

although no definite proof exists.[1-4] Insoluble lipid leaking through a thinned arterial wall from atheromatous plaques is believed to induce an autoimmune response with secondary formation of fibrosis.

Since 1970 the Department of Vascular Surgery, Rigshospitalet, has focused on the combined phenomenon,[5] known as perianeurysmal fibrosis (PF). This survey reports our experience during the period 1969–1990.

Patients and Methods

The present sample comprised all 1,004 patients admitted with AAA during the 22-year period 1969–1990. Rigshospitalet is the primary hospital for approximately 1 million people and the secondary referral center for another 1.5 million in Denmark.

Results

PF was found in 27 (2.7%–95% confidence limits: 1.8–3.9%) patients, of whom 5 have previously been reported.[5] The incidence did not change from the first to the last period under observation (Table 20.1). The age and sex distribution of patients with PF was similar to that of patients without PF (Table 20.2).

Preoperative CT was performed in all 13 patients in the 1987–1990 sample and in 6 of 14 patients representing the 1969–1986 sample. A preoperative diagnosis of PF was made in 18 of the 19 patients who had a preoperative computed tomographic (CT) scan (Fig. 20.1). In the remaining 9 cases the

TABLE 20.1. Abdominal aortic aneurysm (AAA) with perianeurysmal fibrosis (PF). A survey of the period 1969–1990 in a Danish University Hospital.

Period	AAA	AAA + PF	Incidence (95% confidence limits)
1969–1986	539	14	2.6%
1987–1990	465	13	2.8%
1969–1990	1,004	27	2.7% (1.8%–3.9%)

TABLE 20.2. Distribution of patients with abdominal aortic aneurysm (AAA) and perianeurysmal fibrosis (PF) according to sex and age.

	No.	Men/women	Median age (years)	Range (years)
AAA	1,004	838:166	67	38–90
AAA + PF	27	22:5	65	47–76

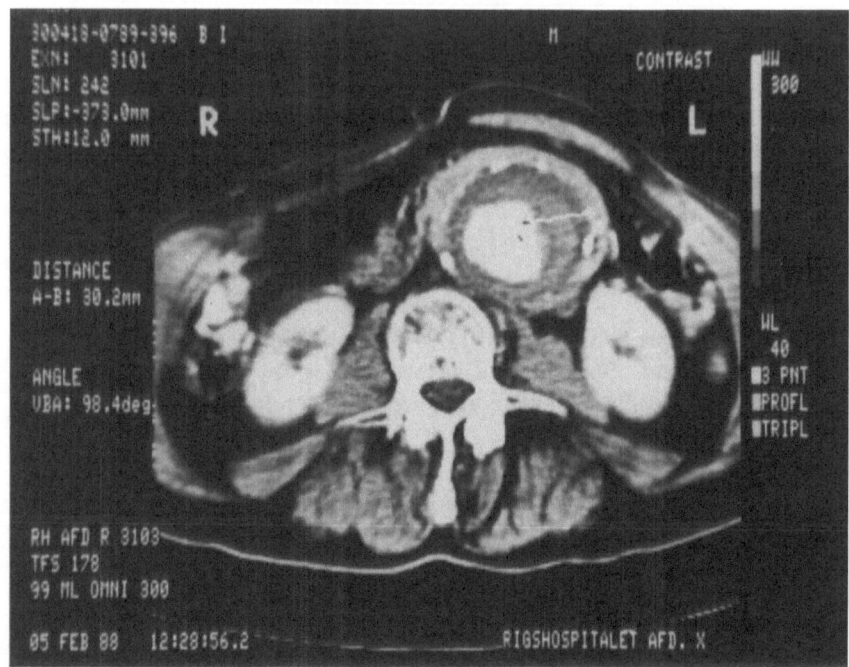

FIGURE 20.1. Preoperative CT scan in a patient with perianeurysmal fibrosis. The fibrosis predominantly covers the anterior wall of the abdominal aortic aneurysm.

diagnosis was established intraoperatively. In 17 patients, one or both ureters were involved in the fibrosis, leading to uremia in 5 patients. Preoperative percutaneous nephrostomy or catheterization with a ureteric J-stent was performed in 10 cases, due to a deterioration of renal function. At the time of surgery, ureterolysis was performed in 14 instances, with intraperitoneal positioning of ureter, and nephrectomy in 1 case.

Emergency surgery was carried out in 3 patients who presented signs of threatened rupture. Surgery involved a standard midline transperitoneal approach with insertion of a tube graft in 7 cases or a bifurcated graft in 18 patients. The remaining 2 patients, treated during the first years of this survey, had only a uterolysis performed. The duodenum was routinely released from the aorta when it was involved in the fibrosis. The intraoperative blood loss was, on average, 2,700 mL (1,000–5,500 mL). The perioperative mortality (30 days) was 3.7%, as one patient died 27 days after surgery due to cardiopulmonary failure.

At the time of follow-up, at a median 60 months postoperatively, 20 patients were still alive. Four patients had died of ischemic heart disease and 2 died of cancer. The last patient died 5 years postoperatively due to hypertension and uremia. This patient was one of the 5 patients who presented with

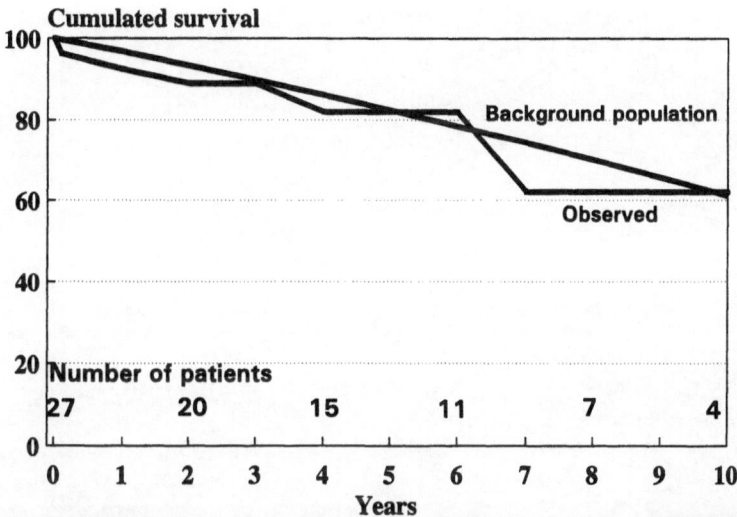

FIGURE 20.2 Cumulative survival for patiens operated on for perianeurysmal fibrosis related to an age- and sex-matched background population.

uremia at the time of diagnosis. Figure 20.2 illustrates the cumulative survival, which did not differ significantly from that of an age- and sex-matched population. The 5- and 10-year survival rates were 82% and 62%, respectively.

During follow-up, renal function remained within normal limits, as assessed by creatinine determination (60–140 mmol/L), with the exception of two patients: the one patient mentioned above, and a second in whom plasma creatinine had doubled, though without signs of ureteric obstruction. CT was performed in 3 patients, 1, 3, and 4 years postoperatively. In all 3 the fibrosis had disappeared (Fig. 20.3). A follow-up is still ongoing, including routine CT scans.

Discussion

This survey represents the experience of one vascular center, in contrast to previous multicenter-based reports. The incidence of PF was 2.7% (95% confidence limits: 1.8%–3.9%) among 1,004 cases of AAA. In the literature, an incidence of up to 15% has been stated.[6] This seeming difference could be due to lack of specific criteria for PF, retrospective data, or small patient series. Our data did not indicate that the incidence changed during the period under study. The age and sex distribution of patients with PF did not differ from those of patients with AAA without PF, in agreement with previous observations.[7-10]

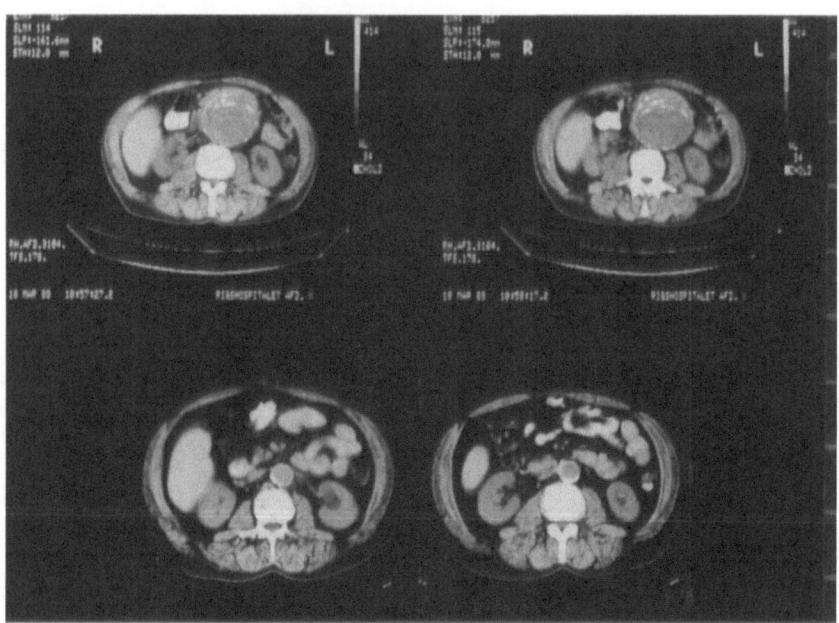

FIGURE 20.3. Pre- and 4-year-postoperative CT scans demonstrating disappearance of perianeurysmal fibrosis.

A transperitoneal versus a left-flank retroperitoneal approach has been discussed, and the latter is preferred by some authors because the aneurysm is approached through the area with the least amount of fibrosis.[11] We find it important with a standard regimen which does not differ from the surgical technique used in the remaining 97% of AAA. Since Pennell et al.[10] reported that 13% of the operations due to PF result in injury to abdominal organs, mobilization of the duodenum has been avoided by more authors.[8,11] We have not changed our policy of disengaging the fibrotic plaque containing the duodenum from the aneurysm. The low mortality and morbidity seen in relation to other reports seems to permit such procedure. [8,10–12] We also performed ureterolysis in case of ureteral fibrosis. This may not be necessary because the fibrosis seems to subside once operation for AAA has been performed, even though only a part of the perianeurysmal tissue has been removed (Fig. 20.3).[9,13] In a Swedish multicenter study, no difference was found in creatinine levels between patients in whom ureterolysis was performed and those patients in whom such procedure was not performed.[8]

In patients with PF it is important to optimize the renal and cardiovascular status before operation. Drainage of hydronephrosis should be done liberally, preferably by percutaneous access guided by ultrasonography. Fortunately, the risk of rupture seems to be lower than in ordinary atherosclerotic aneurysm. In this material, only 3 of 27 patients had rupture of the aneurysm, which is in agreement with other reports.[8–10,12,14]

Laboratory data were not systematically collected in our series. Erythrocyte sedimentation rate (ESR) has been found to be elevated in connection with fibrosis but has no predictive value in itself.[3,8] Whether creatinine, ESR, and orosomucoid could be used as indicators for the level of activity of the fibrosis is doubtful. A reliable diagnosis on the basis of symptoms and clinical examination or of blood samples is not possible. CT scan is the only way to establish the diagnosis. In spite of a preoperative CT examination, Lindblad et al.[8] and Pennell et al.[10] reported that the diagnosis was correctly identified preoperatively in only 10 of 50 patients and 7 of 14 patients, respectively. In our 1987–1990 material, the diagnosis was suspected in all but one case based on a preoperative CT scan. The discrepancy may be due to improved imaging quality with newer CT scanners as well as a larger experience obtained in a single center, as opposed to the experience obtained in centers seeing barely one case every year. In typical cases the scan will reveal a periaortic mass surrounding the aneurysmatic aorta (Fig. 20.1). The clue to the diagnosis is the presence of calcifications central to the periatoric mass. Intravenous contrast helps the interpretation in addition to allowing evaluation of the upper urinary tract.

The survival of patients operated on for AAA and PF did not differ from that of an age and sex-matched group (Fig. 20.2). These figures were in agreement with the theory of regression of fibrosis when the AAA has been operated on.[8,9,15]

We conclude that PF affected the group of patients with the predominance of atherosclerotic diseases. No symptoms or laboratory data were unique for PF, but the combination of AAA and postrenal obstruction is highly suggestive. A high-quality CT scan allows for a preoperative diagnosis. PF should be managed in centers with the necessary experience, because it is mandatory for a successful course of AAA complicated by perianeurysmal fibrosis. A careful follow-up is recommended, despite the apparently rather benign clinical course after operation.[8,10,15,16]

References

1. Bullock N. Idiopathic retroperitoneal fibrosis. Now known to be allergic reaction to insoluble lipid leaking through arteries. BMJ 1988;297:240–241.
2. Mitchinson MJ. Retroperitoneal fibrosis revisited. Arch Pathol Lab Med 1986; 110:784–786.
3. Mitchinson MJ. Some clinical aspects of idiopathic retroperitoneal fibrosis. Br J Surg 1972;59:58–60.
4. Parums DV, Brown DL, Mitchinson MJ. Serum antibodies to oxidized low-density lipoprotein and ceroid in chronic periaortitis. Arch Pathol Lab Med 1990;114:383–387.
5. Lorentzen JE, Sørensen IN, Brun B, Laursen K, Kristensen JK. Abdominal aortic aneurysm in combination with retroperitoneal fibrosis. Acta Chir Scand 1980; 502:94–97.
6. Fitzgerald EJ, Blackett RL. Inflammatory abdominal aortic aneurysm. Clin Radiol 1988;39:247–251.

7. Olsen PS, Schroeder TV, Perko MJ, et al. Mortality and survival in patients operated for abdominal aortic aneurysm. Ugeskr Læger 1991;153:1273–1276.

8. Lindblad B, Almgren B, Bergqvist D, Eriksson l, et al. Abdominal aortic aneurysm with perianeurysmal fibrosis. J Vasc Surg 1991;13:231–237.

9. Almgren B, Eriksson I, Forsberg JO, Norlinder H. Abdominal aortic aneurysm with perianeurysmal fibrosis: A clinical entity. Acta Chir Scand 1981;147:539–543.

10. Pennell RC, Hollier LH, Lie JT, et al. Inflammatory abdominal aortic aneurysms: A thirty year review. J Vasc Surg 1985;2:859–869.

11. Fiorani P, Faraglia V, Speziale F, Lauri D, Massucci M, De Santis F. Extraperitoneal approach for repair of inflammatory abdominal aortic aneurysm. J Vasc Surg 1991;13:692–697.

12. Goldstone J, Malone JM, Moore WS. Inflammatory aneurysms of the abdominal aorta. Surgery 1978;83:425–430.

13. Wright FW, Sanders RC. Is retroperitoneal fibrosis a self-limiting disease? Br J Radiol 1971;44:511–514.

14. Walker DI, Bloor K, Williams G, Gillie I. Inflammatory aneurysms of the abdominal aorta. Br J Surg 1972;59:609–614.

15. Plate G, Forsby N, Stigsson L, Sälström J, Thörne J. Management of inflammatory abdominal aortic aneurysm. Acta Chir Scand 1988;154:19–24.

16. Baker LRI, Mallinson WJW, Gregory MC, et al. Idiopathic retroperitoneal fibrosis. A retrospective analysis of 60 cases. Br J Urol 1988;60:497–503.

21
Vasospasm and Ruptured Aneurysmal Surgery

HWAN YUNG CHUNG

Summary

Aneurysmal surgery was performed in 243 cases, and delayed ischemic neurologic deficit (DIND) developed in 52 cases (21.4%). Consecutive computed tomographic (CT) checking revealed cerebral infarction in 20 cases (38.5%) out of 52. The ocurrence of DIND seemed to be proportional to severity of subarachnoid hemorrhage in CT findings except in cases of intracerebral or intraventricular blood clots. The incidence of DIND was higher 7–14 days after subarachnoid hemorrhage. Early aneurysmal surgery did not alter the incidence of DIND despite removal of blood clots as completely as possible in my series.

Introduction

Vasospasm in neurosurgical practice may result in delayed ischemic neurologic deficit (DIND), which is diagnosed if a patient has progressive decline in neurologic condition during the first 2 weeks after subarachnoid hemorrhage.[1-3] From the point of view of surgical timing, these ischemic conditions can be divided into pre- and postoperative ischemic deficit after subarachnoid hemorrhage. A total of 243 operations for aneurysm were performed, and 52 (21.4%) cases of DIND were encountered. The purpose of this study is to investigate factors affecting clinical features of this condition.

Clinical Materials and Methods

The 243 patients who underwent aneurysmal surgery at Hanyang University Hospital from January 1981 to December 1991 were investigated. The location of the aneurysm, timing of surgery, pre- and postoperative onset of DIND, age, sex, symptoms, signs, laboratory findings, and amount of subarachnoid blood clots were considered as well as outcome. Age and sex distribution of the operated cases and those with DIND are shown in Table 21.1.

TABLE 21.1. Age and sex distribution in DIND.

Age	Total op cases			DIND		
	M	F	Total (%)	M	F	Total (%)
20–29	8	2	10 (4.1)		1	1 (1.9)
30–39	15	18	33 (13.6)	2	2	4 (7.7)
40–49	45	35	80 (32.9%)	9	8	17 (32.8)
50–59	23	52	75 (30.9)	7	12	19 (36.5)
60–69	18	25	43 (17.7)	4	6	10 (19.2)
70	2		2 (0.8)	1		1 (1.9)
Total	111	132	243	23	29	52
	(45.6)	(54.4)	(100)	(44.2)	(55.8)	(100)

TABLE 21.2. Location of aneurysm and DIND.

Location	Operated cases	DIND (%)
Aco A–ACA	115	29 (25.2)
MCA	56	14 (25.0)
ICA	59	8 (13.6)
VBA	4	
Multiple	9	1 (11.1)
Total	243	52 (21.4)

Results

DIND was observed in 52 (21.4%) out of 243 operated cases. The locations of the aneurysms were anterior communicating aneurysm and anterior cerebral artery (AcoA-ACA) aneurysm (115 cases), middle cerebral artery (MCA) aneurysm (56), internal carotid artery (ICA) aneurysm (59), vertebrobasilar artery (VBA) aneurysm (4), and multiple aneurysms (9). DIND developed as shown in Table 21.2.

The timing of surgery after subarachnoid hemorrhage was classified into 4 groups: within 24 hours, 24–72 hours, 4–10 days, and more than 11 days. The numbers of preoperative and postoperative DINDs developed are shown in Table 21.3.

The onset of DIND after subarachnoid hemorrhage developed prior to surgery appeared as shown in Table 21.4. The onset of DIND after subarachnoid hemorrhage was classified arbitrarily into 4 groups: 4–6 days, 7–10 days, 11–14 days, and 15 days.

The incidence of DIND following surgery was higher up to 72 hours postoperatively (Table 21.5).

The symptoms, signs, and laboratory findings in 52 cases of DIND were investigated, and the notable findings are shown in Table 21.6.

TABLE 21.3. Timing of surgery and DIND.

Timing	No. (%)	Preoperative no. (%)	Postoperative no. (%)	Total
24 hr	25		6 (25.0)	6 (25.0)
24–72 hr	79		16 (20.2)	16 (20.2)
4–10 days	52	5 (9.6)	5 (9.6)	10 (19.2)
>11 days	87	14 (16.1)	6 (6.8)	20 (22.9)
Total	243	19 (7.8)	33 (13.6)	52 (21.4)

TABLE 21.4. Onset of DIND prior to surgery.

Onset after subarachnoid hemorrhage	No. of cases (%)
4–6	3 (15.7)
7–10	8 (42.1)
11–14	6 (31.5)
15	2 (10.5)
Total	19 (100)

TABLE 21.5. Onset of DIND following surgery.

Timing of surgery	No. of cases	Onset (post-op days)					Total (%)
		3	4–6	7–10	11–14	15	
24 hr	25		1	3	2		6 (24.0)
24–72 hr	79		6	5	3	2	16 (20.2)
4–10 days	52		3		1		5 (9.6)
>11 days	87		3		1		6 (6.9)
Total	243	3	13	8	7	2	33

The outcome was compared between DIND and non-DIND cases by the Hunt and Hess grading classification (Table 21.7). Regardless of the preexisting neurologic deficit, the outcome of the non-DIND cases was superior to that of the DIND cases, except for grade V.

The relationships between subarachnoid blood and DIND were evaluated in 209 cases of positive CT findings (Table 21.8). Subarachnoid blood was classified according to Fisher's system[5] which classified subarachnoid blood into four grades.

Group I: No blood detected

Group II: A diffuse deposition or thin layer with vertical layers of blood less than 1 mm thick

Group III: Localized clots and/or vertical layers of blood 1 mm or more

TABLE 21.6. Symptoms, signs and laboratory findings in 52 cases of DIND.

Findings	No. of cases (%)
Progressive decline (neurology)	52 (100)
Fever	20 (385)
Increasing	
Neck stiffness	19 (36.5)
Leukocytosis	16 (30.7)
Hyponatremia	33 (63.5)

TABLE 21.7. Outcome and DIND.

Hunt & Hess	DIND Total no. (%)	DIND Good recovery no. (%)	DIND Disabled no. (%)	Nonischemic Total	Nonischemic Good recovery no. (%)	Nonischemic Disabled no. (%)
I	13	7 (53.8)	3 (23.1)	29	26 (96.5)	1 (7.6)
II	10	4 (40.0)	4 (40.0)	74	62 (83.8)	4 (5.4)
III	14	4 (28.6)	4 (54.8)	38	25 (65.8)	5 (13.2)
IV	11	2 (18.2)	9 (81.9)	29	4 (13.8)	8 (27.6)
V	14	1 (25.0)	1 (25.0)	11	2 (18.2)	3 (27.6)
Total	52	18 (34.7)	25 (48.1)	19	135 (70.1)	21 (10.9)

TABLE 21.8. Subarachnoid blood and DIND.

Fisher's group	No. of cases	DIND (%)
I	6	1 (16.7)
II	78	11 (14.1)
III	86	28 (32.6)
IV	36	8 (20.5)
Total	209	48 (22.9)

Group IV: Diffuse or no subarachnoid blood, but with intracerebral or intraventricular clots

Cerebral infarction was detected in repeated CT checking in 20 out of 52 DIND cases.

Discussion

DIND seemed to develop proportionally in cases of severe subarachnoid hemorrhage in most instances,[4-6] but this was not always so in my series. DIND developed less often in cases of Fisher's group IV than in group III.

This suggests that intracerebral or intraventricular clots are less likely to produce DIND in comparison with localized clots and/or vertical layers of blood 1 mm of group III. The incidence of DIND prior to surgery was higher during days 7–14 than in the other periods. Removal of subarachnoid blood clots before the onset of DIND has been suggested as a promising method to prevent delayed ischemic effects after rupture of cerebral aneurysms.[3, 7–11] However, there is no definite evidence that development of DIND could be eliminated by surgery performed shortly after subarachnoid hemorrhage. In my series, early removal of subarachnoid blood did not alter the occurrence of DIND, despite removal of blood clots as completely as possible.

References

1. Adam HP, Kassell NF, Torner JC, et al. Predicting influence of clinical condition, CT results and antifibrinolytic therapy. A report of the cooperative aneurysmal study. Neurology 1987;37:1586.
2. Barker FG, Jr, Heros RC. Clinical aspects of vasospasm. In: Mayberg MR (ed.). *Cerebral Vasospasm.* Neurosurgery Clinics of North America 1990;1:277–288.
3. Hijdra A, van Gijn J, Nagelkerke NJD, et al. Prediction of delayed cerebral ischemia, rebleeding and outcome after aneurysmal subarachnoid hemorrhage. Stroke 1988;19:1250.
4. Allcoke JM, Drake CG. Postoperative angiography in cases of ruptured intracranial aneurysms. J Neurosurg 1963;20:752–759.
5. Fisher CM, Robertson GH, Ojemann RG. Cerebral vasospasm with ruptured saccular aneurysm—the clinical manifestations. Neurosurgery 1977;1:245–248.
6. Fisher CM, Kistler JP, Davis JM. Relation of cerebral vasospasm to subarachnoid hemorrhage visualized by computerized tomographic scanning. Neurosurgery 1980;6:1–9.
7. Hugenholz H, Elgie RG. Considerations in early surgery on good-risk patients with ruptured intracranial aneurysms. J Neurosurg 1982;56:180–185.
8. Johnson RJ, Potter JM, Reid RG. Arterial spasm in subarachnoid haemorrhage: Mechanical considerations. J Neurol Neurosurg Psychiat 1958;21:68 (Abstract).
9. Ljunggren B, Brandt I, Kagstroem E, et al. Results of early operations for ruptured aneurysms. J Neurosurg 1981;54:473–479.
10. Saito I, Ueda Y, Sano K. Significance of vasospasm in the treatment of ruptured intracranial aneurysms. J Neurosurg 1977;47:412–429.
11. Taneda M. The significance of early operation in the management of ruptured intracranial aneurysms. An analysis of 251 cases hospitalized within 24 hours after subarachnoid hemorrhage. Acta Neurochir 1982;63:201–208.

22
Aneurysm of the Abdominal Aorta Associated with Aortocaval Fistula: A Case Report

Duck Jong Han and Young Soon Hyun

Aortocaval fistula has been reported as an unusual complication of abdominal aortic aneurysm. Due to intraoperative massive bleeding and perioperative high morbidity and mortality, preoperative awareness of this condition, proper monitoring and fluid management, and careful handling of the aneurysm are mandatory for a successful recovery.

We successfully treated an aortocaval fistula in a 64-year-old female patient who showed typical physical manifestations such as pulsating abdominal mass, thrill, audible bruit, and venous hypertension.

Abdominal aortic aneurysms are not uncommon in Western populations. However, their incidence is increasing in Korea, where vascular diseases as well as abdominal aortic aneurysms are much rarer than in Western countries. Abdominal aortic aneurysm associated with aortocaval fistula is a rare complication of abdominal aortic aneurysm. Aortocaval fistula arising from an abdominal aortic aneurysm shows peculiar manifestations, such as pulsating abdominal mass, thrill, audible bruit, and venous hypertension. Once the diagnosis is made, surgical intervention is mandatory due to acutely progressing congestive heart failure.

Recently we had a female patient with an abdominal aortic aneurysm complicated with aortocaval fistula who was successfully treated surgically.

Case Report

A 64-year-old Korean woman was admitted in October 1989 with a history of right lower abdominal and back pain that developed 10 days prior to admission.

She had noticed a pulsatile abdominal mass 8 years ago without specific symptoms. Since then, she had felt intermittent abdominal pain without other gastrointestinal or respiratory symptoms until admission. She denied any history of abdominal trauma.

On physical examination, blood pressure was 110/70, pulse was 84, and central venous pressure was 23 cmH$_2$O. Venous engorgement was easily shown in the neck. There was no abnormality in the chest. Abdominal examination revealed an adult fist-sized pulsating mass in the subumbilical area. A bruit with an entire systolic and early diastolic component was heard in the entire abdomen with palpable thrill over the palpable mass. All the pulses of the extremities were present without leg swelling. In laboratory findings, blood gas analysis showed pH 7.410, pCO_2 31.7 mm Hg, pO_2 61.7 mm Hg, and HCO_3 20.1 meQ/L. Electrocardiogram showed sinus tarchycardia. Chest x-ray revealed cardiomegaly with the findings of mild congestive heart failure.

Abdominal x-ray showed fusiform soft tissue density (10 × 10 cm in size) delineated by a calcified rim in the lower mid-abdomen. Abdominal angiogram showed the infrarenal abdominal aortic aneurysm and visualization of inferior vena cava suggesting aortocaval fistula (Fig. 22.1)

Emergency laparotomy was performed. The aneurysm, involving the abdominal aorta and both common iliac arteries (10 × 8 × 5cm), was exposed through a midline abdominal incision. The aneurysmal sac was opened following the occlusion of both proximal aorta and distal iliac arteries. Profuse bleeding was noticed from the fistula opening (1 × 1.5 cm) located right posterior and just above the aortic bifurcation (Fig. 22.2). By finger compression

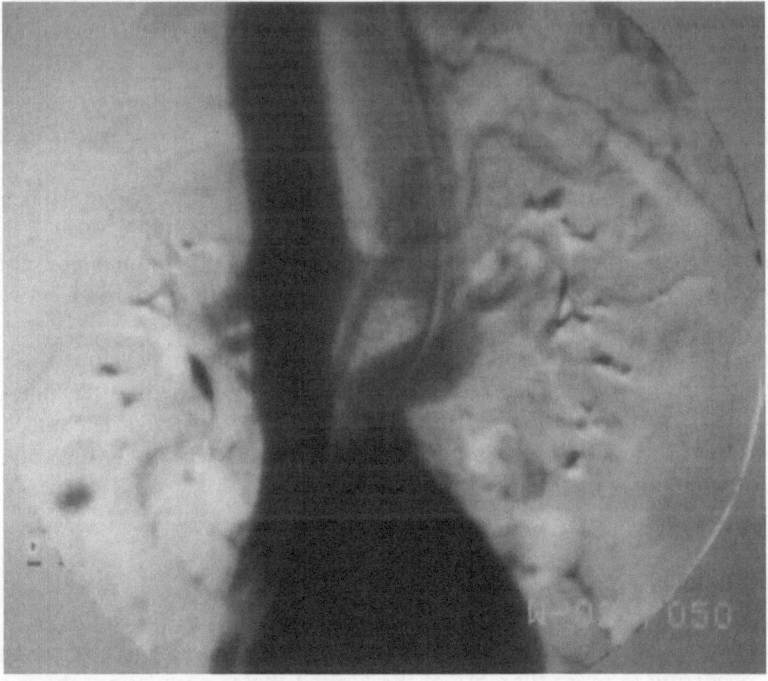

FIGURE 22.1. Abdominal angiogram showing the inferior vena cava and the tortuous abdominal aorta.

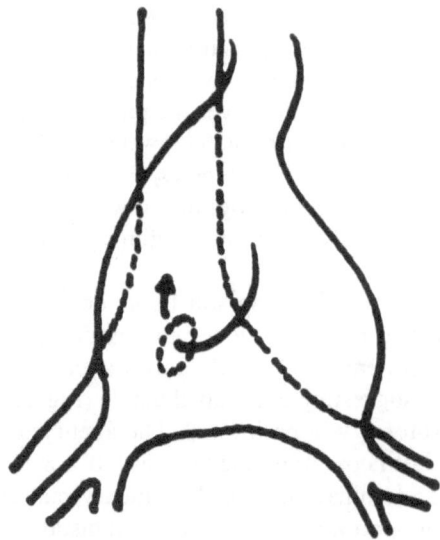

FIGURE 22.2 The fistula is located at the posterolateral wall of the aneurysm.

of the fistula opening, continuous closure of the defect was performed with 3–0 Prolene suture. During the procedure, about 3,500 cc of blood was lost. After closure, central venous pressure (CVP) decreased from the preoperative 25 cmH$_2$O to 5 cmH$_2$O postoperatively. After removal of atheroma from the aortic wall, the aorta was reconstructed end-to-end proximally to the infrarenal aorta and end-to-side distally to the external iliac artery using the Gore-Tex bifurcating graft (Fig. 22.3).

During the operation the total amount of blood loss was about 6,400, cc.

The postoperative course was not eventful until the 16th day, when a high fever developed accompanied by abdominal pain. Abdominal computed tomography (CT) showed the fluid collection mixed with air shadow between the graft and aneurysmal sac (Fig. 22.4).

Reoperation was performed when perigraft infection developed. After opening the aneurysmal sac, turbid fluid was evacuated with atheroma debris. After irrigation of the perigraft space, a drain was inserted. The infecting organism was found to be staphylococcus. The patient was discharged on the 20th postoperative day in good condition.

Discussion

Abdominal aortic aneurysm is not an uncommon disease in Western countries, occurring in more than 5% of the United States population above the age of 60 years. Compared with Western countries, abdominal aortic aneurysm is a rare disease in Korea, with only about 100 operations reported in the Korean Vascular Surgical Society up to now.

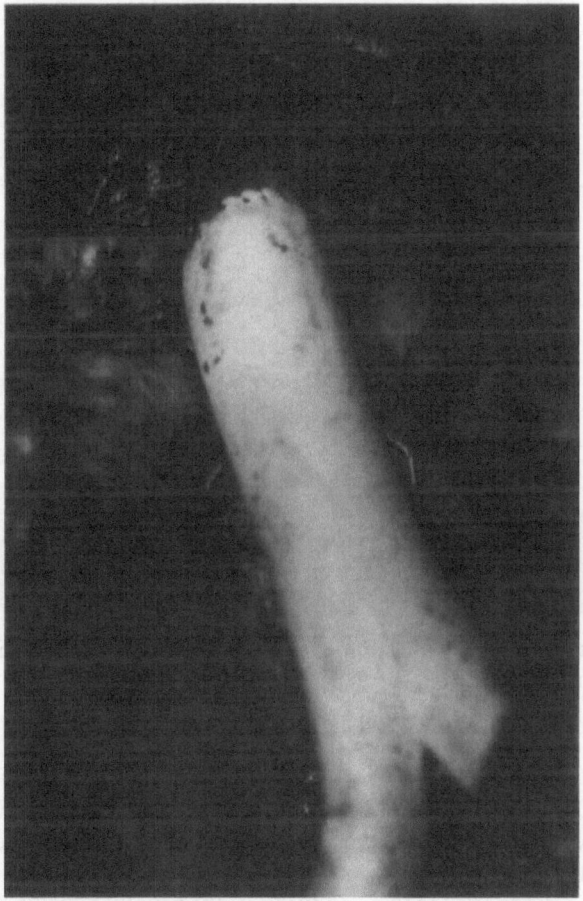

FIGURE 22.3 Reconstructed abdominal aorta with the bifurcating PTFE graft.

Aortocaval fistula presents a challenge to vascular surgeons. Due to its location in a high-flow system, blood flow shunted via fistula could be massive, resulting in high perioperative morbidity and mortality. Aortocaval fistula is a rare condition, reported sporadically in 0.15–2% of abdominal aortic aneurysms and 4% of ruptured abdominal aortic aneurysms.[1-3] After the initial report of this disease by Syme, the first surgical approach was done in 1955 by Eiseman.[4] Hemodynamic instability induced by inflow of high-flow aortic blood into the low-resistant vena cava causes acutely progressive congestive heart failure which is not amenable to medical treatment. Initially, shunting of aortic blood into the vena cava causes the hypovolemic state, but later, hypervolemic status causes a completely different situation, which becomes a risk factor for the patient perioperatively.

The etiology of aortocaval fistula can be classified as congenital or acquired,[5-8] in which atherosclerotic aortic aneurysm is the major cause fol-

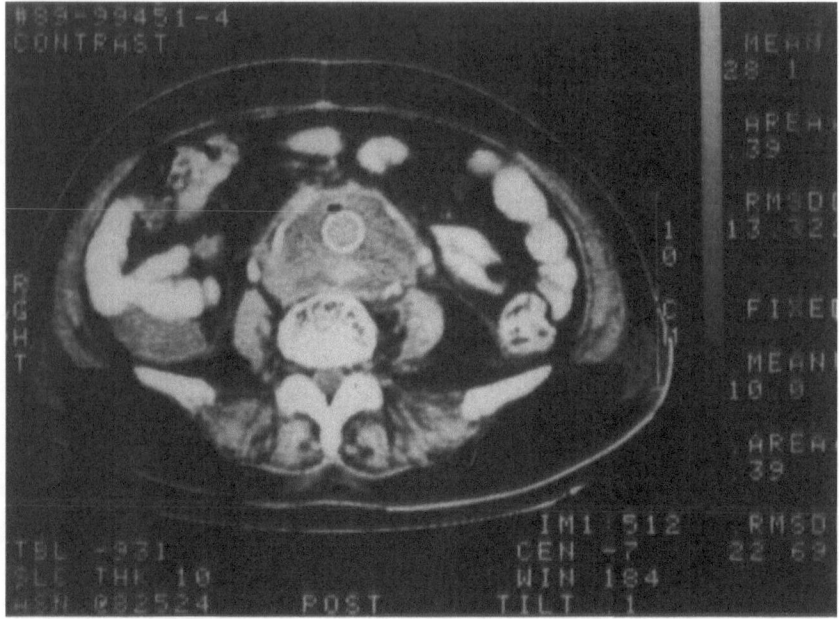

FIGURE 22.4. Abdominal CT illustrating fluid and air collection between the PTFE graft and the aneurysmal sac.

lowed by trauma,[9] operative injury of herniated intervertebral disc, tumor situated between the aorta and the vena cava,[10] and other diseases causing weakness of the aortic wall.[11,12]

Preoperative diagnosis for this condition is not usually difficult, but it may escape routine examination due to its low incidence. Only one or two of six patients were diagnosed preoperatively.[1,13] Diagnosis can be done by a high index of suspicion in the clinical setting of high-output cardiac failure of recent onset associated with a palpable aneurysm and continuous bruit over the aorta, but the typical physical signs are recognized in only half of the patients due to occlusion of the fistula by clots.[5,14]

Other than the above signs, rapidly progressive swelling of the lower extremities, distended veins over the legs and abdomen from venous hypertension, and arterial insufficiency are present. Sometimes bleeding from the rectum or bladder results, probably from increased venous pressure which is transmitted to the pelvic veins causing their subsequent rupture. From the hypotension and decreased renal plasma flow, oliguria or anuria and consistent azotemia may be present associated with distal arterial insufficiency.

Objective confirmation of the presence of the fistula has been achieved by transfemoral catheterization with a Swan-Ganz or other catheter determining increased inferior vena cava pressure and step-ups in oxygen saturation. Definite visualization of aortocaval fistula can be done by abdominal aortography as shown here for this patient. Interestingly, influx of contrast material into the vena cava revisualizes the aorta and its fistula site due to recirculation.

The time from onset of symptoms to diagnosis varies from hours to weeks. Once aortocaval fistula in suspected, immediate operation is indicated. The major aims of surgery are closure of the fistula and restoration of vascular continuity. Careful manipulation of the aneurysm is essential for the prevention of dislodgement of debris and massive bleeding from the fistula site. The fistula site is usually the right posterolateral wall of the aneurysm just above the aortic bifurcation.

Various techniques are suggested to decrease blood loss during operation, such as caval compression with sponge sticks, digital pressure, or balloon catheter. Unavoidable massive bleeding from the fistula site of the vena cava, due to hypervolemia and venohypertension, led surgeons to develop an auto-transfusion device.[15] Blood loss is reported in the range of 3,000–15,000 mL in the literature.[11,15] In our case, the fistula was repaired from inside the aorta, and 3,500 mL of blood was lost during the fistula closure.

Occasionally, when the vein is so friable that repair cannot be accomplished, proximal and distal ligation of the vena cava can be performed with controllable postoperative peripheral edema. After fistula closure, aortic wall reconstruction can be done by replacing the aneurysm with a prosthetic graft.[16]

The complications around the surgery are difficulty with fluid management, intraoperative embolization of intraaortic debris, and massive hemorrhage and its complications. As a result, continuous monitoring of systemic arterial and left atrial pressure, avoidance of great changes in cardiac output, and adjustment of fluid volume replacement are mandatory.

Perioperative mortality is high due to hemodynamic disturbance, massive bleeding during the control of fistula opening, and pulmonary embolism. Around 10%–50% mortality (3/6) is reported compared with 4.7% in patients with nonruptured aneurysm. Other morbidity includes acute tubular necrosis, duodenal ulcer bleeding, and wound dehiscence.

At postoperative day 16, this patient was found to have graft infection, usually a great threat to life and maintenance of the graft. By debridement and drainage of perigraft debris and infected fluid, the graft can be saved without removal of the prosthesis and extraanatomic bypass graft, which has been known as a necessary step for survival of the patient.

Graft infection may be controlled by using polytetrafluoroethylene graft material (PTFE) in which fewer bacteria may seed, treating infection around the perigraft space saving the suture line from infection, and early management of infection by both surgical and medical treatment with the proper use of CT.

This situation cannot be predicted at any time, so prudent care of a complicated aortic aneurysm is required during the entire perioperative period.

References

1. Baker WH, Sharzer LA, Ehrenhaft JL. Aortocaval fistula as a complication of abdominal aortic aneurysms. Surgery 1972;72:933.
2. Burke AM, Jamieson GG. Aortocaval fistula associated with ruptured aortic aneurysm. Br J Surg 1983;70:431.
3. Ivert T, Lie M, Lunde P. Non invasive diagnosis of fistula from abdominal aortic aneurysm to the inferior vena cava. Case report. Acta Chirurg Scand 1988;154: 669.
4. Eiseman B, Hughes RH. Repair of an abdominal aortic vena cava fistula caused by rupture of an atherosclerotic aneurysm. Surgery 1956;39:498.
5. Epstein DH, Higgins WL. Atypical spontaneous aortocaval fistula: CT appearance. Comput Radiol 1986;10:189.
6. Gregson RH, Sutton D, Brennan J, et al. Spontaneous aorta-caval fistula. Clin Radiol 1983;34:683.
7. Harrington EB, Schwartz M, Haimov M, et al. Aorto-caval fistula: A clinical spectrum. J Cardiovasc Surg 1989;30:579.
8. Kazmier FJ, Harrison CE. Acquired aortocaval fistulas. Am J Med 1973;55:175.
9. Krishnasastry KV, Friedman SG, Deckoff SL, Doscher W. Traumatic juxtarenal aortocaval fistula and pseudoaneurysm. Ann Vasc Surg 1990;4:378.
10. Crawford ES, Turell DJ, Alexander JK. Aorto-inferior vena caval fistula of neoplastic origin—hemodynamic and coronary blood flow studies. Circulation 1963; 27:414.
11. Brewster DC, Cambria RP, Moncure AC, et al. Aortocaval and iliac arteriovenous fistulas: Recognition and treatment. J Vasc Surg 1991;13:253.
12. Rutherford RD. *Vascular Surgery*. 3rd ed. Philadelphia: WB Saunders, 1989, p. 1069.
13. Dardik H, Dardik I, Stran MG, Attai I, et al. Intravenous rupture of arteriosclerotic aneurysms of the abdominal aorta. Surgery 1976;80:647.
14. Taheri SA, Plonka AJ. Aortocaval fistula: Diagnosis and treatment: Case studies. Angiology 1986;37:314.
15. Dorty DB, Coright CB, Lamberth WC, Sporto G, Garrelt WV, Cram AE. Aortocaval fistula associated with aneurysm of the abdominal aorta: Current management using autotransfusion technique. Surgery 1978;84:250.
16. Moore WS, Chvapil M, Seiffert G, et al. Development of an infection-resistant vascular prosthesis. Arch Surg. 1981;116:1403.

23
Management of Coronary Disease in Patients with Abdominal Aortic Aneurysm

J. Ernesto Molina, Fredy Abed, and Michael G. Petty

Mortality after aortic aneurysm repair is most commonly related to atherosclerotic coronary disease. [1-9] In fact, the leading cause of death postoperatively is myocardial infarction.[4-10] Several studies show that when the aneurysm reaches 7 cm, 90% of the patients have significant coronary disease. [1,2,7,11]

Therefore, the current recommendation is for patients to undergo cardiac evaluation before any operation for an abdominal aneurysm or for peripheral vascular disease. With such an evaluation, several studies show a decrease in morbidity and mortality.[10-14] If the patient is indeed found to have coronary disease, the question remains: How severe should the coronary component be in order to postpone the aneurysm operation and first solve the coronary problem?

Some publications indicate that, even with coronary disease, the patient can safely undergo resection of the abdominal aneurysm with no increase in morbidity or mortality.[15] However, it has been shown repeatedly[4,8,16] that if coronary artery obstruction is significant [as defined by a positive stress test, positive thallium perfusion scan, impaired ventricular function, 2-D echo assessment, or multiple uptake gated acquisition (MUGA) exams], the patient should undergo coronary arteriography evaluation before surgery. Furthermore, if the coronary arteriography shows significant stenosis of a major coronary vessel (i.e., 50% or more) then the patient should have this treated before the aortic aneurysm is repaired.

We compared, during two periods at our institution, operations for abdominal aortic aneurysms, analyzing the degree of cardiac involvement at the time.

Materials and Methods

Between 1981 and 1991, we operated on 260 patients for atherosclerotic abdominal aortic aneurysms. Within this 10-year span, our approach to cardiac evaluation differed: group I, 1981 to 1986, and group II, 1987 to 1991. Of 218 elective cases, 101 were in group I and 117 in group II. Excluded from

TABLE 23.1. Incidence of abdominal aortic aneurysm

Age (decades)	No.	%
40	3	1.3
50	30	12
60	92	35
70	98	38
80	35	13
90	2	0.7
Total	260	100

TABLE 23.2. Repair for aortic infrarenal aneurysm

Type of graft	No.	%
Straight	111	43
Aortobiilac	100	38
Aortobifemoral	42	16
Aortoiliacfemoral	7	3
Total	260	100

this analysis were 42 cases of acute ruptured aortic aneurysms, since the urgency of the operation precluded any type of cardiac evaluation.

In both groups, routine preoperative workup included a chest x-ray and electrocardiography. We also determined any history of angina, myocardial infarction, arterial hypertension, or diabetes. We assessed signs of old myocardial infarction by electrocardiography. In group I, if a patient had no current symptoms of angina, we did no further cardiac workup.

In group II, in all patients, we used MUGA scans, dipyridamole thallium scans, or 2-D echo to assess left ventricular function and detect any coronary disease. In addition, in 50% of the cases, we did a treadmill exercise test. If any test was positive, we did cardiac catheterization to evaluate the status of the coronary circulation.

Our study had 214 males and 46 females (4.6:1 ratio). The age ranged from the mid-forties to the nineties with a peak incidence in the sixties and seventies (Table 23.1). All operations used a transabdominal approach. The aorta was replaced with a synthetic graft: either a straight or a bifurcated tube, depending on the extent of the aneurysm (Table 23.2).

Cardiovascular Risk Factors

We analyzed five variables as significant of cardiac involvement: angina, hypertension, peripheral vascular disease, diabetes, and history of myocardial infarction. The most significant risk factor was arterial hypertension—a predominant finding in 50% of the cases. Next was peripheral vascular disease, in 33% of the patients. A history of myocardial infarction was found in 20% of the patients; of angina, in 12.6%. Diabetes was not a predominant risk factor; it was only found in 3.3% of the entire group.

Postoperative Cardiac Events

We monitored the patients for 24 to 48 hours in the intensive care unit. After they were transferred out of the intensive care unit, they were maintained on the cardiac monitor (for a total of 7 days). Any patient with any abnormality detected on the cardiac monitor had an electrocardiogram (ECG) and 12-lead ECG obtained before discharge.

We considered cardiac events of significance to be atrial fibrillation, supraventricular tachycardia, ventricular fibrillation, hemodynamic instability, signs of heart failure, angina, electrocardiographic evidence of ischemia, or clear myocardial infarction. For all patients with any of the above cardiac events, we measured cardiac isoenzymes daily for 3 days.

Morbidity and Mortality

We monitored complications related to the operation for up to 1 month postoperatively. Death within 1 month was considered to be related to the operation.

Location and Size of Aneurysms

All of the aneurysms reported in this study were infrarenal; 30% extended into the iliac arteries (unilaterally or bilaterally). Implant of an aortic bifurcation graft (Table 23.2) was required in 57%. We measured the size of the aneurysm by computed tomographic (CT) scan in 75% of the cases, and by ultrasound and/or aortogram in the remaining 25%.

The diameter of the aneurysms ranged from 4.4 to 11.8 cm. Some patients underwent more than one exam to determine the exact size and location.

Results

Operative mortality was 5.5% overall (6.9% in group I, and 4.2% in group II). There were 4 cases of graft infection in both groups combined (1.8%). All infections occurred in bifurcated grafts: 2 connected to the femoral arteries and 2 to the iliac arteries. There were 2 cases of questionable colitis or ischemia of the large bowel; both these patients survived. We reimplanted the inferior mesenteric artery in only 3 cases. In conjunction with the aneurysm repair, we did other procedures: renal artery endarterectomy in 4 patients, left nephrectomy in 1, bilateral renal artery bypass in 1, and autotransplantation of the right kidney in 1. In 15 patients, we did a cholecystectomy during the same operation after the aneurysm repair had been reperitonealized.

Group I

In this group, 19 patients experienced postoperative cardiac events (19%): 7 developed postoperative myocardial infarction, and 2 of them died as a result. These 2 patients died very rapidly: one suddenly collapsed, the other developed cardiogenic shock from which he could not be rescued. The other 5 patients, who survived the infarction, underwent cardiac evaluation 6 weeks after the aneurysm repair: 4 had coronary bypass surgery, and 1 had coronary balloon angioplasty with a percutaneous approach. Ten patients developed arrhythmia postoperatively, but no infarction was proven: 2 of them developed sinus bradycardia and atrioventricular block, and underwent implant of a pacemaker system. In addition, in 2 patients with a history of angina, it recurred postoperatively, but with no infarction.

Group II

As a result of the routine cardiac workup implemented in group II, 17 patients were found to have significant coronary disease (14.5%). All of them had a positive dipyridamole thallium scan, treadmill exercise test, or 2-D echo showing areas of hypokinesis. Coronary arteriography was performed in all 17 of these patients, and showed significant coronary vascular obstructive disease in each instance.

One patient in this group, however, had a ventricular ejection fraction of less than 20% and was considered a candidate for cardiac transplantation. Two patients had symptomatic angina at the time the abdominal aneurysm was evaluated, and both underwent coronary arteriography as well.

Twelve patients were referred for coronary bypass surgery. This operation was done before repairing the abdominal aneurysm. Two patients were satisfactorily treated with percutaneous balloon angioplasty, and subsequently underwent abdominal aneurysm repair. The 1 patient with very poor left ventricular function underwent cardiac transplantation, then 6 weeks later, a successful abdominal aneurysm repair. The 2 patients who had symptomatic angina at the time of evaluation underwent simultaneous coronary bypass operations, then aneurysm repair during the same operation (Table 23.3). Both survived and are doing well, 7 (group I) and 3 (group II) years later.

None of the patients undergoing coronary bypass and then abdominal aortic aneurysm repair died, in either group I or II. Comparing the groups, only 5 patients in group I had coronary arteriography and coronary bypass before undergoing aortic aneurysm repair. In contrast, in group II, the 17 patients reported above required this approach; none of them experienced

TABLE 23.3. Management of coronary disease in AAA patients (218 elective cases)

	Group I (1981–86)	Group II (1987–91)
No.	101	117
Workup for CAD	19	117
AAA repair only	95	100
PTCA before AAA repair	0	2
CAB first—AAA later	5	12
Heart TX first—AAA later	0	1
CAB & AAA simultaneously	1	2
Postop cardiac events	19	1
Postop MI	7	0
Cardiac death	5	1

CAD, Coronary artery disease; AAA, abdominal aortic aneurysm; PTCA, percutaneous coronary angioplasty; CAB, coronary artery bypass; TX, transplant; MI, myocardial infarction.

morbidity or mortality. There was one cardiac death in a patient considered not to need cardiac surgery.

Discussion

Some patients with coronary disease are able to withstand an abdominal aortic aneurysm repair and survive without complications. But which patients will do well is unpredictable, unless a screening cardiac evaluation is done before surgery. It is clear, if cardiac complications occur after aneurysm surgery, that the results can be disastrous (as in group I).

Routine full cardiac evaluation of every patient undergoing elective surgery for aortic abdominal aneurysm would significantly minimize the risk.[4,8,16–18] If severe coronary disease is found by coronary arteriography, our results show that performing the cardiac operation first and repairing the aortic aneurysm later is a safe approach, with no mortality or morbidity.

Occasionally, patients symptomatic of either condition will require a simultaneous operation for their coronary disease and their abdominal aneurysm.[8,16] This approach is seldom necessary. But if needed, it can also be safe: by doing the coronary bypass surgery first, and then during the same operation, repairing the aortic aneurysm.

References

1. Hertzer NR, Beven EG, Young JR, et al. Coronary artery disease in peripheral vascular patients: A classification of 1000 coronary angiograms and results of surgical management. Ann Surg 1984;199:223–233.

2. Young AE, Sanberg GW, Couch NP. The reduction of mortality of abdominal aortic aneurysm resection. Am J Surg 1977;134:585–590.
3. Taylor LM, Jr, Yeager RA, Moneta GL, McConnell DB, Porter JM. The incidence of perioperative myocardial infarction in general vascular surgery. J Vasc Surg 1992;15:52–59.
4. Pelissier FT, Lehot JJ, George M, Villard J. Effects of coronary insufficiency on the early and late results in patients surgically treated for aneurysm of the subrenal abdominal aorta. J Mal Vasc 1990;15:339–343.
5. Hollier LH, Taylor LM, Ochsner J. Recommended indications for operative treatment of abdominal aortic aneurysms. J Vasc Surg 1992;15:1046–1056.
6. Fraedrich G, Wollschlager H, Schonbach B, Schlosser V. Reduction of the risk of surgery for abdominal aortic aneurysms by extended coronary diagnostics and therapy. Thorac Cardiovasc Surg 1991;39:255–257.
7. Nevitt MP, Ballard DJ, Hallett JW. Prognosis of abdominal aortic aneurysms: A population-based study. N Engl J Med 1989;321:1009–1014.
8. Golden MA, Whittmore AD, Donaldson MC, Mannick JA. Selective evaluation and management of coronary artery disease in patients undergoing repair of abdominal aortic aneurysms. A 16 year experience. Ann Surg 1990;212:415–420.
9. Raby KE, Barry J, Creager MA, Cook EF, Weisberg MC, Goldman L. Detection and significance of intraoperative and postoperative myocardial ischemia in peripheral vascular surgery. JAMA 1992;268:222–227.
10. Chadwick L, Galland RB. Preoperative clinical evaluation as a predictor of cardiac complications after infrarenal aortic reconstruction. Br J Surg 1991;78:875–877.
11. Yeager RA, Weigel RM, Murphy ES, McConnell DB, Saski TM, Vetto RM. Application of clinically valid cardiac risk factor to aortic aneurysm surgery. Arch Surg 1986;121:278–281.
12. Bunt TJ. The role of a defined protocol for cardiac risk assessment in decreasing perioperative myocardial infarction in vascular surgery. J Vasc Surg 1992;15:626–634.
13. Whittmore AD, Clowes AW, Hechtman HS, Mannick JA. Aortic aneurysm repair reduced operative mortality associated with maintenance of optimal cardiac performance. Ann Surg 1989;192:414–421.
14. Boucher CA, Brewster DC, Darling RC, Okada RD, Strauss HW, Pohost GM. Determination of cardiac risk by dipyridamole–thallium imaging before peripheral vascular surgery. N Engl J Med 1985;312:389–394.
15. Hollier LH, Reigel MM, Kazmier FJ, Pairolero PC, Cherry KJ, Hallett JW, Jr. Conventional repair of abdominal aortic aneurysm in the high-risk patient: A plea for abandonment of nonresective treatment. J Vasc Surg 1986;3:712–717.
16. Acinapura AJ, Rose DM, Kramer MD, Jacobowitz IJ, Cunningham JN, Jr. Role of coronary angiography and coronary artery bypass surgery prior to abdominal aortic aneurysmectomy. J Cardiovasc Surg (Torino) 1987;28:552–557.
17. Johnson KW, Scobie TK. Multicenter prospective study of nonruptured abdominal aortic aneurysms. Population and operative management. J Vasc Surg 1988;7:69–81.
18. Ruby ST, Whittmore AD, Couch NP, Collins JJ, Cohn L, Shemin R, Mannick JA. Coronary artery disease in patients requiring abdominal aortic aneurysm repair. Selective use of a combined operation. Ann Surg 1985;201:758–764.

24
Management of Thoracoabdominal Aneurysm and Difficult Aneurysmal Problems of the Aorta

SAMUEL R. MONEY AND LARRY H. HOLLIER

Introduction

The repair of thoracoabdominal aortic aneurysms is a challenge for the vascular surgeon. Not only does mortality vary between 5% and 20%, but serious complications occur quite frequently.[1-3] Paraplegia is perhaps the most devastating complication, with serious physical, emotional, and financial sequelae. Paraplegia has been reported to occur in between 4% and 40% of cases.[1,4]

The etiology of paraplegia secondary to aortic surgery is related to spinal cord ischemia which begins during aortic cross-clamping and may continue over the next few days due to secondary factors.[5] Since the rates of paraplegia have been reported to be as high as 40%,[1] multiple attempts to reduce this problem have been made. Monitoring of somatosensory-evoked potentials or motor evoked potentials has been advocated as a technique for identifying the group of patients who develop neurologic deficits during thoracoabdominal aortic replacement.[6] This safe and simple technique has one major limitation: the monitoring does not prevent paraplegia but simply indicates those patients who are at greatest risk of ischemia and require rapid cord revascularization. The use of heparin-bonded shunts, femorofemoral bypass, and atriofemoral bypass also have been advocated for reducing paraplegia. These shunts reduce the paraplegia risk in some patients, but other complications have been reported to increase.[4] Included among the risks are air embolism, aortic wall injury, and hemorrhagic complications.

The types of paraplegia that occur are varied. Patients can awaken from anesthesia following what was believed to be an uneventful procedure and be totally paralyzed. Other patients do well for the first few days postoperatively and then develop what is termed "delayed-onset paraplegia." The exact etiology of both early and delayed-onset paraplegia is probably multifactorial.[7] Figure 24.1 describes what we believe to be some of the causes of spinal cord ischemia following thoracoabdominal aortic replacement.

In an attempt to reduce the rate of both early and late neurologic complications, we have developed a multimodality perioperative protocol (Table

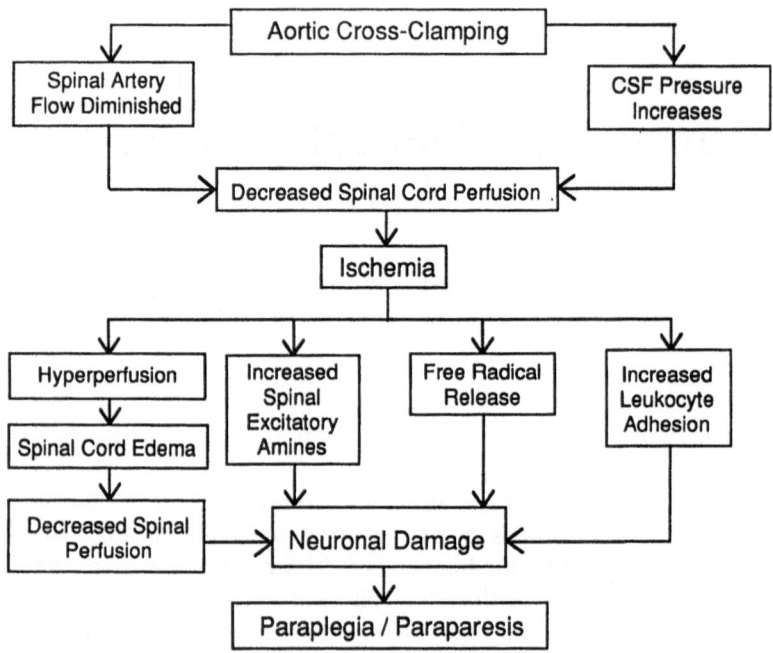

FIGURE 24.1. Cascade of effects on the spinal cord secondary to thoracoabdominal aortic cross-clamping.

24.1).[4] In a recent review of our results, spinal cord dysfunction was reduced from 6% to 0%. Overall, our paraplegia/paralysis rate is 4% (170 patients). This protocol involves efforts to limit the severity of ischemia to the spinal cord during surgery while reducing the metabolic requirements of the spinal cord and minimizing the effects of postischemic reperfusion injuries.

Spinal Cord Blood Supply

The major blood supply to the spinal cord is carried by the anterior and posterior spinal arteries. These are supplied by multiple sources. The anterior spinal artery supplies the majority of blood to the cord and supplies most of the blood to both the gray and white matter; of importance in this are the major motor tracts of the cord. There are few, if any, interconnections between the anterior and posterior arteries. The major arteries that supply the anterior spinal artery derive blood from the vertebral artery, the intercostals of the thoracic aorta, the lumbar arteries, and branches of the hypogastric artery. The largest of the intercostal arteries (radicular arteries), the artery of Adamkiewicz, provides a significant amount of blood flow to the anterior spinal artery. This artery usually originates between T-8 and L-2. When the

TABLE 24.1. Adjunctive measures utilized to reduce the incidence of spinal cord dysfunction occurring secondary to thoracoabdominal aortic replacement.

I. Decrease spinal cord ischemia
  a. Complete cord revascularization
  b. Minimize aortic cross-clamp time
  c. CSF drainage
  d. Proximal hypertension
II. Reduce metabolic rate
  a. Hypothermia
  b. Barbiturates
  c. Avoid hyperglycemia
III. Limit reperfusion injury
  a. Mannitol
  b. Steroids

---

artery of Adamkiewicz arises below the thoracic aorta, another major radicular artery can frequently be found high up in the mid to upper thoracic region.[8]

Perioperative Protocol

After the induction of general anesthesia, an intrathecal catheter is placed through the second or third lumbar interspace. Cerebrospinal fluid (CSF) pressure is monitored and, in addition, CSF is aspirated perioperatively for the first 48–72 hours. The catheter is attached to a transducer with the CSF pressure kept below 10 mmHg via a special "pop-off" valve mechanism. Arterial pressure is monitored via indwelling arterial cannulae. During the procedure the blood pressure is kept within the normal range prior to cross-clamping. Intravenous vasodilators are started as required. The patient is volume loaded with crystalloid at the time of the skin incision. No solutions containing dextrose are used, and hyperglycemia is avoided. If blood glucose levels exceed 220 mg/dl, regular insulin is administered intravenously to normalize the blood glucose levels. During aortic cross-clamping, blood pressure is increased 15–20% above baseline to increase collateral blood supply to the potentially ischemic spinal cord.

The operating room is cooled to 15°C and the patient receives room temperature fluids in an attempt to passively cool the core body temperature to 32–34°C. The reduction of core temperature is confirmed by both an indwelling bladder catheter with a thermistor attachment and by the pulmonary artery catheter thermistor attachment. High-dose steroids are administered at the start of the procedure. Prior to aortic cross-clamping, 10 mg/kg of thiopental is administered. Mannitol is given both prior to aortic cross-clamping and just prior to unclamping.

Obviously, rapid surgical repair tends to minimize cord ischemic time. We routinely reimplant all intercostal arteries into the graft if technically possible. The three techniques of reimplantation we mainly use are direct reimplantation as a Carrel-type patch, direct incorporation into the anastomosis, or use of a separate interposition graft. In order to reduce the hypotension which accompanies declamping, clamps are removed slowly. Blood and fluid are infused via a Rapid Infusion Device (Haemonetics®, Braintree, Massachusetts, USA). Patients frequently develop a mild coagulopathy and require multiple transfusions of fresh frozen plasma, cryoprecipitate, and platelets. It is our policy to keep the hematocrit above 35 in the postoperative period to maximize oxygen delivery. If fibrinolysis occurs, intravenous Amicar (aminocaproic acid) is given over 4–8 hours.

Discussion

The protocol outlined above is the one presently being used at our institution. We are constantly modifying the protocol based on basic research carried out by ourselves and others. In addition, different clinical problems with which certain patients present dictate some modifications of the procedure.

It is evident that spinal cord injury following thoracoabdominal aortic replacement is probably not entirely preventable.[1-4] The risk of spinal cord injury has been reduced by the use of the adjunctive measures outlined in this article.[4] It is our hypothesis that paraplegia/paraparesis occurs due to the interaction of multiple interrelated variables. These variables include the extent of the ischemic insult to the cord, the metabolic rate of the spinal cord at the time of ischemia, and the rate of extent of reperfusion injury which occurs. It is our belief that any attempt to reduce spinal cord injury should be directed towards each of these three mechanisms of injury.

Rapid and complete spinal cord revascularization is an obvious technical consideration that will limit the severity of ischemia. The pre- or intraoperative identification of critical spinal cord blood supply is difficult. Kieffer[9] demonstrated that selective preoperative angiography could identify these arteries, but these efforts were not entirely successful and, therefore, did not prevent paraplegia. We favor routine complete revascularization of all intercostals when technically feasible. As described above, by increasing the proximal arterial blood supply by 15%–20% above baseline, we believe we increase the collateral blood flow to the spinal cord. This mechanism will, to some extent, reduce some neuronal injury that occurs at the time of aortic cross-clamping. We routinely use CSF drainage in cases of thoracoabdominal aortic surgery. In our laboratory and others,[10,11] multiple animal studies have demonstrated the benefit of CSF drainage in improving spinal cord perfusion and protecting against neurologic complications during aortic occlusion. Both the production and the pressure of the CSF are increased during aortic cross-clamping. By reducing the CSF pressure, spinal cord perfusion is therefore increased. In a prospective study, Crawford and co-workers[1] could not show any significant decrease in neurologic complications following thoracoabdominal aortic aneurysm repair in patients who had CSF drainage compared to the control group who did not. However, certain flaws did exist in this study. Firstly, CSF drainage was limited to a volume of 50 cc and postoperative drainage was not utilized at all. Only the patients who were at highest risk (type I and type II aneurysms) were tested. In this group they had an overall neurologic deficit rate approaching 30%. Furthermore, CSF drainage reduced the risk of neurologic complications in their highest risk patients, that small subgroup of patients who required reoperation or had postoperative hypotension ($p = 0.07$). It is our belief that CSF drainage is effective if it is directed at reducing spinal cord pressure and not simply at reducing a certain amount of CSF volume. It is not unusual for us to drain 300–500 cc of CSF during the perioperative period. Also, we believe that perioperative drainage is quite important in the prevention of some of the delayed-onset deficits that occur secondary to late spinal cord edema. One of our patients who developed delayed paraparesis had his paraparesis resolve following removal of an additional 40 cc of CSF. Furthermore, Crawford's group of patients with type I and type II aneurysms, 40% of which were caused by aortic dissection, was a group at extremely high risk of spinal cord dysfunction, since extensive intercostal revascularization may be required and is extremely difficult in this group. The marginal benefit of CSF drainage along may, in these patients, be inadequate to protect against neurologic deficit. However, in those patients at lesser risk, we feel that CSF drainage does reduce the severity of ischemia of the spinal cord and may help reduce the risk of postoperative neurologic dysfunction.

Hypothermia and barbiturate coma both serve to reduce the rate of spinal cord metabolism. Hypothermia can reduce the oxygen consumption of neural tissue by approximately 6% for each degree of temperature below 37°C.[12] This results in an increase in the safe time of ischemia that the spinal cord can tolerate. The increase is approximately 5–6 minutes for each degree Celsius the temperature of the cord is reduced. Thiopental reduces the central nervous system (CNS) metabolic rate and relaxes the vascular smooth muscle of the CNS. Relaxation of the vascular smooth muscle results in an augmentation of blood flow; in addition, reducing the metabolic rate also reduces the oxygen demand.[13] Another important mechanism in the protective effect of thiopental is its property of lowering CSF pressure. Decreasing CSF pressure increases cerebral cord perfusion and blood flow, and therefore the long-term formation of edema will decrease. Previously in our laboratory we demonstrated the protective effect of thiopental in the rabbit model.

Hyperglycemia has been demonstrated in multiple animal models to increase the risk of neuronal injury.[14] This may relate to the concentration of energy substrate (glucose) that is available to the spinal cord, therefore resulting in an increased production of oxygen-derived free radicals during the period of aortic cross-clamping. Another potential theory is that by avoiding hyperglycemia the cord metabolic rate is kept within the normal limits. Whatever the mechanism may be, we believe that the avoidance of hyperglycemia is easily accomplished by administering fluids without dextrose and by the use of exogenous insulin when required.

The clinical observations of delayed-onset neurologic deficits suggest that a reperfusion injury may be occurring.[7] This phenomenon is poorly understood. It has been suggested that delayed-onset paraplegia can simply be accounted for by hypotension or other hemodynamic compromises in the postoperative period. In the three cases we have observed, no such mechanism was identified and no periods of hypotension were noted. In our laboratory we have demonstrated that there is an intermediate degree of spinal cord ischemia that is too great to avoid any spinal cord injury, but not severe enough to cause acute paraplegia.[15] This model can result in a high incidence of delayed-onset neurologic deficits. From experimental observations, we believe that reperfusion injury is a causal factor in the etiology of delayed-onset neurologic deficits.

Steroids are given prior to aortic occlusion, since they act at a cellular and subcellular level. They have been shown to work as stabilizers of both cellular and lysosomal membranes.[4] Another measure employed to reduce reperfusion injury is intravenous mannitol. Aside from its benefit in renal perfusion, it has also been shown to have potential beneficial effects as an oxygen-derived free radical scavenger. More effective free radical scavengers exist but are not yet available for human use. Steroids and mannitol are used largely empirically at this point. We believe that more research in this field is needed to delineate the exact role of these two pharmacologic agents.

No single intervention can eliminate the risk of spinal cord injury associated with thoracoabdominal aortic surgery. However, it is our belief that a multimodality protocol directed at reducing the severity of ischemia, reducing the rate of metabolism of the spinal cord during the period of ischemia, and the prevention of reperfusion injury can significantly reduce the risk of spinal cord dysfunction following thoracoabdominal aortic replacement. Hopefully, with additional investigation, spinal cord injury from aortic surgery can be minimized.

References

1. Crawford ES, Svensson LG, Hess KR, et al. A prospective randomized study of cerebrospinal fluid drainage to prevent paraplegia after high-risk surgery on the thoracoabdominal aorta. J Vasc Surg 1990;13:36–46.
2. Crawford ES, Walker HSJ, Saleh SA, et al. Graft replacement of aneurysm in descending thoracic aorta: Results without bypass or shunting. Surgery 1981;89: 73–85.

3. Hollier LH, Symmonds JB, Pairolero PC, et al. Thoracoabdominal aortic aneurysm repair. Arch Surg 1988;123:871–875.
4. Hollier LH, Money SR, Naslund TC, et al. Risk of spinal cord dysfunction in patients undergoing thoracoabdominal aortic replacement. Am J Surg 1992;164: 210–214.
5. Hollier LH. Protecting the brain and spinal cord. J Vasc Surg 1987;5:524–528.
6. Laschinger JC, Cunningham JN, Jr, Cooper MM, et al. Monitoring of somatosensory evoked potentials during surgical procedures on the thoracoabdominal aorta. J Thorac Cardiovasc Surg 1987;94:260–265.
7. Moore WM, Jr, Naslund TC, Hollier LH. Neurologic outcome following transient spinal cord ischemia during thoracoabdominal aortic aneurysm repair. In: Cohen JR (ed.). *Vascular Surgery 2000*. Austin, TX: R. G. Landes Company, 1991, pp. 84–90.
8. Hollier LH, Procter CD, Sr, Naslund TC. Spinal cord ischemia. In: Bernhard VM, Towne JB (eds.). *Complications in Vascular Surgery*. St. Louis: Quality Medical Publishing, 1991, pp. 153–159.
9. Kieffer E, Richard R, Chivas J, et al. Preoperative spinal cord arteriography in aneurysmal disease of the descending thoracic and thoracoabdominal aorta: Preliminary results in 45 patients. Ann Vasc Surg 1989;3:34–46.
10. Granke K, Hollier LH, Zdrahal P, et al. Longitudinal study of cerebral spinal fluid drainage in polyethylene glycol-conjugated superoxide dismutase in paraplegia associated with thoracic aortic cross-clamping. J Vasc Surg 1991;13:615–621.
11. McCullough JL, Hollier LH, Nugent M. Paraplegia after thoracic aortic occlusion: Influence of cerebrospinal fluid drainage. J Vasc Surg 1988;7:153–160.
12. Michenfelder JD. Anesthesia and the brain: Clinical, functional metabolic and vascular correlates. New York: Churchill Livingstone, 1988.
13. Naslund TC, Hollier LH, Money SR, et al. Protecting the ischemic spinal cord during aortic clamping: The influence of anesthetics and hypothermia. Ann Surg 1992;215:409–415.
14. Drummond JC, Shapiro HM. Cerebral physiology. In: *Miller RD (ed.)*. *Anesthesia*. New York: Churchill Livingstone, 1990, pp. 621–658.
15. Moore WM, Jr, Hollier LH. The influence of severity of spinal cord ischemia in the etiology of delayed-onset paraplegia. Ann Surg 1991;213:427–432.

25
Inflammatory Abdominal Aortic Aneurysms

HIROSHI OUCHI, MASATAKA ICHIKI, KICHIYA OKUYAMA, AND
SHUZO KAMIOKI

Summary

From January 1980 to March 1992, a total of 203 patients with abdominal
aortic aneurysms were operated on in our department. We encountered
10 cases (5%) with inflammatory abdominal aortic aneurysms. The most
common chief complaints were abdominal pain and/or lumbago. Positive
C-reactive protein (CRP) and increased erythrocyte sedimentation rate
(ESR) and Mantle sign by computed tomography (CT) and magnetic resonance imaging were noted in 90% of cases. In 40% of cases, hydroureter was
present.

For graft implantation, the inclusion technique was used in 60% of patients
and thromboexclusion in 40%. Postoperatively, CRP became negative and
ESR returned to normal. There were 2 early deaths, 1 cerebral and 1 cardiac.
One late death from aortoduodenal fistula was seen. The remaining 7 individuals have survived. Histopathological examination revealed atherosclerosis in 90% and cystic medionecrosis in 10%. Medial atrophy and/or degeneration and fibrosis were detected. The adventitia was relatively well preserved,
but with lymphoplasmacytic inflammatory infiltrate mainly at the thickened
perivascular portion.

Introduction

The exact etiology of inflammatory abdominal aortic aneurysm is still unknown, although numerous relevant etiological factors have been reported.
The present communication deals with our experience of inflammatory abdominal aortic aneurysm at the Department of Surgery of Sendai Hospital
of the East Japan Railway Company, Sendai, Japan. We describe signs and
symptoms, laboratory findings, diagnostic procedures, operative methods
employed, histopathology, and outcome. We also discuss etiological factors
in the English literature.

Clinical Materials

From January 1980 through March 1992, a total of 203 patients with abdominal aortic aneurysms were operated on in our hospital. We encountered 10 cases (5%) with inflammatory abdominal aortic aneurysms.

The illustrative case is a 59-year-old man with a history of hypertension, diabetes mellitus, and hyperlipidemia of 16 years duration. On the July 18, 1988, he suddenly noted persistent abdominal pain with lumbago. He was seen by a physician who noted a pulsatile mass in the abdomen. The patient was referred to our surgical department. Dynamic Computed Tomography (CT) revealed rapid luminal enhancement and slightly delayed enhancement of the outer layer (Fig 25.1). Five layers were identified: enhanced lumen, nonenhanced thrombus, a focally calcified layer, nonenhanced aortic wall, and enhanced periaortic layer. This is called Mantle sign, which is characteristic of inflammatory abdominal aortic aneurysm. The erythrocyte sedimentation rate (ESR) was 84 mm for 1 hour and 150 mm for 2 hours with positive C-reactive protein (CRP). Intravenous digital subtraction angiography (Fig. 25.2) demonstrated a saccular-type infrarenal aortic aneurysm. A renogram

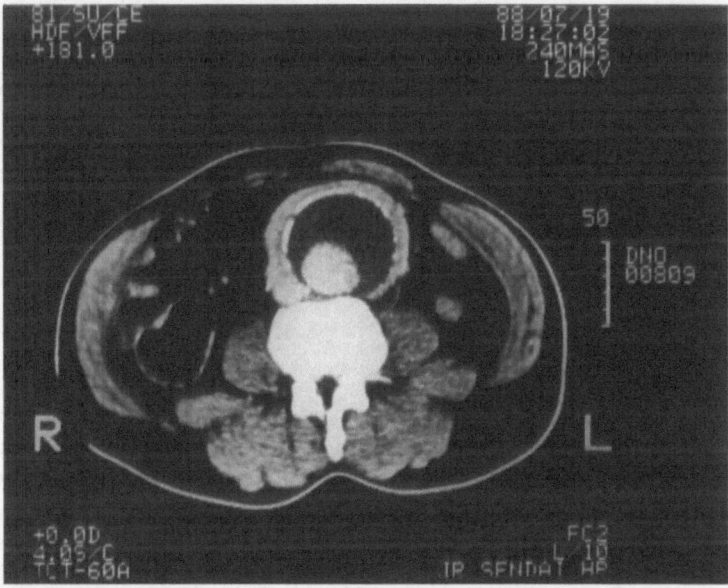

FIGURE 25.1. A dynamic CT scan reveals rapid luminal enhancement and slightly delayed enhancement of the outer layer, as well as the layering of the Mantle sign, which is the most characteristic evidence of IAAA. The patient in all these figures is a 59-year-old man with a history of hypertension, diabetes mellitus, and hyperlipidemia of 16 years' duration.

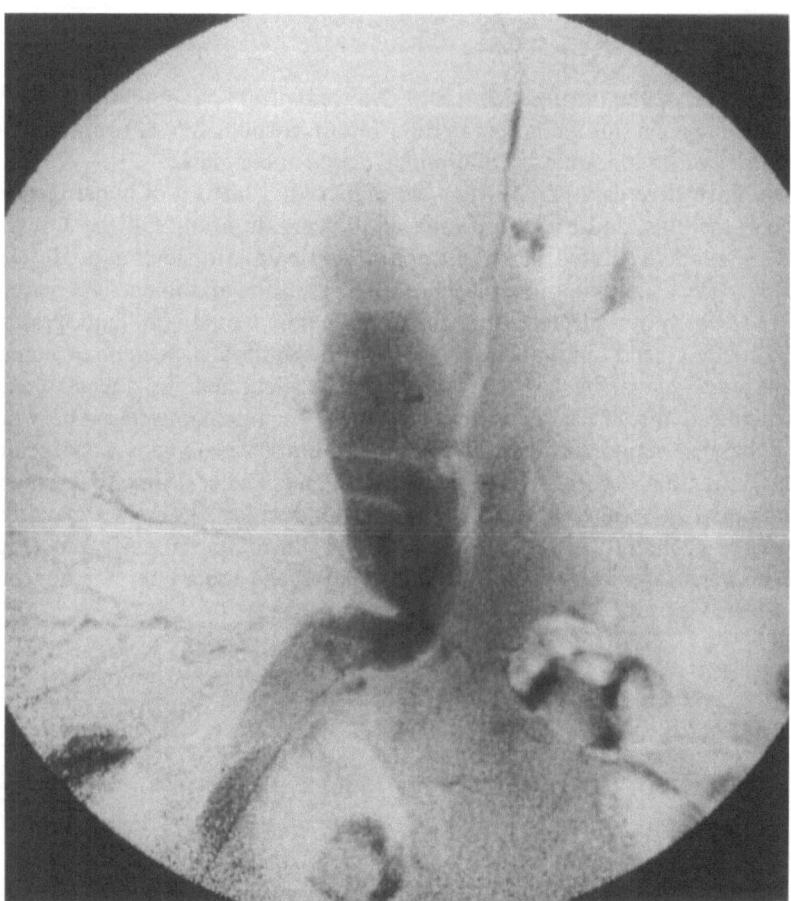

FIGURE 25.2. Digital subtraction angiography demonstrates a saccular-type infrarenal aortic aneurysm.

showed excretory prolongation of the left kidney (Fig. 25.3). The preoperative drip infusion pyelogram (Fig. 25.4) indicated narrowing of the left ureter at its midportion and hydronephrosis. Hypofunction of the left kidney was noted on the renoscintigram. At operation, a glittering, whitish-colored aneurysm was found, to which the duodenum was adhered. This is a typical view of inflammatory abdominal aortic aneurysm (Fig. 25.5). With minimal dissection, an Ochsner bifurcation graft was implanted by an inclusion technique (Fig. 25.6). The graft was covered with the aneurysmal wall (Fig. 25.7). A CT scan taken 20 days after operation demonstrated patency of both limbs of the graft implanted within the aneurysm (Fig. 25.8). ESR returned to normal during the postoperative period of $1\frac{1}{2}$ months. One cannot see the thickening of the outer layer of the aortic wall in the CT scan taken 1 year after opera-

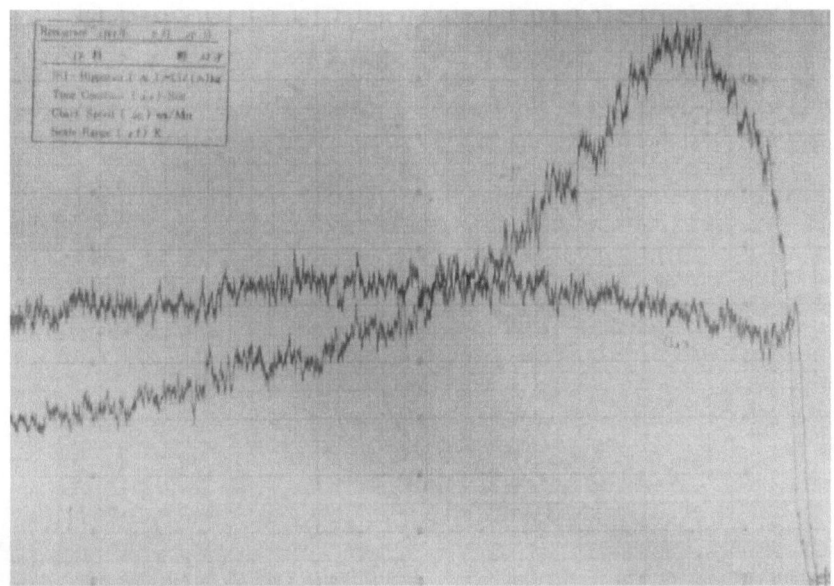

FIGURE 25.3. The renogram shows excretory prolongation of the left kidney.

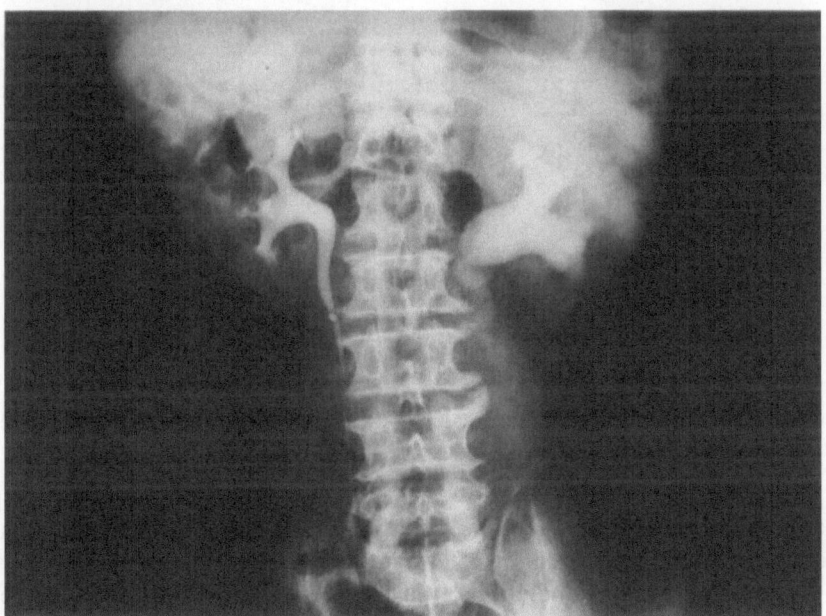

FIGURE 25.4. The preoperative drip infusion pyelogram indicates narrowing of the left ureter at its midportion and hydronephrosis.

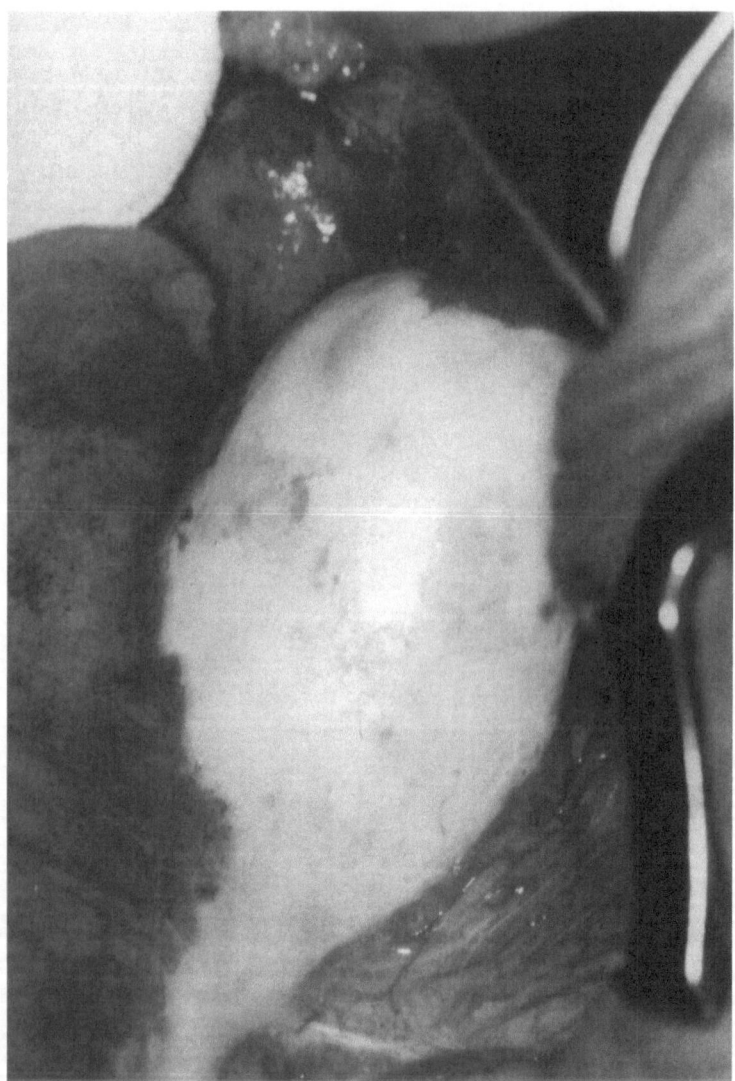

FIGURE 25.5. The renoscintigram reveals a typical view of inflammatory abdominal aortic aneurysm.

tion, the evidence of disappearance of inflammatory process. The patient is doing well 4 years and 2 months after operation.

Histopathological examination revealed atheromatous change within the aneurysmal lumen and foam cells, an appearance consistent with athero-sclerosis. The medial coat, however, nearly completely disappeared, adjacent to which markedly thickened adventitial and/or perivascular layer was pre-sent. The outer layer was granulomatous with abundant lymphoplasmacytic inflammatory infiltrate and lymph follicle formation (Fig. 25.9).

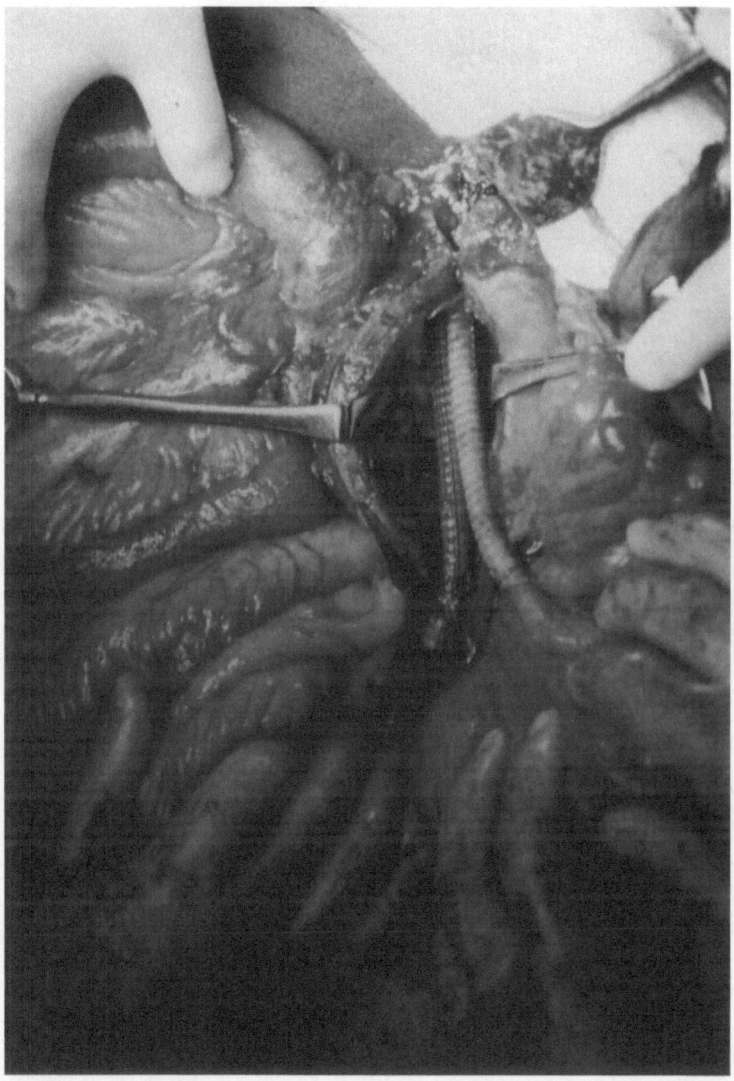

FIGURE 25.6. An Ochsner bifurcation graft that has been implanted by an inclusion technique.

Signs and Symptoms

Signs and symptoms of the present series of 10 individuals are shown in Table 25.1. Abdominal pain, lumbago, abdominal distension, claudication, and hematuria have been seen. Among these symptoms, claudication is the result of accompanying arterial occlusion. Increased ESR with positive CRP is common. This sign of inflammation has spontaneously subsided after graft replacement. Hydroureter is frequent, which has become ameliorated after

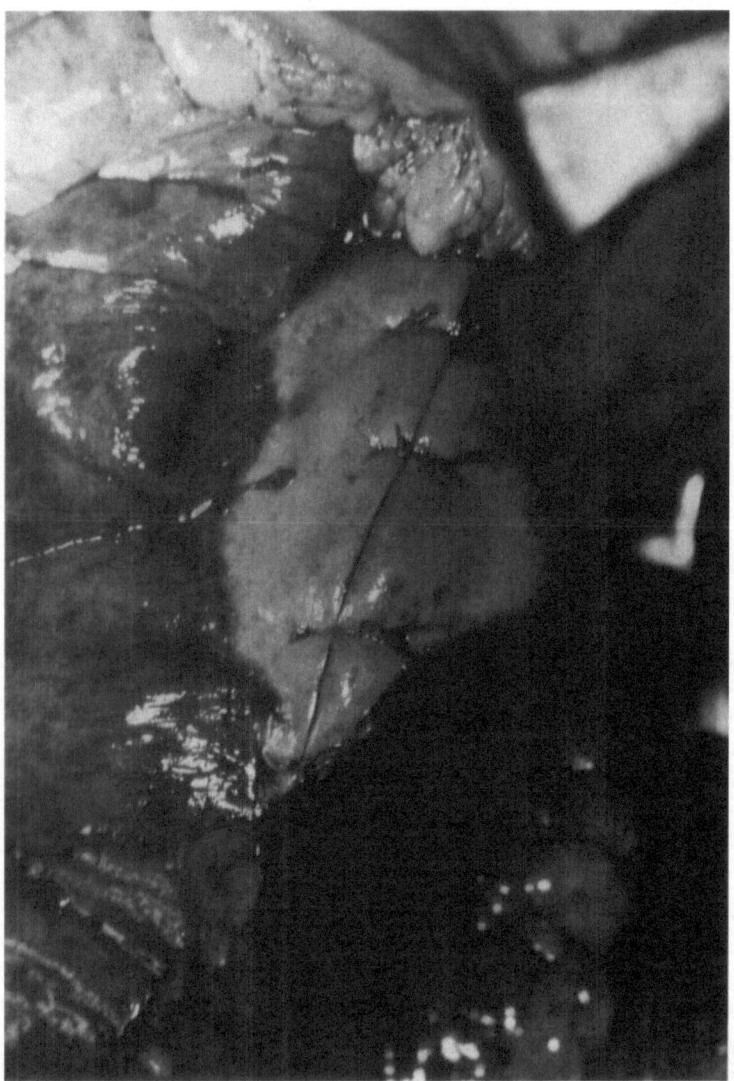

FIGURE 25.7. The graft has been covered with the aneurysmal wall.

graft replacement. Mantle sign on CT scan is the most characteristic evidence of inflammatory abdominal aortic aneurysm. Magnetic resonance imaging (MRI) is also a useful tool for demonstration of Mantle sign (Fig. 25.10).

Operative Methods

The inclusion technique was utilized in 60% of operations and thrombo-exclusion in the remaining 40% (Table 25.2). As a supportive measure, particularly for the proximal anastomotic site, Dacronfelt wrapping was performed

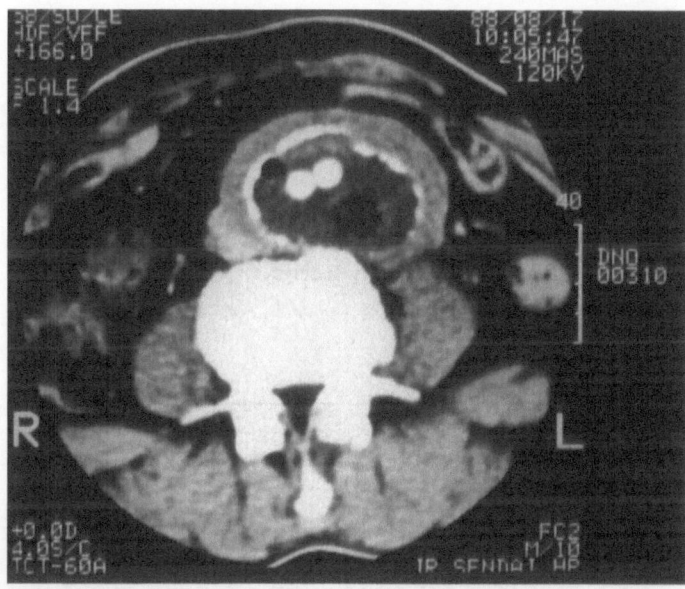

FIGURE 25.8. A 20-day-postoperative CT scan demonstrates patency of both limbs of the graft.

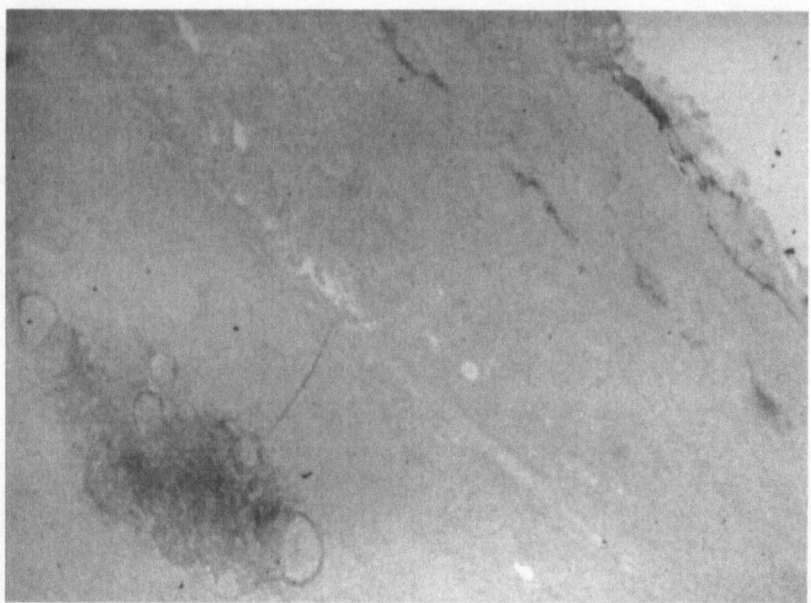

FIGURE 25.9. Histopathological examination reveals atheromatous change within the aneurysmal lumen and foam cells.

TABLE 25.1. Diagnosis of inflammatory abdominal aortic aneurysms

Signs and symptoms	% of patients
Abdominal pain	50
Lumbago	20
Abdominal distension	10
Claudication	10
Hematuria	10
Clinical and laboratory findings	
Positive CRP	80
Increased ESR	90
Hydroureter	40
Mantle sign	90

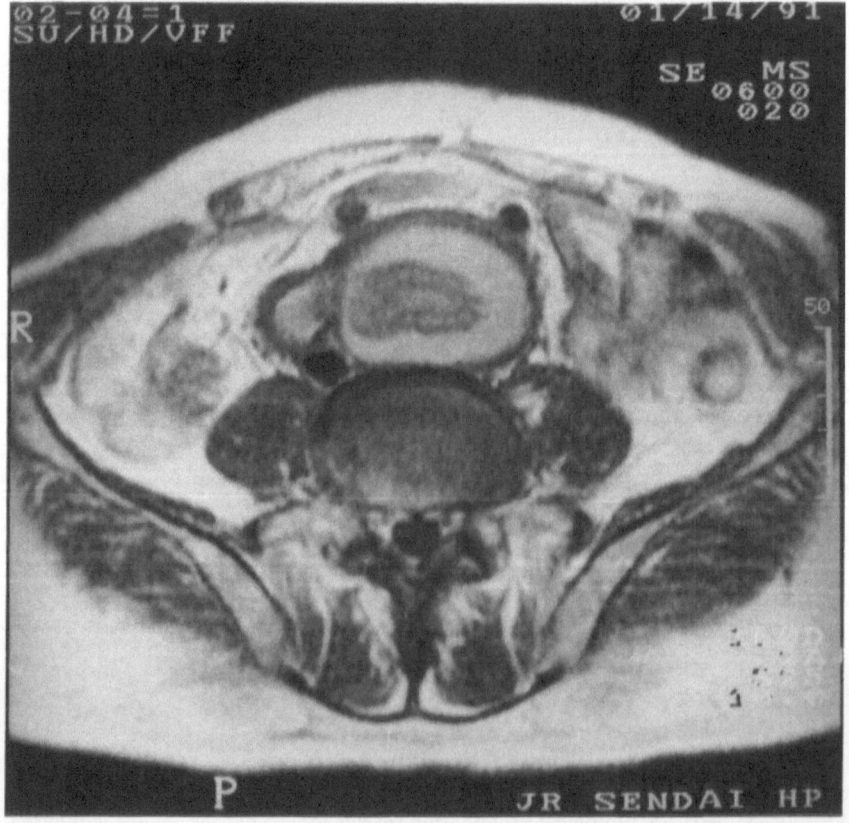

FIGURE 25.10. The MRI is also a useful tool for demonstration of the Mantle sign.

TABLE 25.2. Inflammatory abdominal aortic aneurysms: Operative methods

Op. method	%	Dacronfelt	%	Graft	%
Inclusion	60	+	70	Cooley	30
Thromboexcl.	40	−	30	Ochsner	70

TABLE 25.3. Inflammatory abdominal aortic aneurysms: Outcome

Death		3/10
Early	Cerebral thrombosis	1
	Cardiac complications	1
Late	Aortoduodenal fistula	1
Surviving		7/10
Range: 10 mos to 5 yrs & 11 mos		
Mean: 3 yrs & 7 mos		

TABLE 25.4. Inflammatory abdominal aortic aneurysms: Histopathology

Findings	%
Atherosclerosis	90
Cystic medionecrosis with moderate atherosclerosis	10
Medial atrophy and/or degeneration and fibrosis	60
Lymphoplasmacytic inflammatory infiltrate, adventitial and perivascular	70

in 70% of the cases. The synthetic grafts utilized were Cooley double velour bifurcation graft in 30% and Ochsner graft in 70%. On one occasion, division and reanastomosis of the left renal vein had to be added to facilitate a proper transection of the infrarenal aorta and implantation of the synthetic graft.

The outcome of 10 cases is summarized in Table 25.3. Early death occurred in 2 patients, 1 cerebral and 1 cardiac. Late death was seen in 1 with complicated aortoduodenal fistula 10 months after graft implantation. He failed to respond to reimplantation, resulting in death 1 year after the initial operation. The remaining 7 individuals have survived after operation, from 10 months to 5 years and 11 months, with a mean of 3 years and 7 months.

Histopathology is summarized in Table 25.4. Atherosclerosis was seen in 90% of the cases. Cystic medionecrosis with moderate atherosclerosis was detected in 10%. Medial atrophy and/or degeneration and fibrosis were demonstrated in 60%. In 70%, lymphoplasmacytic inflammatory infiltrate was predominant in the adventitial and/or perivascular layer.

Comment

The history of inflammatory abdominal aortic aneurysm dates back to 1935, when James[1] first described the disease. In 1955 DeWeerd and associates[2] performed the first surgical operation. Bilateral nephrostomy and uretrolysis were done without graft implantation. In the same year Shumacker and Garrett[3] reported a case of graft replacement and bilateral ureterolysis. On the other hand, Walker and associates[4] first named inflammatory aortic aneurysm. They reported 19 patients. Rupture was seen in 15% and overall mortality was 31%. In 1977 Clyne[5] found that the steroids were effective for control of inflammation and relief of ureteral obstruction.

In 1992 Kazmier[6] from the Ochsner Clinic accumulated a large number of patients comprising 2,816 cases subject to aortic grafting for abdominal aortic aneurysms. Among these, there were 127 abdominal aortic aneurysms of the inflammatory type, indicating an incidence of 4.3%. Ureteral compression was detected in 20%. The symptoms were abdominal pain, weight loss, ureteric colic, tenderness, and (in 37.0% of patients) associated arterial occlusion. In 1985 Crawford and associates[7] stated that inflammation was found at the thoracic or thoracoabdominal aorta. Kazmier[6] has commented on similar lesions. Duodenal adhesion is most frequent.

In regard to theories of inflammation, in 1972 Mitchinson[8] proposed that spasm-induced ischemic damage to the aortic wall led to leakage of atheromatous material into the media and adventitia, causing an immune-mediated reaction and resulting in periaortitis with characteristic lymphoplasmacytic infiltrate. In 1983 Haust[9] postulated that the intimal thickening and atheroma deposition caused reduction of transintimal penetration of nutrients into the aortic media, resulting in reactive proliferation of vasa in normally avascular media. In 1988 West[10] reported that local hypoperfusion due to histologically confirmed atheroemboli to vasa arterioles induced ischemia or infarction of the media with resultant disappearance or thinning of the medial coat and periaortitis.

Preoperative diagnosis is not difficult with the use of sophisticated modern diagnostic tools such as CT, MRI, and echography in conjunction with laboratory data showing increased ESR and positive CRP. The first Japanese report on this surgical entity, by Yasuda and associates,[11] appeared in 1987.

To avoid injury to the surrounding tissues and organs during operation, minimal dissection is mandatory. Following graft replacement, the inflammatory process will subside. Ureterolysis is not required, since spontaneous relief or amelioration of ureteral obstruction can be expected.

References

1. James TGI. Uremia due to aneurysm of the abdominal aorta. Br J Urol 1935;7: 157.
2. DeWeerd JH, Ringer MG, Jr, Pool TL, Cambill EE. Aortic aneurysm causing bilateral ureteral obstruction: Report of case. J Urol 1955;74:78–81.

3. Shumacker HB, Jr, Garrett R. Obstructive uropathy from aortic aneurysm. Surg Gynecol Obstet 1955;100:785–761.
4. Walker DI, Bloor K, Williams G, et al. Inflammatory aneurysms of the abdominal aorta. Br J Surg 1972;59:609.
5. Clyne CAA, Abercrombie GF. Perianeurysmal retroperitoneal fibrosis: Two cases responding to steroids. Br J Urol 1977;49:463–467.
6. Kazmier F. Inflammatory abdominal aortic aneurysm. Presented at the 20th Annual Congress of Japan Society for Vascular Surgery, Sapporo, Japan. July 1, 1992.
7. Crawford JL, et al. Inflammatory aneurysms of the aorta. J Vasc Surg 1985;2: 113–124.
8. Mitchinson MJ. Aortic disease in idiopathic retroperitoneal and mediastinal fibrosis. J Clin Pathol 1972;25:287–293.
9. Haust MD. Atherosclerosis-lesions and sequelae. In: Silver MD (ed.). Cardiovascular Pathology. London: Churchill Livingstone, 1983, pp. 191–315.
10. West AB, Path MRC, Ryan PC. Inflammatory aortic aneurysm: Report of a case suggesting athero-ischemic aetiology. J Cardiovasc Surg 1988;29:213–215.
11. Yasuda K, Sakuma M, Go K, et al. Surgical treatments for inflammatory abdominal aortic aneurysm. J Jpn Surg Soc 1987;88:1503 (in Japanese).

26
Inflammatory Aneurysms of the Abdominal Aorta

Keishu Yasuda, Makoto Sakuma, Yoshiro Matsui, and
Tatsuzo Tanabe

The term "inflammatory abdominal aortic aneurysm" (IAAA.) was coined by Walker et al.[1] in 1972 describing a group of 19 patients with an abdominal aortic aneurysm (AAA) with excessive mural thickening and adherence of structures adjacent to the aneurysm. The cases represented 10% of their total series of AAAs. The operative mortality rate in these cases was 31%. Goldstone et al.[2] in 1978 described in detail their most recent consecutive 200 patients with AAA. They summarized the pathologic and clinical features of the disease and suggested technical modifications to make graft operation safer, including minimal dissection of the tissue adjacent to the aneurysm, clamping the aorta above the level of the duodenum, and graft insertion with the inclusion technique. IAAAs constitute 2.5% to 15% of all AAAs.[3-5] Despite this prevalence, signs and symptoms and diagnostic findings of IAAAs are not well understood and etiology is speculative.[6,7] We report here our experience at Hokkaido University Hospital concerning clinical presentation, severity of the inflammatory process, and operative management of IAAA.

Clinical Material and Methods

The records of 263 patients who underwent repair of an AAA from 1986 to 1991 were reviewed. Twenty-nine (11%) were women and 234 (89%) were men. Eleven (10 men and 1 woman) were diagnosed as cases of IAAA based on the intraoperative presence of perianeurysmal fibrosis, marked thickening of the aneurysmal wall, and adherence of adjacent structures to the aneurysm.

Results

Profiles and Symptoms in Patients with IAAA

Eleven patients (4.2%, 1 woman and 10 men) of 263 patients with AAA had IAAA. These patients ranged in age from 53 to 75 years, the mean age being

65 years. In our study, the range of age for patients with typical atherosclerotic AAA was 52 to 84 years, with an average age of 68 years.

Nine patients with IAAA were hypertensive, 1 was diabetic, 3 had renal dysfunction, 3 had coronary artery disease, 2 had cerebrovascular disease, and 1 had occlusive disease of the lower extremity. The striking feature of IAAA was that most of the patients were symptomatic and the condition may be confused with ruptured or expanding AAA. Ten of the patients with IAAA presented with abdominal, back, or flank pain or abdominal tenderness. Weight loss had occurred in 6 patients (Tables 26.1 and 26.2)

Laboratory Data

Preoperative laboratory data are given in Table 26.3. Slight elevation in temperature was noted in 4/11 patients. Erythrocyte sedimentation rate (ESR) was elevated in 5/5 patients. Eighty percent of the patients were C-reactive protein (CRP) positive. Serologic tests for syphylis were negative (Table 26.3).

TABLE 26.1. Profile of patients with AAA

	Inflammatory	Noninflammatory
No. of patients	11 (4.2%)	252 (95.8%)
Age (years)	65 (53–75)	68 (52–84)
Sex		
Male	10 (91%)	224 (89%)
Female	1 (9%)	28 (11%)
Pain	9 (82%)	25 (10%)
Ruptured	0 (0%)	29 (12%)
Symptomatic	11 (100%)	214 (81%)
Asymptomatic	0 (0%)	38 (19%)

TABLE 26.2. Symptoms of patients with IAAA ($n = 11$)

Abdominal pain	6(55%)
Back pain	1(10%)
Flank pain	1(10%)
Tenderness	2(20%)
Weight loss	6(55%)
Fever	3(27%)

TABLE 26.3. Preoperative laboratory data

ESR elevation	5/5(100%)
CRP positive	4/5(80%)
Syphilis	0/6(0%)
Rheumatoid arthritis	0/3(0%)

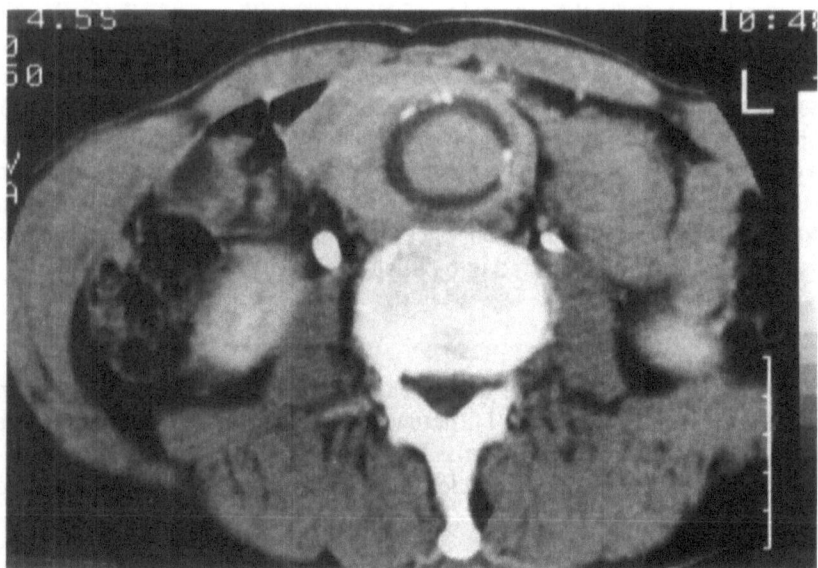

FIGURE 26.1 CT scans of a patient with IAAA. The contrast enhancement of the thickened aneurysm wall is diagnostic of the inflammatory process. (a) CT scan performed before steroid therapy showed typical enhanced inflammatory mass (23 April 1987). (b) CT scan performed 3 months after steroid therapy showed regression of the inflammatory mass (24 July 1984). (c) CT scan performed 4 years after steroid therapy showed regression of the enhanced inflammatory mass.

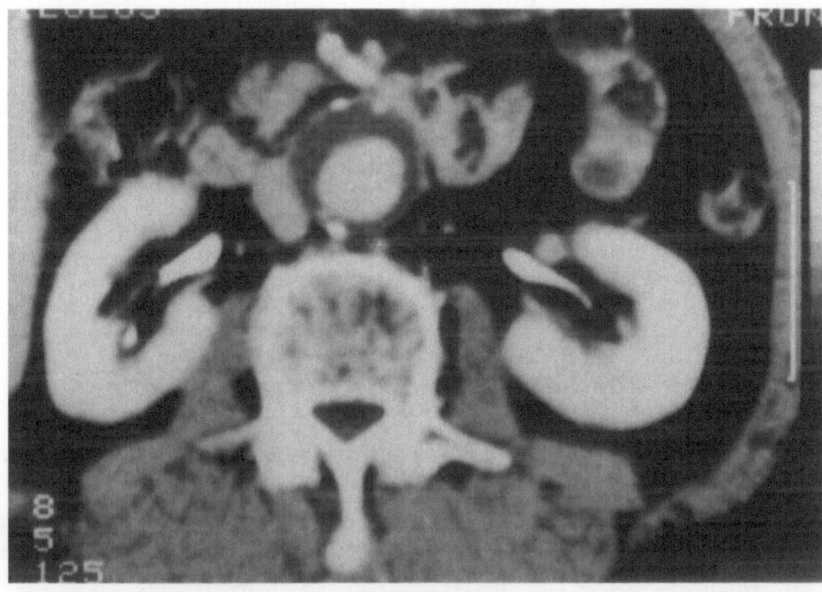

C

FIGURE 26.1 (*continued*)

Radiological Findings

Preoperative diagnostic studies included computed tomographic (CT) scan in 11 patients, sonography in 6, and angiography in 9 patients. The size of the aneurysm ranged from 53 to 76 mm (mean 61.8 mm). Diagnosis was immediately suspected when the CT scans showed a contrast-ehnancing thickened inflammatory wall lying outside the lucent rim of the intima and subintima (mantle core sign) (Fig. 26.1). The mantle core sign was recognized in all 11 patients. Abdominal ultrasound detected a sonolucent halo and thickening of the aortic wall. In 2 patients a second or third CT examination was performed prior to surgery, and resolution of the inflammatory process was evident (Fig. 26.1 and 26.2)

Ureteric stenosis and compression of the inferior vena cava were seen in two patients

Operative Findings

All 11 patients had perianeurysmal inflammation, with thick, dense, glistening fibrous tissue that often involved adjacent structures (Fig. 26.3). In one patient, fibrosis was particularly marked in tissues around the duodenum and the common iliac vessels. Resection of the aneurysm was abandoned because of exposure difficulties and visceral arterial involvement. This patient is alive 5 years after laparotomy. CT scan done 4 years after operation showed resolution of the inflammatory process (Fig. 26.1). Control of the

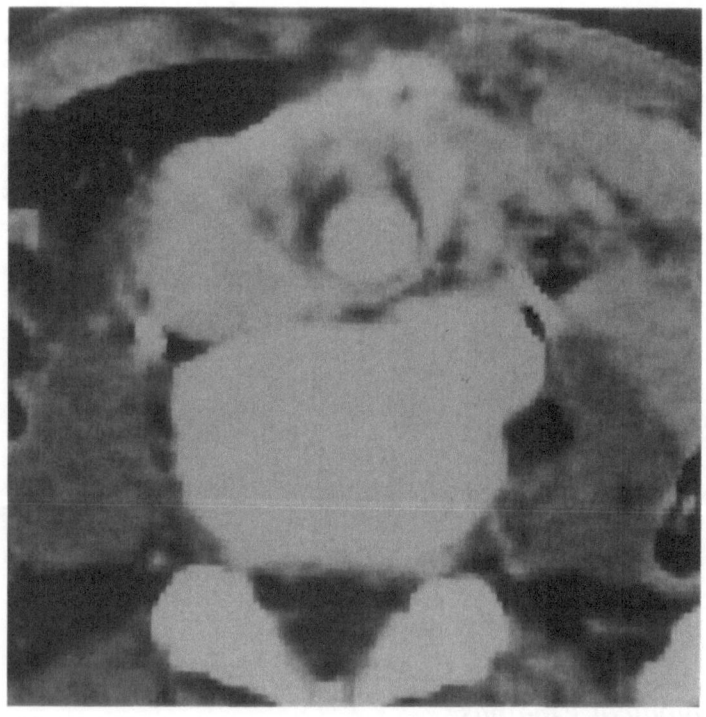

A

FIGURE 26.2. CT scans of a patient with IAAA. CT scans showed typical enhanced inflammatory mass. After 5 months of treatment with steroid, a regression of the enhanced inflammatory mass was seen, but the CT revealed a marked increase in the size of the aneurysm. (a) 8 March 1990; (b) 6 April 1990; (c) 9 July 1990.

aorta was obtained through the infarenal arteries in 9 patients and the supra-renal arteries in 2. In 10 patients, aneurysms were resected and the aorta was reconstructed with a prosthetic graft. A bifurcated graft was placed in 8 patients, and a tube graft was used in 2 cases.

Pathology

There was marked intimal proliferation and fibrosis with cholesterol cleft and foci of mononuclear cells. The media showed loss of smooth muscle, inflammatory infiltration, and collagenization. The adventitia was markedly thickened and was infiltrated with numerous aggregates of lymphocytes (Fig. 26.4).

Operative Results

All 11 patients survived the operation (30 days). Transient renal failure not requiring hemodialysis occurred in 2 patients. Pneumonia and gastrointesti-nal bleeding occurred in 1 patient.

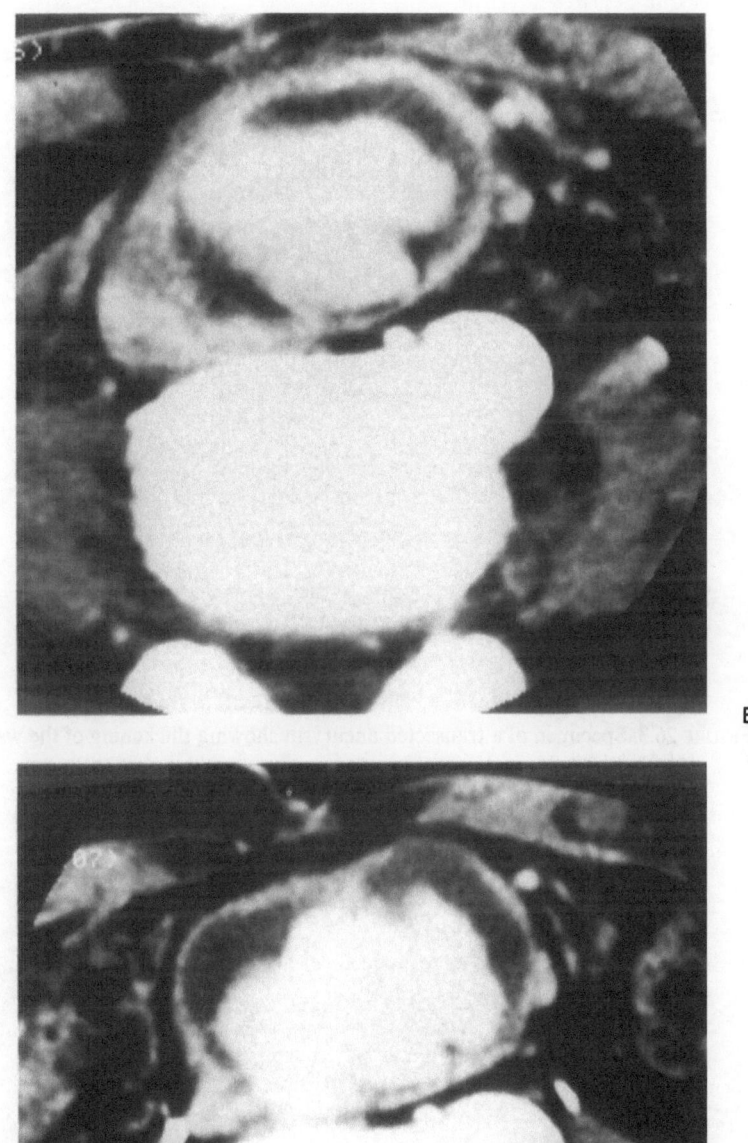

B

C

FIGURE 26.2 (*continued*)

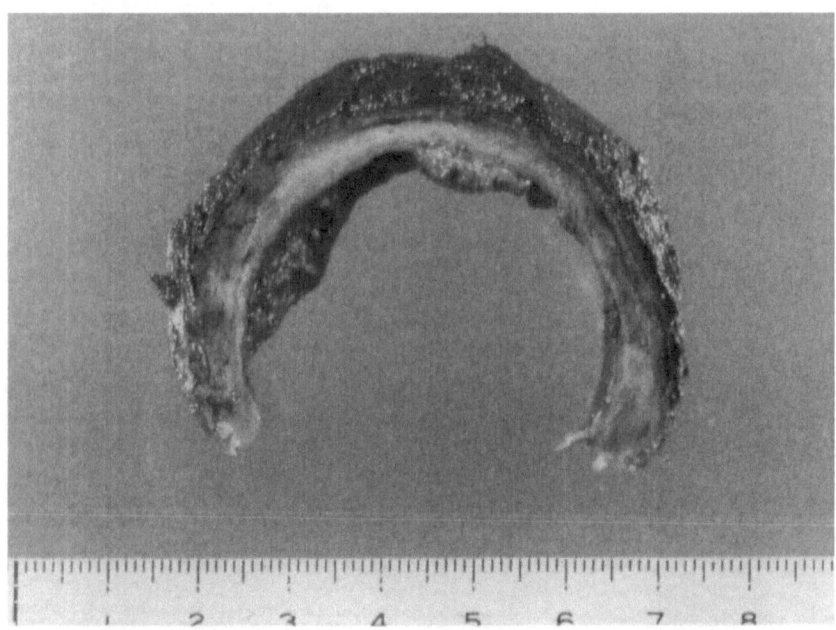

FIGURE 26.3. Specimen of a transected aneurysm showing thickening of the wall.

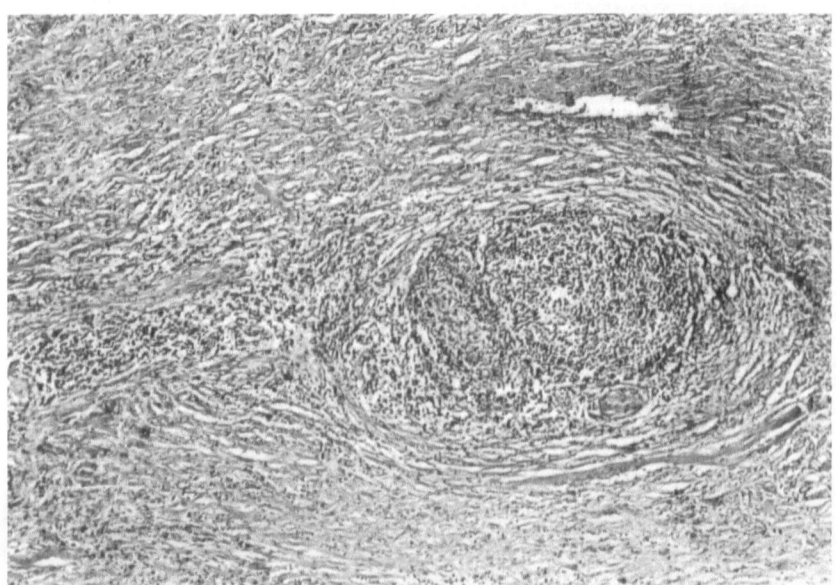

FIGURE 26.4. Photograph of aortic wall from resected specimen showing chronic inflammatory cell focus (hematoxylin and eosin × 100).

TABLE 26.4. Operative results of 11 patients with
IAAA

Survivors	11
Complications	
Renal failure (transient)	1
Pneumonia and GI bleeding	1
Follow-up: 2 months to 8 years (mean 25 months)	
Deaths	2
Pneumomia (2 months p.o.)	
Rupture of TAA (2 years p.o.)	

The length of follow-up of the 11 patients was from 2 months to 8 years
(mean 25 months). Of the 11 patients who survived surgery, one died of
pneumonia 2 months after operation, and another who had separate inflammatory aneurysms of the descending thoracic aorta and the infrarenal
abdominal aorta died 2 years after AAA operation due to rupture of the
thoracic arota. One patient who underwent exploratory surgery and who
was treated with a steroid remains alive 5 years later. Nine patients are alive
up to 8 years after the operation (Table 26.4).

Case Report

Case 1

A 67-year-old man was admitted because of an AAA. There was a 3-month
history of abdominal pain and claudication of the left calf. Ct scan revealed
a 42-mm AAA with the appearance of an inflammatory aneurysm with a
thickened aneurysmal wall. At surgery, extensive fibrotic adhesions between
the aneurysm and the duodenum were visible, and mobilization of the duodenum was difficult. Surgery was abandoned and the patient was treated with
prednisone. Two months later he was free of pain and fever was down.

Four years later there was no increase in size of the aneurysm. A CT scan
performed 5 years after the first examination showed resolution of the inflammatory process (Fig. 26.1).

Case 2

A 65-year-old man had a 5-month history of abdominal pain, weight loss,
and slight fever. Examination revealed a elevated ESR and a positive CRP.
CT scan revealed a 58-mm AAA with typical IAAA. Prednisone was prescribed for 5 months, and after this treatment, while he was free from abdominal pain, the CT revealed a marked increase in size of the aneurysm (Fig.
26.2). Five months later surgery was performed, and he remains well 5 years
after this surgery.

Comment and Summary

IAAA should be considered a clinical and anatomical entity separate from atherosclerotic aneurysm, because of involvement of adjacent structures and of different therapeutic implications. The incidence of IAAA in the literature is 2.5% to 15%.[3-5] The etiology is uncertain, but it is evident both macroscopically and microscopically that IAAA differs from atherosclerotic AAA.[2,5-8]

Until recently, the diagnosis of this type of aneurysm was not made before surgery. Symptoms of abdominal pain, weight loss, and elevated ESR in a patient with AAA are highly suggestive of an inflammatory aneurysm. Characteristic CT scans with contrast and exhibiting periaortic inflammation or involvement of adjacent structures seem to be the most reliable diagnostic test.[5,9-12]

Resection of the aneurysm with prosthetic graft replacement is recommended, but graft replacement in these patients is often difficult and is associated with increase in morbidity and mortality. At surgery, no attempt should be made to mobilize adjacent viscera in order to avoid injury. Arterial control should be obtained with minimal dissection. Some authors have described effective steroid therapy which resolved the inflammatory process and alleviated the symptoms; however, surgery remains the treatment of choice.[5,13]

A retrospective review of 263 patients who underwent repair of AAA in Hokkaido University Hospital revealed 11 (4.2%) aneurysms considered to be inflammatory. The symptoms included severe abdominal, back, or flank pain and abdominal tenderness, suggesting rupture or leakage. The diagnoses were based on findings of CT scans and clinical symptoms in all 11 patients. Ten patients underwent aneurysm resection and graft replacement. Exploratory surgery was performed in one patient because of exposure difficulties and visceral arterial involvement. Treatment with prednisone was prescribed. Three of 10 patients were emergency cases because of severe abdominal pain, but there was no evidence of ruptured aneurysm. All patients had characteristic gross findings of a densely inflamed retroperitoneal mass with a white, glistening area centrally with surrounding injection of neovascularity and puckering of the adjacent mesentery. All 10 patients who underwent aneurysm resection and 1 patient who underwent exploratory operation survived. Two patients died after surgery, 1 after 2 months and 1 after 2 years. Nine patients are alive.

Conclusions

1. IAAA is considered a clinical and anatomic entity separate from atherosclerotic aneurysm because of involvement of adjacent structures and because of different therapeutic implications.

2. The diagnosis of IAAA can be made preoperatively by the presence of symptoms and elevated ESR in a patient with AAA.
3. CT scan with contrast exhibiting periaortic inflammation or involvement of adjacent structures is the most reliable diagnostic test.
4. Resection of the aneurysm with prosthetic graft replacement is recommended and can be performed with excellent results.
5. Steroids may reduce the inflammatory process, but they should not be used as a substitute for surgery.

References

1. Walker DI, Bloor K, Williams G, et al. Inflammatory aneurysms of the abdominal aorta. Br J Surg 1972;59:609.
2. Goldstone J, Malone JM, Moore WS. Inflammatory abdominal aortic aneurysms of the aorta. Surgery 1978;83:425.
3. Pennel RC, Hollier LH, Lie JT, et al. Inflammatory abdominal aortic aneurysms: A thirty-year review. J Vasc Surg 1985;2:859.
4. Crawford JL, Stowe CL, Safi HJ, et al. Inflammatory aneurysms of the aorta. J Vasc Surg 1985;2:113.
5. Cullenward MJ, Scanlan KA, Pozniak MA, et al. Inflammatory aortic aneurysms (periaortic fibrosis). Radiologic Imaging. Radiology 1988;159;75.
6. Abbott DK, Skinner DG, Yalowitz PA, et al. Retroperitoneal fibrosis associated with abdominal aortic aneurysms: An approach to management. J Urol 1973;109.
7. Rose AG, Dent DM. Inflammatory variant of abdominal aortic aneurysms. Arch Pathol Lab Med 1981;105:409.
8. Almgren B, Eriksson I, Forsberg JO, et al. Abdominal aortic aneurysm with retroperitoneal fibrosis. A clinical entity. Acta Chir Scand 1981;147:539.
9. Henry LG, Doust B, Korns ME, et al. Abdominal aortic aneurysm and retroperitoneal fibrosis. Ultrasonic diagnosis and treatment. Arch Surg 1978;113:1456.
10. Bundy AL, Ritchie WGM. Inflammatory aneurysm of the abdominal aorta. J Cardiovasc Ultrasonogr 1984;12:102.
11. Vint VC, Usselman JA, Warmanth MA, et al. Aortic perianeurysmal fibrosis: CT density enhanced and ureteral obstruction. Am J Roentgenol 1980;134:577.
12. Degesys GE, Dunnick NR, Silverman PM, et al. Retroperitoneal fibrosis. Use of CT in distinguishing possible causes. AM J Roentgenol 1986;146:57.
13. Bainbridge ET, Woodward DAK. Inflammatory aneurysms of the abdominal aorta with associated ureteric obstruction or medial deviation. J Cardiovasc Surg 1982;23:365.

27
Treatment of Consumption Coagulopathy Complicated with Abdominal Aortic Aneurysm

Haruo Aramoto, Hiroshi Shigematsu, Toshiyuki Kubo, and Tetsuichiro Muto

Introduction

Disseminated intravascular coagulation (DIC) has been described as an occasional complication of abdominal aortic aneurysm (AAA). However, the mechanism of DIC caused by AAA differs from that of DIC caused by sepsis, carcinoma, or leukemia, and apparently involves chronic and local consumption coagulopathy in the aneurysm or on the surface of the mural thrombus. The definitive treatment for DIC is removal of the underlying cause, i.e., removal of AAA. However, hemorrhage often complicates surgery. In the present article, we examine the effect of a protease inhibitor (nafamostat mesilate; Futhan) on coagulopathy accompanying AAA.

Materials and Methods

Patients (Table 27.1)

From 100 patients who underwent AAA repair from January 1988 to September 1991, we studied 58 patients with unruptured AAA and normal liver function whose coagulative and fibrinolytic function could be followed perioperatively. These patients were divided into two groups (group A and group N) preoperatively on the basis of the criteria for coagulation abnormalities in the "Diagnostic Criteria of DIC" proposed by the Ministry of Health and Welfare of Japan in 1988 (Table 27.2). Group A was further divided into two subgroups [subgroup A(+) and subgroup A(−)], according to the need for preoperative control of the bleeding disorder by the protease inhibitor.

Administration of Nafamostat Mesilate

Nafamostat mesilate was administered only preoperatively for 4 to 12 days in doses ranging from 60 to 80 mg per day. The total amount administered ranged from 300 to 720 mg (mean 450 mg).

TABLE 27.1. Patient groups.

Normal group	Patients failing to meet any of the criteria of coagulation abnormalities in diagnostic criteria of DIC (group N; $n = 32$)
Abnormal group	Patients satisfying 1 or more of the criteria of coagulation abnormalities (group A; $n = 26$)
Subgroup A($+$)	Patients who required preoperative administration of Futhan ($n = 6$)
Subgroup A($-$)	Patients who did not require preoperative control ($n = 20$)

TABLE 27.2. Diagnostic criteria of DIC (proposed by the Ministry of Health and Welfare of Japan in 1988)

				Score
I Cause			$+$	1
			$-$	0
II Clinical symptoms	1) Bleeding disorder		$+$	1
	2) Organ dysfunction		$-$	0
			$+$	1
			$-$	0
III Criteria of coagulation abnormalities				
1) Serum FDP level(μg/ml)		$40 \leqq$		3
		$20 \leqq$	< 40	2
		$10 \leqq$	< 20	1
		$10 >$		0
2) Platelet count($\times 10^3/\mu$l)		$50 \geqq$		3
		$80 \geqq$	> 50	2
		$120 \geqq$	> 80	1
		$120 <$		0
3) Plasma level of fibrinogen(mg/dl)		$100 \geqq$		2
		$150 \geqq$	> 100	1
		$150 <$		0
4) Prothrombin time(ratio)(%)		$60 \geqq$		2
		$80 \geqq$	> 60	1
		$80 <$		0

Total score $7 \leqq$: DIC; 6: DIC suspected; $5 \geqq$: DIC nearly denied

FDP, Fibrin/fibrinogen degradation products.

Coagulative and Fibrinolytic Parameters

We measured intraoperative blood loss and surgical duration, and performed coagulation tests on admission, before surgery and at the first, seventh, and fourteenth postoperative day. The coagulation tests were as follows: platelet count (Plt), prothrombin time (PT), activated partial thromboplastin time (aPTT), fibrinogen (Fbg), plasminogen activity (Plg), fibrin/fibrinogen degradation products (FDP), antithrombin III activity (AT-III), and α-2-plasmin inhibitor (α-2-PI). In addition, we also calculated the DIC score of each group on admission and after drug administration by comparing these parameters to the Diagnostic Criteria of DIC.

Statistical Analysis

Group laboratory data were expressed as mean or mean ± standard deviation (s.d.). The differences between groups were analyzed by Student's unpaired t-test. PT, Plg, AT-III, and α-2-PI are shown as percentages versus normal mixed plasma from 10 healthy individuals.

Results

There was no significant difference between the mean duration of surgery in groups N and A (294.3 ± 57.5 vs. 358.9 ± 126.9 min, respectively). However, there was a significant difference between the mean intraoperative blood loss (1,186.1 ± 832.9 g in group N vs. 2,146.7 ± 1,164.4 g in group A; $p < 0.01$) (Fig. 27.1).

Figure 27.2 shows the preoperative levels of various parameters in subgroups A(+) and A(−). On admission, the mean AT-III in subgroup A(−) was more than 70% of normal activity. However, the mean AT-III of subgroup A(+) was significantly lower [66.8 ± 14.8 vs. 86.0 ± 7.4% in subgroups A(−) and A(+), respectively; $p < 0.05$], and three patients had baseline activity levels below 70%. After administration of Futhan, the mean value in subgroup A(+) significantly increased to 84.3% ($p < 0.05$). The mean Plt in subgroup A(+) was lower than that in subgroup A(−)(17.1 ±

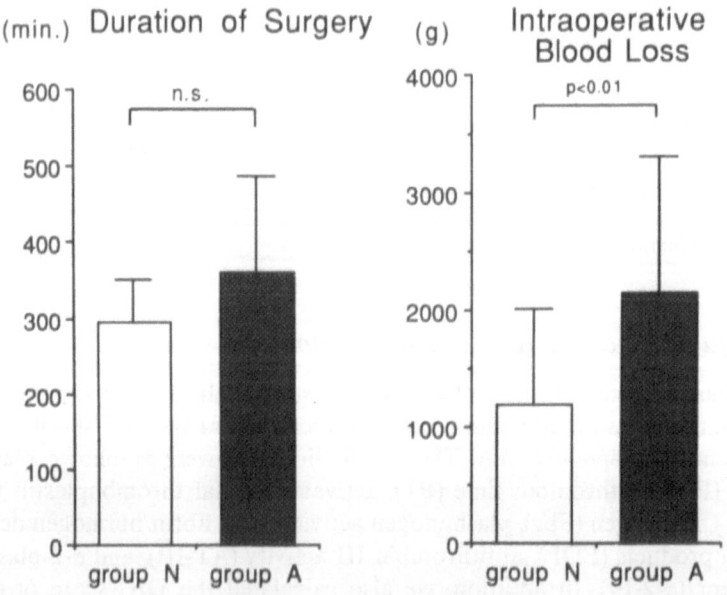

FIGURE 27.1. Duration of surgery and intraoperative blood loss in each patient group. □, Mean values in group N; ■, mean values in group A.

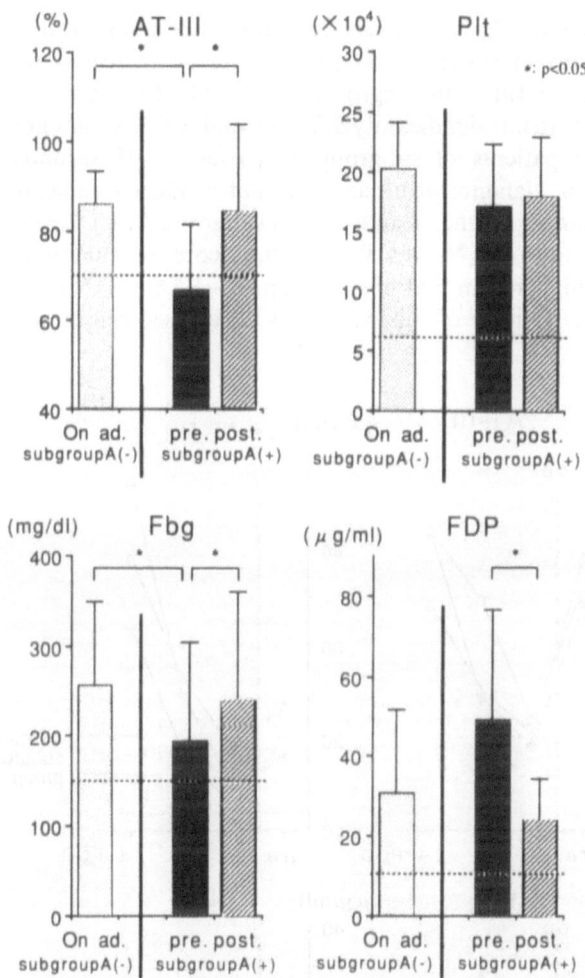

FIGURE 27.2. Preoperative levels of AT-III, Plt, Fbg, and FDP in each subgroup. ▨, Mean values in subgroup A(−); ■, mean values in subgroup A(+) before Futhan infusion; ▨, mean values in subgroup A(+) after infusion. The dotted horizontal lines represent the threshold level of each parameter; On ad. = on admission; pre. = before infusion of Futhan; post. = after infusion of Futhan.

5.2 vs. $20.2 \pm 3.9 \times 10^4$, respectively; not significant) on admission and showed no apparent change despite the infusion of nafamostat mesilate. On admission, the mean Fbg in subgroup A(+) was lower than that in subgroup A(−)(194 ± 110.7 vs. 256 ± 93.6 mg/dL, respectively; $p < 0.05$), but rose to 239 mg/dL ($p < 0.05$) after Futhan therapy. The mean FDP in subgroup A(−) was 31 μg/mL, ($p < 0.05$) as a result of administration of nafamostat mesilate. The mean preoperative PT ratios in subgroups A(−) and A(+)

were 97.1% and 67.3%, respectively. However, after administration of Futhan, the mean ratio in subgroup A(+) significantly increased to 77.7%. On admission, aPTT values in subgroups A(−) and A(+)(36.1 ± 4.9 vs. 37.0 ± 6.1 seconds) were not significantly different, and aPTT values greater than 40 seconds in 2 patients of subgroup A(+) fell to 35 seconds after drug administration. Nafamostat mesilate did not produce significant changes in either the mean Plg or the mean α-2-PI in subgroup A(+). On admission, the DIC score of group N was 0, and the score of subgroup A(+) was significantly higher than that of subgroup A(−)(5.6 vs. 2.8; $p < 0.05$). Before surgery, the DIC score of subgroup A(+) decreased significantly to almost

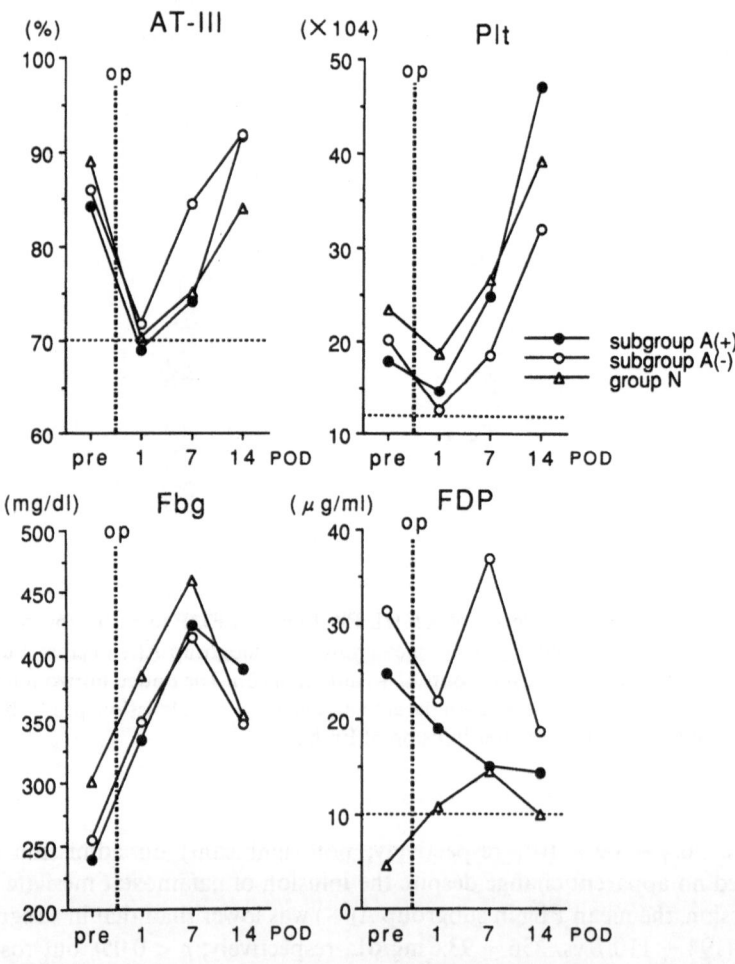

FIGURE 27.3. Perioperative changes in AT-III, Plt, Fbg, and FDP in each group. The dotted horizontal lines represent the threshold level of each parameter; pre = before surgery; op = operation; POD = postoperative day.

the same level as that seen in subgroup A(−)(2.9 vs. 2.8) as a result of preoperative Futhan therapy.

Figures 27.3 and 27.4 show the perioperative changes in the parameters of the three groups. Mean AT-III in all of the groups declined as a result of surgery, but soon recovered to more than 80% of normal activity by the fourteenth postoperative day. The mean Plt in all of the groups transiently decreased after AAA repair but soon recovered, rising to a value appreciably

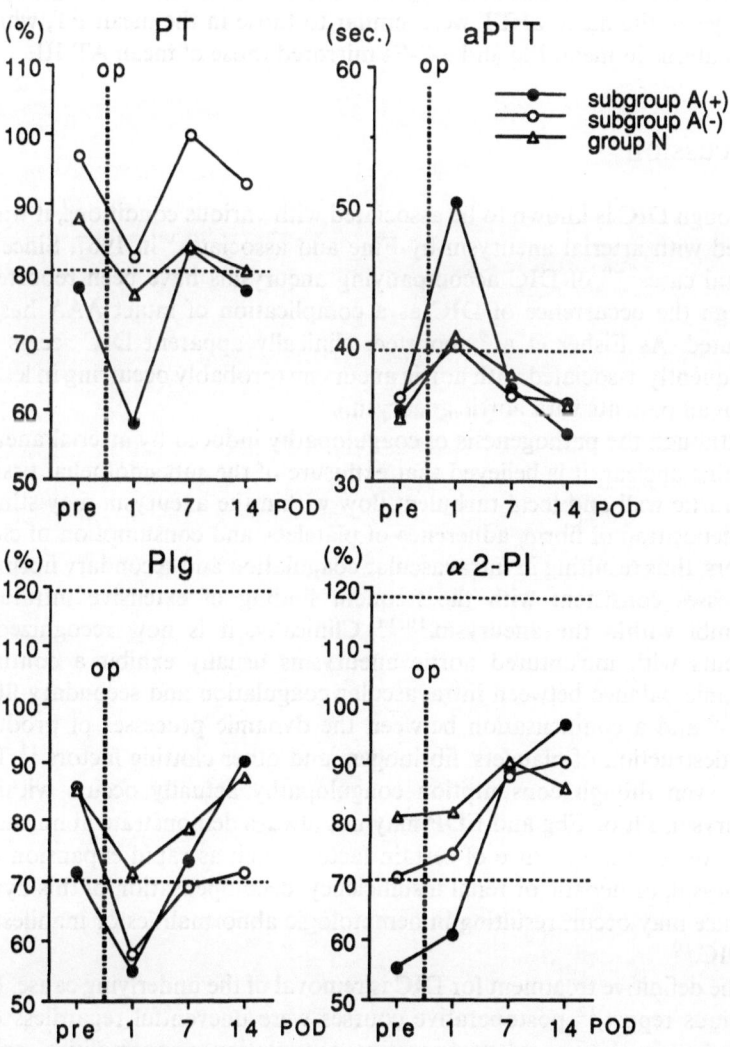

FIGURE 27.4. Perioperative changes in PT, aPTT, Plg, and α 2-PI in each group. The dotted horizontal lines represent the threshold level of each parameter; pre = before surgery; op = operation; POD = postoperative day.

higher than the mean preoperative count 14 days after surgery. Fbg rapidly rose above 200 mg/dL in all of the groups, and after the seventh postoperative day, these values remained at levels greater than 150 mg/dL. There was no significant intergroup difference in Fbg values postoperatively. In all of the groups, FDP either remained at high values or rose gradually until 7 days after surgery. By the fourteenth postoperative day, these levels had declined. Although the mean PT was prolonged in all of the groups 1 day after surgery, by the seventh postoperative day, it had partially recovered and showed no significant intergroup differences. In all of the groups, the changes in the mean aPTT were similar to those in the mean PT, while the fluctuations in mean Plg and α-2-PI mirrored those of mean AT-III.

Discussion

Although DIC is known to be associated with various conditions, it was first linked with arterial aneurysm by Fine and associates[1] in 1967. Since then, several cases[2-9] of DIC accompanying aneurysms have been reported, although the occurrence of DIC as a complication of intact AAA has been disputed. As Fisher et al.[9] reported, clinically apparent DIC seems to be infrequently associated with aortic aneurysm (probably occurring in less than 5% of all patients with aortic aneurysm).

Although the pathogenesis of coagulopathy induced by arterial aneurysm remains unclear, it is believed that exposure of the subendothelial tissues of the aortic wall and local turbulent flow within the aneurysm may stimulate the deposition of fibrin, adherence of platelets, and consumption of clotting factors, thus resulting in intravascular coagulation and secondary fibrinolysis processes consistent with the frequent finding of extensive intraluminal thrombi within the aneurysm.[10,11] Clinically, it is now recognized that patients with unruptured aortic aneurysms usually exhibit a continuous dynamic balance between intravascular coagulation and secondary fibrinolysis[10] and a compensation between the dynamic processes of production and destruction of platelets, fibrinogen, and other clotting factors.[11] Therefore, even though consumption coagulopathy actually occurs within the aneurysm, Plt or Fbg and FDP may not always demonstrate abnormalities. However, in the presence of certain factors, such as rapid expansion of the aneurysm, or hepatic or renal insufficiency, decompensation of this dynamic balance may occur, resulting in hematologic abnormalities or manifestation of DIC.[10]

The definitive treatment for DIC is removal of the underlying cause. In our previous report,[12] postoperative courses were uneventful regardless of the presence or absence of preoperative coagulation abnormalities, and the changes in hematologic indices did not differ significantly. Moreover, these indices returned to nearly normal ranges 14 days after AAA repair. Therefore, once a diagnosis is made and other contributory factors have been excluded or treated, aneurysmectomy should be aggressively applied.

Although hemorrhage may complicate the surgical repair and worsen the postoperative course, there is no consensus as to whether an attempt should be made preoperatively to correct the coagulopathy. Several authors have noticed spontaneous correction of the coagulation disorder.[7,13] As Fisher et al[9]. suggested, aneurysm repair may succeed without any preoperative therapy, but transfusion of adequate blood components during surgery and careful surgical technique at all stages are required. In practice, the anticoagulant heparin has been reported to be useful for controlling preoperative consumption coagulopathy and for correction of the hypercoagulable stage. Many authors have used this agent in doses usually ranging from 300 to 600 units per hour and have improved coagulative function.[5,7,10,14,15] However, others[8,9,16] have avoided heparin for fear that it would lead to excessive blood loss and that it could be of no use when AT-III is low or when activation of fibrinolysis is predominant over activation of coagulation.

Synthetic protease inhibitors, which can block serine proteases, such as trypsin, kallikrein, thrombin, and plasmin, may be used to treat pancreatitis and prevent activation of coagulation factors and development of DIC, if administered properly. Although the synthetic protease inhibitors that are currently used in clinical applications, such as gabexate mesilate (FOY)[11] and nafamostat mesilate,[17,18] do not have the same spectrum of action, they may be superior to heparin, and do not require AT-III for their activities because of competitive inhibitors of coagulative enzymes. The half-time of these agents in human circulating blood is usually less than several minutes and less than that of heparin.

For treatment of DIC, nafamostat mesilate may be administered by continuous intravenous infusion at doses ranging from 0.06 to 0.20 mg/kg/hr.[19] According to in vitro studies,[17,18,20,21] nafamostat mesilate is believed to have a more potent inhibitory effect on the coagulation-fibrinolysis system than gabexate mesilate. Nafamostat mesilate has a longer half-time than gabexate mesilate, and produces pain and phlebitis at the infusion site less frequently than gabexate mesilate. In order to treat coagulopathy while preventing fatal rupture, AAA should be aggressively resected. Meticulous surgical repair, as well as proper preoperative control of the bleeding disorder with a protease inhibitor or heparin together with replacement of the blood components during surgery, might be effective in reducing blood loss associated with aneurysmectomy.

References

1. Fine NL, Applebaum J, Elguezabal A, et al. Multiple coagulation defects in association with dissecting aneurysm. Arch Intern Med 1967;119:522–526.
2. Mulcare RJ, Royster TS, Weiss HJ, et al. Disseminated intravascular coagulation

as a complication of abdominal aortic aneurysm repair. Ann Surg 1974;180:343–349.

3. Collins GJ, Rich NM, Scialla, S, et al. Pitfalls in peripheral vascular surgery: Disseminated intravascular coagulation. Am J Surg 1977;134:375–380.

4. Satiani B, Savrin R, Evans W. Consumption coagulopathy associated with arterial aneurysms. J Cardiovasc Surg 1979;20:273–278.

5. Keagy BA, Pharr WF, Bowes DE. Unusual presentations of abdominal aortic aneurysms. J Cardiovasc Surg 1981;22:41–46.

6. Fouser LS, Morrow NE, Davis RB. Platelet dysfunction associated with abdominal aortic aneurysm. Am J Clin Pathol 1980;74:701–705.

7. Bieger R, Vreeken J, Stiebe J, et al. Arterial aneurysm as a cause of consumption coagulopathy. N Engl J Med 1971;285:152–154.

8. Rhodes GR, Cox CB, Silver D. Arteriovenous fistula and false aneurysm as the cause of consumption coagulopathy. Surgery 1973;73:535–540.

9. Fisher DF, Yawn DH, Crawford ES. Preoperative disseminated intravascular coagulation associated with aortic aneurysm. A prospective study of 76 cases. Arch Surg 1983;118:1252–1255.

10. Thompson RW, Adams DH, Cohen JR, et al. Disseminated intravascular coagulation caused by abdominal aortic aneurysm. J Vasc Surg 1986;4:184–186.

11. Mukaiyama H, Shionoya S, Ikezawa T, et al. Abdominal aortic aneurysm complicated with chronic disseminated intravascular coagulopathy: A case of surgical treatment. J Vasc Surg 1987;6:600–604.

12. Aramoto H, Shigematsu H, Hatakeyama T, et al. Perioperative change in coagulative and fibrinolytic function during aneurysmectomy of the abdominal aorta. Suppl to JAMA SEA MAY: 30–36, 1992.

13. Macneily AE, Graham AM. Coagulopathy induced by aortoiliac aneurysms. Can J Surg 1988;31:27–30.

14. Siebert WT, Natelson EA. Chronic consumption coagulopathy accompanying abdominal aortic aneurysm. Arch Surg 1976;111:539–541.

15. Goto H, Kimoto A, Kawaguchi H, et al. Surgical treatment of abdominal aortic aneurysm complicated with chronic disseminated intravascular coagulopathy. J Cardiovasc Surg 1985;26:280–282.

16. Miyata T, Tada Y, Takagi A, et al. Disseminated intravascular coagulation caused by abdominal aortic aneurysm. J Cardiovasc Surg 1988;29:494–497.

17. Fujii S, Hitomi Y. New synthetic inhibitors of Clr, Cl esterase, thrombin, plasmin, kallikrein and trypsin. Biochim Biophys Acta 1981;661:342–345.

18. Aoyama T, Ino Y, Ozeki M, et al. Pharmacological studies of FUT-175, Nafamostat Mesilate. I. Inhibition of protease activity in in vitro and in vivo experiments. Jpn J Pharmacol 1984;35:203–227.

19. Aramoto H, Saito H, Shigematsu H, et al. Synthetic protease inhibitors in the treatment of DIC. Nippon Rinsho 1993;51:93–98.

20. Ino Y, Suzuki K, Sato T, et al. Comparative studies of nafamostat mesilate and various serine protease inhibitors in vitro. Folia Pharmacol Japan 1986;88:449–455 (Abs. in English).

21. Hitomi Y, Ikari N, Fujii S. Inhibitory effect of a new synthetic protease inhibitor (FUT-175) on the coagulation system. Haemostasis 1985;15:164–168.

28
Abdominal Aortic Aneurysms and Surgical Management

Takeshi Ueyama

Recent advances in various examination methods have enabled precise diagnosis of abdominal aortic aneurysms (AAA). The information obtained by these examinations allows surgical management of AAA to become daily procedure. However, as the number of patients with AAA has increased, the number of high-risk patients has also increased. This fact prevents further improvement in surgical results. The rate of hospital death after surgery remains at least 2–5%.[1] Some patients initially judged as being at too high a risk to undergo surgery are later required to undergo surgical treatment because of impending rupture or ruptured aneurysm.

Despite the advances in diagnostic technology, the number of patients detected with ruptured AAA has not decreased. The results of surgery for ruptured aneurysm depend on the presence or absence of shock, the type of rupture, the volume of blood loss, and the time from rupture to surgery. The rate of death for patients with ruptured AAA remains high (about 50%).[2,3] We have not yet developed effective surgical management to reduce the rate of death from ruptured AAA in these patients.

This chapter reports the results of 205 cases of AAA that we have encountered since 1980.

Prevalence

Between 1980 and 1990, 192 cases of AAA were encountered at the Toyama Medical and Pharmaceutical University Hospital (Table 28.1). The average number of patients per years was 17.5 for the entire period, but it rose to 21 during the last 5 years. Toyama Prefecture has a population of about 1.05 million. According to statistics in 1989, the mean life expectancy was 72.2 years for males and 81.7 years for females. Even when patients treated at other hospitals in this prefecture are excluded, at least 20 of 1 million people in this prefecture have this disease, which is indicated for surgery. According to the report of Brickestaff[4] in Minnesota, USA, in 1984, the number of patients with AAA per 100,000 population was 21.1, which is 10 times the

TABLE 28.1. Cases of AAA (1980–90).

	1980	81	82	83	84	85	86	87	88	89	90	Total
Total	8	17	9	15	15	23	23	24	13	19	26	192
Male	4	16	8	11	13	19	18	18	12	13	24	152
Female	4	1	1	4	2	4	5	6	1	6	2	36
Ruptured	1	1	0	1	1	3	5	1	3	1	3	20

prevalence of this disease in Toyama prefecture. This comparison suggests that the actual number of patients with AAA in Japan may be much higher than the numbers shown by statistics.

Of the 192 cases of AAA encountered at our hospital, 20 cases (10.4%) showed ruptured AAA. The number of males with nonruptured aneurysms was 4.3 times that of females with nonruptured aneurysms. The number of males with ruptured aneurysms (13 cases) was only 1.62 times that of females with ruptured aneurysms (8 cases). Thus, ruptured aneurysms tended to be more frequently seen in females than in males.

Materials

The mean age for the 156 males was 68.9 years (range 49–88 years), and that for the 35 females was 71.3 years (50–80). Of the 205 patients, 178 underwent an elective operation. Of these 178 patients, 5 (2.8%) died in the hospital. Their mean age was 77.8 years, and their mean postoperative survival was 48.8 days (Table 28.2). All these 5 patients were elderly with many sclerotic lesions, which were responsible for death. The frequently encountered coronary and cerebrovascular diseases were not responsible for any of these 5 deaths, reflecting our care and management of cases with these diseases. In the future, satisfactory preoperative assessment and postoperative manage-

TABLE 28.2. Patients with elective operation.

178/205 = 86.8%
Operative mortality 5/178 = 2.8%
Mean age 77.8 years (72–81)
Mean postoperative days 48.8 days (3–131)

Case 1	postop.	3D	occlusion of celiac artery
Case 2		19D	bleeding, MOF
Case 3		31D	continued DIC
Case 4		60D	renal failure
Case 5		131D	intestinal perforation

MOF = multiple organ failure
DIC = disseminated intravascular coagulation

TABLE 28.3. Patients with ruptured AAA.

Operative mortality 8/20 = 40%		
Mean age 69.3 years (50–78)		
Mean postoperative days 6.8 days (0–8)		
Case 1	on the op. table	bleeding
Case 2	postop. 1D	MOF
Case 3	1D	bleeding
Case 4	2D	MOF
Case 5	3D	celiac occlusion
Case 6	4D	intestinal necrosis
Case 7	6D	MOF
Case 8	8D	cerebral embolism

MOF = multiple organ failure

ment for all type of lesions will be important.[5] The mean age of patients with ruptured aneurysms was 69.7 years (53–78) in males and 68.4 years (50–77) in females. Of 20 patients with ruptured aneurysms, 8 patients (40%) died in the hospital. The mean age for these 8 patients was 69.3 years (Table 28.3). In all of these 8 patients, death was attributed to rupture-related collapse of the circulation system. All of them showed persistent hypotension, and 3 were admitted under mechanically assisted ventilation because of respiratory arrest.

Twelve patients did not undergo surgery. Their mean age was 77.3 years (70–88). According to our criteria, surgery is indicated in all patients with AAA except for those who can stand and walk without assistance and patients who are expected to die within 1 year because of an accompanying disorder. Among the patients of this study, the reason for not performing surgery was dementia in 4, advanced malignant tumor in 3, severe ischemic heart disease in 2, right leg necrosis induced by thrombotic aneurysm in 1, cor pulmonale from lung tuberculosis in 1, and refusal in 1.

Surgical Management

According to our standard surgical procedure for AAA, an aneurysm is first opened and the proximal and distal segments of the aneurysm are cut completely, followed by end-to-end anastomosis with insertion of an artificial graft. In the cases where the branch of the Y-shaped graft is anastomosed to the femoral artery due to the presence of obstructive disease in the iliac artery, we use end-to-side anastomosis. This anastomosis was used with 19 arteries. Replacement with a Y-graft was perfomed in 149 cases, and replacement with a straight graft in 35 cases. Thus, Y-graft replacement was used 4.25 times more frequently than straight-graft replacement. To improve surgical results, the following procedures were performed.

Reconstruction of the Inferior Mesenteric Artery (IMA) and the Internal Iliac Artery (IIA)

It has been reported that ligation of the patent IMA during surgery for AAA does not often cause complication or sequelae. Since arterial blood flow is more deficient in the sigmoid colon than in the other parts of the intestine, colon ischemia is likely to be caused by postoperative hypotension, hypoxia, and a reduced blood velocity.[6] Hamanaka[7] measured serosa blood flow on the mesenteric side of the sigmoid colon using a laser Doppler velocimeter. In this study, occlusion of the IMA reduced blood flow to 40.1 ± 9.8%, suggesting that the IMA plays an important role in maintaining blood flow in this region. Since the point where the IMA branches from the aorta tends to be markedly sclerotic, we cut 2–3 cm distally from the point, and then the stump was anastomosed to the graft (Figs. 28.1 and 28.2). In early cases, we anastomosed a graft at a point immediately distal to the patent IMA or used oblique anastomosis, for the purpose of preserving the IMA. However, since

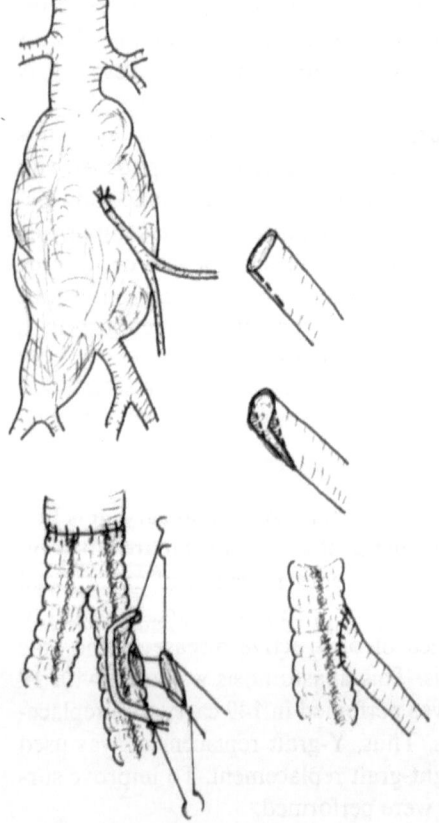

FIGURE 28.1. Our method of reconstructing the IMA.

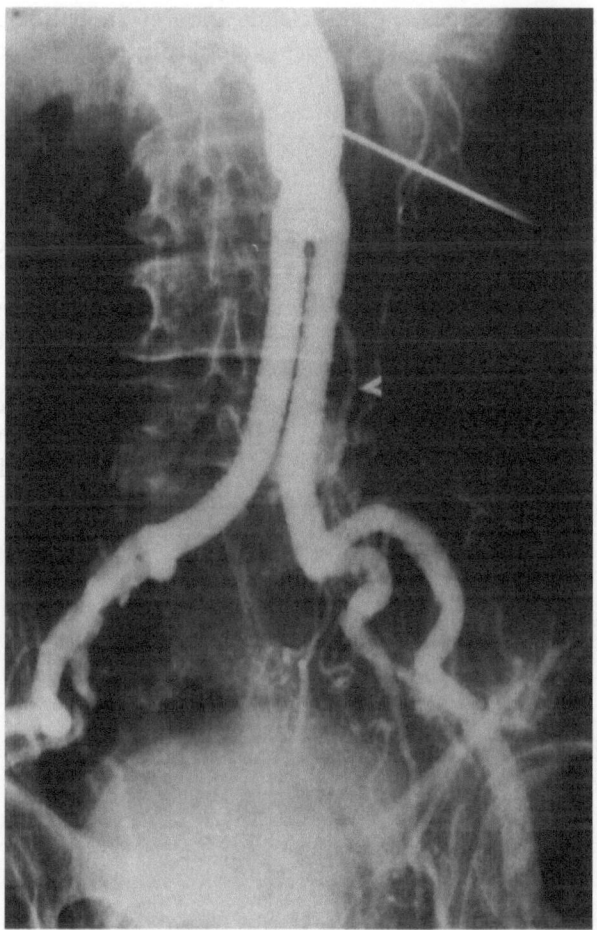

FIGURE 28.2. Postoperative angiogram. White arrow indicates reconstructed IMA.

this region is often involved in aneurysms, and because it often shows marked sclerotic change, we now make it a rule to anastomose at a point closer to the renal artery and to later reconstruct the IMA. In 93 patients, we anastomosed the IMA to the side of a graft. Thus, we have achieved successful reconstruction in 50.5% of all patients after graft replacement. After these procedures came into use, we have experienced no case of severe complication associated with colonic ischemia.

The IIA has also been reconstructed by various methods, if it was patent. Even when the IIA was occluded on both sides, the blood flow through the sigmoid colon decreased only by 30% or less. Therefore, the IIA does not seem to be closely related to colonic ischemia.[7] However, since this artery has been reported to be associated with claudication of the buttocks, vascular impotence, and paraplegia,[8,9] we attempted to reconstruct all preoperatively patent arteries as much as possible.

Exclusion of Abdominal Aortic Aneurysms

The volume of blood lost during surgery of huge aneurysms, including ruptured aneurysms, adversely affects the prognosis. Therefore, it is necessary to minimize intraoperative blood loss. For this purpose, Tomikawa developed the exclusion technique (Fig. 28.3). With this technique, the aneurysm is completely excluded from the blood flow system.[10] Since 1981, this technique has been used in 15 cases (including 5 cases of ruptured aneurysms). This technique prevents massive bleeding during aneurysmotomy and reduces the preparation area of the retroperitoneum, thus resulting in less invasive surgery. Even in cases of ruptured aneurysms, this technique reduced the blood pressure within aneurysms and produced cessation of bleeding from the rup-

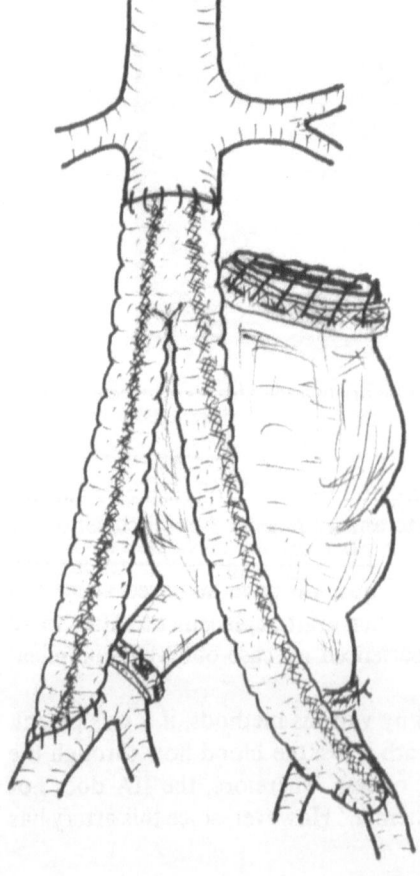

FIGURE 28.3. Schema of the exclusion technique and anatomical reconstruction.

tured point, resulting in a reduction of the size of the aneurysms and the extent of anatomical reconstruction. The mean volume of blood lost during surgery with the exclusion technique (705 mL) was about 500 mL less than that with aneurysmotomy (1,200 mL). On the other hand, after surgery with the exclusion technique, the aneurysms can rapidly develop thrombi, increasing the risk of hemorrhage due to a sharp decrease of platelets. For this reason, the platelet count of patients after surgery with this technique needs to be frequently checked. If a decrease in platelet count is noted, transfusion of platelets or fresh blood needs to be performed without delay. In our patients, the platelet count was normalized in 5.4 days on the average (3–11 days). Although all patients were in the high-risk group, only one died in the hospital.

Delayed Surgery to Ruptured Aneurysms

In cases of ruptured aneurysms, emergency surgery has been thought to be the only means of saving the life of patients. However, as we have previously reported, rupture of aneurysms tends to cause persistent shock, resulting in respiratory arrest, loss of conciousness and disseminated intravascular coagulation (DIC), suggesting a hemorrhagic tendency already upon arrival at the hospital. In such cases, surgery is not effective. Based on such experiences, in 1984 we began conservative therapy, lasting for 2 to 50 days (mean 18.3 days) after hospital admission for the 7 patients who were judged as being at high risk for emergency surgery.[11] None of these 7 patients died before surgery. Only one patient (14.2%) died after surgery. This patient died of necrosis of the small intestine due to occlusion of the superior mesenteric artery 4 days after surgery, which was performed after 3 days of conservative treatment. The death rate for these 7 patients was lower than that for the patients who underwent emergency surgery (Table 28.4). When the disease history of patients with ruptured aneurysms was examined in detail, they did not develop shock after the first bleeding. Instead, they developed massive bleeding after recurrence of vague abdominal pain and back pain. Furthermore, once

TABLE 28.4. Results of delayed surgery.

Cases of ruptured AAA	20
Emergency surgery	13
Aneurysmotomy	12 (7 dead)
Exclusion	1
Mortality	7/13 = 53.8%
Delayed surgery	7
Aneurysmotomy	4 (1 dead)
Exclusion	3
Mortality	1/7 = 14.2%

rupture caused acute circulatory failure, the functional failure of major organs could not be recovered by blood transfusion within short periods. Considering the serum enzyme reaction, renal function, and clotting function, at least 3 days are need for the function of these organs to recover. Therefore, it seems necessary to modify the conventional thought that patients with ruptured aneurysms always require emergency surgery, and that death despite emergency surgery has to be accepted as an unavoidable outcome. We believe that delayed operation is occasionally useful in cases of ruptured aneurysms.

Conclusion

In 200 cases of AAA that we have encountered since 1980, we report our efforts to reduce the postoperative morbidity and mortality, accompanied by presentation of the statistics of this disease in Toyama Prefecture, Japan. As surgical results improve, the indications for surgery have expanded, and it has become necessary to struggle with more difficult complications which have not been experienced before. To improve surgical results for ruptured aneurysms by using a delayed operation, intensive pre- and postoperative patient management is required. Continued efforts will further improve surgical prognosis for this disease.

References

1. Scott A, Smith A, Baillie CT, Bowyer RC, Sutton GL. Audit of 200 consecutive aortic aneurysm repairs carried out by a single surgeon in a district hospital: Results of surgery and factors affecting outcome. Ann R Coll Surg Engl 1992;74: 205–210.
2. Gloviczki P, Pairolero PC, Mucha P, Jr, Farnell MB, Hallett JW, Jr, Ilstrup DM, Toomey BJ, Weaver AL, Bower TC, Bourchier RG, Cherry KJ, Jr. Ruptured abdominal aortic aneurysms: Repair should not be denied. J Vasc Surg 1992;15: 851–857.
3. Harris LM, Faggioli GL, Fiedler R, Curl GR, Ricotta JJ. Ruptured abdominal aortic aneurysms: Factors affecting mortality rates. J Vasc Surg 1991;14:812–818.
4. Bickerstaff LK, Hollier LH, Van Peenen HJ, Melton LJ III, Pairolero PC, Cherry KJ. Abdominal aortic aneurysms: The changing natural history. J Vasc Surg 1984;1:6–12.
5. Lachapelle K, Graham AM, Symes JF. Does the clinical evaluation of the cardiac status predict outcome in patients with abdominal aortic aneurysms? J Vasc Surg 1992;15:964–970.
6. Van Vroonhoven TH JMV, Verhagen HJM, Broker WFH, Janssen IMC. Transmural ischaemic colitis following operation for ruptured abdominal aortic aneurysms. Neth J Surg 1991;43:56–59.
7. Hamanaka H, Tomikawa M, Ueyama T. A study of colonic ischemia during abdominal aortic surgery. J Jpn Coll Angiol 1991;31:161–167.

8. Gloviczki P, Cross SA, Stanson AW, Carmichael SW, Bower TC, Pairolero PC, Hallett JW, Jr, Toomey BJ, Cherry KJ. Ischemic injury to the spinal cord or lumbosacral plexus after aorto-iliac reconstruction. Am J Surg 1991;162:131–136.
9. Hands LJ, Collin J, Lamont P. Observed incidence of paraplegia after infrarenal aortic aneurysm repair. Br J Surg 1991;78:999–1000.
10. Tomikawa M, Ueyama T, Nagai A, Miyazawa H, Yokokawa M, Ohba Y, Yamaguchi T, Yamamoto K. Total exclusion technique and anatomical reconstruction for the treatment of abdominal aortic aneurysms. In: *Modern Vascular Surgery. Vol. 3.* New York: PMA Publishing Corp., pp. 215–229.
11. Ueyama T, Tomikawa M. Delayed surgery to ruptured abdominal aortic aneurysms. Operation (Japanese) 1986;40:1115–1120.

IX
Aortic Surgery

29
Clinical Application of Deep Hypothermia and Total Circulatory Arrest for Treatment of Aortic Disease

Wan Ki Baek and Hyuk Ahn

As Bigelow[1] predicted in his landmark experimented work in 1950, deep hypothermia and total circulatory arrest became a widely used technique in a number of cardiovascular operations with the advance of extracorporeal circulation. Especially in the treatment of aortic lesions, it is a valuable adjunct in that it prevents ischemic injury of the brain while maintaining a bloodless, clean surgical field.

Here we report our experience of deep hypothermia and circulatory arrest in the treatment of lesions involving the thoracic aorta since 1988 at Seoul National University Hospital.

Materials and Methods

Between January 1988 and December 1991, 34 adult patients with aortic disease underwent surgical repair using deep hypothermia and total circulatory arrest. There were 16 males and 18 females. The mean age at operation was 47.4 ± 1.9 years with a range of 17 to 65 years. The disease entities included aortic dissection in 26, ascending aortic aneurysm with or without aortoannuloectasia in 5, arch aneurysm in 2, and descending aortic aneurysm in 1 patient (Table 29.1).

Marfan's syndrome was seen in 5 patients. Syphilitic aneurysm was found in 2 patients; one in the ascending aorta, and the other presenting as multiple lesions along the descending thoracic aorta and abdominal aorta.

One case of arch aneurysm turned out to be a pseudoaneurysm with contained rupture. As for aortic dissection, acute dissection (less than 14 days) was present in 18 patients, DeBakey type I in 15, type II in 2, and type III in 1. Chronic aortic dissection was present in 8 patients: type I in 6 and type III in 2 (Table 29.2).

One patient with chronic type III dissection had recurrent dissection of the descending aorta 6 years after successful ascending aorta replacement with intraluminal ringed graft for type I dissection.

Twenty patients were operated on an emergency basis. Cardiac tampon-

TABLE 29.1. Disease entities (I).

	No.
Aortic dissection	26
Ascending aortic aneurysm with/without aortoannuloectasia	5
Arch aneurysm	2
Descending aortic aneurysm	1
Total	34

TABLE 29.2. Disease entities (II).

	Acute dissection	Chronic dissection
DeBakey		
Type I	15	6
Type II	2	0
Type III	1	2
Total	18	8

TABLE 29.3. Operative procedures.

	No.
Ascending aortic replacement ($\pm$partial arch replacement)	18
Modified Bentall operation	9
Descending aortic graft interposition	4
Aneurysmectomy and onlay patch	2
Total arch replacement	1
Total	34

ade was present in 8 cases. A patient with acute type I dissection came to the operation theater in a state of cardiac arrest. He survived the operation but he never regained consciousness and subsequently died.

The surgical procedures employed were ascending aorta replacement (with or without partial arch replacement) in 18 cases, modified Bentall operation (Cabrol's modification) in 9, graft interposition in descending thoracic arota in 4, aneurysmectomy and onlay patch repair in 2, and total arch replacement in 1 patient (Table 29.3).

The concomitant procedures included aortic valve resuspension in 4, suture repair of intimal tear in arch in 3, arch vessel reconstruction in 2, left pneumonectomy for intractable tracheal bleeding with patch angioplasty of right coronary ostium in 1, and mitral valve exploration for suspected mitral regurgitation in 1 (Table 29.4).

Most patients were operated on using median sternotomy. Left thoracotomy or thoracoabdominal incision was used in the patients with lesions

TABLE 29.4. Concomitant procedures.

	No.
AV resuspension	4
Repair 26 intimal tear	3
Arch vessel reconstruction	2
Pneumonectomy	1
MV exploration	1
Total	10

AV, Aortic valve; MV, mitral valve.

involving the descending aorta. Transsternal bilateral anterior thoracotomy was used in two patients with arch aneurysm.

Cardiopulmonary bypass was established in most cases by femoral artery cannulation and two-stage single venous cannulation into the right atrium for venous drainage. In the case of huge aneurysm with imminent rupture or if dense adhesion to adjacent structure was anticipated, the chest was opened after instituting femorofemoral bypass. After opening the chest, an additional venous line was established at the right atrium to guarantee enough venous return to maintain an adequate flow rate.

Since 1989, right axillary dissection and axillary artery cannulation have been performed at the same time as femoral dissection to maintain cerebral blood flow that might be impaired at the beginning of bypass by squelching of arch vessels because the arterial flow is in the retrograde direction (Fig. 29.1).

Both surface and core cooling was started after the initiation of bypass, and not until the nasopharyngeal temperature reached 18–20°C was total circulatory arrest initiated. Vasodilators were used liberally to achive even cooling and even rewarming during cardiopulmonary bypass. In addition, methylprednisolone sodium succinate (25 mg/kg) and thiopental sodium (50 mg/kg) were given just before the institution of circulatory arrest to protect the brain from ischemic injury.

In cases requiring left thoracotomy, an additional venous line was established to the right ventricle via the main pulmonary artery. After the construction of a proximal anastomosis, cardiopulmonary bypass and cerebral circulation were reestablished by a sidearm attached to the graft beforehand to shorten the arrest time (Fig. 29.2).

Results

Ten of the 34 patients did not survive the operation (overall hospital mortality was 29.4%). Brain damage was responsible for death in 5 patients. The other causes of death were bypass weaning failure in 3, renal failure in 1, and unexplained sudden death in 1 patient.

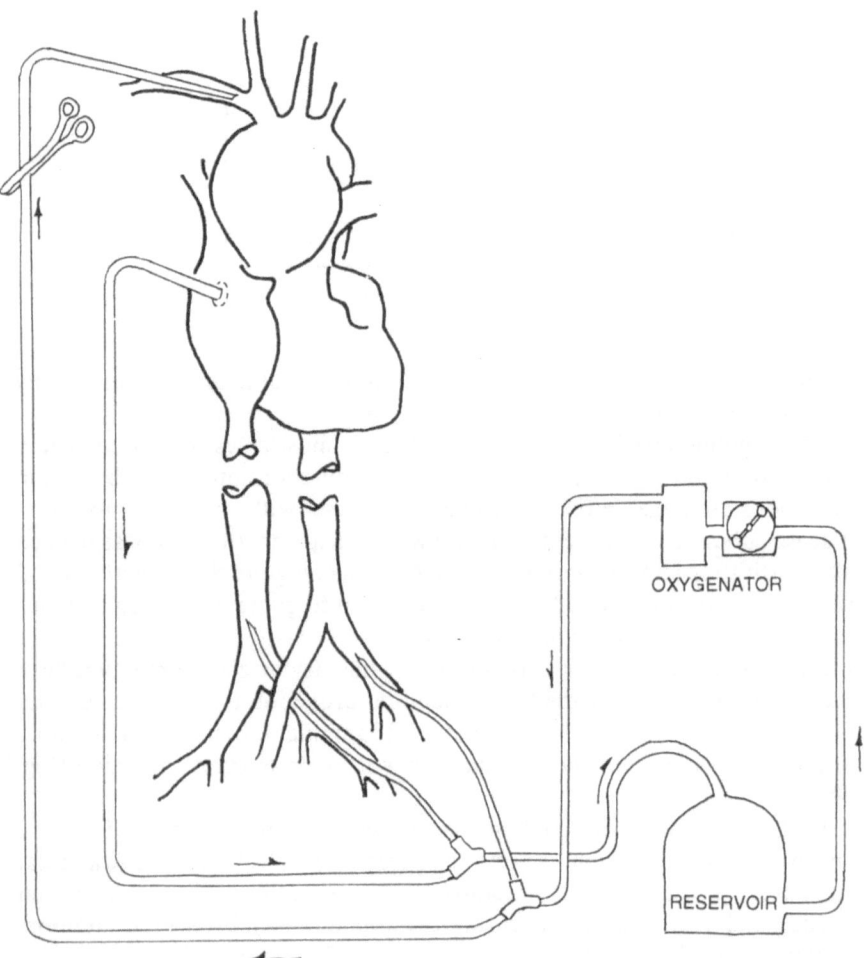

FIGURE 29.1. Cardiopulmonary bypass circuit.

The mean bypass time was 153.9 ± 39.1 minutes with a range of 83 to 279 minutes except for three cases of cardiopulmonary bypass weaning failure and subsequent death. The ischemic time ranged from 4 to 134 minutes (mean 50.2 ± 30.0). The mean cooling and rewarming times were 47.5 ± 15.4 minutes and 83.0 ± 24.5 minutes, respectively. Total circulatory arrest was maintained for periods of 2 to 86 minutes (mean 35.4 ± 3.1 minutes).

All survivors regained consciousness within 4 hours to 20 days. Excluding the cases exhibiting neurologic dysfunction postoperatively, the mean interval of consciousness recovery was 5.5 ± 1.6 hours.

Seven patients out of 24 survivors experienced postoperative neurologic dysfunction: slow to wake up in 5; psychosis, hallucination, personality change,

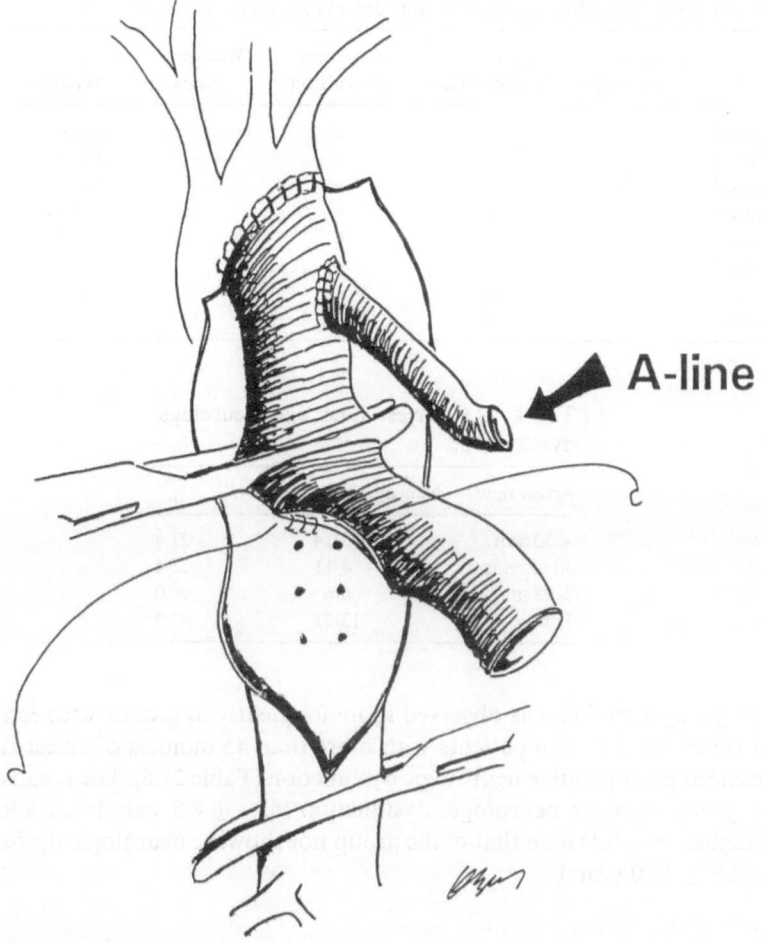

A-line

FIGURE 29.2. Cerebral circulation is maintained through side arm during distal anastomosis.

and/or memory loss in 5; twiching or convulsion in 3; and hemiparesis in 1 patient. All but one patient showing left-side weakness recovered completely without sequelae (Table 29.5).

Twenty-three patients were followed up postoperatively with a mean follow-up period 19.4 ± 2.4 months. There were no late deaths. All are in good clinical condition, except for one patient with recurrent dissection and aortic regurgitation.

The arrest time of the group showing neurologic dysfunction (47.2 ± 16.7 minutes) was significantly different from that of the group not showing neurologic dysfunction (25.9 ± 12.7 minutes) ($p < 0.05$).

When the patients were grouped by length of arrest time, postoperative

TABLE 29.5. Neurologic complications among survivors (7/24, 29.2%).

	Slow to wake up	Psychosis/ hallucination	Twitching/ convulsion	Weakness/ plegia	Sequelae
Case 1	+	−	+	+	None
Case 2	+	+	+	−	None
Case 3	+	−	−	−	None
Case 4	+	+	+	+	Lt paresis
Case 5	+	+	−	−	None
Case 6	−	+	−	−	None
Case 7	−	+	−	−	None
Total	6	5	3	1	1

TABLE 29.6. Arrest time and neurologic dysfunction.

Arrest time	Neurologic dysfunction	%
< 30 min	3/14	21.4
30–45 min	4/11	36.4
> 45 min	6/6	100.0
Total	13/31	41.9

neurologic dysfunction was observed more frequently in groups with longer arrest times. In fact, all 6 patients with more than 45 minutes of arrest time experienced postoperative neurologic dysfunction (Table 29.6). The mean age of the group showing neurologic dysfunction (52.4 ± 8.6 years) was somewhat higher ($p < 0.1$) than that of the group not showing neurologic dysfunction (42.9 ± 12.0 years).

Discussion

The technique of deep hypothermia and total circulatory arrest for the surgical repair of aortic lesions was introduced by Borst and associates[2] in 1964. It soon became a widely used technique in the treatment of a variety of cardiac and aortic diseases, especially disease involving the aortic arch, because interruption of cerebral blood flow is inevitable in arch repair and consequently some form of brain protection is mandatory.[3-10] The well-known advantages of total circulatory arrest are: 1) it provides a bloodless, dry field; 2) there is no need for obstructing cannulas and clamps, which minimizes surgical difficulties from clouding and crowding of the field and enables a precise operation to be accomplished in a shorter time; 3) it shortens total bypass time. The additional advantages of total circulatory arrest for aortic lesions are: 1) clamp injury and resultant further propagation of dissection can be avoided; 2) it enables thorough inspection of the inner aspect of the aorta, including the arch, and as a result, helps to estimate the extent of the lesion and make correct decisions; 3) it enables more secure anastomosis and less suture line bleeding; 4) no arch vessel cannulation is needed, and thus possible injury of the arch vessel is avoided and the risk of thromboembolic disease of the brain is decreased.[3,7,9,11]

It is well known that the oxygen consumption of the body decreases as the temperature is lowered, and the safety duration of total circulatory arrest is inversely proportional to oxygen consumption. Yet there is no clear consensus as to the most appropriate level of hypothermia and safety duration at that temperature. According to animal experiments, 30 minutes of total circulatory arrest at 18–20°C is known to be safe. The possibility of brain damage is anticipated to increase sharply as the arrest time exceeds 45 minutes.[12,13] In clinical practice, usually 45 to 60 minutes of total circulatory arrest is accepted as within the safety margin at body temperature 18°C.[14-16] In our series, all 6 patients in whom arrest time was more than 45 minutes died or experienced neurologic dysfunction postoperatively.

Despite its advantages, total circulatory arrest has been less commonly employed in adult patients than in infants or children, probably due to the longer time necessary for cooling and rewarming in adults and to difficulties in achieving even cooling leading to unpredictability of the safety duration.

Coselli and associates[17] reported no reliable relationship of peripheral body temperature and cerebral (brain) temperature. They monitored the electroenoephalogram well throughout the operation and defined the isoelectric state with no cerebral electric activity as electrocerebral silence (ECS). They also proposed that the metabolic inactivity of the brain is better reflected by ECS than by peripheral temperature.

Since 1989, in cases of aortic dissection, we have routinely prepared an additional arterial line in the right axillary artery through the right axillary dissection so as to establish separate cerebral perfusion after the painful experience of cerebral flow disturbance at the start of bypass via the femoral approach. The additional advantages of axillary artery cannulation are: 1) it prevents propagation of dissection by influx of retrograde pump flow into the reentry site; 2) it permits isolated cerebral perfusion when the arrest time is prolonged; 3) it helps to obliterate the false lumen and consequently reduce suture line bleeding and facilitate bypass weaning after the repair owing to antegrade arterial flow.

The fact that the mean age of the group that exhibited neurologic dysfunction postoperatively was higher than that of the group that did not exhibit neurologic dysfunction correlates with the other reports that total circulatory arrest might be risky in the elderly[18,19] We think that the higher rate of postoperative neurologic problems after employing circulatory arrest in the elderly is mainly due to degenerative changes in small vessels that prevent even cooling of the brain parenchyme. Atheromatous emboli or previous subclinical cerebral infarcts with areas of increased vulnerability to ischemic insult might contribute to postoperative neurologic problems as well.

In conclusion, the principle of deep hypothermia and total circulatory arrest could be applied in adult patients with acceptable risk. Although more clinical experiences and studies are needed to weigh the risk–benefit ratio of total circulatory arrest, we think better clinical results can be anticipated with judicious selection of patients.

References

1. Bigelow WG, Lindsay WK, Grenwood WF. Hypothermia—its possible role in cardiac surgery: An investigation of factors governing survival in dogs at low body temperature. Ann Surg 1950;132:849.
2. Borst HG, Schanding A, Rudolph W. Arteriovenons fistula of the aortic arch: Repair during deep hypothermia and circulatory arrest. J Thorac Cardiovasc Surg 1964;48:443.
3. Culliford AT, Ayvaliotis B, Shemin R, et al. Aneurysm of the ascending aorta and transverse arch: Surgical experience in 80 patients. J Thorac Cardiovasc Surg 1982;83:701.
4. Massimo CG, Presenti LF, Marranci P, et al. Extended and total aortic resection in the surgical treatment of acute type A aortic dissection: Experience with 54 patients. Ann Thorac Surg 1988;46:420.
5. Massimo CG, Presenti LF, Favi PP, et al. Excision of the aortic wall in the surgical treatment of acute type A aortic dissection. Ann Thorac Surg 1990;50: 274.
6. Crawford ES, Coselli JS, Safi HJ. Partial cardiopulmonary bypass, hypothermic circulatory arrest, and posterolateral exposure for thoracic aortic aneurysm operation. J Thorac Cardiovasc Surg 1987;94:824.
7. Crepps JT, Jr, Allmandinger P, Ellison L, et al. Hypothermic circulatory arrest in the treatment of thoracic aortic lesions. Ann Thorac Surg 1987;43:644.
8. Coselli JS, Crawford ES. Surgical treatment of aneurysms of the intrathoracic segment of the subclavian artery. Chest 1987;91:704.
9. Mahfood S, Foazi A, Garcia J, et al. Management of aortic arch aneurysm using profound hypothermia and circulatory arrest. Ann Thorac Surg 1985;39:412.
10. Crawford ES, Crawford JL, Stowe CL, et al. Total aortic replacement for chronic aortic dissection occurring in patients with and without Marfan's syndrome. Ann Surg 1983;199:358.
11. Graham JM, Stinnett DM. Operative management of acute aortic dissection using profound hypothermia and circulatory arrest. Ann Thorac Surg 1987;44: 192.
12. Kramer RS, Sanders AP, Lesage AN, et al. The effect of profound hypothermia on preservation of cerebral ATP content during circulatory arrest. J Thorac Cardiovasc Surg 1968;56:699.
13. Treasure T, Naftel DC, Conger KA, et al. The effect of hypothermic circulatory arrest time on cerebral function, mortality and biochemistry. J Thorac Cardiovasc Surg 1983;86:761.
14. Wells FC, Coghill S, Caplan HL, et al. Duration of circulatory arrest does influence the psychological development of children after cardiac operations in early life. J Thorac Cardiovasc Surg 1983;86:823.
15. Messmer BJ, Schallberger U, Gattiker R, et al. Psychomotor and intellectual

development after deep hypothermia and circulatory arrest in early infants. J Thorac Cardiovasc Surg 1976;72:495.

16. Clarkson PM, MacArthur BA, Barrat-Boyes B, et al. Development progress after cardiac surgery in infancy using profound hypothermia and circulatory arrest. Circulation 1980;62:855.

17. Coselli JS, Crawford ES, Beall AC, Jr, et al. Determination of brain temperatures for safe circulatory arrest during cardiovascular operation. Ann Thorac Surg 1988;45:638.

18. Cooley DA, Ott DA, Frazier OH, et al. Surgical treatment of aneurysm of the transverse aortic arch: Experience with 25 patients using hypothermia technique. Ann Thorac Surg 1981;32:261.

19. Livesay JJ, Cooley DA, Reul GJ, et al. Resection of aortic arch aneurysm: A comparison of hypothermic techniques in 60 patients. Ann Thorac Surg 1983; 36:19.

30
Results of Concomitant Renal Artery Reconstruction in Abdominal Aortic Surgery

Masashi Inaba, Tadahiro Sasajima, Yoshihiko Kubo, Yuhichi Izumi, and Kazutomo Goh

This paper presents the latest results on the effects of concomitant renal artery reconstruction to preserve renal function in abdominal aortic and iliac artery surgery.

Materials and Methods

Between November 1976 and January 1992, we performed abdominal aortic and iliac artery surgery in 353 patients; 213 had arteriosclerosis obliterans (ASO) and 140 had abdominal aortic and iliac artery aneurysms (AAA). Concomitant renal artery reconstructions in abdominal aortic surgery were performed in 36 (10.2%) of these. Aortic involvement included 15 AAAs and 21 ASOs. The renal artery lesions consisted of one aneurysm and 35 atheromatous stenoses greater than 50%.

AAA Group

There were 10 men and 5 women whose mean age was 68.1 (range 48 to 77 years). Preoperative risk factors were hypertension in 10 patients, ischemic heart disease in 3, renal dysfunction (serum creatinine level $\geq$ 1.8 mg/dL) in 3, thoracic aortic aneurysm in 3, hyperlipidemia in 2, hemiplegia in 1, and diabetes in 1. Of the 10 hypertensive patients, 4 had diastolic blood pressure readings of 100 mm Hg or more. Abdominal aortic aneurysms were treated by resection and replacement in 8 patients, and by exclusion and bypassing in 7. Y-shaped Dacron ® prostheses were used in all patients (8 aortobiiliac, 3 aortobifemoral, and 4 aortoiliac and femoral bypasses). The renal revascularization techniques were 13 aortorenal bypasses (bilateral 2, unilateral 9), 3 patch angioplasties, 1 splenorenal anastomosis, and 1 splenorenal bypass. Bilateral renal artery reconstructions were performed in 3 cases (20%). One patient had contralateral renal occlusion with irreversible atrophy of the kidney. The graft materials used for all renal revascularizations were autogenous saphenous veins. Other associated procedures performed during the

278

TABLE 30.1. Renal artery reconstruction in AAA:15 cases.

Operative procedures	
Abdominal aorta	
Resection and replacement	8
Exclusion and bypassing	7
Renal artery (18 arteries)	
Aortorenal bypass	13 (vein 13)
Patch angioplasty	3 (vein 3)
Splenorenal bypass	1 (vein 1)
Splenorenal anastomosis	1
Bilateral reconstruction	3 (20%)
Unilateral reconstruction	12
Associated procedures	
Femoropopliteal bypass	1 ⎤
Femorotibial bypass	2 ⎦ 20%
Reconstruction of inferior mesenteric artery	7

same operation included 1 femoropopliteal bypass, 2 femorotibial bypasses, and 7 reconstructions of the inferior mesenteric artery (Table 30.1).

ASO Group

There were 19 men and 2 women whose mean age was 63.1 (range 50 to 74 years), significantly lower than the AAA patients ($p < 0.05$). Twenty-one patients had preoperative hypertension, and 8 of them had diastolic blood pressure readings of 100 mm Hg or more. Five patients (24%) had preoperative renal dysfunction (serum creatinine level $\geq$ 1.8 mg/dL). The other preoperative risk factors included cerebral infarction in 4 patients, hemiplegia in 2, ischemic heart disease in 2, arrhythmia in 5, diabetes in 3, gastroduodenal ulcer in 3, and respiratory dysfunction in 2. The aortoiliac occlusive lesions were treated by aortofemoral bypass in 19 cases (bilateral 15, unilateral 4), by aortobiiliac bypass in 1 case, and by aortofemorofemoral bypass in 1. Dacron® prostheses were used in all cases. All renal artery lesions were atheromatous stenoses greater than 50%, and unilateral renal artery occlusions were seen in 3 cases. The renal revascularization techniques were 18 aortorenal bypasses (bilateral 2, unilateral 14) and 8 patch angioplasties. Bilateral renal artery reconstructions were performed in 5 cases (24%). Of the 18 renal artery bypass grafts, autogenous veins (saphenous vein 14, basilic vein 1) were used in 15 (83%), polytetrafluoroethylene (PTFE) in 2, and Biograft® in 1. Of the 8 renal artery patch angioplasties, saphenous vein was used in 7 and Dacron® prosthesis was used in 1. Other associated procedures during the same operation included 16 femoropopliteal bypasses, 2 femorotibial bypasses, 2 profundaplasties, 2 superficial femoral artery reconstructions, and 1 patch angioplasty of the subclavian artery. The outflow procedures were performed in 14 of 21 patients (67%) simultaneously (Table 30.2).

TABLE 30.2. Renal artery reconstruction in ASO: 21 cases.

Operative procedures	
Abdominal aorta	
Aortofemoral bypass	19 (15 bilateral, 4 unilateral)
Aortofemorofemoral bypass	1
Aortoiliac bypass	1 (1 bilateral)
Renal artery (26 arteries)	
Aortorenal bypass	18 (vein 15, PTFE2, Biograft® 1)
Patch angioplasty	8 (vein 7, Dacron® 1)
Bilateral reconstruction	5 (24%)
Unilateral reconstruction	16
Associated procedures	
Femoropopliteal bypass	16 ⎤
Femorotibial bypass	2 ⎥
Reconstruction of SFA	2 ⎬ 67%
Profunda plasty	2 ⎦
Patch angioplasty of subclavian artery	1

PTFE, Polytetrafluoroethylene; SFA, superficial femoral artery.

Results

AAA Group

One patient died of sepsis during the perioperative period, and the operative mortality rate was 6.7%. Postoperative complications included bleeding in 2 cases, ischemic colon necrosis in 2 cases, and liver dysfunction in 3 cases. Postoperative renal failure (BUN $\geq$ 80 mg/dL, creatinine $\geq$ 6 mg/dL) was seen in 3 cases (20%). All cases required hemodialysis. One of these 3 patients had preoperative renal dysfunction. One patient died (operative death), but the remaining 2 patients recovered from renal failure. The 14 surviving patients were followed 1 to 98 months, with a mean follow-up of 36.1 months. One patient (6.7%) died 4 years after operation, but the cause of death was unknown. The 5-year cumulative survival rate was 72.2 $\pm$ 21.9% (Fig. 30.1). Of the 4 patients with preoperative hypertension (diastolic blood pressure $\geq$ 100 mm Hg), 2 recovered completely and 2 experienced improvement. Of the patients who had preoperative renal dysfunction, 2 improved and 1 remained stable. There were no postoperative occlusions of the renal revascularization procedures, but in the patient with splenorenal anastomosis, splenic artery and anastomotic stenosis was found 1 year after operation (Fig. 30.2A).

ASO Group

One patient died of sepsis during the perioperative period, and the operative mortality rate was 4.8%. Postoperative complications included bleeding in 2

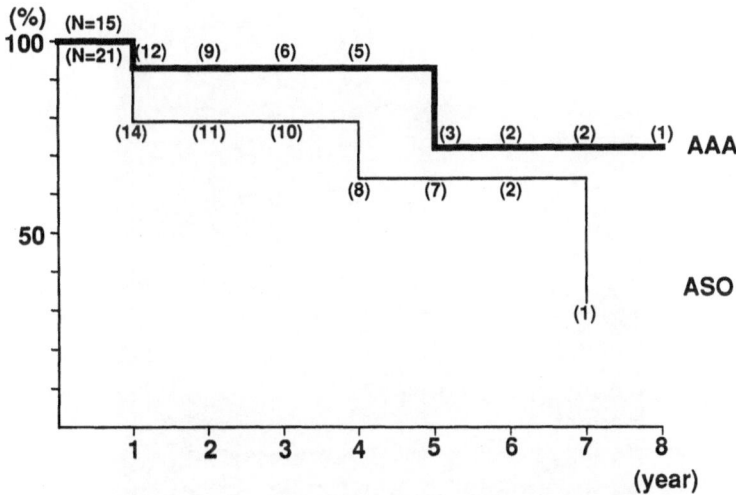

FIGURE 30.1. Cumulative survival curve.

cases, graft infection (femoropopliteal bypass) in 1 case, ischemic colon necrosis in 1 case, liver dysfunction in 2 cases, and ileus in 1 case. Five patients (24%) had renal dysfunction postoperatively, and 2 of 5 patients (9.5%) experienced renal failure (BUN $\geq$ 80 mg/dL, creatinine $\geq$ 6 mg/dL). One patient required hemodialysis. The 20 surviving patients were followed 1 to 84 months, with a mean follow-up of 35.4 months. Six patients (28.6%) died, 3 during the first year, the other at 3 (2 patients) and 6 years. The 5-year cumulative survival rate was 63.6 $\pm$ 13.5% (Fig. 30.1). The causes of death included rupture of thoracic aortic aneurysm in 1 case, pancreatic cancer in 1 case, stroke in 1 case, cardiac failure in 2 cases, and unknown in 1 case. Of the 8 patients with preoperative hypertension (diastolic blood pressure $\geq$ 100 mm Hg), 2 recovered completely, while 5 experienced improvement, for an overall favorable result in 86% (7/8) of cases. Of the 5 patients who had preoperative renal dysfunction, one improved, 3 remained stable, and 1 was aggravated (operative death). Two patients without preoperative renal dysfunction had moderate degradation of renal function postoperatively. There were no postoperative occlusions of renal revascularization procedures, but 1 venous aneurysmal change was found at the proximal anastomotic site 1 year after operation (Fig. 30.2B). The incidence of postoperative bleeding (38%) and renal dysfunction (50%) was significantly higher among patients with bilateral renal artery reconstructions than among those with unilateral reconstructions (3.6%, 14.3%) ($p < 0.01$, $p < 0.05$) (Table 30.3). In addition, there were 2 operative deaths (25%) in bilateral reconstruction group, but there were no operative deaths in the unilateral reconstruction group at all ($p < 0.05$).

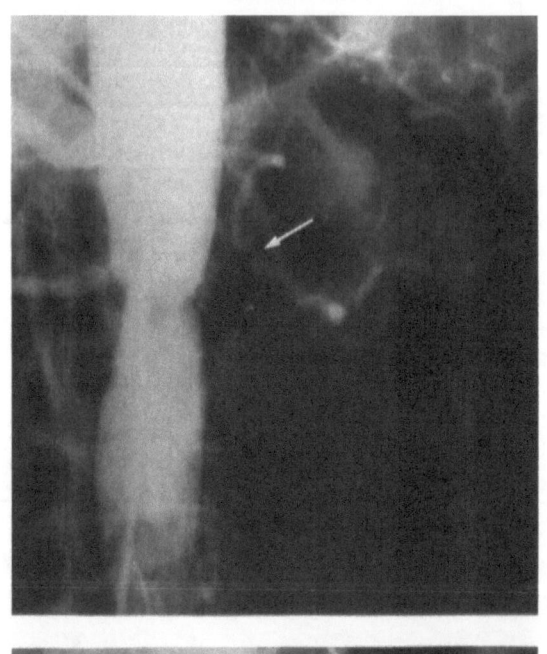

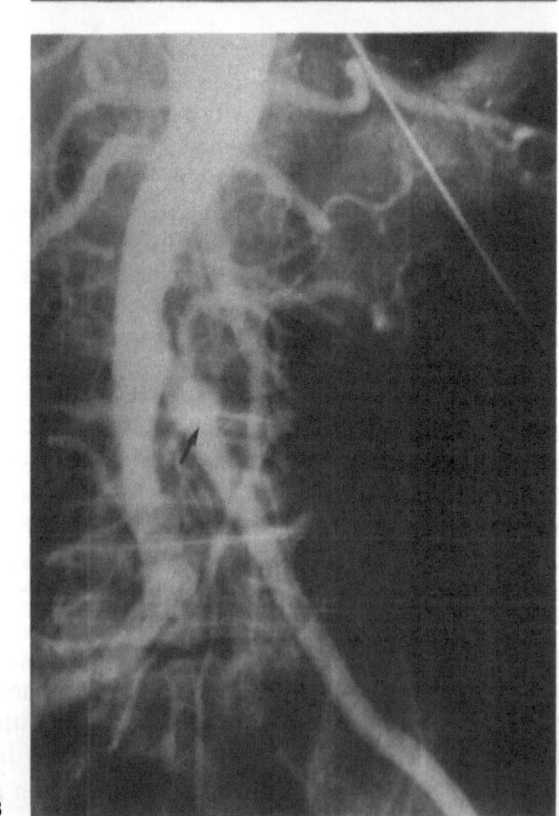

FIGURE 30.2. Postoperative angiography. (A) Spleno-left renal anastomosis performed in a 75-year-old patient. Graft stenosis is found at anastomotic site (white arrow) 1 year after operation. (B) Aortorenal vein bypass performed in a 59-year-old patient. Aneurysmal change is seen at proximal anastomotic site (black arrow) 1 year after operation.

TABLE 30.3. Correlation between renal artery reconstruction and operative mortality.

	Postoperative complication			
	Bleeding	Renal dysfunction	Colon necrosis	Operative mortality
Bilateral ($n = 8$)	3 (38%)	4 (50%)	2 (25%)	2 (25%)
	$p < 0.01$	$p < 0.05$	n.s.	$p < 0.01$
Unilateral ($n = 28$)	1 (3.6%)	4 (14.3%)	1 (3.6%)	0

Discussion

In recent years, with an increasing number of elderly patients indicated for abdominal aortic surgery and with progress of operative technique, simultaneous reconstructions of associated vascular lesions have increased. We have performed concomitant renal artery reconstructions in abdominal aortic surgery to preserve renal function. Simultaneous renal artery reconstructions are indicated when greater than 50% stenoses are visualized in angiography because of the progress of renal artery lesion[1] and the difficulties of a second operation. However, these patients usually have many risk factors, such as coronary artery disease, cerebral infarction, and renal dysfunction. In addition, in our series, outflow procedures were required in 14 of 21 ASO cases (66.7%) to improve patency of proximal aortofemoral bypasses and to improve the quality of the patient's life. So it is meaningful to simplify the aortic reconstruction procedures to decrease operative invasion. In AAA operations, high-risk patients with extensive aortoiliac aneurysms or large internal iliac aneurysms can be successfully treated by exclusion and bypassing procedure.[2] Isolated renal artery stenosis (< 75%) at the proximal site is preferably treated by transaortic endarterectomy and patch angioplasty using an autogenous vein or Dacron® patch. Autogenous vein graft is recommended for distal segmental stenotic lesions. Prosthetic graft can be selected if atrophy of the kidney is not found. In bypass procedures, we routinely proceed to construct a composite graft with vein graft and Dacron® prosthesis (Fig. 30.3). We usually perform renal artery reconstructions after aortic restoration. Core cooling of the kidney is achieved using a perfusate of 450 mL lactated Ringer's solution, 50 mL mannitol, 500 mg hydrocortisone, and 1,000 units heparin at 4°C. After clamping a renal artery, 150 mL of this perfusate is infused immediately. We consider core cooling of the kidney to be effective when the renal collateral flow is very limited and clamping time of a renal artery is more than 30 minutes. In our series of 36 patients who underwent concomitant renal artery reconstructions in abdominal aortic surgery, there were 2 operative deaths (5.6%). The 5-year cumulative survival rate was 72.2% in AAA and 63.6% in ASO, and there were no significant differences

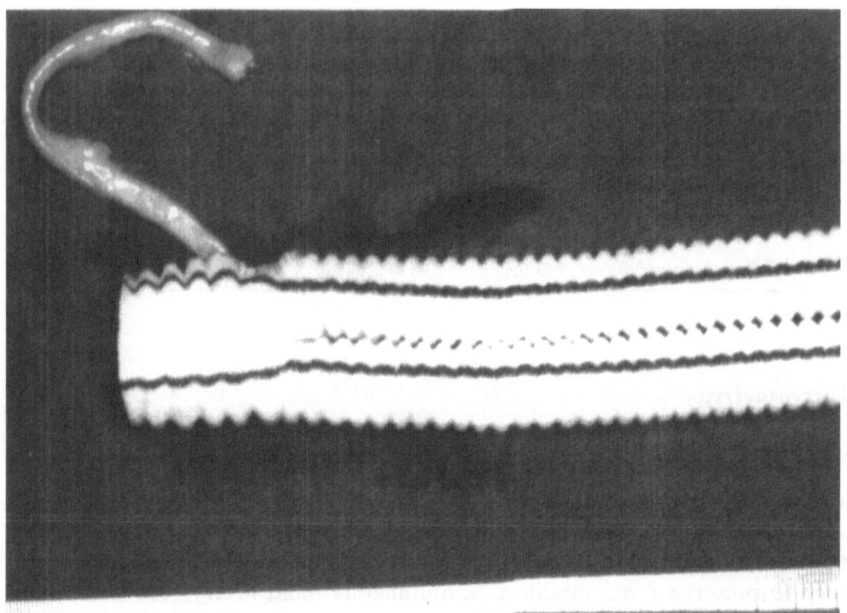

FIGURE 30.3. A composite graft constructed vein graft and Dacron® prosthesis.

between the two groups. The outcome was favorable in 92% of the cases with preoperative hypertension (diastolic blood pressure $\geq$ 100 mm Hg) (11/12) and in 88% of the cases with preoperative renal dysfunction (7/8). No patient has required chronic dialysis during a mean follow-up period of 35.7 months. These results are comparable to recent published data.[3–10] However, the rate of postoperative bleeding and operative mortality is significantly high in bilateral renal artery reconstruction.

In conclusion, the results of concomitant renal artery reconstructions in abdominal aortic surgery are good. If the degree of renal artery stenosis is greater than 50%, it should be treated simultaneously to preserve renal function.

References

1. Tollefson DF, Ernst CB. Natural history of atherosclerotic renal artery stenosis associated with aortic disease. J Vasc Surg 1991;14:327–331.
2. Masashi I. Experimental and clinical studies on the exclusion and bypassing operation for abdominal aortic and iliac artery aneurysms. J Jpn Surg Soc 1989; 12:2044–2049.
3. Kessler AR, Mulherin JL, Edwards WH. Combined aortic and renal arterial reconstruction. South Med J 1984;77:155–158.
4. Bickerstaff LK, Hollier LH, Van Peenen HJ, et al. Abdominal aortic aneurysm

repair combined with a second surgical procedure—Morbidity and mortality. Surgery 1984;95:487–491.

5. Stewart MT, Smith RB, Fulenwider JT, et al. Concomitant renal revascularization in patients undergoing aortic surgery. J Vasc Surg 1985;2:400–405.

6. Tarazi RY, Hertzer NR, Beven EG, et al. Simultaneous aortic reconstruction and renal revascularization: Risk factors and late results in eighty-nine patients. J Vasc Surg 1987;5:707–714.

7. Huffman AD, Johnson RC. Renal artery reconstruction: Extended indications. South Med J 1988;81:440–443.

8. O'Mara CS, Maples MD, Kilgore TL, et al. Simultaneous aortic reconstruction and bilateral renal revascularization: Is this safe and effective procedure? J Vasc Surg 1988;8:357–366.

9. Cooper GG, Atkinson AB, Barros AA. Simultaneous aortic and renal artery reconstruction Br J Surg 1990;77:194–198.

10. Brancherean A, Espinoza H, Magnan PE, et al. Simultaneous reconstruction of infrarenal abdominal aorta and renal arteries. Ann Vasc Surg 1992;3:232–238.

31
Complications Following Aortic Reconstructive Surgery

Jang Sang Park, Wook Kim, and Yong Bok Koh

Since the report of successful repair of abdominal aortic aneruysm using the first prosthetic graft, Vinyon-N cloth tubes,[1] improvement in operative techniques and refinements in perioperative care have resulted in progressive decline of mortality and morbidity rates. Despite these many advances in technique and prosthetic graft, postoperative complications still continue to occur.

Aortoiliac reconstruction has a better patency and a relatively low incidence of complications compared with peripheral reconstruction.[2,3] The reported immediate patency rate of aortic replacement surgery is 98.9%, and the cumulative 5-year and 10-year patency rates are, respectively 80% and 62%.[4] the 5-year patency rate for aortoilialfemoral reconstruction is about 85% in the first 5 years after operation according to other published literature.[5]

Thrombosis of a graft continues to be the most common complication of aortoiliac or aortofemoral bypass surgery. Other complications include false aneurysm, graft infection, graft-enteric fistula, and wound infection.[5] Haiart[3] reported in 1991 that the commonest complication following aortic surgery was graft occlusion due to thrombosis, occurring in 56% of cases; other problems were false aneurysm in 22%, aortoenteric fistula in 18%, and graft infection in 4%. The high mortality rate of 37% at 10 years has been reported after aortofemoral bypass for occlusive disease, and therefore there are a large number of patients at risk of such late complications.[4]

Many patients have associated cardiac, renal or pulmonary disease, hypertension, peripheral occlusive arterial disease, or diabetes mellitus. These factors must be carefully assessed preoperatively by a cardiologist and anesthetist. Intensive cardiac evaluation, renal assessment, and mechanical bowel preparation are all essential, and perioperative antibiotic prophylaxis is routine in arterial reconstruction.

Complications and Etiology

Thrombosis with Graft Occlusion

The causes of graft failure can be divided into the following: 1) deficiency of inflow. 2) problem inherent within the graft, 3) hypercoagulability, and 4) inadequacy of the outflow tract (the most common problem).[6-9] Inflow problems are rare, accounting for no more than 5% of graft failure, but inflow could be impeded to a degree that would promote thrombosis only in the limb with more severely reduced outflow while the other limb remains patent.

All synthetic grafts are thrombogenic, with minimal advantages in patency of different materials.[10] The incidence of hypercoagulability is not well known but may be as high as 9.5% in vascular surgery.[11]

The most important factor causing graft occlusion is almost always a technical problem due to inadequate outflow. Two-thirds of the patients with aortofemoral reconstruction have associated femoropopliteal occlusive disease according to Dunn et al,[12] and Bernhard and Cottrell.[13]

Excellent outflow into the femoral system should be provided, including good profunda outflow, either by profundaplasty at the orifice or distal profundaplasty, which may be accomplished with an onlay patch using the occluded superficial femoral artery or long saphenous vein or prosthetic patch graft. Many published experiences suggest that providing good outflow at the initial operation will provide better long-term patency.[14-17]

Reduced graft flow resulting from decreased cardiac output or hypovolemia may be a primary or contributing factor to graft limb thrombosis. Other causes for aortic graft thrombosis include emboli from the heart or proximal arteries that lodge distally and obstruct outflow. Too large a graft or dilatation of the prosthesis may lead to stasis and thrombus formation.[13]

Distal Thrombosis or Embolization

Distal thrombosis and embolization has occurred more commonly following surgery for occlusive disease than in aneurysmal disease, and it may occur under the condition of severe occlusive disease with poor collateralization. This complication can be reduced with adequate systemic heparinization administered intravenously by the anesthetist.

The most common cause of distal ischemia is embolization, and it is important to clamp the femoral arteries early before clamping the aorta to reduce the incidence of this complication. Distal thrombosis or embolization is usually manifested by digital ischemia after operation.

Graft Infection

Infection remains the most dangerous complication of the aortic bypass operation. Most graft infections present late, although the contamination probably occurs at the time of the initial operation.[18,19] It is most important to eradicate any source of infection prior to arterial surgery.

Pulmonary, urinary tract, bowel, or skin infections should be treated before proceeding. Meticulous operative technique with extensive wound irrigation with saline before closure will minimize local contamination. Perioperative antibiotic prophylaxis probably will contribute to a reduction in wound infection. Lymphatic fistula may cause groin wound breakdown with secondary infection, and this can best be prevented by ligation of lymphatics.

Anastomotic Aneurysms

Femoral anastomotic aneurysm following aortofemoral bypass is a rare but known complication.[20] Like femoral anastomotic aneurysm, aortic anastomotic aneurysm is rare.[21,22] In a collective review of false aneurysms following arterial reconstruction, Satiani[23] found that aortic anastomotic aneurysm occurred in 10.5% of 444 surgically repaired false aneurysms.

There are several factors causing the formation of anastomotic false aneurysms: suture material, weakness of host tissue, arterial prosthetic compliance mismatch, and infection.[24-26]

Aortoenteric Fistula

Aortoenteric fistula occurs in two forms. The most common type (approximately 90%) is a communication with the lumen of a reconstructed aorta, most commonly at the suture line of a prosthetic replacement. A less common type is paraprosthetic sinus, which develops between the graft body and the bowel.[27] In this form, a chronically infected graft is partially bathed in digestive juices.

The incidence of aortoenteric fistula is quite low, and it is difficult to get accurate data on its exact incidence. A recent report from the Cleveland Clinic suggested an incidence of 0.36% (13 of 3,652 grafts) over a 25-year period.[28]

The pathogenesis of aortoenteric fistula is not completely understood, but it seems to be a combination of mechanical and infectious processes. Most authorities agree that the mechanical component is most important.[29-31] The exact role of infection as a primary or secondary factor in the pathogenesis of this disease is still unknown.

The other complications following aortic surgery are sexual dysfunction, bowel ischemia, and distal ischemia.

Diagnosis and Management

Most patients with acute thrombosis of a limb of a bifurcation graft will present with abrupt return of ischemic symptoms and absence of the femoral pulse. Eighty-one percent of patients in a recently reported series presented with severe limb ischemia.[6] The absence of both femoral pulses indicates complete graft occlusion and suggests that the precipatating cause is either systemic or an inflow problem such as progressive disease above the graft or a large embolus.

Reduced high-thigh Doppler pressures will confirm the diagnosis of acute thrombosis. If limb viability is not immediately threatened, arteriography should be obtained before intervention. It usually shows the proximal aortic anastomotic area, inflow problems, the contralateral limb for outflow anastomotic stenosis, or pseudoaneurysm.

Computed tomography (CT) is valuable to evaluate pathologic findings that otherwise may not be suspected, such as proximal or distal pseudoaneurysms, severe graft dilatation or focal graft aneurysm, extrinsic compression of the graft, or perigraft fluid suggesting an infection. CT scan also demonstrates proximal thrombus in the upper aorta or the aortic portion of the graft.

The patient who presents with absent Doppler flow and loss of motor function and sensation requires immediate exploration to restore perfusion based on clinical and Doppler findings alone. The performance of arteriography can be omitted in order to minimize the delay in restoring limb perfusion.

Management strategies should be designed to reestablish limb circulation, and the severity of ischemia will dictate the urgency of revascularization.

As soon as acute occlusion has been identified by physical examination, heparin should be administered while other diagnostic procedures are performed. Heparin administration will prevent further propagation of the thrombus and help to maintain patency in low-flow distal vessels that may be prone to thrombosis.

Late patency of grafts that underwent either inflow graft replacement or thrombectomy without complementary outflow procedure was nil.[9] By contrast, those patients in whom both inflow and outflow procedures were performed had a late patency rate of 77%.

The role of local intraarterial thrombolytic therapy for unilateral graft limb occlusion is not well known. Occasionally lytic therapy will allow better preoperative definition of the distal vasculature.

However, surgical intervention will be required in most patients to restore adequate runoff regardless of the method. The most commonly performed surgical procedure for this problem is graft thrombectomy and profundaplasty. If preoperative angiography was not obtained or visualization of the profunda femoris and distal limb vasculature was inadequate, intraoperative angiography may be obtained. It is most important to visualize adequately the profunda femoris. If the profunda femoris appears inadequate, it may be essential to expose the popliteal artery and repeat angiogram to visualize the infrageniculate circulation for possible bypass. For outflow procedures, various methods of profundaplasty may be required. If the profunda femoris is occluded or diseased in its distal portion, bypass to the popliteal or tibial vessels is essential.[15-17] Inflow is usually obtained by retrograde thrombectomy.[32,33]

Distal thrombosis or embolization is usually not recognized until after operation and is manifested by digital ischemia. In most experiences, reoperation is not useful and most patients recover with minimal tissue loss as long as the major vessels of the lower extremity remain patent.

When infection of an aortofemoral graft is confined to the groin, it usually presents with signs and symptoms such as localized groin pain, erythema, swelling, tenderness, a pulsatile mass, and/or drainage.

When doubt of graft infection exists, diagnostic maneuvers can include sinography, which can also diagnose the extent of proximal infection along the graft, ultrasound, and CT scan. Prophylactic antibiotic therapy is routinely administered.

Experiences at Catholic University

We reviewed 71 patients who had aortic reconstructive surgery in our hospital, especially with regard to the complications of aortofemoral and aortoiliac procedures. Thirty-two patients underwent aortofemoral or aortoiliac Dacron bypass for aortoiliac occlusive disease, and 39 patients for aortic aneurysmal disease from January 1983 to December 1991. Most of the patients were men. There were 64 men and 7 women of mean age 61.3 years (range 12-79 years) (Table 31.1 and Fig. 31.1). Cardiovascular disease was the most frequently associated disease, and other diseases including diabetes, hypertension, pulmonary tuberculosis, and peptic ulcer were commonly associated (Table 31.2).

In 32 patients the original pathology was occlusive disease with ischemic pain, nonhealing ulcer, and gangrene, causing claudication in 29. The other 39 patients had aneurysmal disease, causing abdominal discomfort in 19.

TABLE 31.1. Age and sex distribution.

| Age (years) | Obstructive disease | | Aneurysmal disease | | Total (%) |
	Male	Female	Male	Female	
0-9	0	0	0	0	0
10-19	0	0	0	1	1 (1.4)
20-29	0	0	0	1	1 (1.4)
30-39	0	0	1	0	1 (1.4)
40-49	2	0	2	1	5 (7.0)
50-59	12	0	6	1	19 (26.8)
60-69	13	0	11	2	26 (36.6)
70-79	4	1	13	0	18 (25.4)
Total (%)	31 (96.9)	1 (3.1)	33 (84.6)	6 (15.4)	71 (100)

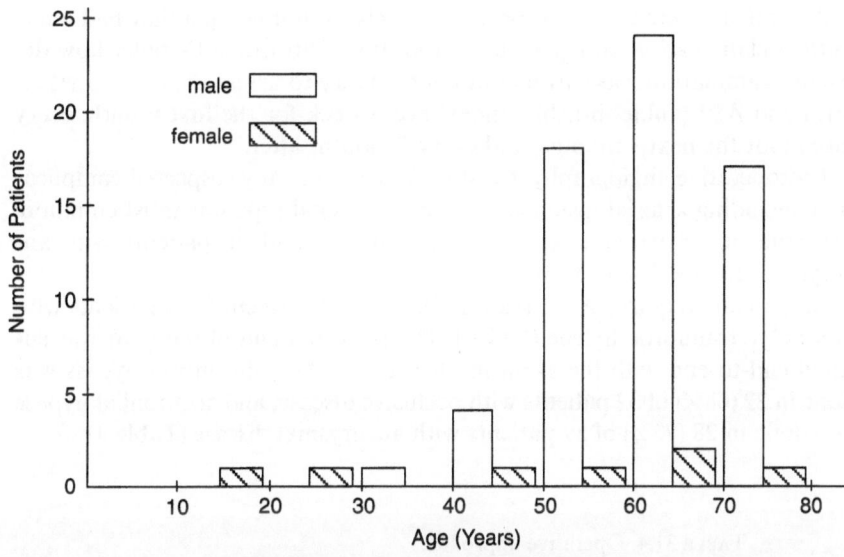

FIGURE 31.1. Age and sex distribution.

TABLE 31.2. Associated disease.

	Occlusive disease	Aneurysmal disease
Cardiovascular disease	9	8
Diabetes mellitus	3	0
Others[a]	4	13

[a] Peptic ulcer, pulmonary tuberculosis, accident, etc.

TABLE 31.3. Type of aortic disease.

	Occlusive disease	Aneurysmal disease
Suprarenal	2	3
Infrarenal	18	26
Juxtarenal	3	1
Thoracoabdominal	0	5
Ruptured[a]	0	4
Mixed[b]	9	0
Total	32	39

[a] Aneurysmal rupture on arrival.
[b] Infrarenal + lower extremity peripheral occlusion.

All patients were evaluated postoperatively for follow-up if they had intermittent claudication, rest pain, and ulceration. Ultrasonic Doppler flow detector examination was carried out after surgery to assess the arterial waveform and ABI (ankle–brachial index) every week for the first month, every month for the next 3 months, and every 3 months after.

Postoperative angiography was done if there was any suspected complication, including arterial insufficiency. The infrarenal type was most common, occurring in 18 patients with occlusive disease and 26 patients with aneurysmal disease (Table 31.3).

All patients required a bifurcation Dacron graft except for 5 patients who had polytetrafluoroethylene (PTFE). The proximal end of the graft was sutured end-to-end with the aorta in all patients. Aortobifemoral bypass was done in 22 (68%) of 32 patients with occlusive disease, and aortobiilial bypass was done in 28 (72%) of 39 patients with aneurysmal disease (Table 31.4).

TABLE 31.4. Operative approach.

	Occlusive disease	Aneurysmal disease
Aortobifemoral	22	5
Aortobiilial	2	28
Tube graft	0	5
Aortofemoral and ilial	1	0
Combined[a]	7	0
Mixed[b]	0	1

[a] Aortobifemoral + peripheral bypass.
[b] Tube graft + aortobiilial bypass.

TABLE 31.5. Complications.

Complication	Number (%)
Thrombosis	12 (16)
Wound infection	1 (2)
Lymphocele	1 (2)
Amputation	1 (2)
Total	15 (22)

TABLE 31.6. Complication rate and interval.

	Occlusive disease	Aneurysmal disease
Number	6 (16.2%)	1 (2.5%)
Interval	26.7 months	30 months

TABLE 31.7. Postoperative mortality rate.

	Occlusive disease	Aneurysmal disease
Number	4 (12.5%)	5 (12.8%)

In Nevelsteen's[4] data the patency rate at 5 years and at 10 years was 80% and 62%, respectively. In our hospital no graft occlusion was noted in aneurysmal disease, and 12 occlusions were found only in occlusive disease. The mean interval between the original operation and the occurrence of complications was 28 months, with a range of 2–180 months (Tables 31.5 and 31.6).

Nine (12.6%) have died of the total group of 71 patients. Postoperative mortality was 12.5% in occlusive disease and 12.8% in aneurysmal disease (Table 31.7). Neither graft–enteric fistula nor false anastomotic aneurysm was found postoperatively in our experiences.

Conclusions

In aortic reconstructive surgery, most complications are usually related to the initial operative procedure. Particular attention must be paid to potential complications for their prevention and management. Vascular surgeons should be aware that the outcome after complications is poor and therefore every precaution must be taken at the time of original surgery. Meticulous operative and perioperative management of properly selected patients can provide the best surgical treatment, with low mortality and morbidity in patients with extensive aortic disease.

When dealing with the patient with a graft limb thrombosis, the surgeon should pay attention to the causes of failure and to reestablishing flow to minimize the risk of limb loss. It is essential to pay particular attention to maximizing runoff in those cases with occlusive disease.

References

1. Voorhees AB, Jr, Jarezki A, Blakemore AH. The use of tubes constructed from Vinyon "N" cloth in bridging arterial defects. Ann Surg 1952;135:332–336.
2. Brewster DC, Darling RC. Optimal method of aortoiliac reconstruction. Surgery 1978;84:739–748.
3. Haiart DC, Callam HJ, Murie JA, Ruckleu CV, Jenkins AM. Reoperations for late complications following abdominal aortic operation. Br J Surg 1991;78:204–206.
4. Nevelsteen A, Suy R. Daenen W, Boel A, Stalpaert G. Aorto-femoral grafting: Factors influencing late results. Surgery 1980; 88:642–653.
5. Crawford ES, Bomberger RA, Glaser DH, Saleh SA, Russel WL. Aortoiliac occlusive disease: Factors influencing survival and function following reconstructive operation over a twenty-five year period. Surgery 1981;90:1055–1067.

 6. Brewster DC, Meier GH III, Darling RC, Moncure AC, SaMuraglia GM, Addott WM. Reoperation for aortofemoral graft occlusion: Optimal methods and long-term results. J Vasc Surg 1987;5:363–374.

 7. Bernhard VM, Ray Ll, Towne JB. The reoperation of choice for aortofemoral graft occlusion. Surgery 1977;82:867–874.

 8. Harris PL. Aorto-iliac-femoral re-operative surgery: Supplementary surgery at secondary operations. Acta Chir Scand 1987;538:51–55.

 9. LeGrand DR, Vermilion DB, Hayes JP, Evans WE. Management of the occluded aortofemoral graft limb. Surgery 1983;93:818–821.

10. Cintora I, Pearce DE, Cannon JA. A clinical survey of aortobifemoral bypass using two inherently different graft types. Ann Surg 1988;208:625–630.

11. Donaldson MC, Weinberg DS, Belkin M, Whittemore A, Mannick JA. Screening for hypercoagulable states in vascular surgical practice: A preliminary study. J Vasc Surg 1990;11:825–831.

12. Dunn DA, Downs AR, Lye CR. Aortoiliac reconstruction for occlusive disease: Comparison of end-to-end and end-to-side proximal anastomoses. Can J Surg 1982;25:382–389.

13. Bernhard VM, Coffrell ED. Diagnosis and management of aortic bifurcation graft limb occlusions. In: Bernhard VM, Towne JB (eds).: *Complications* in *Vascular Surgery*. St. Louis: Quality Medical Publishing, 1991, pp. 204–215.

14. Malone J, Moore WS, Goldstone J. The natural history of bilateral aortofemoral bypass grafts for ischemia of lower extremities. Arch Surg 1975;110:1300–1306.

15. Flanigan PD, Quinn T, Kraft RO. Selective management of high risk patients with an aortic aneurysm. Surg Gynecol Obstet. 1980;150:171–179.

16. Berguer R, Hiffins RF, Calton LT. Hemetry: Blood flow and reconstruction of the deep femoral artery. Am J Surg 1975;130:68–73.

17. Ward AS. Morris-Jones W. The role of the profunda femoris in aorto-iliac surgery. Br J Surg 1978;65:308–312.

18. Darling RC, Brewster DC. Elective treatment of abdominal aortic aneurysms. World J Surg 1980;4:661–667.

19. Szilagy DX, Smith RF, Elliot JP, Varanderic MP. Infection in arterial reconstruction with synthetic graft. Ann Surg 1972;176:312–319.

20. Yao JST, Flinn WR, Rizz RJ, Park JS, Bergan JJ. Recurrent aortic and anastomotic aneurysms. In: Bergan JJ, Yao JST (eds.): *Aortic Surgery*. Philadelphia: WB Saunders, 1989, pp. 305–316.

21. John JH, Joseph SL, Paul NJ. A study of anastomotic aneurysms following aortobifemoral prosthetic bypass. Ann Surg 1980;192:69–75.

22. Plate G, Hollier LA, O'Brien P, et al. Recurrent aneurysms and late vascular complications following repair of abdominal aortic aneurysm. Arch Surg 1985; 120:590–594.

23. Satiani B. False aneurysms following arterial reconstruction. Surg Gynecol Obstet 1981;152:357–363.

24. Downs AR, Lye CR, Mackean G. Graft infections in Aorto-iliac arterial reconstructions. Can J Surg 1983;26:328–334.

25. Knox GW. Peripheral vascular anastomotic aneurysms. Ann Surg 1976;183:120–126.

26. Szilagy DZ, Smith RF, Elliot JP. Anastomotic aneurysms after vascular reconstruction: Problems of incidence, etiology and treatment. Surgery 1975;78:800–809.

27. Brennaman BM, Shepard AD, Ernst CB. Aortoenteric and caval fistulae. In: Bergan JJ, Yao JST (eds.) *Aortic Surgery*. Philadelphia: WB Saunders, 1989, pp. 497–510.
28. O'Hara PJ, Hertzer NR, Beven EG, Krajewski LP. Surgical management of infected abdominal aortic grafts: Review of a 25 year experience. J Vasc Surg 1986;3: 725–731.
29. Busuttil RW, Rese W, Baker JD, Wilson SE. Pathogenesis of aortoduodenal fistula: Experimental and clinical correlates. Surgery 1979;85:1–13.
30. Ikonomopoulos DC, Spanos PK, Lazarides DP. Pathogenesis of aorto enteric fistula. An experimental study. Int Angiol 1986;5:33–37.
31. DeWeese MS, Fry WJ. Small bowel erosion following aortic resection. JAMA 1962;179:882–885.
32. Strandness DE. Functional results after revascularization of the profunda femoris artery. Am J Surg 1970;119:240–246.
33. Hills DA, Jamieson CW. The results of arterial reconstruction utilizing the profunda femoris artery in the treatment of rest pain and gangrene. Br J Surg 1977;64: 359–363.

32
Cardiovascular Changes After Infrarenal Aortic Cross-Clamping in Clinical and Animal Studies

Kazuro Sugi, Akira Furutani, Takayuki Kuga, Kentaro Fujioka, Hidetoshi Tuboi, and Kensuke Esato

Introduction

Previous studies[1-3] have demonstrated a fall in cardiac output during aortic cross-clamping in patients without assisted circulation, particularly in those with coronary artery disease or cardiac failure. Such cardiac dysfunction was thought to be due to an increased afterload of the left ventricle during clamping. Recent studies also point to a significant reduction in cardiac failure following aortic declamping associated with the reperfusion of the ischemic lower torso.[4]

To assess these two mechanisms used to explain the myocardial depression associated with aortic cross-clamping, we evaluated cardiac contractility during and after 1 hour of infrarenal aortic cross-clamping in human and dog studies.

Methods

Preparation and Protocol in the Clinical Study

In 15 patients (mean age 67 ± 8 years, 11 males and 4 females) with aortic abdominal aneurysm, a Swan-Ganz thermal dilution catheter (model 93A-131-7F, Edwards Labs., USA) was preoperatively inserted in the pulmonary artery via the internal jugular vein. The patients were anesthetized with 1% or 2.5% isoflurane throughout the operation. Maintenance fluid was infused at a rate of 15 ± 1 ml/kg/hr throughout the operation to maintain cardiac output at the normal level. Following abdominal median laparotomy, heparin 0.5 or 1 mg/kg was introduced. The infrarenal abdominal aorta was clamped for 63 ± 16 minutes to replace the infrarenal abdominal aorta with a graft. Data were recorded during clamping and over the following 2 hours. Aortic and pulmonary wedge pressures were measured with transducers (MK 12030US, Baxter, Japan). Cardiac output was measured using the thermal dilution technique with a Swan-Ganz catheter and a cardiac output computer (Model 9520, Edwards Labs., USA).

Preparation and Protocol in the Animal Study

Adult mongrel dogs ($n = 11$), mean body weight 13.2 ± 0.5 kg, were prepared for this study. Catheters were placed in the thoracic aorta and inferior vena cava via carotid arterial and femoral venous cut-downs. A Swan-Ganz thermal dilution catheter (model 93A-131-7F, Edwards Labs., USA) was positioned in the pulmonary artery via the external jugular vein. Left thoracotomy was performed through the sixth intercostal space for implantation in the heart of a pulse transit ultrasonic dimension transducer (LMT-53, Crystal Biotech, USA). Matched ultrasonic transducers were sutured to the anterior and posterior epicardium in the plane of the minor axial circumference. A tip manometer (TCP1, Sanei Denki Inc., Japan) was placed in the left ventricle via a stab incision made through the apex (Fig. 32.1). Following abdominal median laparotomy, the infrarenal abdominal aorta was prepared for clamping. The study was conducted after hemodynamics had stabilized.

The animals were anesthetized with 1% or 2% halothane throughout the experiment. After 0.5 mg/kg heparin administration into a venous line, baseline measurements were obtained. The animals were divided into two groups. In the clamp group ($n = 6$), the infrarenal abdominal aorta was clamped for 1 hour. Data were recorded 5 minutes after clamping, 5 minutes before declamping, and then 5 and 30 minutes and 1 and 2 hours after removal of the clamp. Lactated Ringer's solution was infused at a rate of 10 ml/kg/hr as maintenance fluid throughout the study. In the control group ($n = 5$), the abdominal aorta was not clamped. Data were obtained as in the clamp group, and lactated Ringer's solution was infused at the same rate.

In both groups, the thoracic aorta was manually occluded for 15 seconds

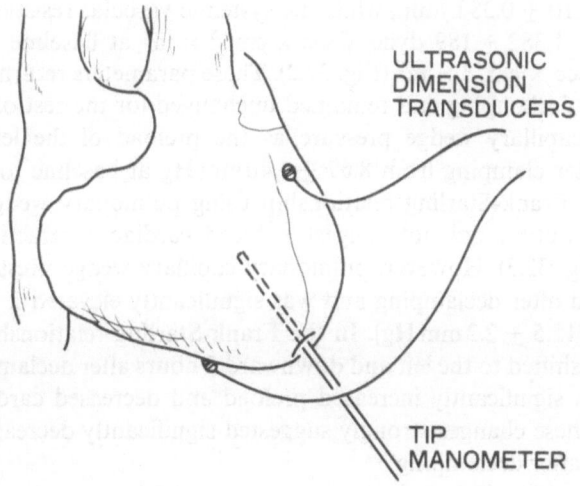

ULTRASONIC
DIMENSION
TRANSDUCERS

TIP
MANOMETER

FIGURE 32.1. Illustration of cardiac instrumentation in animal study.

to obtain the end-systolic pressure–volume relationship (E_{max}) for the left ventricle at each measurement.[5]

An ultrasonic transducer was connected to a polygraph system (Amplifier Case 7746, Sanei Denki Inc., Japan) and continuously monitored on an oscilloscope (LBO-522, Sanei Denki Inc., Japan). Aortic, pulmonary, and wedge pressures were measured with transducers (MK 12030US, Baxter, Japan). Cardiac output was measured using the thermodilution technique with a Swan-Ganz catheter and a cardiac output computer (Model 9520, Edwards Labs., USA).

Simultaneously determined left ventricular pressure and diameter were used to calculate the end-systolic pressure–volume relationship for the left ventricle. E_{max} of the left ventricle was calculated by linear regression performed with the end-systolic pressure (y axis) and dimension (x axis) data.

Statistical Analysis

Data were expressed as mean $\pm$ standard error of the mean (SEM). The significance of the differences between groups and from baseline was analyzed using Dunnett's test and analysis of variance. The level of statistical significance was set at $p < 0.05$.

Results

Clinical Study

The cardiac output was reduced after clamping from 5.15 ± 0.48 L/min at baseline to 4.10 ± 0.38 L/min, while the systemic vascular resistance was increased from $1,382 \pm 189$ dyne $\times$ sec $\times$ cm^{-5} $\times$ m^2 at baseline to $1,775 \pm 258$ dyne $\times$ sec $\times$ cm^{-5} $\times$ m^2 (Fig. 32.2). These parameters returned to baseline levels at declamping and remained unchanged for the rest of the study. Pulmonary capillary wedge pressure as the preload of the left ventricle decreased after clamping from 8.67 ± 1.40 mm Hg at baseline to 7.67 ± 1.4 mm Hg. The Frank-Starling relationship using pulmonary wedge pressure and cardiac output did not suggest reduced cardiac contractility during clamping (Fig. 32.3). However, pulmonary capillary wedge pressure gradually increased after declamping and was significantly elevated 2 hours after declamping (12.5 ± 2.2 mm Hg). In the Frank-Starling relationship, cardiac contractility shifted to the left and downward 2 hours after declamping, associated with a significantly increased preload and decreased cardiac output (Fig. 32.3). These changes strongly suggested significantly decreased cardiac contractility after declamping.

There was no significant change in mean arterial pressure, heart rate, and mean pulmonary arterial pressure throughout the operation (Table 32.1).

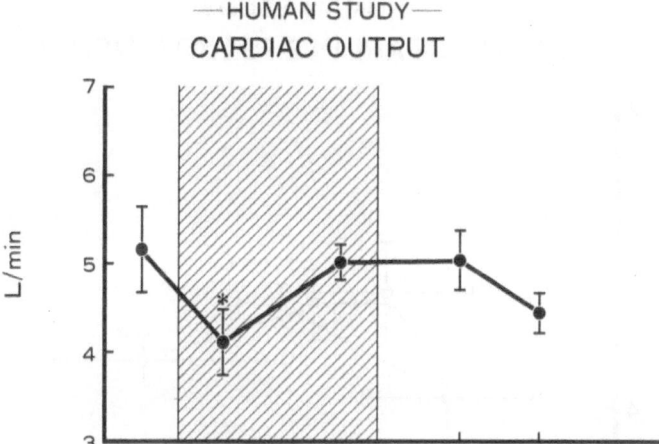

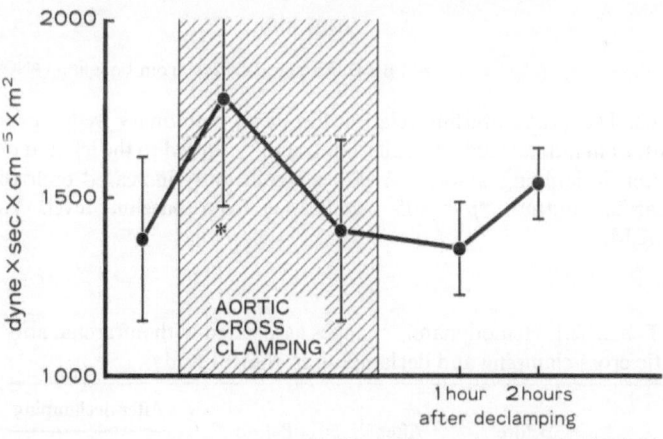

FIGURE 32.2. Changes in systemic vascular resistance and cardiac output in human study. Cardiac output was reduced after clamping from 5.15 ± 0.48 L/min at baseline to 4.10 ± 0.38 L/min, while systemic vascular resistance was increased from $1,382 \pm 189$ dyne $\times$ sec $\times$ cm^{-5} $\times$ m^2 at baseline to $1,775 \pm 258$ dyne $\times$ sec $\times$ cm^{-5} $\times$ m^2. $*p\,0.05$ significance from baseline level (ANOVA). Values are means $\pm$ SEM.

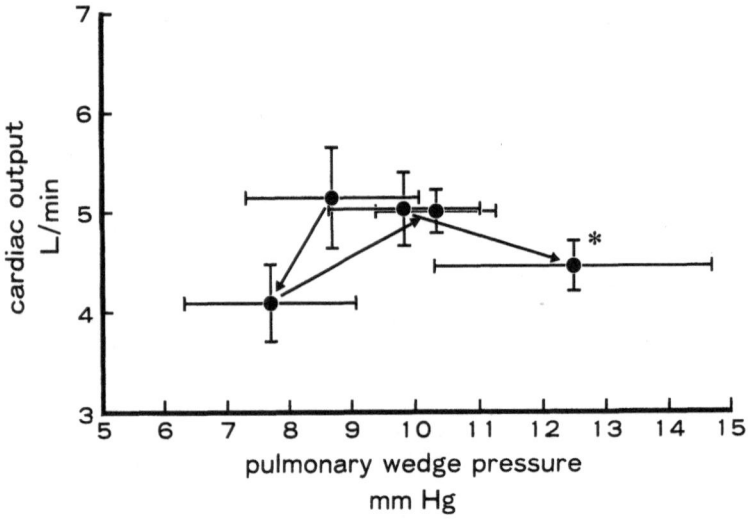

FIGURE 32.3. The Frank-Starling relationship using pulmonary wedge pressure and cardiac output in human study. Cardiac contractility shifted to the left and downward 2 hours after declamping, associated with a significantly increased preload and decreased cardiac output. *$p < 0.05$ significance from baseline level. Values are means ± SEM.

TABLE 32.1. Hemodynamic changes associated with infrarenal aortic cross-clamping and declamping in clinical study.

	Before clamping	After clamping	Before declamping	After declamping	
				60′	120′
MAP	89 ± 2	91 ± 3	88 ± 3	85 ± 3	85 ± 3
HR	80 ± 4	75 ± 3	76 ± 2	77 ± 3	76 ± 3
PAP	14 ± 1	13 ± 1	14 ± 1	15 ± 2	13 ± 1

MAP, Mean arterial pressure (mm Hg); HR, heart rate (beats/min); PAP, pulmonary arterial pressure (mm Hg). All values are mean ± SEM. There was no significant difference from baseline level.

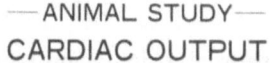

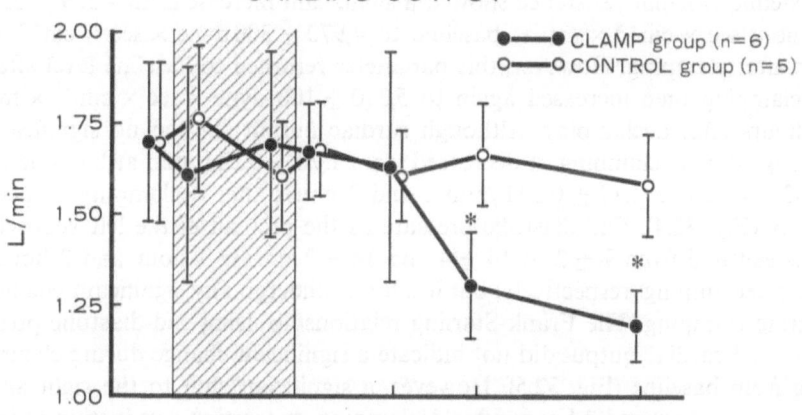

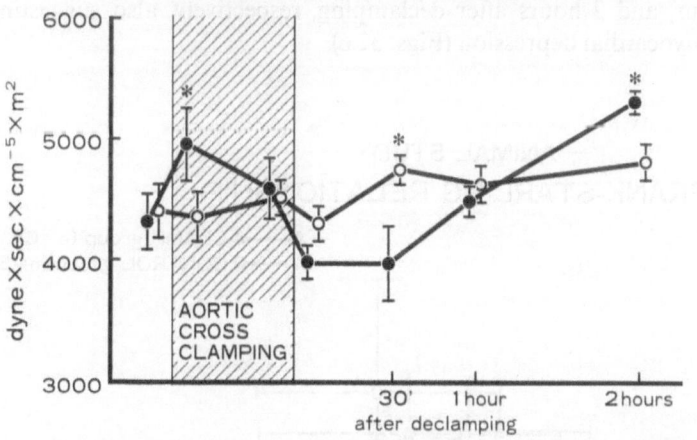

FIGURE 32.4. Changes in systemic vascular resistance and cardiac output in animal study. Systemic vascular resistance showed a significant increase after clamping from $4{,}329 \pm 220$ dyne $\times$ sec $\times$ cm^{-5} $\times$ m^2 at baseline to $4{,}970 \pm 300$ dyne $\times$ sec $\times$ cm^{-5} $\times$ m^2 after the clamping in the clamp group. It increased again 2 hours after declamping to $5{,}310 \pm 100$ dyne $\times$ sec $\times$ cm^{-5} $\times$ m^2. Cardiac output decreased from 1.70 ± 0.22 L/min at baseline to 1.30 ± 0.14 and 1.19 ± 0.10 L/min 1 and 2 hours after declamping, respectively.

Animal Study

Systemic vascular resistance showed a significant increase from $4,329 \pm 220$ dyne $\times$ sec $\times$ cm^{-5} $\times$ m^2 at baseline to $4,970 \pm 300$ dyne $\times$ sec $\times$ cm^{-5} $\times$ m^2 after clamping. However, this parameter returned to baseline level after declamping then increased again to $5,310 \pm 100$ dyne $\times$ sec $\times$ cm^{-5} $\times$ m^2 2 hours after declamping. Although cardiac output showed no significant change during clamping, it decreased from 1.70 ± 0.22 L/min at baseline to 1.30 ± 0.14 and 1.19 ± 0.10 L/min 1 and 2 hours after declamping, respectively (Fig. 32.4). End-diastolic pressure as the preload of the left ventricle was elevated from 7 ± 2 to 14 ± 4 and 14 ± 3 mm Hg 1 hour and 2 hours after declamping, respectively, but it did not undergo any significant change during clamping. The Frank-Starling relationship using end-diastolic pressure and cardiac output did not indicate a significant change during clamping from baseline (Fig. 32.5). However, a significant shift to the right and downward occurred 2 hours after declamping, suggesting a reduction in intrinsic myocardial contractility (Fig. 32.5). E_{max} decreased from 29.7 ± 6.3 mmHg/mm at baseline to 18.1 ± 3.6, 16.5 ± 4.6, and 17.2 ± 3.5 at 30 minutes, 1 hour, and 2 hours after declamping, respectively, also suggesting significant myocardial depression (Figs. 32.6).

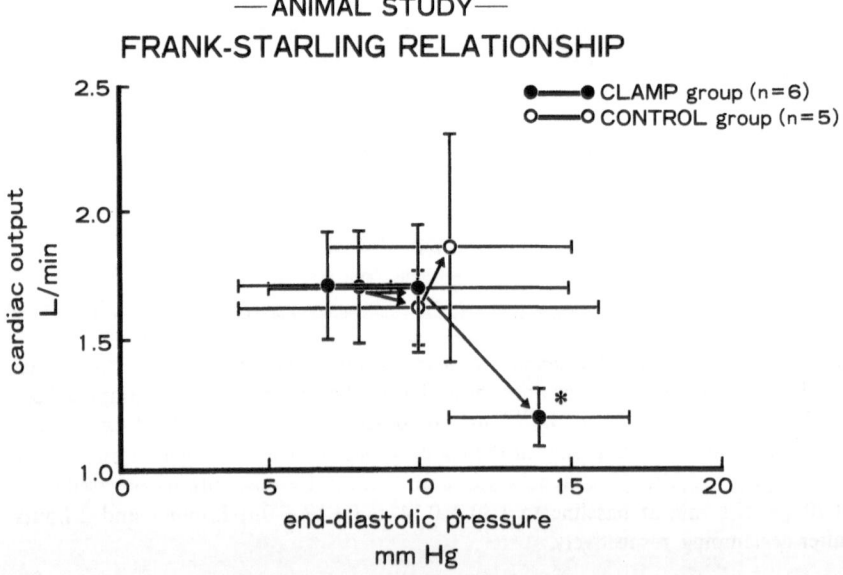

FIGURE 32.5. The Frank-Starling relationship using end-diastolic pressure and cardiac output in animal study. A significant shift to the right and downward occurred 2 hours after declamping, suggesting a reduction in intrinsic myocardial contractility.

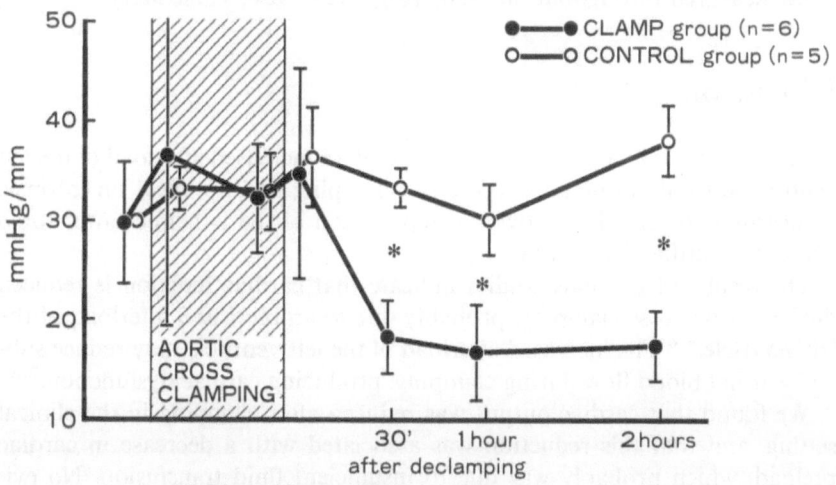

FIGURE 32.6. Change in end-systolic pressure–volume relationship of the left ventricle (E_{max}). It decreased from 29.7 ± 6.3 mm Hg/mm at baseline to 18.1 ± 3.6, 16.5 ± 4.6, and 17.2 ± 3.5 mm Hg/mm at 30 minutes, 1 hour, and 2 hours after declamping, respectively. *$p < 0.05$ between groups, as determined by Dunnett's test. Values are means $\pm$ SEM.

TABLE 32.2. Hemodynamic changes associated with infrarenal aortic cross-clamping and declamping in animal study

Group	Before clamping	After clamping	Before declamping	After declamping			
				5′	30′	60′	120′
MAP							
Clamp	99 ± 15	107 ± 24	107 ± 18	90 ± 19	89 ± 7	87 ± 16	93 ± 14
Control	102 ± 11	101 ± 4	101 ± 9	95 ± 10	109 ± 5	106 ± 8	108 ± 8
HR							
Clamp	129 ± 11	130 ± 11	138 ± 10	122 ± 10	123 ± 11	122 ± 11	129 ± 8
Control	121 ± 13	119 ± 13	126 ± 11	122 ± 8	113 ± 7	119 ± 21	112 ± 14
PAP							
Clamp	20 ± 3	22 ± 2	22 ± 5	18 ± 2	24 ± 3	23 ± 3	21 ± 3
Control	25 ± 3	24 ± 2	22 ± 5	23 ± 4	23 ± 4	22 ± 5	23 ± 3

Clamp group, $n = 6$; control group, $n = 5$. MAP, Mean arterial pressure (mm Hg), HR, heart rate (beats/min); PAP, pulmonary aterial pressure (mm Hg). All values are mean $\pm$ SEM. $p < 0.05$ between groups.

Mean arterial pressure, heart rate, and mean pulmonary arterial pressure were unchanged throughout the experiment in the clamp group (Table 32.2).

There was no significant change in the control group in any of the variables measured throughout the study (Figs. 32.4–32.6, Table 32.2).

Discussion

In clinical and animal studies, we found that an increased afterload of the left ventricle during infrarenal aortic cross-clamping had no effect on intrinsic myocardial contractility. However, reperfusion of the ischemic lower torso led to myocardial depression.

The results of previous studies indicate that cardiac function is reduced during aortic cross-clamping, probably due to an increased afterload of the left ventricle.[4,6] The increased afterload of the left ventricle may reduce subendocardial blood flow during clamping, producing cardiac dysfunction.[7,8]

We found that cardiac output was reduced after clamping in the clinical setting, and that this reduction was associated with a decrease in cardiac preload, which probably was due to insufficient fluid transfusion. No evidence of a reduction in intrinsic cardiac contractility during clamping was seen. This finding well agrees with the results of Brusoni et al.,[9] who found no significant change in cardiac index even during cross-clamping of the thoracic aorta.

It has been reported that significant cardiac dysfunction, so-called declamp shock, occurs soon after removal of the aortic cross-clamp. Recent studies have reported another type of cardiac dysfunction that develops at a late phase after declamping. Anner et al.[4] showed that the cardiac index declined to 44% of the baseline value 4 hours after reperfusion of infrarenal aortic cross-clamping. Kouchoukos et al.[10] also observed that after removing the cross-clamp from the descending thoracic aorta, systemic pressure returned to baseline but cardiac index remained below the baseline value. The mechanisms of the late-phase myocardial depression that followed declamping were not apparent. However, Anner et al.[4] reported that a fall in cardiac output following aortic declamping is related to ischemia-induced thromboxane. In our study, intrinsic myocardial contractility was significantly reduced following declamping.

In the clinical setting, a fall in cardiac output after the declamping was not usually seen. In this study, cardiac output was maintained at almost the same level with the baseline level after the declamping. It is important to note that a higher preload of the left ventricle with fluid transfusion was needed to prevent cardiac dysfunction following the declamping.

In conclusion, reperfusion of the ischemic lower torso led to myocardial depression in human and animal studies. An increased afterload of the left ventricle during infrarenal aortic cross-clamping had no effect on intrinsic cardiac contractility in either study. Sufficient fluid transfusion during the operation could prevent a fall in cardiac output to compensate for the reduction in cardiac contractility.

References

1. Carroll R, Laravuso R, Schauble JF, et al. Left ventricular function during aortic surgery. Arch Surg 1976;111:740–743.
2. Dunn E, Prager RL, Frey W, et al. The effect of abdominal aortic cross-clamping on myocardial function. J Surg Res 1977;22:463–468.
3. Perry M. The hemodynamics of temporary abdominal aortic occlusion. Ann Surg 1968;168:193–200.
4. Anner H, Kaufman RP, Jr, Kobzik L, et al. Pulmonary hypertension and leuko-sequestration after lower torso ischemia. Ann Surg 1987;206:642–648.
5. Suga H, Sagawa K, Shoukas AA. Load independence of the instantaneous pressure-volume ratio of the canine left ventricle and effects of epinephrine and heart rate on the ratio. Circ Res 1973;32:314–322.
6. Mandelbaum I, Webb MK. Left ventricular function during cross-clamping of the descending thoracic aorta. JAMA 1963;186:229–231.
7. Attia RR, Murphy JD, Snider M, et al. Myocardial ischemia due to infrarenal aortic cross-clamping during aortic surgery in patients with severe coronary artery disease. Circulation 1976;53:961–965.
8. Longo T, Marchetti G, Vercellio G. Coronary hemodynaic changes induced by aortic cross-clamping. J Cardiovasc Surg 1969;10:36–42.
9. Brusoni B, Colombo A, Merlo L, et al. Hemodynamic and metabolic changes induced by temporary clamping of the thoracic aorta. Eur Surg Res 1978;10:206–216.
10. Kouchoukos NT, Lell WA, Karp RB, et al. Hemodynamic effects of aortic clamping and decompression with a temporary shunt for resection of the descending thoracic aorta. Surgery 1979;85:25–30.

33
Surgical Management of Aortoiliac Occlusive Disease

JOHN B. CHANG

Introduction

When patients present with ischemia requiring revascularization, caused by occlusive disease limited to the aortoiliac segment, the vascular surgeon has only to deal with various surgical options available for the treatment of aortoiliac occlusive disease and need not be concerned about the treatment of infrainguinal occlusive disease. Thus there are no concerns about which segment is primarily responsible for the ischemia. The treatment choices in isolated aortoiliac disease have evolved from the traditional aortofemoral bypass or endarterectomy to include extraanatomic bypass such as axillofemoral and femorofemoral bypasses and, more recently, balloon angioplasty.[1]

It is evident that this surgical evolution is multifactorial. Careful attention to each aspect of patient management is crucial to a successful outcome. Operative difficulty, increased morbidity and mortality, and graft failure may be avoided by anticipating those situations that have yielded poor results or caused problems in the past. A thorough knowledge of the surgical pitfalls that may be encountered in aortoiliac reconstruction will help avoid surgical misadventure and result in safer, longer-lasting reconstruction. When significant aortoiliac disease is present, disabling claudication, rest pain, and tissue necrosis (including ischemic ulceration and gangrene) are recognized indications for reconstructive surgery.

Proper patient selection, choice of appropriate surgical approach, and correct technical methods of aortic reconstruction remain the principal determinants of success and consistently good results.[2] There are, however, certain historical pitfalls, particularly with regard to symptoms and signs of degenerative arthritis (particularly of the hip), intervertebral disc disease, spinal cord disease, other types of degenerative neurovascular diseases, and situations in which nonvascular conditions must be ruled out. Careful analysis of the symptomatology and physical findings usually yields correct diagnosis in these diseases. Patterns of aortoiliac disease may be grouped into three categories based on anatomy and clinical manifestations[3]:

Type I, or truly segmental aortoiliac disease, occurs in only 5% to 10% of the patients. These patients are commonly younger and are smokers. Half are women, and they frequently have elevated blood lipids. With localized bifurcation disease, they characteristically have symptoms of thigh or buttock claudication. Impotence is common in males (Leriche's syndrome).

Type II, with atherosclerotic involvement of the distal aorta and iliac arteries, comprises an additional group of approximately 25% of the patients. Involvement is still confined to the abdomen, without significant distal disease. Due to collateral circulation in the pelvis, claudication is the most common presenting symptom in such patients, and advanced distal ischemia is unusual.

Type III, with diffuse, multilevel disease, comprises 65% to 75% of the patients. It involves the infrainguinal arterial tree as well as the aortoiliac system. Associated occlusive disease in these patients most commonly involves the superficial femoral artery, popliteal or runoff vessels, and/or the profunda origin. There is a clearly male predominance (7 to 1) in this group. Many of the patients have diabetes and hypertension, as well as other sites of atherosclerotic involvement, such as in the carotid and coronary vessels. Symptoms of more advanced ischemia, including rest pain and tissue necrosis, are often the presenting complaints in this category. The choice and timing of surgical intervention remain especially problematic in type III patients with multilevel occlusive disease. It is wise to avoid doing only distal reconstruction, such as femoropopliteal bypass, if hemodynamically significant aortoiliac disease is present, since inadequate inflow may be an important cause of early failure of distal grafts. Nor can routine proximal reconstruction for all patients with lower extremity occlusive disease be supported, as many patients will not have adequate relief of ischemic symptoms if aortoiliac disease is not primarily responsible for impaired blood flow to the legs.

When iliac disease is localized to a short segment and is causing a stenosis rather than an occlusion, balloon angioplasty is probably most often indicated.[1] However, certain factors make success more likely and include the indication for revascularization (claudication versus salvage), site of the disease, severity of the lesion (stenosis versus occlusion), and runoff. If there is an isolated degree of stenosis causing claudication, the patient should have a very good response to balloon angioplasty. Johnston[4] has shown in a large follow-up study that balloon angioplasty of the iliac arteries has a 60% success rate at 5 years.

Balloon angioplasty can be applied in both good-risk and poor-risk patients who are good candidates for the procedure. In higher-risk patients, angioplasty is employed more liberally. For more severe disease, especially in good-risk patients, surgical intervention is required. In this latter group, the operation chosen depends on the operative risk of the patient and the location of the disease.

Preoperative Assessment

All patients with symptoms of aortoiliac artery occlusive disease are evaluated with a careful history, clinical examination, and noninvasive vascular study. Most of those patients, depending on the severity of the symptoms, are treated conservatively by changing their life style. This includes complete stopping of smoking, and diet and weight control. Some patients are given medical regimentation including exercise programs with hemorrheological agents. If the patient's symptoms are significant, with dissevering claudication, frequent nocturnal symptoms, rest pain, and/or tissue necrosis, he or she is prepared for full evaluation, including angiography studies. At the time of surgical consideration, the patient is also evaluated for other vascular problems including coronary artery heart disease and carotid artery stenosis. Following these initial and follow-up evaluations, the surgeon then chooses a suitable management plan for the given patient. The following options are available:

Aortofemoral Bypass

Aortofemoral Dacron reconstruction for aortoiliac occlusive disease was instituted almost 40 years ago. Following the original publications, its efficacy was soon recognized and it became probably the most widely employed arterial reconstruction. Consequently, numerous reports dealing with successes and pitfalls of this operation have been published. Nonetheless, research extending beyond the first postoperative decade is rarely mentioned.[5-12]

One large series of aortofemoral bypass graft procedures had late patency rates of 74% and 70% after 10 and 15 years, respectively.[13] Operative mortality rates of 2%, 2.9%, and 4.5% have been reported.[2,13,14]

One study shows that aortobifemoral bypass is the preferred operation for extensive iliac artery occlusive disease that is hemodynamically significant only on the symptomatic side unless specifically contraindicated by prohibitive risk or abdominal disease. This is particularly true in the face of superficial femoral artery occlusion.[15]

Angiography

Most of our angiographies have been performed on an outpatient basis, utilizing the digital subtraction angiography (DSA) technique. Whenever clinically indicated, on the basis of evaluation and noninvasive studies, distal runoff studies are performed at the same time. In case of a stenotic lesion, the pressure gradient is measured over the stenotic lesion for hemodynamic studies at the time of angiography. If the transfemoral route is not technically feasible, the transaxillary or brachial approach is used (Figs. 33.1–33.4).

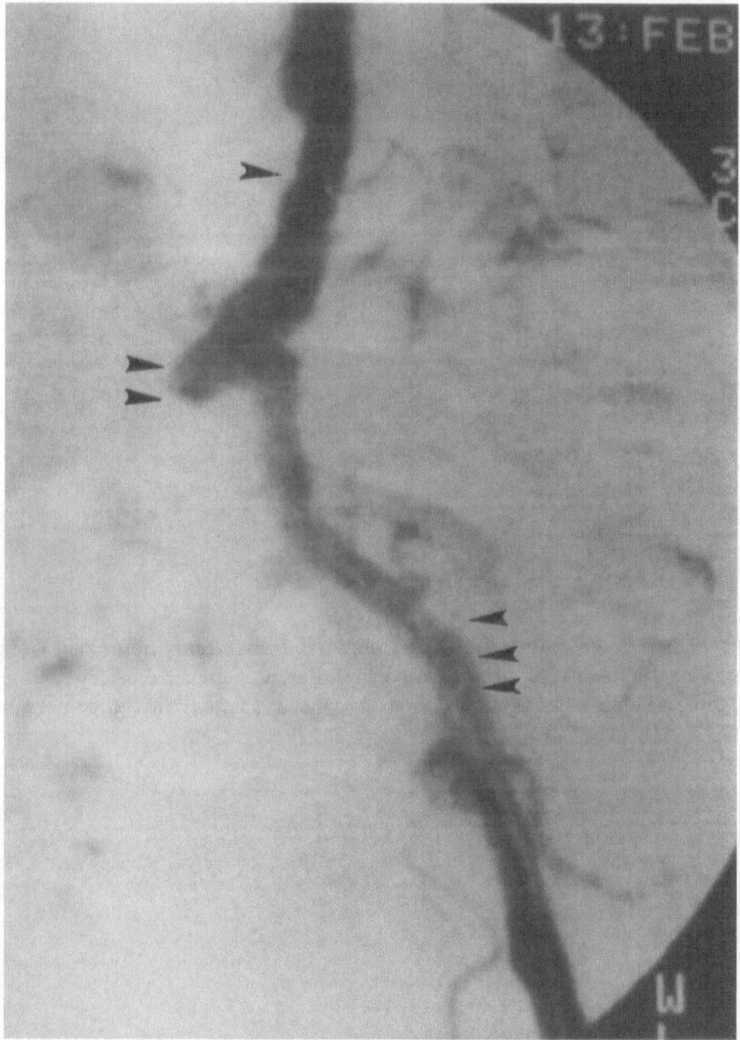

FIGURE 33.1. Transfemoral angiography using DSA technique. Arteriosclerotic disease noted at the abdominal aorta (arrowhead). Right common iliac artery is completely occluded at the origin (two arrowheads). Patent left iliac artery system (three arrowheads).

Surgical Technique

Transabdominal Approach

This approach is most commonly used for the aortofemoral bypass procedure in our practice, as well as by many other surgeons. A midline incision is made extending from the xiphoid process down to the pubic bone, removing

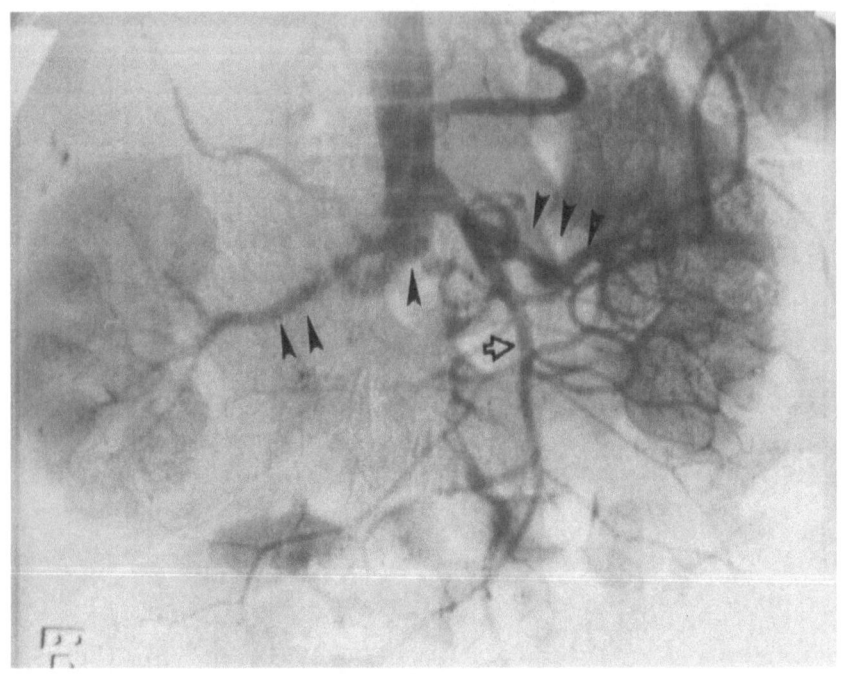

FIGURE 33.2. Angiography using DSA technique, transaxillary approach. Complete occlusion at the juxtarenal aorta (arrowhead). Patent right renal artery (two arrowheads) and left renal artery system (three arrowheads). Patent SMA (open arrow).

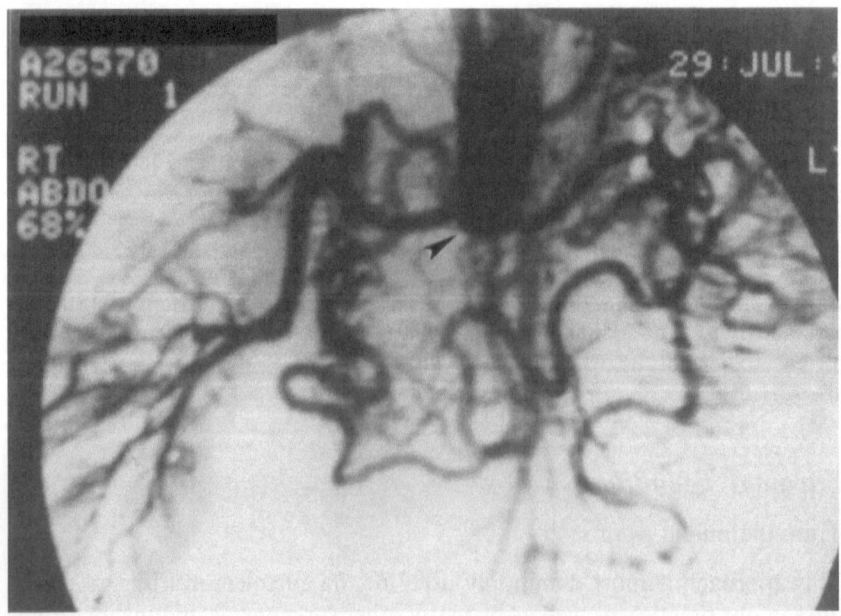

FIGURE 33.3. Transaxillary aortography showing complete occlusion at the juxtarenal aorta (arrowhead) with extensive collaterals.

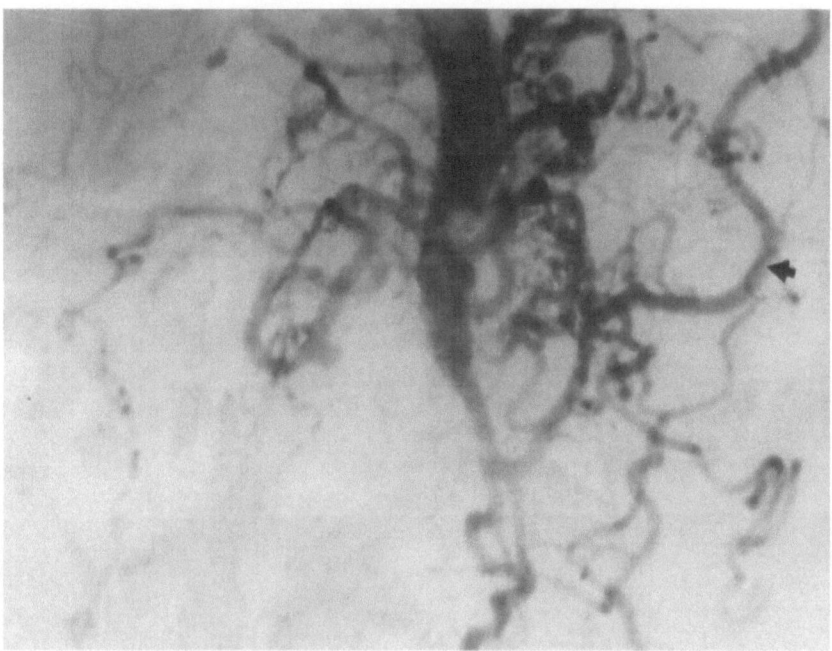

FIGURE 33.4. Angiography with occlusion at the distal aorta, infrarenal with meandering mesenteric artery (arrow).

the umbilicus, at the time of midline incision, in order to eliminate a potential source of contamination from the umbilicus. Dissection is carried out with sharp dissection at the midline. Following abdominal exploration, the transverse colon and small intestines are eviscerated onto the right side of the abdominal wall or within the right side of the abdominal cavity using self retractor devices. The retroperitoneal space is entered. The abdominal aorta proximal to the disease and slightly below the renal artery is routinely used for proximal anastomosis. In the event the proximal aorta has extensive disease and/or juxtarenal aortic occlusive process, temporary aortic clamping is done above the renal artery origin for infrarenal aortic endarterectomy. Following the infrarenal or juxtarenal endarterectomy, aortic clamps are then safely moved on the infrarenal aorta for the proximal anastomosis. It is the author's practice to do proximal anastomosis at the most proximal end at the infrarenal portion of the proximal aorta.

In most cases, particularly with extensive proximal disease, the proximal aorta is transected for true end-to-end anastomosis. If, however, there are good segments of proximal aorta in a young male patient, the author prefers to do end-to-side proximal anastomosis.

The distal anastomoses are chosen, most of the time, on the femoral arteries. At the time of femoral artery anastomosis history, if the patient has occlusive or stenotic disease at the profunda femoral artery with an occluded

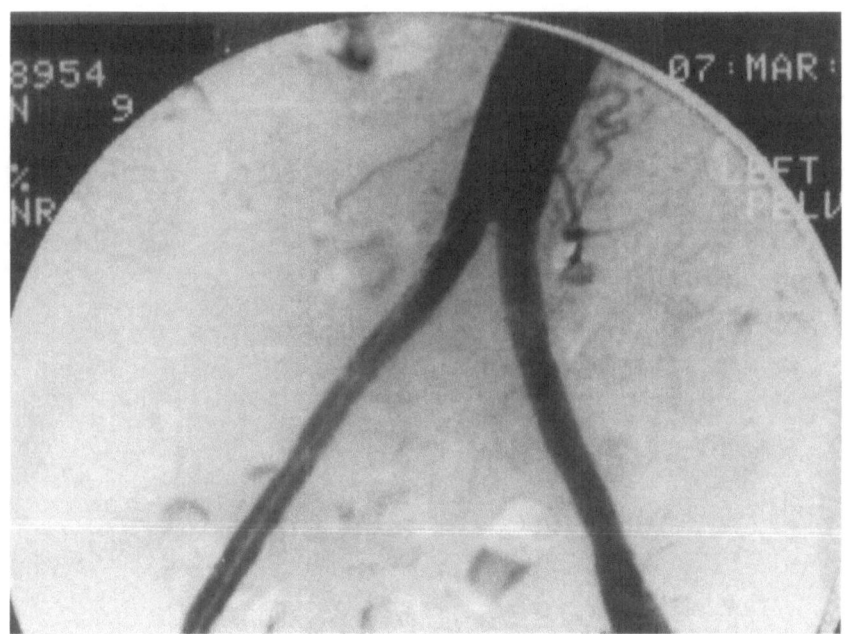

FIGURE 33.5. Ten-year-old aortofemoral Dacron graft.

superficial femoral artery system, the author's preferred choice would be profundaplasty at the time of distal anastomosis with or without endarterectomy. At the time of endarterectomy, we use liberal dissection into the distal profundafemoral artery beyond the diseased point to insure that proper reconstruction is accomplished (Figs. 33.5 and 33.6).

In most cases, double velour Dacron Y graft, No. 18, is used. In the small aorta, particularly in female patients, No. 16 PTFE Y graft has been utilized (Fig. 33.7). The prosthesis is completely covered using vascularized pedicle of omentum.[16]

Retroperitoneal Approach

Retroperitoneal aortic reconstruction has been performed successfully since Robb[17] in 1962, reporting on 500 aortic reconstructions performed through the retroperitoneal approach, listed the benefits to be less ileus, atelectasis, and pain; reduced incidence of wound dehiscence; easier anesthesia; a shorter stay in bed and in the hospital; and a faster return to work.

Certain pitfalls of retroperitoneal aortic reconstruction deserve comment. These include injury to the vena cava, which is very difficult to manage through the retroperitoneal approach. Vigorous retraction in the upper aspect of the operative field may lead to unrecognized splenic trauma. This should be minimized by using self-retaining retractors. The lumbar branch of

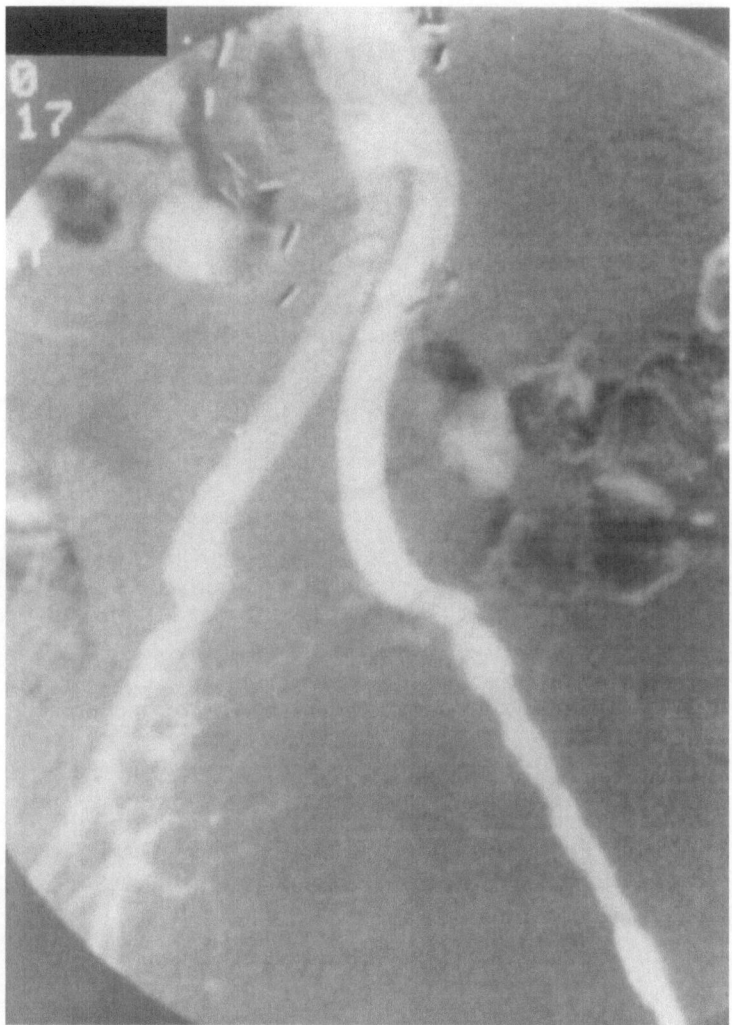

FIGURE 33.6. Ten-year-old aorto bilateral iliac artery bypass Dacron graft.

the left renal vein must be identified not only because it serves as a marker to the left renal artery, but to avoid injuring it as well.

Similarly, although rarely, a retroaortic left renal vein or circumaortic left renal vein may cause problems if not recognized. During mobilization of the retroperitoneum, it is important to identify the left gonadal vein so that, during the course of sweeping the retroperitoneum anteriorly, the gonadal vein is not avulsed from the left renal vein. A left pneumothorax may occur and be unrecognized, particularly if the left 11th intercostal space incision is not made carefully. Both the inferior mesenteric artery (IMA) and the left

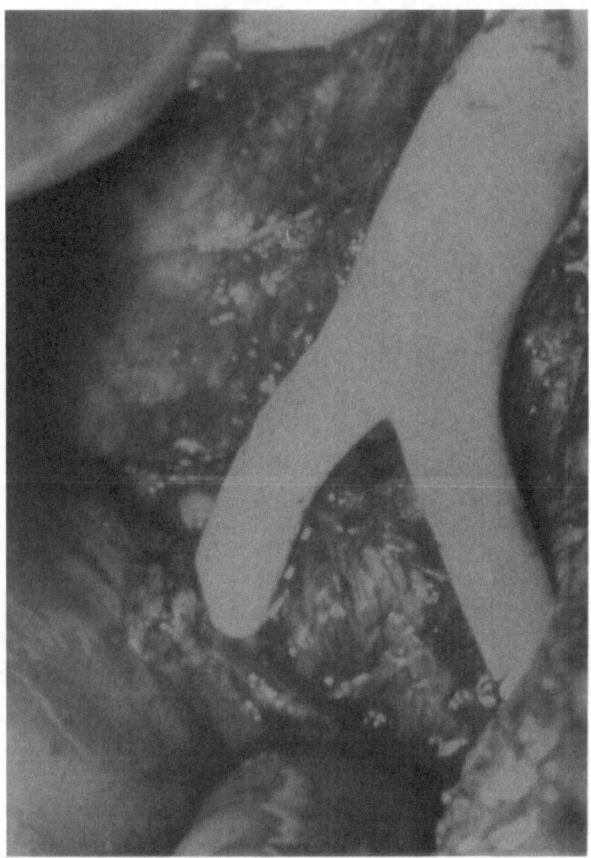

FIGURE 33.7. No. 16 PTFE Y-graft (in position).

renal artery are swept anteriorly when retrorenal dissection is performed and must be identified to prevent injury.

Proper positioning of the patient is important. The left thorax is elevated 45 to 60 degrees, while the hips should lie as flat as possible to allow access to the right groin should that become necessary. The patient's position is secured by placement on a vacuum styrofoam bean bag. The midpoint between the patient's left costal margin and iliac crest is centered over the table flexion point, so that flexing the operating table causes the incision to spiral open. Wound closure is facilitated by flattening the operating table. The surgeon stands to the left of the patient. Rotation of the table away from the surgeon facilitates retroperitoneal dissection, while rotation towards the surgeon facilitates groin dissection.

An oblique left flank incision is used starting midway between the umbilicus and symphysis pubis and extending from the lateral margin of the left rectus sheath into the 11th intercostal space for 8 to 10 cm. The abdominal wall and intercostal muscles are divided in the line of the incision, taking care not to injure the 11th and 12th dorsal neurovascular bundles. Damage to these nerves denervates the abdominal wall leading to muscle weakness, manifest as an asymmetric abdominal contour with unsightly bulging.

The retroperitoneal space is entered at the tip of the 12th rib, and with blunt dissection, the anterior peritoneum is dissected away from the transversalis fascia as far as the rectus sheath. Dissection medial to the rectus is not necessary for exposure. Also, this prevents tearing the peritoneum where it is firmly attached at the lateral border of the rectus.

Posterolaterally, the plane of the flank musculature, psoas, and diaphragm are followed as the peritoneal sac and its contents are dissected and retracted anteromedially. This plane is developed along the lumbodorsal fascia behind the left kidney, mobilizing the kidney and urethra anteriorly. Alternatively, dissection can be performed anterior to the left kidney and ureter, but an advantage of the retroperitoneal approach is lost, since the left renal vein obscures the juxtarenal aorta. However, dissection anterior to the kidney is useful when exposure of the superior mesenteric artery beyond its origin is required for endarterectomy or when endarterectomy of the pararenal aorta is anticipated.

The aorta is easily exposed from above the renal artery to the aortic bifurcation. To prevent injury to the left renal artery, its identification is important. The artery can usually be identified behind the lumbar branch of the left renal vein, which is a fairly constant structure. Ligation of this lumbar branch, which crosses over the aorta, provides good exposure of the aorta and origin of the left renal artery.

Lymphatics and fat overlying the aorta are ligated to minimize lymphorrhea. Blunt dissection of the aorta, anteriorly and posteriorly, either above or below the renal artery, is performed to allow placement of the proximal clamp. Circumferential aortic dissection is not required as long as the tip of the clamp can reach beyond the aortic wall. Inferior vena cava injury is not a concern, as it is not immediately adjacent to the aorta at this level.

If suprarenal aortic control is required, dissection is carried out cephalad, with longitudinal division of the diaphragmatic crus. Suture ligation of the areolar tissue surrounding the origin of the superior mesenteric artery (SMA) minimizes potential lymphatic leaks. With the need for supraceliac exposure, dissection proceeds further cephalad. Investing fascia around the aorta is incised and blunt dissection anteriorly and posteriorly creates tunnels to accommodate the jaws of an aortic clamp. Supraceliac control is often easier to obtain than juxtarenal control because of the relative paucity of lymphatics and fat at the paraceliac level. If juxtarenal or supraceliac aortic clamping is anticipated preoperatively, a 9th or 10th intercostal space incision is recommended.

Distal exposure of the iliac arteries is accomplished by blunt dissection of the peritoneal sac out of the iliac fossa. The left iliac artery can be exposed easily over its entire length. Exposure of the right iliac artery is more challenging. Minimal dissection of the distal aorta is required when managing occlusive disease and the inferior mesenteric artery is preserved.

Anastomoses to the right distal common or external iliac arteries are difficult through the left retroperitoneal approach. Some authors have advocated extending the abdominal incision across the midline into the right lower quadrant to facilitate right iliac arterial exposure. A right lower quadrant counter incision a few centimeters above the inguinal ligament with extraperitoneal dissection of the iliac vessels provides excellent exposure for right external iliac artery anastomoses. This avoids groin dissection with its small but real risk of infection, even though one should not hesitate to make a groin incision if necessary.[14,17,18]

Aortoiliac Endarterectomy

Thoughtful selection of patients for aortoiliac endarterectomy is crucial. This procedure should be considered primarily in the 5% to 10% of patients in whom disease is localized to the aortic bifurcation (type I). Although the procedure is technically demanding, it offers several advantages. No prosthetic material is used, so the infection rate is virtually nil. Inflow to the hypogastric arterial network may be better preserved than with a bypass method; it may even be increased. Improved hypogastric inflow in turn may better maintain or restore erectile function in the male.[19]

The technical success of aortoiliac endarterectomy depends on the proper plane of dissection at the level of the external elastic lamina. This dissection can be done even in the presence of extensive calcification in the wall of the aorta or the proximal common iliac arteries. A secure end point to prevent flaps in subintimal dissection is necessary. One or more tacking sutures of 5–0 or 6–0 Prolene placed in a mattress fashion across the distal end point are often required to hold the distal intima in place. When disease is localized to the larger common iliac vessels, this is possible under direct vision. Endarterectomy becomes a suboptimal procedure when atherosclerotic disease extends beyond the bifurcation of the common iliac vessles. Extension of endarterectomy distally into the external iliac artery makes the operation longer and more difficult. It is often technically less satisfactory, due to the more difficult exposure, the small size of the external iliac artery, and adherence of the intima to the more muscular vessel. Distal extension of aortoiliac endarterectomy is associated with a decrease in long-term patency, with the late failure rate climbing to 25% at 5 years.[2]

The most common cause of failure after endarterectomy is progression of disease distal to the endarterectomized segment.[2,8,20] It is important to remember, then, that angiographic evidence or an operative finding of occlusive disease extending beyond the iliac bifurcation favors bypass grafting. Moreover, endarterectomy is frankly contraindicated whenever there is evidence of aneurysmal disease, because the endarterectomized vessel is prone to continued aneurysmal degeneration. Similarly, total occlusion of the infrarenal aorta is best handled by simple transection of the aorta within several centimeters of the renal arteries, with thrombectomy of the aorta cuff and subsequent graft insertion. This is more expedient then endarterectomy and is associated with better long-term function.[21]

The follow-up results of aortoiliac endarterectomy, accumulated and tabulated in the same manner as described for the bypass procedure, disclosed a patency rate of 88.8% at the end of the first year of observation. Thereafter, the rate showed a deterioration closely comparable to that seen for the bypass operations, namely a deterioration of nearly 3% per year. Again, the 15-year patency rate was just below 50%, and the late cumulative mortality rate was 36.8%.[22]

In one institution's 15-year study of aortoiliac endarterectomy, there was no operative mortality and an early patency rate of approximately 98% with a 66% 15-year patency rate. Limb salvage was 92% and 79% at the 5th and 10th years, respectively.[23]

Combined Aortoiliac and Infrainguinal Occlusive Disease

When the patient presents with multilevel occlusive disease causing ischemia requiring revascularization, the traditional approach has been to address the proximal disease prior to any consideration of therapy for the infrainguinal disease. Arteriography historically has been the primary method of determining the significance of aortoiliac disease. Although this diagnostic technique is the gold standard in many areas of vascular surgery, its inadequacy in the area of aortoiliac disease has been well documented. Moore and Hall[24] have nicely demonstrated how single-plane arteriography can miss significant aortoiliac lesions.

Accurate assessment of hemodynamic significance requires physiological measurements. Knowledge of physiological changes accompanying arteriographically demonstrated aortoiliac lesions is of great importance in the surgical decision-making process in patients with combined aortoiliac and femoropopliteal disease. Significant common femoral artery outflow obstruction and/or superficial femoral artery occlusion frequently coexists with aortoiliac disease and may necessitate distal bypass surgery to maintain graft patency and limb salvage. The profunda femoris artery, through its many branches, forms extensive communication with the popliteal artery at the knee and the tibial vessels in the calf. In the presence of superficial femoral artery occlusion, the profunda femoris artery provides the major collateral circulation through which blood reaches the distal limb.[25]

Although arteriosclerosis does not affect the profunda femoris artery as severely as the superficial femoral artery, a review of angiographic evaluation of ischemic limbs showed atheroma in the ostium of the profunda femoris artery in 39% of the cases.[26] The atheromatous lesion affecting the profunda femoris artery was confined to the ostium or proximal segment in 74% of the cases, but affected the mid and distal segments in 26%.[27]

In the presence of coexisting aortoiliac occlusive disease and common femoral artery outflow obstruction, use of the profunda femoris artery as the outflow vessel in aortofemoral bypass will optimize the collateral circulation and may lessen the need for distal bypass. Standard aorta–common femoral artery and aorta–profunda femoris bypass provide cumulative patency and limb salvage exceeding 90% at 5 years. Concomitant or subsequent distal

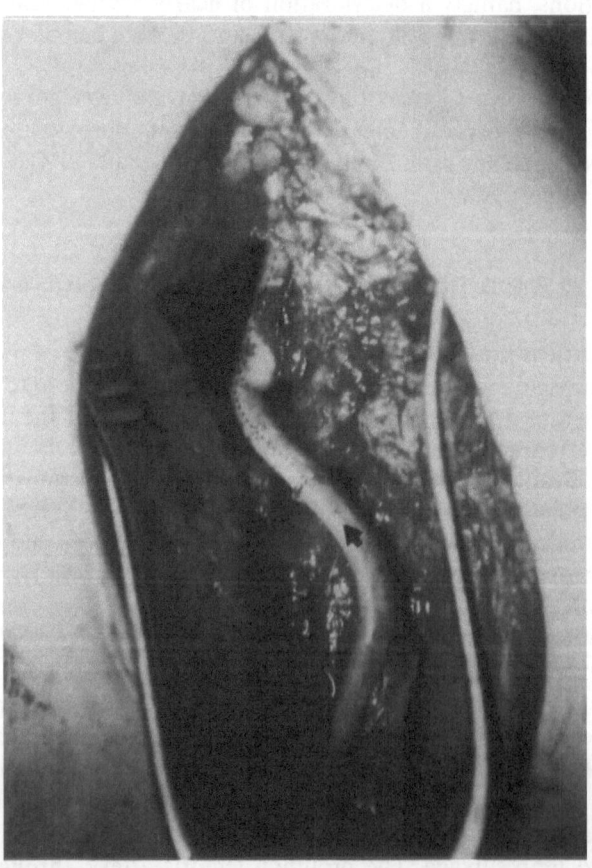

FIGURE 33.8. PTFE graft for common femoral-above knee popliteal artery bypass (arrow).

bypass was required in 12% of the limbs undergoing aorta–profunda femoris bypass. Both proximal and distal profunda femoris arteries provide a durable outflow tract when aortoiliac and femoropopliteal occlusive disease are combined.[25]

As indicated in another study, in patients with poorly developed deep femoral artery (DFA) collateral flow with severe ischemia [gangrene and/or an ankle–brachial index (ABI) under 0.30], and in patients in whom an angiographically occluded or severely diseased below-knee (BK) popliteal artery is demonstrated, adding a synchronous femorodistal bypass is essential.[28]

In our practice, in addition to the angiographic and physiological evaluation, the patient is offered distal bypass if there is tissue necrosis or extensive occlusive disease in the profunda femoris artery or popliteal arterial system at the time of aortofemoral bypass grafting or subsequent to that operation,

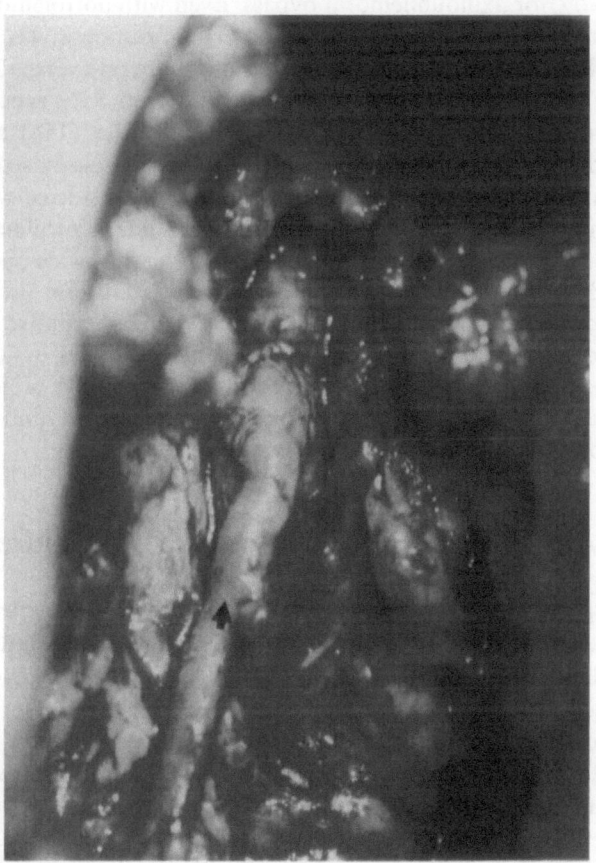

FIGURE 33.9. Common femoral artery-above knee popliteal artery bypass with autogenous vein.

depending upon the clinical setting. When distal anastomosis can be performed at the above-knee popliteal segment polytetrafluoroethylene (PTFE) (Fig. 33.8) or autogenous vein graft (Fig. 33.9) can be utilized. If distal bypass grafting is necessary, autogenous vein graft is preferable, either by in situ technique (Figs. 33.10 and 33.11) or reverse saphenous vein technique. In the cases where autogenous vein graft is utilized, the author prefers proximal anastomosis of that vein graft at the artery distal to the aortofemoral bypass anastomosis, rather than making anastomoses through the prosthesis. To accomplish this, one has to do extended distal dissection to free the distal segment of the profunda femoris artery for proximal vein anastomosis. If the autogenous vein graft is not available in its entirety, composite grafts have been used (Figs. 33.12–33.14).

In one study, the patency of the aortobifemoral bypass was reduced from 90% to 76% by superficial femoral artery (SFA) occlusion, compared to reduction from 92% to 52% for femorofemoral, 92% to 41% for axillobifemoral, and 54% to 0% for axillounifemoral bypass. Even with aortofemoral bypass, where patency was not so affected, hemodynamic response was affected by SFA occlusion; there was a 29% hemodynamic failure rate versus 2% in those without SFA occlusion. This can be predicted (with 85% accuracy) from preoperative consideration of the thigh–brachial index (TBI) and ankle–brachial index (ABI). Synchronous distal bypass, particularly sequential extension to an above-knee popliteal artery, should be considered when hemodynamic failure can be predicted, when the profunda geniculate collateral system and its reentry into a patent popliteal artery is not wide open distal to the profunda orifice, or when advanced ischemic lesions are present in the foot. Extended profundaplasty may provide a viable alternative in selected cases, particularly if performed with autogenous tissue, but limited profundaplasty (extending a tongue of the graft into the profunda orifice) did not improve pressure transmission to the ankle or improve graft limb patency. It is justified only for orificial profunda stenosis.[29]

Balloon Angioplasty and Endovascular Procedures

In managing patients with peripheral arterial occlusive disease, percutaneous transluminal angioplasty (PTA) provides an important alternative. An improved balloon dilating catheter was described by Gruntzig and Hopff in 1974[30] (Figs. 33.15–33.17).

In a large series, the 5-year patency rate of PTA on common iliac artery stenosis with a good runoff was 63%; with a poor runoff, it was 51%. Occluded common iliac artery with a good runoff had a 48% PTA patency rate in 5 years. However, in poor runoff cases, the 5-year patency was 33%. These were cases where the PTA was performed with claudication as indication. Where salvage was the indication for PTA, common iliac artery stenosis with a good runoff had a 50% 5-year patency rate, with a 36% rate in poor runoff

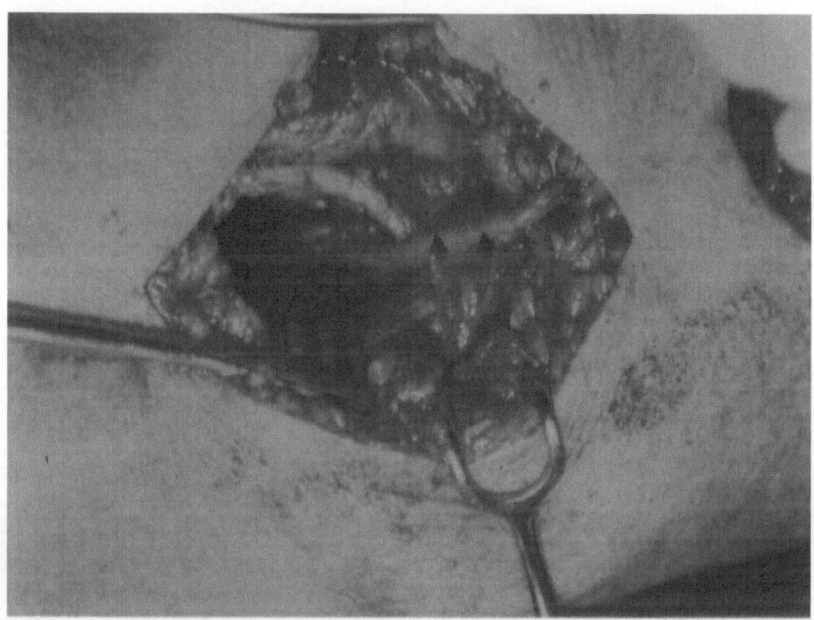

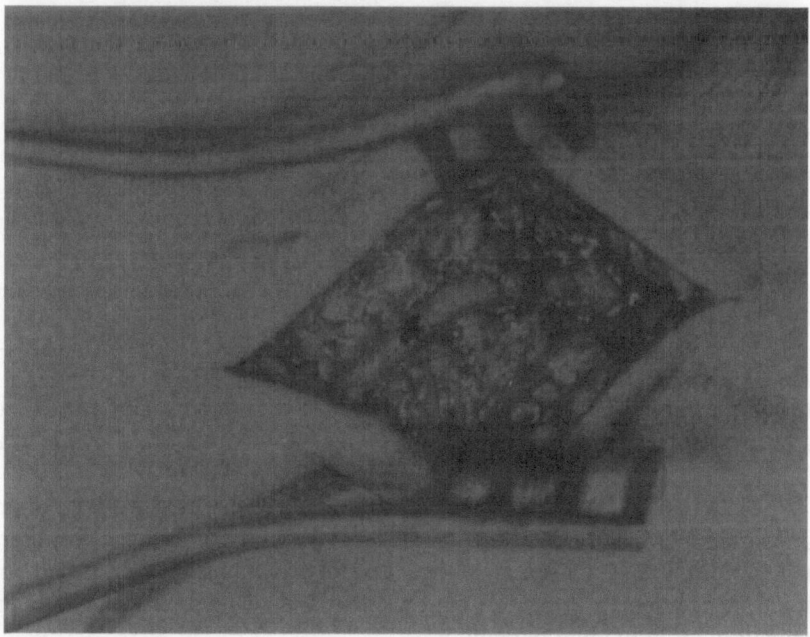

FIGURE 33.10 (top) and 33.11 (bottom). Femoral-distal posterior tibial artery bypass with in situ (two arrows at Figure 33.10, indicating proximal portion of the in situ greater saphenous vein graft). Arrow at Figure 33.11 showing the distal end of the in situ greater saphenous vein graft at the posterior tibial artery.

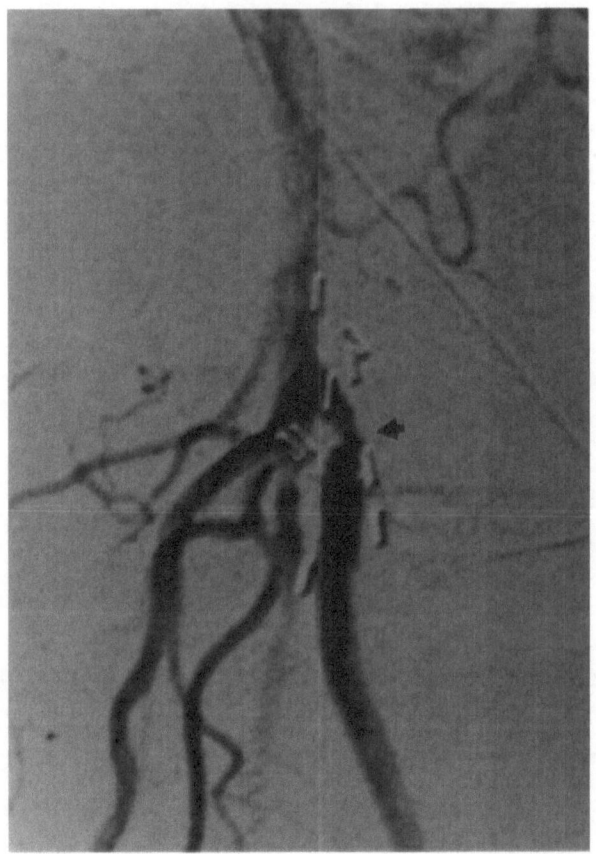

FIGURE 33.12 (above), 33.13, and 33.14 (following pages). Right common femoral artery to distal popliteal artery bypass using composite graft, 6 mm PTFE, and small segment of the greater saphenous vein. Six years old. Proximal anastomosis in Figure 33.12 (one arrow).

cases. If the common iliac arteries were occluded with good runoff, the 5-year patency was 32%; with a poor runoff in the same situation, the rate was 19%.[31]

When an iliac dilatation failed, the clinical grade was worse in 10.3% of the patients and the ankle–brachial systolic blood pressure ratio fell by more than 0.20 in 9.5%.[32] The advantage and disadvantage of the procedure should be considered in determining whether PTA is indicated in the management of an individual patient.[33]

PTA has a low cost and the morbidity and mortality rates are low in the hands of an experienced operator. If it fails, the procedure can usually be repeated and does not preclude future vascular reconstructive surgery.

There are disadvantages to PTA. The extent of improvement following a

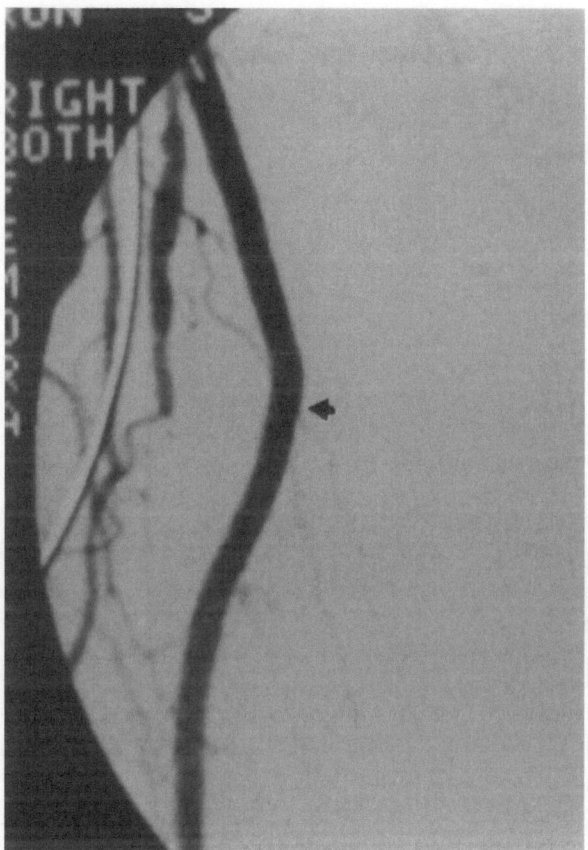

FIGURE 33.13. PTFE portion of the graft (arrow).

successful PTA is less dramatic than that following surgery. The morbidity of the PTA is quite high if the operator is not experienced with the technique.

PTA may be used as an adjunct or as an alternative to surgery. It can be used to improve inflow prior to a distal arterial repair or a femoral crossover graft. PTA is an alternative to surgery in approximately 25% of cases. The patient should be considered for the procedure only if the arterial disease is localized (i.e., the lesion is less than 10 cm in length and the adjacent vessels are relatively free of disease), the operator is experienced with the technique, and the risk–benefit ratio of PTA is favorable relative to conservative therapy and surgery. One study identified the risks of PTA as mortality, 0.4%; serious complications requiring an operation, 1.1%; and major complications delaying hospital discharge, 3.4%. Fortunately, if the PTA fails, the patient is not usually significantly worse. The benefits of PTA (i.e., the chances of success) can be predicted from knowledge of four interrelated variables: the indication for the procedure, the site of the PTA, the severity of the lesion,

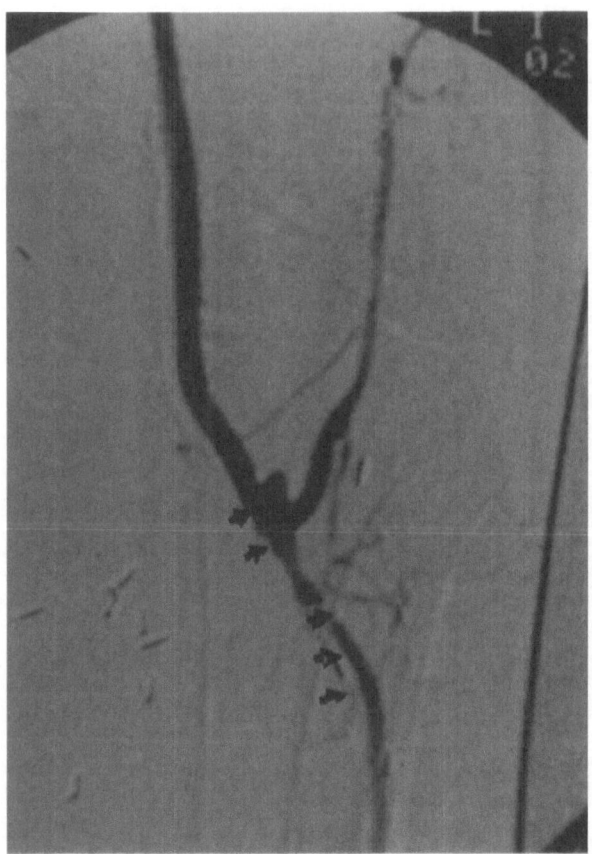

FIGURE 33.14. Small piece of autogenous vein distal to the PTFE graft and proximal to the popliteal segment (two arrows). Anterior tibial artery runoff (three arrows).

and the runoff. Results are best if the patient has claudication, common iliac artery stenosis, and good runoff. Even in the ideal patient with no distal disease, mild persistent symptoms are frequent after successful PTA, and the ankle–brachial blood pressure ratio often remains abnormal.[31]

There is a need for internal support, or endoskeleton, to improve the results from PTA in two general areas: to improve early technical results and to correct or prevent problems with restenosis. In 1985, Palmaz[34] first reported a canine experiment using a balloon-expandable stent. Even though PTA has been an accepted modality for localized occlusive iliac artery disease, the reported success rate at 1 year ranged between 50% and 93%.[4,35–39] This may be the result of an immediately unsuccessful attempt at PTA (6–15%)[35–38,40] or of a recurrent disease process.[4,35–37,40,41]. The introduction of a stent to mechanically maintain the opening made by balloon angioplasty seems logical in those patients otherwise destined for failure.

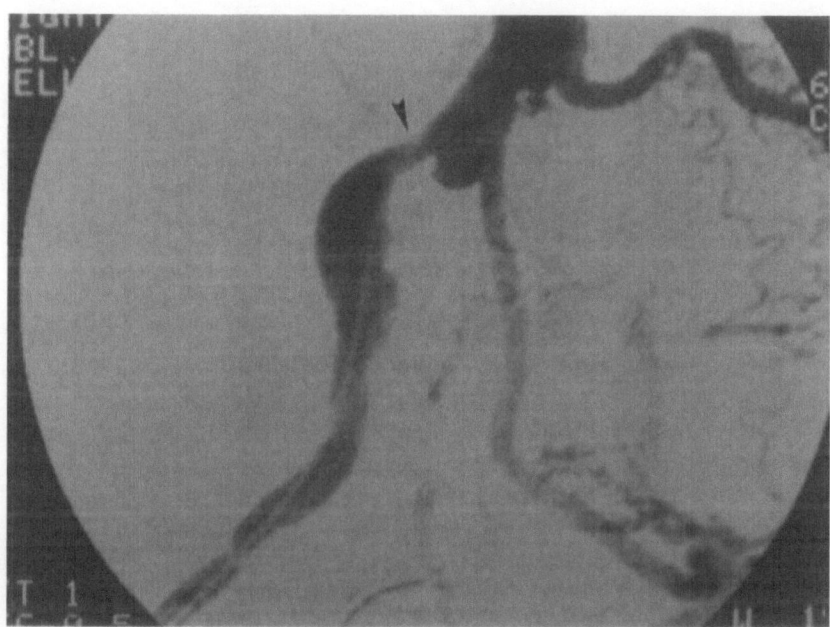

FIGURE 33.15. Angiography showing stenotic lesion at the right common iliac artery (arrowhead).

Early experience with the Palmaz expandable intraluminal stent suggests that it can be valuable in salvaging PTA cases that might otherwise be initial failures. PTA-induced dissection, elastic recoil, and technically unsuccessful PTA attempts can be corrected with acceptable results. PTA restenosis may also be favorably addressed by the use of stents, although longer follow-up is required to fully clarify this issue. There is significant morbidity and mortality reported in the initial learning experience with a stent. These problems may improve with experience and technological advances, but presently these factors must be considered in the overall risk–benefit decisions for any given patient. In the final analysis, greater experience and more extensive follow-up will solidify the role of the stent in the treatment of iliac artery occlusive disease.[42]

Extraanatomic Bypasses

Since 1963, when Blaisdell[43] introduced axillofemoral bypass as an alternative reconstructive procedure for aortoiliac occlusive disease, a number of techniques have been described. The primary purposes of the extraanatomic bypasses are to reduce operative risks, to overcome the problem with infec-

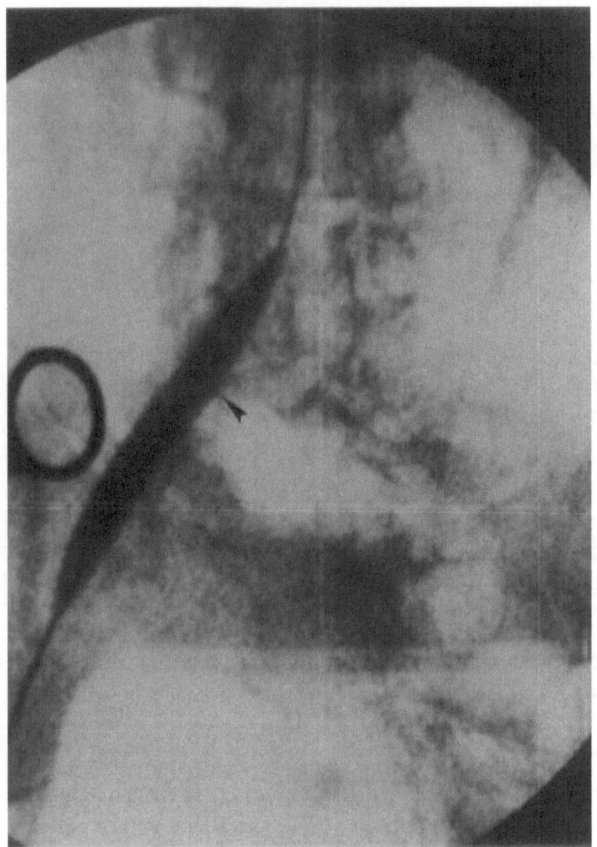

FIGURE 33.16. Patient in Figure 33.15, balloon angioplasty in progress with a dilated balloon (arrowhead).

tion at the primary surgical site, or to achieve other medical and surgical aims.

Chang and his group have reported their experience with axillofemoral bypass[44] and the current state of extraanatomic bypass in 1986.[45]

Axillary–Femoral Artery Bypass

The first description of this procedure was published in 1963.[46] Since then, extensive reports have been available in the literature.[44,45,47–52] There are many different indications for this type of revascularization. Axillobilateral femoral artery bypass grafts have a primary patency rate of approximately 75% at the 5th year. With appropriate measures, net limb salvage can be accomplished in 84% of the surviving patients at the 5th year.

Some reports indicate that the life table primary patency for those opera-

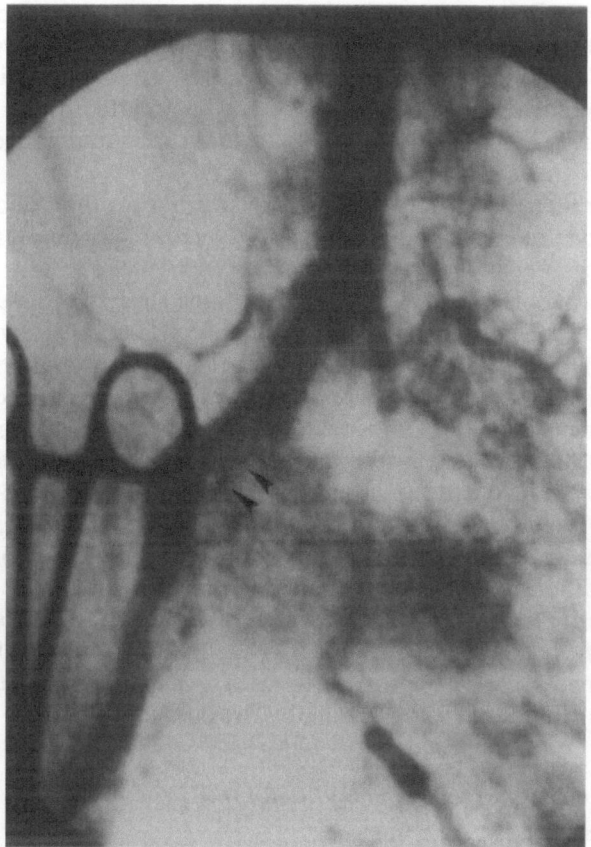

FIGURE 33.17. Successful outcome of balloon angioplasty of the right common iliac artery (two arrowheads) on the patient shown in Figure 33.15.

tions with axillobifemoral bypass grafts using externally supported PTFE prostheses showed a primary patency rate of 85% after 4 years. The patency results achieved in these series are sufficiently satisfactory to warrant use of axillobifemoral bypass graft in an expanding number of patients with high operative risk and need for bypass of aortoiliac occlusive disease.[53] Lewis[54] was the first to describe the use of an upper extremity artery as the inflow donor for a lower extremity bypass graft. His patient had a rupture of an abdominal aortic aneurysm complicated by aortic dissection. A nylon graft was placed from the left subclavian artery to the abdominal aorta. The graft was tunneled subcutaneously along the chest wall, gaining an intraperitoneal location at the xiphoid.

As previously indicated, Blaisdell et al.[55] were the first to describe the use of an extraanatomic bypass graft in the treatment of an infected aortic prosthetic graft. Efforts to explain the decreased patency of axillounilateral femoral grafting compared to axillobifemoral bypass grafting have centered on the use of bilateral versus unilateral grafts, the type of prosthetic material used, and the possible effect of the subcutaneous location of the grafts. Increasing opinion has favored an axillobifemoral configuration over the axillounifemoral graft.

The 5-year secondary patency rates were superior for the axillobifemoral grafting versus axillounifemoral grafting, 74% versus 37% in one series,[56] and similar findings were noted in other studies.[43,44,57]

In doing axillobifemoral bypass grafting, some suggest aggressive use of the profunda femoris artery in the face of superficial femoral artery occlusion to achieve optimal results.[58] When axillofemoral bypass grafting was performed for acute vascular occlusion, there was a higher incidence of perioperative complications (63% versus 26%, $p = 0.001$), perioperative mortality (26% versus 3%, $p < 0.05$), lower graft patency at 1 year (60% versus 90%, $p < 0.05$), lower rate of freedom from reoperation in the 1st year (50% versus 82%, $p < 0.01$), and lower rates of limb salvage (76% versus 94%, $p < 0.05$) than patients undergoing axillofemoral bypass grafting for chronic symptoms or conditions. These two groups did not differ in any of the other risk factors or perioperative characteristics examined. Therefore, the authors of this study concluded that axillofemoral bypass grafting performed for indications other than acute vascular occlusion is associated with acceptable morbidity, mortality, graft patency, and limb salvage rate.[59]

Femoral–Femoral Artery Bypass Graft

Since Vetto[60] reported in 1962, there have been reports of favorable results.[47,61,62] The long-term patency rate of this bypass graft was 85% at 5 years and 75% at 10 years in my own series[45] (Fig. 33.18)

With the proper indication and sound surgical technique, this bypass procedure will give optimum results.[48–51,61] To achieve successful results, it is crucial that the patient be evaluated preoperatively with noninvasive vascular studies and excellent angiography evaluation. One of the major contraindications to this procedure used to be stenotic lesion at the donor site of the iliac artery. The new improvements in technology using transluminal balloon angioplasty permit treatment of some limited cases with extremely high risk; with a combination of ipsilateral percutaneous or transluminal balloon angioplasty of the donor site of the iliac artery, one can still proceed with femorofemoral artery bypass rather than the conventional aortofemoral or iliofemoral bypass procedure. Distal extension of the bypass has to be based on the condition of the individual patient. It is advisable to extend distal bypass grafting in multilevel disease with tissue necrosis at the foot. It is my policy to revascularize in maximum degree for limb salvage purposes in cases with multilevel occlusive process and tissue necrosis. After proper selection

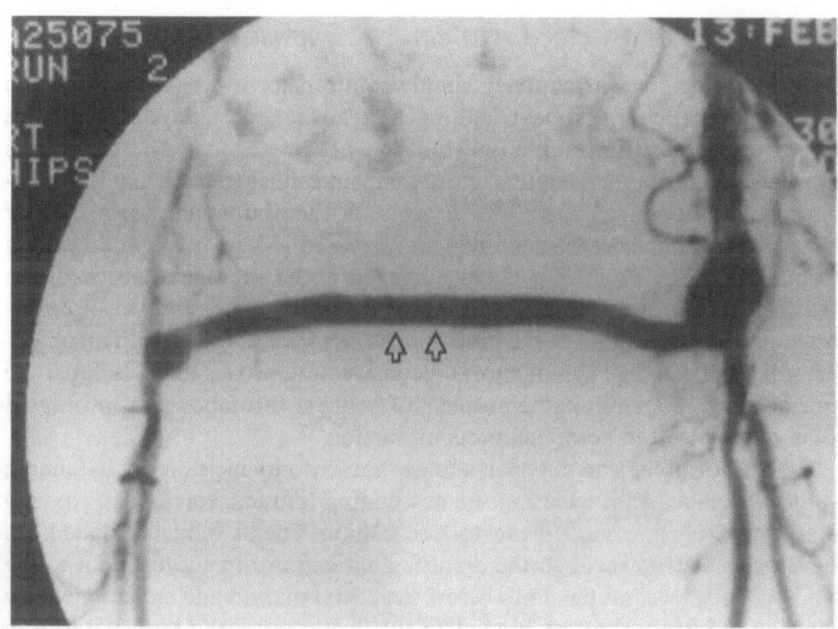

FIGURE 33.18. Functioning left femoral–right femoral artery bypass PTFE graft, 8 years old (two arrows).

of the donor site and the receiving site of the arterial system, the tunnel is made over the pubic bone, subcutaneously, in S shape, inverted U shape, or straightforward U shape. I avoid straight grafting in T shape in order to avoid friction or tension with different postures of the hip joint.

Ascending Aortofemoral Artery Bypass

This is another alternative for treatment of aortofemoral occlusive process in good-risk patients with intraabdominal sepsis or other conditions prohibiting standard aortofemoral bypass grafting.[63–65]

Iliofemoral Artery Bypass Graft

Ipsilateral iliofemoral bypass through a retroperitoneal incision may be preferable to femorofemoral artery bypass if the occlusive disease is limited to the external iliac artery because it can avoid violating the opposite groin and a normal femoral artery.[29] Ipsilateral iliofemoral bypass, with or without distal extension, has been one of the preferred choices in aortoiliac occlusive disease management in the author's experience.

Descending Thoracic Aortofemoral Bypass Graft

This technique gives a relatively simple solution to several complex aortic problems in patients who have had repeated aortic graft failure or who have had extensive gastrointestinal and biliary tract procedures. The use of this approach avoids possible injury to the gastrointestinal tract during the exposure of the abdominal aorta. Encasement of the abdominal aorta by scar tissue is common. There is definitely an increased risk involved in dissection around the aorta. Following elective division of the abdominal aorta for the treatment of an aortic graft-to-duodenal fistula or after removal of an infected graft, arterial flow to the limb is routinely reestablished with an axillofemoral bypass. While axillofemoral reconstruction proves to be useful at the time of initial reoperation, the problem of frequent thrombosis has prompted some centers to seek permanent reconstruction.[52]

The author prefers an anterior-lateral thoracotomy incision not extending to the abdomen. After isolating the descending thoracic aorta, the proximal anastomosis is performed in end-to-side fashion. Then a tunnel is made from the left chest cavity through the diaphragmatic insertion and brought to the subcutaneous level on the flank below the costal margin and subcutaneously down to the femoral artery medial to the iliac crest. Long-term patency of this graft is encouraging. The most commonly used graft material in my practice is PTFE with a size ranging from 6 to 10 mm.

Conclusion

In managing aortoiliac occlusive disease, surgeons now have many choices other than standard aortofemoral bypass procedure. To choose the proper procedure for a given patient, the vascular surgeon should be familiar with all the available alternative procedures. By understanding these alternatives, the risks and benefits of the procedures, and the long-term results of each procedure, and by having the technical ability to apply the procedures as necessary, the surgeon can assure that the patient will have the best protection with a long-term successful outcome.

References

1. Flanigan DP. Management of aortoiliac occlusive disease with/without infrainguinal occlusion. In: Chang JB (ed.): *Modern Vascular surgery. Vol 4.* California: PMA Publ. Corp., 1991, pp. 179–187.
2. Von Gryska P, Brewster DC. Surgical treatment of aortoiliac occlusive disease: Surgical pitfalls. In: Chang JB (ed.): *Modern Vascular Surgery. Vol 2.* New York: PMA Publ. Corp., 1987, pp. 54–68.
3. Darling RC, Brewster DC, Hallett JW, Jr, Darling RC III. Aorta-iliac reconstruction. Surg Clin North Am 1979;59:565–579.

4. Johnston WK, Rae M, Hogg-Johnston SA, et al. Five-year results of a prospective study of percutaneous transluminal angioplasty. Ann Surg 1987;206:403–413.
5. Szilagyi DE. Ten years experience with aorta-iliac and femoro-popliteal arterial reconstruction. J Cardiovasc Surg 1964;5:502–509.
6. Hansteen V, Lorentsen E, Sivertsseb E, Bergan F. Long-term follow-up of patients with peripheral arterial obliterations treated with arterial surgery. Acta Chir Scand 1975;141:725–730.
7. Malone JM, Moore WS, Goldstone J. The natural history of bilateral aortofemoral bypass grafts for ischemia of the lower extremities. Arch Surg 1975;110:1300–1306.
8. Brewster DC, Darling RC. Optimal methods of aortoiliac reconstruction. Surgery 1978;84:739–748.
9. Nevelsteen A, Suy R, Daenen W, Boel A, Stalpaert G. Aortofemoral grafting: Factors influencing late results. Surgery 1980;88:642–653.
10. Crawford ES, Bomberger RA, Glaeser DH, Saleh SA, Russell WL. Aortoiliac occlusive disease: Factors influencing survival and function following reconstructive operation over a twenty-five-year period. Surgery 1981;90:1055–1067.
11. Poulias GE, Polemis L, Skoutas B, Doundoulakis N, Papaloannou K, Ershaid B, Sendekeya S. Bilateral aorta-femoral bypass in the presence of aorta-iliac occlusive disease and factors determining results: Experience and long term follow-up with 500 consecutive cases. J Cardiovasc Surg 1985;26:527–538.
12. Szilagyi DE, Elliott JP, Smith RF, Reddy DJ, McPharlin M. A thirty-year survey of the reconstructive surgical treatment of aortoiliac occlusive disease. J Vasc Surg 1986;3:421–436.
13. Nevelsteen A, Wouters L, Suy R. Aortofemoral Dacron reconstruction for aorta-iliac occlusive disease: A 25-year survey. Eur J Vasc Surg 1991;5:19–186.
14. Tollefson DFJ, Ernst CB. Retroperitoneal aortic reconstruction: Indications and pitfalls. In: Chang JB (ed.) Modern Vascular Surgery. Vol. 5. New York: Springer-Verlag, 1992, pp. 126–131.
15. Piotrowski JJ, Pearce WH, Jones DN, et al. Aortobifemoral bypass: The operation of choice for unilateral iliac occlusion? J Vasc Surg 1988;8:211–218.
16. Chang JB. Surgical treatment of aorta-iliac artery disease. Angiology 1981;32:73–105.
17. Rob C. Extraperitoneal approach to the abdominal aorta. Surgery 1963;53:87.
18. Sicard GA, Freeman MB, VanderWoude JC, et al. Comparison between the transabdominal and retroperitoneal approach for reconstruction of the intrarenal abdominal aorta. J Vasc Surg 1987;5:19.
19. Wylie EJ, Olcott C IV, String ST. Aortoiliac thrombo-endarterectomy. In: Varco RL, Delaney JP (eds.). Controversy in Surgery. Philadelphia: WB Saunders, 1976, pp. 437–350.
20. Crawford ES, Manning LG, Kelly TF. "Redo" surgery after operations for aneurysm and occlusion of the abdominal aorta. Surgery 1977;81:41–52.
21. Corson JD, Brewster DC, Darling RC. The surgical management of infrarenal aortic occlusion. Surg Gynecol Obstet 1982;155:369.
22. Szilagyi DE. Surgical management of aortoiliac occlusive disease. In: Chang JB (ed.). Vascular Surgery. New York: Spectrum Publications, 1985, pp. 105–112.
23. Imparato AM, Riles TS, Weintraub N. Aortoiliac femoral endarterectomy: A reappraisal. Circulation 1984;70:136.

24. Moore WS, Hall AD. Unrecognized aortoiliac stenosis: A physiologic approach to the diagnosis. Arch Surg 1971;103:633–638.
25. Prendiville EJ, Burke PE, Colgan MP, et al. The profunda femoris: A durable outflow vessel in aortofemoral surgery. J Vasc Surg 1992;16:23–29.
26. Beales JSM, Adcock FA, Frawley IS, et al. The radiological assessment of disease of the profunda-femoris artery. Br J Radiol 1971;44:854–859.
27. Martin P, Frawley JE, Barabas AP, Rosengarten DS. On the surgery of atherosclerosis of the profunda femoris artery. Surgery 1972;71:182–189.
28. Sterptetti AV, Feldhaus RJ, Schultz RD. Combined aortofemoral and extended deep femoral artery reconstruction: Functional results and predictors of need for distal bypass. Arch Surg 1988;123:1269–1273.
29. Rutherford RB. Management of aortoiliac disease with and without infrainguinal occlusion: Indications and technique. In: Chang JB (ed.). *Modern Vascular Surgery. Vol. 3.* New York: PMA Publ. Corp., 1989, pp. 201–204.
30. Gruntzig A, Hopff H. Perkutane rekanalisation chronischer arterieller verschulusse mit einem neuen dilationskatheter modifikation der Dotter-technik. Dtsch Med Wochenschr 1974;99:2502–2507.
31. Johnston KW. Percutaneous balloon angioplasty and long-term results. In: Chang JB (ed.). *Modern Vascular Surgery. Vol. 4.* California: PMA Publ. Corp., 1991, pp. 287–295.
32. Kalman PG, Johnston KW. Outcome of a failed percutaneous transluminal dilatation. Surg Gynecol Obstet 1985; 161:43–46.
33. Casarella WJ. Noncoronary angioplasty. Curr Probl Cardiol 1986;11:141–174.
34. Palmaz JC, Sibbitt RR, Reuter SR, et al. Expandable intraluminal graft: A preliminary study. Radiology 1985;156:73–77.
35. Spence RK, Freiman DB, Gatenby R, et al. Long-term results of transluminal angioplasty of the iliac and femoral arteries. Arch Surg 1981;116:1377–1386.
36. Wilson SE, Wolf GL, Cross AP. Percutaneous transluminal angioplasty versus operation for peripheral arteriosclerosis. J Vasc Surg 1989;9:1–9.
37. Stokes KR, Strunk JM, Campbell DR, et al. Five-year results of iliac and femoropopliteal angioplasty in diabetic patients. Radiology 1990;174:977–982.
38. Kadir S, White RI, Kaufman SL, et al. Long-term results of aortoiliac angioplasty. Surgery 1983;94:10–14.
39. Walden R, Siegel Y, Rubinstein ZJ, et al. Percutaneous transluminal angioplasty. J Vasc Surg 1986;3:583–590.
40. Cambria RP, Faust G, Gusberg R, et al. Percutaneous angioplasty for peripheral arterial occlusive disease. Arch Surg 1987;122:238–287.
41. Glover JL, Bendick PJ, Dilley RS, et al. Efficacy of balloon catheter dilatation for lower extremity atherosclerosis. Surgery 1982;91:560–565.
42. Dalsing MC, Ehrman KO, Cikrit DF, et al. Current experience with angioplasty and stents in the iliac artery. In: Chang JB (ed.). *Modern Vascular Surgery. Vol. 5,* New York: Springer-Verlag, 1992, pp. 220–236.
43. Blaisdell FW, Hall AD. Axillary-femoral artery bypass for lower extremity ischemia. Surgery 1963;54:563–568.
44. Chang JB, Chan F. Axillo-bifemoral bypass. Vasc Surg 1986;20:27–35.
45. Chang JB. Current state of extraanatomic bypasses. Am J Surg 1986;152:202–205.
46. Myers WO, Lawton BR, Sautter RD. Axilloaxillary bypass graft. JAMA 1971; 217:826.

47. Chang JB. Surgical treatment of aorta-iliac artery disease. Angiology 1981;32:73–105.
48. Blaisdell FW. Extraanatomical bypass procedures. World J Surg 1988;12:798–804.
49. Rutherford RB, Patt A, Pearce WH. Extra-anatomic bypass: A closer view. J Vasc Surg 1987;6:437–446.
50. Hepp W, deJonge K, Pallua N. Late results following extra-anatomic bypass procedures for chronic aortoiliac disease. J Cardiovasc Surg 1988;29:181–185.
51. Pietri P, Pancrazio F, Adovasio R, et al. Long term results of extra anatomical bypasses. Int Angiol 1987;6:429–433.
52. Chang JB. Extraanatomic bypasses. In: Chang JB (ed.). *Modern Vascular Surgery. Vol. 4.* California: PMA Publ. Corp., 1991, pp. 189–227.
53. Harris EJ, Jr, Taylor LM, Jr, McConnell DB, et al. Clinical results of axillobifemoral bypass using externally supported polytetrafluoroethylene. J Vasc Surg 1990;12:416–421.
54. Lewis CD. A subclavian artery as the means of blood-supply to the lower half of the body. Br J Surg 1961;48:574–575.
55. Blaisdell WF, DeMattei GA, Gauder PJ. Extraperitoneal thoracic aorta to femoral bypass graft as replacement for an infected aortic bifurcation prosthesis. Am J Surg 1961;102:583–585.
56. LoGerfo FW, Johnson MC, Corson JD, et al. A comparison of the late patency rates of axillobilateral femoral and axillounilateral femoral grafts. Surgery 1977; 81:33–40.
57. Eugene J, Goldstone J, Moore WS. Fifteen-year experience with subcutaneous bypass grafts for lower extremity ischemia. Ann Surg 1977;186:177–183.
58. Kalman PG, Hosang M, Cina C, et al. Current indications for axillounifemoral and axillobifemoral bypass grafts. J Vasc Surg 1987;5:828–832.
59. Agee JM, Kron IL, Flanagan T, Tribble C. The risk of axillofemoral bypass grafting for acute vascular occlusion. J Vasc Surg 1991;14:190–194.
60. Vetto RM. The treatment of unilateral iliac artery obstruction with a transabdominal, subcutaneous femorofemoral graft. Surgery 1962;52:342–345.
61. Deruyter L, Caes F, Van den Brande P, et al. Femorofemoral bypass grafting in high-risk patients. Acta Chir Belg 1986;86:271–276.
62. Fahal AH, McDonald AM, Marston A. Femorofemoral bypass in unilateral iliac artery occlusion. Br J Surg 1989;76:22–25.
63. Chang JB, Rao GN, Thomson, NB, Jr. Ascending aorta to bilateral femoral artery graft. Vasc Surg 1961;82:831.
64. Chang JB. Extracranial revascularization. In: Chang JB (ed.): *Vascular Surgery.* New York: Spectrum Publications, 1985, pp. 31–83.
65. Chang JB. Extra-anatomic bypasses and their long-term results. In: Chang JB (ed.). *Modern Vascular Surgery. Vol. 2.* New York: PMA Publ. Corp., 1987, pp. 45–53.

X
Iliofemoral Occlusive Disease

34
Treatment of Iliofemoral Stenosis and Occlusion by Means of Modified Gianturco Expandable Metallic Stents

BYUNG SUK ROH, SEE SUNG CHOI, SEON KWAN JUHNG, CHANG GUHN KIM, AND JONG JIN WON

Introduction

Percutaneous transluminal angioplasty (PTA) is a well-accepted modality in the therapy for atheromatous lesions of peripheral occlusive vascular disease. The primary success rate has been very high due to improvements in equipment and methods. PTA is particularly effective for the treatment of short, concentric lesions but is less effective for long, irregular stenoses and occlusions, and in patients with diabetes mellitus and poor runoff vessels. Recent reports of a large series of iliac angioplasties indicate an average 5-year success rate of only 55%.[1]

The mechanism of restenosis is still debated; restenosis occurs within the first 5 months after dilatation. The causes of acute and early restenosis that occurs during or after PTA include spasm with or without thrombosis, dissection with complete closure, and elastic recoil. In an attempt to improve on the apparent limitations of conventional balloon angioplasty, self or balloon expandable metallic intraluminal stents were permanently implanted in areas of atherosclerotic stenosis and occlusion.

We inserted the modified Gianturco expandable metallic stents into the iliofemoral arteries of 5 patients to prevent restenosis after PTA. In this report, we present our initial and follow-up results.

Materials and Methods

Five patients (all men) were treated percutaneously with implantation of self-expanding intravascular stents for stenosis or occlusion in the iliac and superficial femoral arteries. (Table 34.1) The age of the patients ranged from 48 to 65 years (mean, 58 years).

The lesions were situated in the common iliac artery ($n = 1$), the external iliac arteries ($n = 2$), and the superficial femoral arteries ($n = 2$). Four patients had claudication, and one patient had gangrenous necrosis at risk for amputation of the great toe.

TABLE 34.1. Summary of cases.

Case	Age	Sex	Location of lesion	Type of lesion	No. of stents	Ankle–brachial index			Remarks
						Before stent placement	After stent placement	At follow-up	
1	65	M	EIA	Occlusion	5 + 5 + 3	0.54	1.23	0.97	Patent
2	48	M	CIA	Stenosis	5 + 6	0.64	1.01	0.91	Patent
3	58	M	SFA	Stenosis	4	0.73	1.05	—	Restenosis
4	61	M	SFA	Stenosis	4	0.61	0.99	0.88	Fibrinolysis Patent
5	56	M	EIA	Occlusion	7	0.61	1.08	1.01	Patent

CIA, common iliac artery; EIA, external illiac artery; SFA, superficial femoral artery.

Three patients had arterial stenoses, one in the common iliac artery and two in the superficial femoral arteries. The length of the stenoses ranged from 3 to 11 cm. For two of the five patients, the arterial occlusions were located in the external iliac arteries. The length of the occluded segments ranged from 5 to 13 cm.

The stents used in this study were constructed of 0.32-mm stainless steel wire bent in a zigzag pattern of 10 bends at each end. The stents were 1 cm in length and 8 or 10 mm in diameter when fully expanded. Several stents were connected in tandem by metallic struts cut from the same wire. We used four connected stents for two cases, and seven connected stents for one case. In one case, we used five connected stents and six connected stents in both common iliac arteries separately with overlapping in the bifurcation area. In one case, five, five, and three connected stents overlapping by 0.5 cm were inserted (Figs. 34.1 and 34.2).

The primary vascular approach was percutaneously performed in an ipsilateral antegrade mannner for lesions of the superficial femoral artery and in a retrograde manner for lesions of the iliac artery. The occluded or stenosed segment was entered by combined use of a 5 Fr polyethylene catheter with a slight bend at the tip and a 0.9-mm guide wire. After the obstruction was passed, angioplasty was performed with 8- to 10-mm balloons for the iliac arteries and 6- to 8-mm balloons for the superficial femoral arteries. Angiograms were obtained after angioplasty to evaluate the response of the lesion and were followed by stent insertion. The diameter of the stents at full expansion was chosen to be about 1.2 times that of the native artery.

A stent was manually compressed and inserted into a 9 Fr sheath, which was positioned across the stenotic segment of the artery. After the stents were introduced at the optimum position within the sheath, the sheath was gradually removed and the stents were expanded and fixed to the arteral wall. The stent was always placed so that the lesion might be completely covered. Side branches were spared, if possible.

Heparin, 5,000 IU, was administered intraarterially during the procedure,

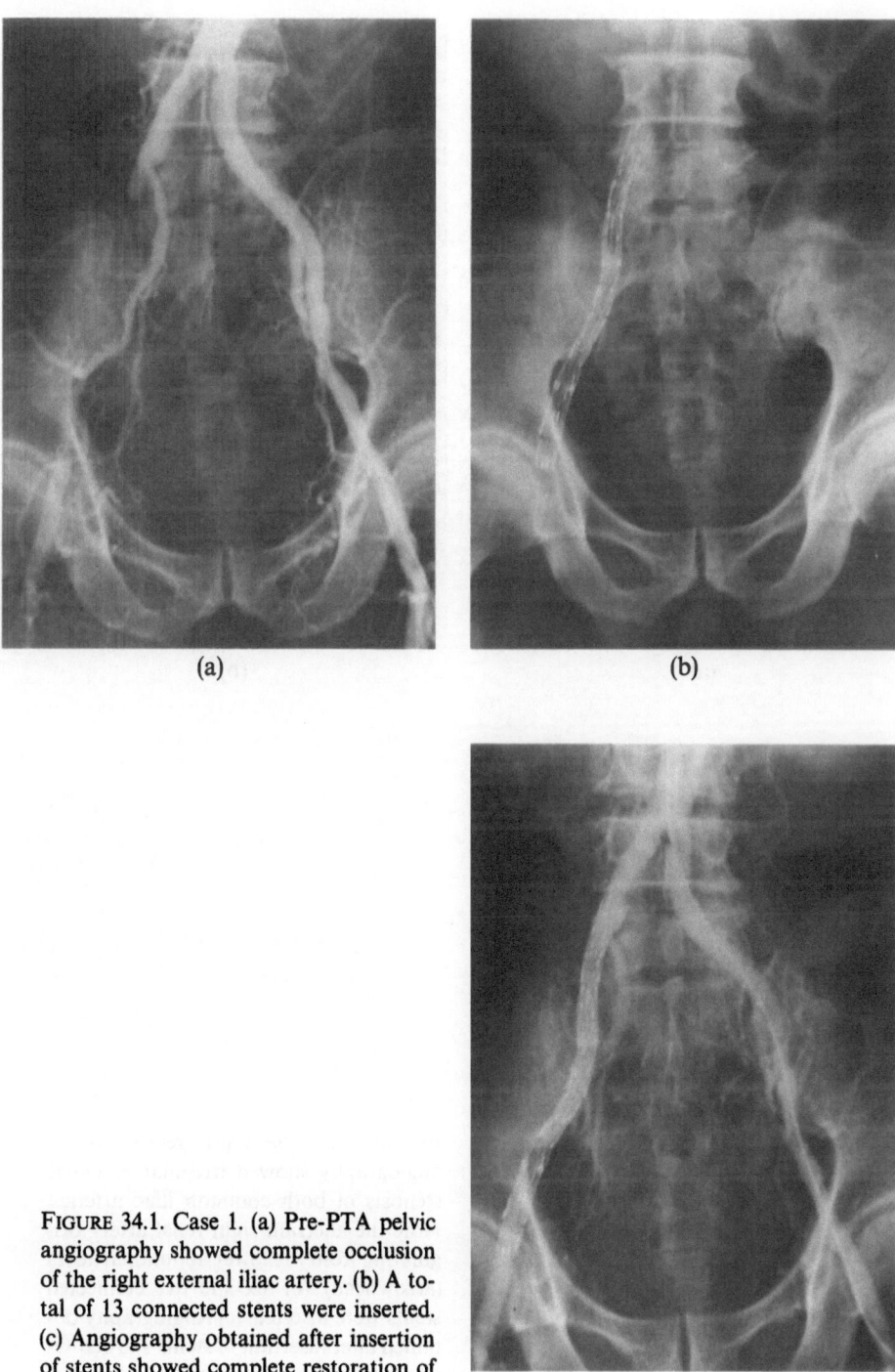

(a)

(b)

(c)

FIGURE 34.1. Case 1. (a) Pre-PTA pelvic angiography showed complete occlusion of the right external iliac artery. (b) A total of 13 connected stents were inserted. (c) Angiography obtained after insertion of stents showed complete restoration of lumen of the artery and good patency.

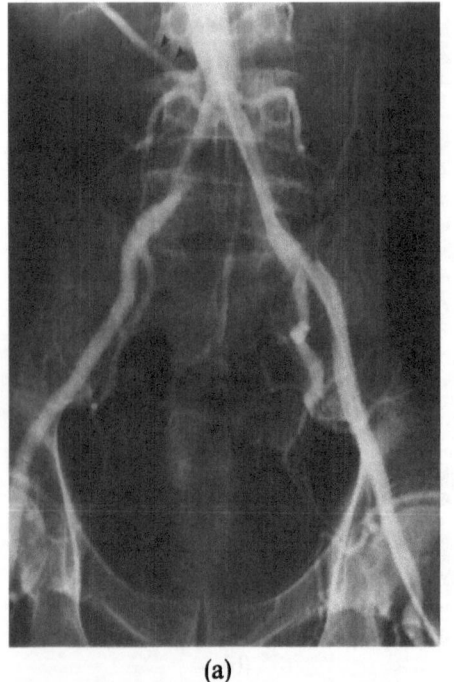

(a)

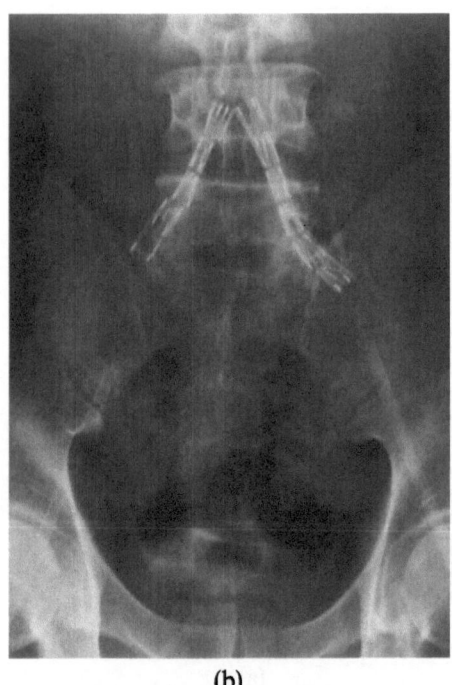

(b)

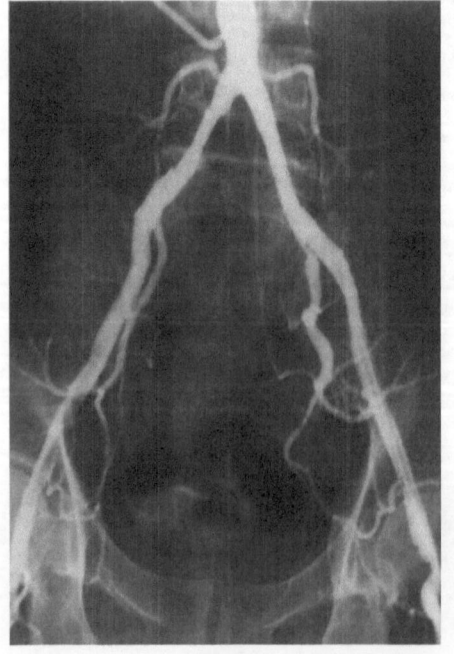

(c)

FIGURE 34.2. Case 2. (a) Pre-PTA pelvic angiography showed irregular eccentric stenosis of both common iliac arteries. Note the aberrant right renal artery originating from the lower abdominal aorta (arrowhead). (b) Six and five connected stents were inserted. (c) Angiography obtained after insertion of stents showed restoration of lumen and good patency of the arteries.

followed by intravenous infusion of 1,000 IU/hr for 24 hours. Oral anticoag-ulation therapy with 100 mg of aspirin and 300 mg of dipyridamole was administered for at least 6 months after stent placement.

The patients were followed up for 2–16 months (mean, 10 months). Clini-cal examination and Doppler ankle–brachial index studies were performed every month. A plain radiograph of the pelvis or thigh was obtained at several days, 1 month, and 3 months after stent placement.

Results

Stent implantation was technically successful in all five cases, and no migra-tion or traumatic dissection occurred. In all patients with inadequate results after angioplasty (two with occlusions and three with eccentric, heavily calci-fied, and severely ulcerated stenoses), stent insertion resulted in an immedi-ately visible improvement in flow. Pressure gradient curves obtained with hemodynamic studies were improved compared with those obtained with angioplasty. In all cases, clinical and Doppler ankle–brachial indexes were improved.

In two patients, the internal iliac artery was bridged by the stent. Despite the bridge, the artery remained patent.

Two complications were observed: thrombosis and restenosis. One throm-bosis in the superficial femoral artery occurred immediately after angioplasty and stent implantation and was successfully treated with low doses of uro-kinase. Among the five patients, one restenosis in the superficial femoral artery appeared 6 months after stent implantation.

Discussion

The concept of intraluminal stenting was first proposed by Charles Dotter[2] in 1969. Extensive investigation of the technique, however, did not begin until 1983, when Dotter[3] and Cragg[4] reported separately a technique for percut-aneous implantation of intraluminal stents. After the first clinical report of intravascular stenting in humans by Sigwart et al.[5] in 1987, recent clinical reports of the balloon-expandable Palmaz or Strecker stent and the self-expandable Gianturco stent or wallstent for treatment of arterial occlusive disease have been published.[6-12]

The Gianturco expandable metallic stent is a stainless steel wire bent in a zigzag configuration. It has a high expansion ratio so that it can be inserted through a relatively small sheath.

Intravascular stent placement after undersized balloon dilation results in a smooth and regular lumen, which decreases or prevents the development of luminal irregularities after angioplasty. Furthermore, the good hoop strength and permanent expansile force opposes elastic recoil of the dilated vessel wall and removes the need for overdilatation.

Intravascular stenting is most often applied in the case of failed or inadequate PTA for the treatment of vascular occlusive disease. In most reports, the clinical failure rate of PTA is in the range of 25–40% over a follow-up interval of approximately 1 year. In less than 5% of the cases, PTA resulted in abrupt closure of the dilated vessel segment. This was usually due to a combination of dissection, intimal flap production, and thrombosis. Another factor in early PTA failure may be the elastic recoil of the dilated vessel. Late restenosis is usually due to accelerated intimal hyperplasia and progression of the atherosclerotic process. The rationale for intervascular stenting is based upon the use of a mechanical intraluminal device that acts to support the artery, reducing the failure rate of angioplasty.

The most important complication in intravascular stenting is early thrombotic occlusion and restenosis or occlusion due to neointimal proliferation. In one case of our series, the stent was placed in an incompletely dilated superficial femoral artery after multiple PTA and was buried in a residual mural thrombus with new thrombus formation after stent placement. Selective intraarterial infusion of low-dose urokinase for 10 hours completely restored the vessel lumen. For prevention of early thrombotic occlusion, we will perform balloon dilatation for to eliminate residual stenosis and give intraarterial fibrinolytic therapy to eliminate the residual thrombus before stent placement.

Intravascular stents may induce intimal hyperplasia to the extent that the vessel becomes occluded. Severe intimal hyperplasia occurred in the superficial femoral artery in one patient in our series. It is too early to conclude that intimal hyperplasia tends to develop more often in the femoral artery than in the iliac artery. Intimal hyperplasia seems to develop more frequently in humans than in animal experiments. To keep intimal hyperplasia to a minimum, we selected a stent diameter about 1.2 times that of the native iliac artery, based on the results of Chae et al.[13]

Other studies with longer follow-up will be required to analyze the results of this new therapy. However, our preliminary study leads us to think that endovascular stent implantation is an important complement to traditional angioplasty, especially for long, eccentric, and irregular lesions.

References

1. Johnston KW, Rae M, Hogg-Johnston SA, et al. 5-Year result of a prospective study of percutaneous transluminal angioplasty. Ann Surg 1987;206:403–413.
2. Dottern CT. Transluminally-placed coilspring endarterial tube grafts: Long-term patency in canine popliteal artery. Invest Radiol 1969;4:329–332.
3. Dotter CT, Buschmann RW, McKinney MK, Rosch J. Transluminal expandable nitinol coil stent grafting: Preliminary report. Radiology 1983;147:259–260.
4. Cragg A, Lund G, Rysavy J, Castaneda F, Castaneda-Zuniga W, Amplatz K.

Nonsurgical placement of arterial endoprostheses: A new technique using nitinol wire. Radiology 1983;147:261–263.

5. Sigwart U, Puel J, Mirkovitch V, Joffre F, Kappenberger L. Intravascular stents to prevent occlusion and restenosis after transluminal angioplasty. N Engl J Med 1987;316:701–706.

6. Raillat C, Rousseau H, Joffre F, Roux D. Treatment of iliac artery stenoses with the wallstent endoprosthesis. Am J Roentgenol 1990;154:613–616.

7. Palmaz JC, Richter GM, Noeldge G, et al. Intraluminal stents in artherosclerotic iliac artery stenosis: Preliminary report of a multicenter study. Radiology 1988; 168:727–731.

8. Rousseau HP, Raillat CR, Joffre FG, Knight CJ, Ginestet MC. Treatment of femoropopliteal stenoses by means of self-expandable endoprostheses: Midterm results. Radiology 1989;172:961–964.

9. Rees CR, Palmaz JC, Garcia O, et al. Angioplasty and stenting of completely occluded iliac arteries. Radiology 1989;172:953–959.

10. Gunther RW, Vorwerk D, Bohndorf K, Peters I, El-Din A, Messmer B. Iliac and femoral artery stenoses and occlusions: Treatment with intravascular stents. Radiology 1989;172:725–730.

11. Kichikawa K, Uchida H, Yoshioka T, et al. Iliac artery stenosis and occlusion: Preliminary results of treatment with Gianturco expandable metallic stents. Radiology 1990;177:799–802.

12. Vorwerk D, Guenther RW. Mechanical revascularization of occluded iliac arteries with use of self-expandable endoprostheses. Radiology 1990;175:411–415.

13. Choe YH, Park JH, Han JK, Han MC, Kim CW. An experimental study on the influence of the intravascular Gianturco type stents on the vascular structures. J Korean Radiol Soc 1991;27:431–439.

XI
Arterial Aneurysm

35
A Profile of Peripheral Arterial Aneurysms in South India

Booshanam V. Moses, Stanley John, R. David Sadhu, and Sunil Agarwal

Introduction

Peripheral arterial aneurysms comprise a relatively uncommon mode of pre-sentation of peripheral vascular disease. Until recently they were considered to be diagnostic curiostities for which the only treatment offered was either proximal arterial ligation or amputation. Now it is possible to surgically excise or exclude these lesions from the general circulation and to restore arterial continuity with gratifying results.

Materials and Methods

This is a descriptive retrospective study of 42 patients with 43 peripheral arterial aneurysms treated over the past 22 years (1970–1991) as inpatients at the Christian Medical College and Hospital, Vellore, South India, to study their distribution, mode of treatment, and outcome.

Selection of Cases

Inpatient records were reviewed and all cases with definitive clinical or/and radiological diagnosis of aneurysm were included. Aneurysms arising inside the chest cavity or cranial cavity or from the abdominal aorta were excluded.

Results

Age Distribution

Most cases occured in the third or fourth decade of life (Table 35.1). The youngest patient, a 9-year-old boy, had a superficial temporal artery aneurysm of traumatic etiology. The oldest patient, a 76-year-old man, had a syphilitic brachial artery aneurysm.

TABLE 35.1. Age distribution of patients.

Age group (years)	No. patients
< 20	4
21–30	12
31–40	9
41–50	7
51–60	5
> 60	5
Total	43 aneurysms in 42 patients

TABLE 35.2. Sites of aneurysms.

Site	No. aneurysms
Superficial temporal	1
Carotid	3
Subclavian	2
Axillary	1
Brachial	4
Ulnar	1
Common iliac	2
External iliac	1
Femoral	13
Popliteal	11
Posterior tibial	4
Total	43

Sex Distribution

All cases encountered were in males. This preponderance could be because men are more prone to atherosclerosis and trauma.

Sites

A total of 43 aneurysms were encountered at almost all known sites in 42 patients (Table 35.2). However, 65% of them originated in the lower extremity.

Multiple Aneurysms

Three patients had more than one aneurysm. One patient had aneurysms of the posterior tibial artery bilaterally. The second patient had aneurysms of the left brachial artery and the abdominal aorta (polyarteritis nodosa). The third patient had aneurysms of the left common iliac artery and the left common carotid artery (atherosclerosis). This carotid artery aneurysm was not included in the present study, as it had been surgically treated $1\frac{1}{2}$ years earlier elsewhere. Also, the aneurysm of the abdominal aorta is not part of our present study of peripheral arterial aneurysm.

Etiology

Trauma (42%) and atherosclerosis (37%) were the commonest etiological factors (Table 35.3). The modes of trauma were 1 blunt injury, 13 stab or gunshot injuries, 1 bull gore injury, and 3 iatrogenic (2 postangiography and 1 postinguinal herniorrhaphy).

Syphilitic aneurysms, now regarded as clinical rareties, were seen in 5 (12%) of cases. Of these, 4 were popliteal artery aneurysms and the 5th was a brachial artery aneurysm.

Associated Disorders

The associated disorders were hypertension, ischemic heart disease, renal failure, and cerebrovascular accidents (Table 35.4). These were seen mainly in patients with atherosclerosis. Four patients (10%) had tuberculosis which was unrelated to the aneurysm. None of the patients had diabetes mellitus.

TABLE 35.3. Etiology of aneurysms.

Etiology	No. aneurysms
Traumatic	18
Atherosclerosis	16
Mycotic	2
Syphilitic	5
Poststenotic	1
Polyarteritis nodosa	1
Total	43

TABLE 35.4. Associated disorders.

Disorder	No. aneurysms
Hypertension	13
Ischemic heart disease	4
Renal failure	3
Cerebrovascular accident	2
Syphilis	5
Tuberculosis	4
Diabetes mellitus	0

TABLE 35.5. Presentation.

Symptoms and signs	No. aneurysms
Painful mass	30
Asymptomatic mass	9
Pressure symptoms	13
Distal ischemia	6
Signs of rupture	6
Diminished or absent distal pulses	15

TABLE 35.6. Diagnostic evaluation.

Method	No. aneurysms
Clinical only	27
Clinical and angiography	15
Clinical and ultrasound	1
Total	43

Presentation

Thirteen patients (30%) had symptoms and signs suggestive of neurovenous compression (Table 35.5). Only 15 of 43 (35%) had diminished or absent pulses distally. Of these, 2 were subclavian, 1 axillary, 1 brachial, 1 common iliac, 2 femoral, and 8 popliteal artery aneurysms. However, only 6 of these 15 patients had symptoms and signs of ischemia, which were seen predominantly in popliteal artery aneurysms. Six patients (14%) had evidence of rupture, of which 3 were popliteal artery aneurysms and 1 each were in the common iliac, external iliac, and posterior tibial arteries.

Diagnostic Evaluation

In view of their superficial location, all 43 of our cases were diagnosed clinically (Table 35.6). Angiography was used as an adjuvant diagnostic measure in 15 patients (35%). The pattern of involvement included segmental arterial block and dilated arterial segment. The outflow tree was satisfactory in the majority of the cases. Ultrasound was used as a diagnostic tool in one patient.

Surgical Procedures

Table 35.7 lists the surgical procedures and figures 35.1–35.5 illustrate them. One patient with an aneurysm of the popliteal artery refused surgery. All the others were treated surgically. One case of posterior tibial artery aneurysm

TABLE 35.7. Surgical procedures.

Procedure	No. aneurysms
Excision	2
Excision with end-to-end anastomosis	4
Partial excision with bypass	19
Excision and closure of defect with or without patch	8
Exclusion	4
Exclusion with bypass	4
Amputation	1
Total procedures	42
Refused surgery	1
Total aneurysms	43

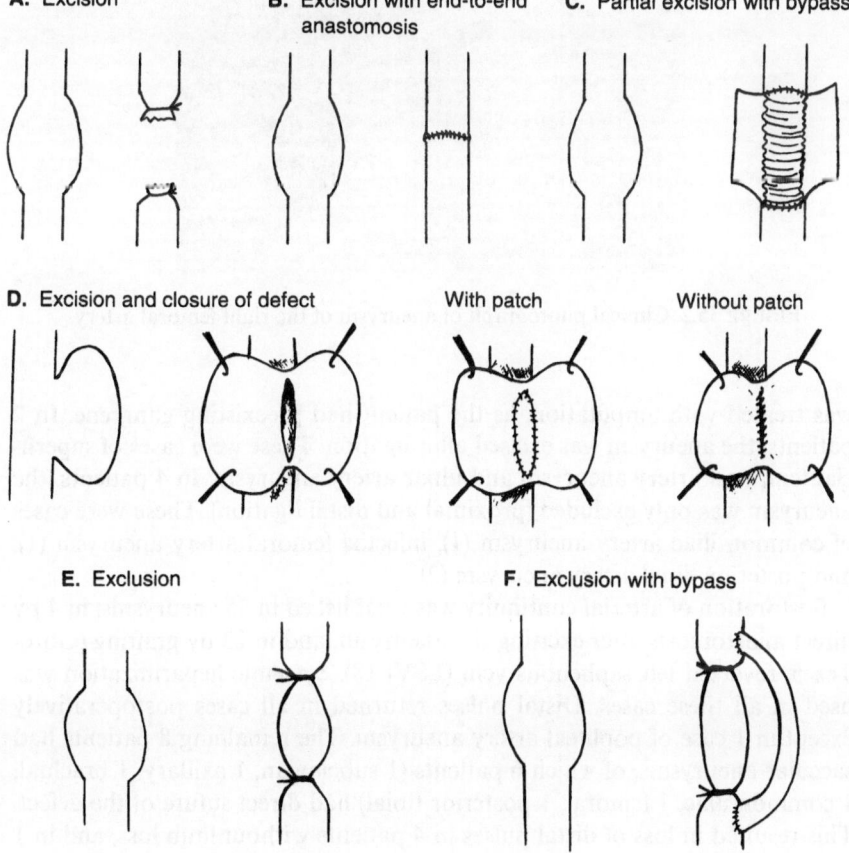

FIGURE 35.1. Surgical treatment.

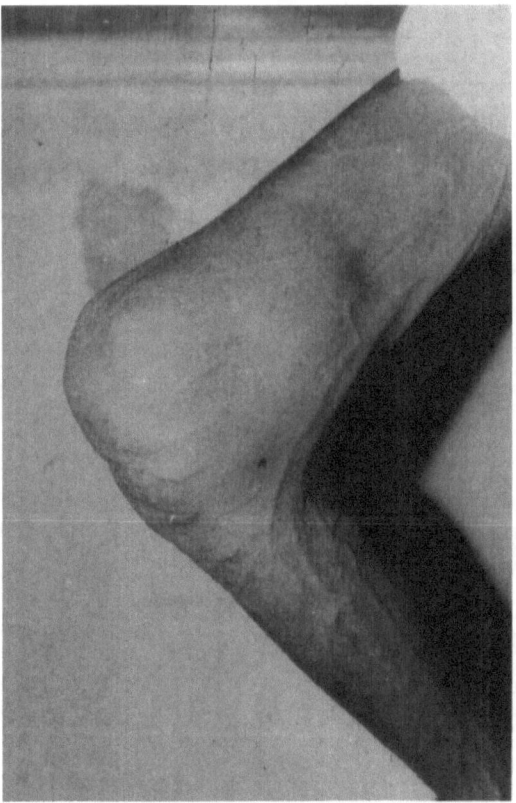

FIGURE 35.2. Clinical photograph of aneurysm of the right femoral artery.

was treated with amputation, as the patient had preexisting gangrene. In 2 patients, the aneurysm was excised after ligation. These were cases of superficial temporal artery aneurysm and ulnar artery aneurysm. In 4 patients, the aneurysm was only excluded (proximal and distal ligation). These were cases of common iliac artery aneurysm (1), infected femoral artery aneurysm (1), and posterior tibial artery aneurysm (2).

Restoration of arterial continuity was established in 35 aneurysms: in 4 by direct anastomosis after excising the aneurysm, and in 23 by grafting (Gore-Tex 5, reversed left saphenous vein (LSV) 18). Systemic heparinization was used in all these cases. Distal pulses returned in all cases postoperatively except in 1 case of popliteal artery aneurysm. The remaining 8 patients had saccular aneurysms, of which 6 patients (1 subclavian, 1 axillary, 1 brachial, 1 common iliac, 1 femoral, 1 posterior tibial) had direct suture of the defect. This resulted in loss of distal pulses in 4 patients without limb loss, and in 1 femoral and 1 posterior tibial aneurysm the pulses returned postoperatively. It seems from the foregoing that direct suturing of the defect tends to occlude

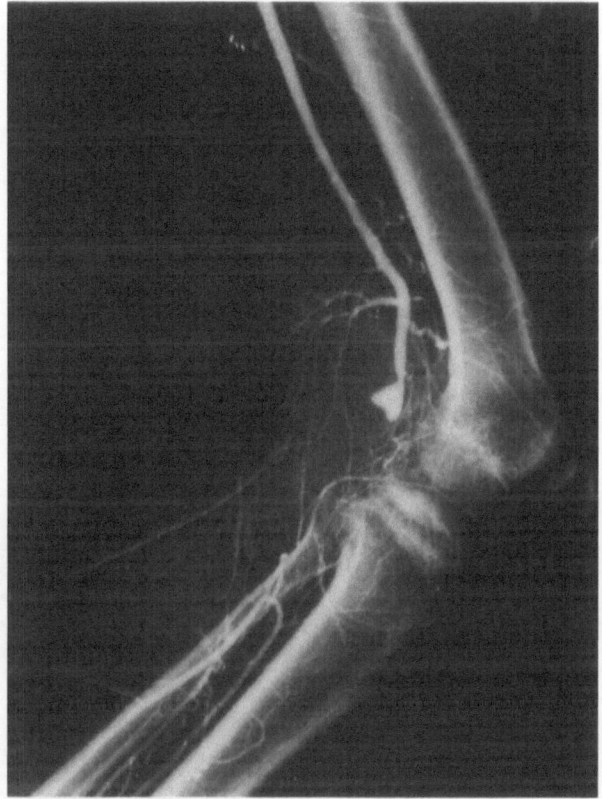

FIGURE 35.3. Arteriogram showing abrupt cutoff in a popliteal artery aneurysm.

the lumen of the vessel. In the other 2 saccular aneurysms, patch angioplasty was done and the distal pulses were well felt postoperatively.

Three patients with popliteal artery aneurysms who had absent pulse preoperatively were treated by bypass graft, the pulses returned postoperatively, indicating that the distal vessels in peripheral aneurysms are usually normal and that bypass surgery is worth attempting.

Morbidity and Mortality

Ten patients had local wound complication. None of them required any further surgical intervention. Three patients had secondary hemorrhage (2 femoral artery aneurysms and 1 popliteal artery aneurysm). All 3 required ligation with a resultant loss of distal pulse. One patient developed anastomotic aneurysm following surgery for femoral artery aneurysm (excision of sac and vein angioplasty). He subsequently underwent exclusion and reversed saphenous vein graft bypass. He did well postoperatively. One patient

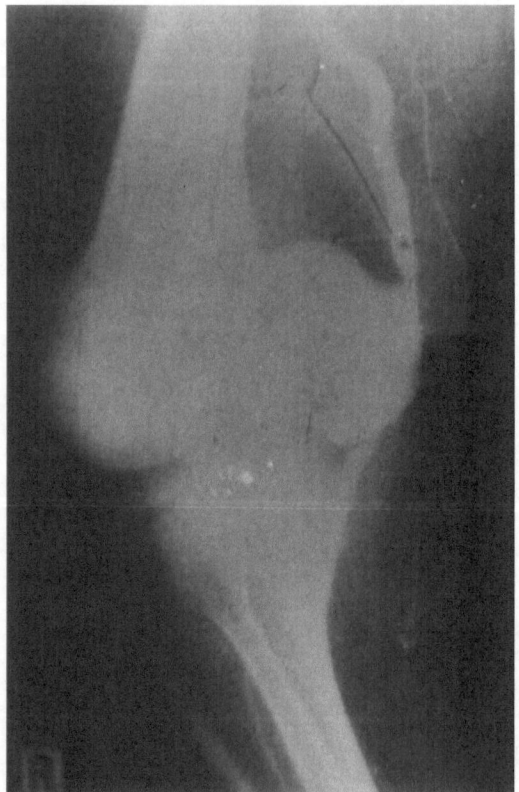

FIGURE 35.4. Arteriogram showing aneurysm of the popliteal artery.

who had popliteal artery aneurysm required regrafting for thrombosis of the graft. None of these complications resulted in limb loss. One patient who had bypass grafting for popliteal arterial aneurysm died in the immediate postoperative period due to septicemia.

Conclusions

1. Peripheral arterial aneurysms are a rare presentation of peripheral arterial disease. They are seen mostly in the third and fourth decades of life and commonly affect the lower extremities. Distal pulses are usually present, except in popliteal artery aneurysms, where they may be diminished or absent.
2. Multiple aneurysms were seen in only 3 patients (7%).
3. Diabetes mellitus does not seem to be an associated factor in peripheral arterial aneurysms.

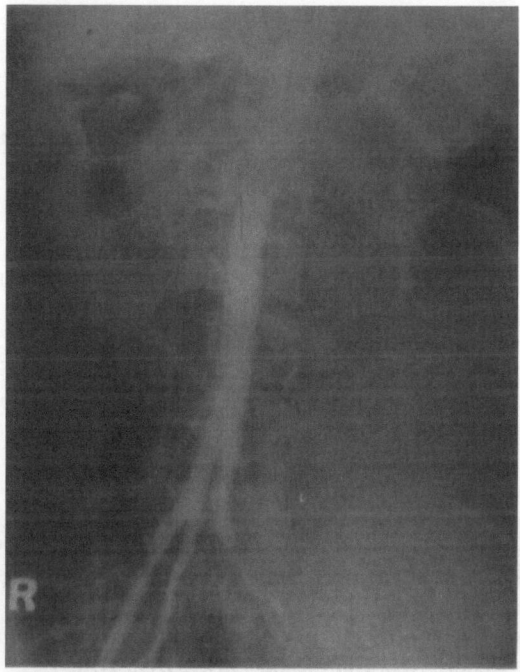

FIGURE 35.5. Arteriogram showing aneurysm of left common iliac artery.

TABLE 35.8. Morbidity and mortality.

Complications	No. aneurysms
Wound infection	6
Wound hematoma	4
Secondary hemorrhage	3
Anastomotic aneurysm	1
Graft thrombosis	1
Limb loss	0
Mortality	1

4. Among the etiological agents, syphilis was common earlier, but now trauma and atherosclerosis are more common.
5. Surgery is the treatment of choice. Restoration of arterial continuity should be the aim of treatment in all cases, even in ruptured aneurysm with absent distal pulses. Results following bypass procedures have been excellent, with return of distal pulses postoperatively, as the distal vessels are usually normal. However, direct suturing of the defect is fraught with the danger of obliterating the lumen, resulting in loss of distal pulses. Exclusion and bypass grafting seems to be the treatment of choice for peripheral aneurysms.

Bibliography

1. Chitwood WR, et al. Popliteal artery aneurysms—Past and present. Arch Surg 1978;113:1078–1082.
2. Chrichlow RW, et al. Treatment of popliteal aneurysms by restoration of continuity—Review of 48 cases. Ann Surg 1966;163:417–426.
3. Railly MK, et al. Aggressive surgical management of popliteal artery aneurysms. Am Surg 1983;145:498–502.
4. Hardy JD, et al. Aneurysms of the popliteal artery. 1975;140:401–404.
5. Whitehouse WM, et al. Limb threatening potential of arteriosclerotic popliteal artery aneurysms. Surgery 1983;93:694–699.
6. Farino C, et al. Popliteal aneurysms. 1989;169:7–13.
7. Wychalis AR, et al. Popliteal aneurysms. Surgery 1970;68:942–952.
8. Vermilion BD, et al. A review of 147 popliteal aneurysms with long term follow-up. Surgery 1981;90:1009–1014.
9. Graham LM, et al. Clinical significance of arterio-sclerotic femoral artery aneurysms. Arch Surg 1980;115:502–507.
10. Hardy DG, et al. Femoral aneurysms. Br J Surg 1972;59:614–616.
11. Adiseshiah M, et al. Aneurysms of the femoral artery. Br J Surg 1977;64:174–176.
12. Hollier LH, et al. Arteriomegaly: Classification and morbid implications of diffuse aneurysmal disease. Surgery 1983;93:700–708.
13. Parra HH, et al. Ruptured atherosclerotic aneurysm of the superficial femoral artery—Case Report. Acta Chir Scand 1989;155:493–494.
14. Grooma GJ, et al. Vascular injury after arterial catheterization. Postgrad Med J 1989;65:86–88.
15. McGready RM, et al. Isolated iliac artery aneurysms. Surgery 1983;93:688–693.
16. Welling RE, et al. Extracranial carotid artery aneurysms. Surgery 1983;93:319–323.
17. Harris EJ. Surgical treatment of distal ulnar artery aneurysm. Am J Surg 1990;159:527–530.
18. Hands LJ, et al. Intrainguinal aneurysms: Outcome for patient and limb. Br J Surg 1991;78:996–998.

XII
Arteritis

36
Surgical Treatment of Takayasu's Arteritis: Report of Clinical Experience of 27 Patients

Yong Bok Koh, Seung Nam Kim, Hae Myung Chun, and In Chul Kim

Introduction

Takayasu's arteritis is a large-vessel vasculitis involving the aorta and its major branches. It has been described as pulseless disease, occlusive thromboaortopathy, aortic arch arteritis, aortitis syndrome, and aortoarteritis. These names imply that this disease entity possesses various patterns and complicated courses.

It is well known that Takayasu's arteritis begins initially as a systemic inflammatory disease with flu-like illness and later is followed by large-vessel vasculitis leading to stenosis or aneurysm. The etiology is still unclear, although a systemic immunologic process seems to be most likely.

Takayasu's arteritis is a rare disease. About 120 cases have been reported in the Korean literature so far,[1-8] although this disease is known to be prevalent in East Asia. Most of the patients have been cared for by physicians, since this disease progresses very slowly with ambiguous general symptoms for years. Only a few cases have been referred to surgeons when typical ischemic symptoms appeared.

The present report does not include all Korean cases but is confined to our surgical experience of 27 patients who underwent vascular surgery.

Patients

From April 1983 through December 1991, 27 patients with Takayasu's arteritis were operated on in the Department of Surgery, Kangnam St. Mary's Hospital. Twenty patients were female and 7 were male. The ages ranged from 12 to 58 years, with a mean of 32.5 years.

Preoperative Symptoms and Signs

Nineteen patients had a history of flu-like illness such as fever, myalgia, joint pain, skin rash, anorexia, and weight loss, but the remaining 8 patients denied past illness. They usually visited the hospital in the late phase with various complaints. The main preoperative problems included headache (16); dizziness (9); syncope (1); impaired vision (3); photophobia (1); hemiplegia due to recent stroke (1); claudication, tingling, numbness, and cold intolerance in the hand (14); weakness of lower extremities (2); painful pulsating mass on neck (2); tinnitus (2); hypertension (9); absent or weak radial pulses (15); bruit over neck (4); and bruit over epigastrium (4).

The mean duration of symptoms before surgery was 22.9 months (range 4 months to 8 years).

Preoperative Workup

Detailed anamnesis was done by interview with patients and their close families. Physical examination included pulse status in four limbs and blood pressure by Doppler examination, auscultation for bruit on neck and epigastrium, and eye fundus examination. Systemic hypertension was defined when the systolic blood pressure was more than 180 mmHg. In 5 patients, the blood pressure measured on one upper extremity was more than 50 mmHg higher than that measured on the lower extremity. Pale fundus was a frequent finding in ophthalmoscopic examination. Laboratory studies consisted of complete blood count (CBC), liver function test (LFT), erythrocyte sedimentation rate (ESR), C-reactive protein (CRP), anti-nucleic acid antibody (ANA), and fibrinogen measurement. None were significant except for ESR and CRP, which were positive in only 16 patients. Arteriography was performed in all patients by the Seldinger technique.

Anatomic classification was made according to the categories outlined by Ueno and Lupi-Herrera: type I, occlusive lesions of the main branches of the aortic arch; type II, occlusive lesions of the thoracoabdominal aorta and its branches; type III, combinations of types I and II; type IV, aneurysmal dilatation of the aorta and its main branches.

Diagnosis

The diagnoses depended on the typical arteriographic findings following close clinical evaluation. Obtaining a biopsy specimen from diseased arterial wall was not always easy because our procedures were done on nondiseased arterial segments. However, confirmative diagnostic findings were available in successful biopsy specimens.

The main pathologic findings included chronic inflammatory cell (mainly lymphocyte) infiltration in the vessel wall, increased perivascular fibrosis, intimal fibrinoid hyperplasia, obliterated vasa vasorum, and some giant cell infiltration (Figs. 36.1 and 36.2).

Arterial lesions were found at arteriography in the left subclavian in 8 patients, right subclavian in 2, bilateral subclavian arteries in 1, subclavian

FIGURE 36.1. Operating view of opened carotid artery showed markedly thickened arterial wall with diffuse intimal hyperplasia.

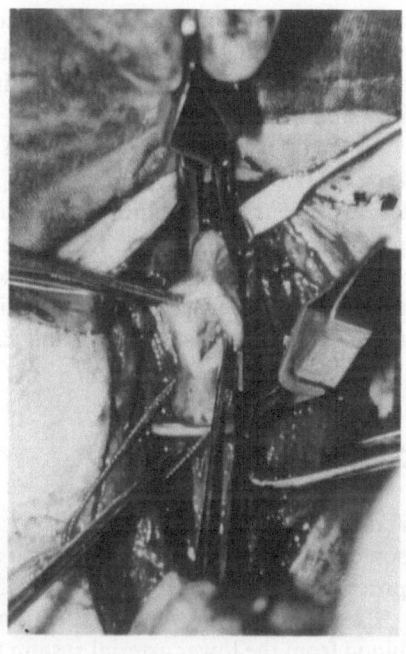

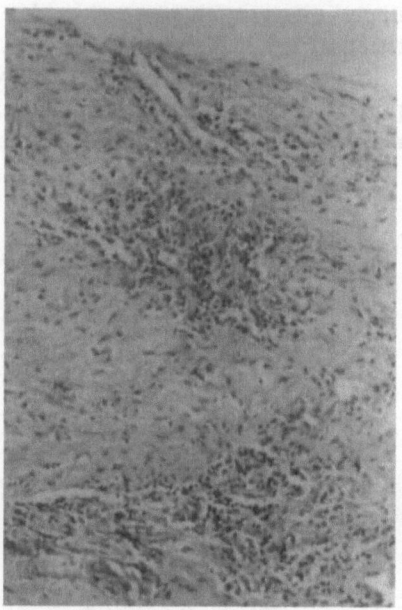

FIGURE 36.2. Microphotography (×100) of surgical specimen of Figure 36.1 showed massive chronic inflammatory cell infiltration, intimal hyperplasia, and obliterated vasa vasorum.

artery with concomitant involvement of brachial artery in 2, left carotid in 5, right carotid in 1, bilateral carotid arteries in 2, innominate artery in 3, descending thoracic aorta in 4, abdominal aorta in 7, left renal in 1, right renal in 4, and bilateral renal arteries in 2.

In the arteriographic classification of our patients, 13 patients (48.1%) had type I, 7 (25.9%) had type II, 5 (18.5%) had type III, and 2 (7.4%) had type IV lesions (aneurysm of innominate and common carotid artery, aneurysm of proximal thoracic aorta). The most common artery involved was the left subclavian artery. The majority of the cases had lesions involving aortic arch takeoff vessels; consequently, presenting symptoms were mostly those of arterial insufficiency of subclavian and carotid arteries.

Surgical Procedures

Axilloaxillary bypasses using 6- to 8-mm polytetrafluoroethylene (PTFE), sometimes with extension to carotid artery or brachial artery, were the main procedures for types I and III (Figs. 36.3 and 36.4).

Concomitantly reverse axillofemoral bypasses were added to bring up blood from the lower arterial system to the axillary artery in cases of multiple brachiocephalic vessel lesions (Figs. 36.5–36.7) and also axilloiliac bypasses to bring down blood from the upper to the lower arterial system in cases of upper extremity hypertension due to thoracoabdominal aortic stenotic lesions (Figs. 36.8 and 36.9).

The type II arterial lesions in this report were mainly confined to the initial portion of renal arteries with minimal involvement of neighboring abdominal aorta. So the surgical procedures for type II were aortorenal bypasses in

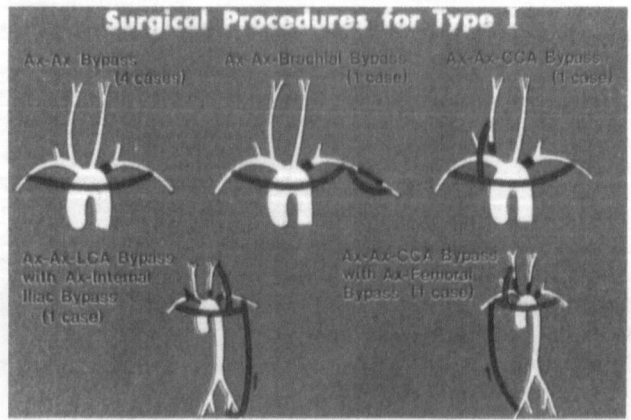

FIGURE 36.3. Schematic illustration of various bypass procedures for type I.

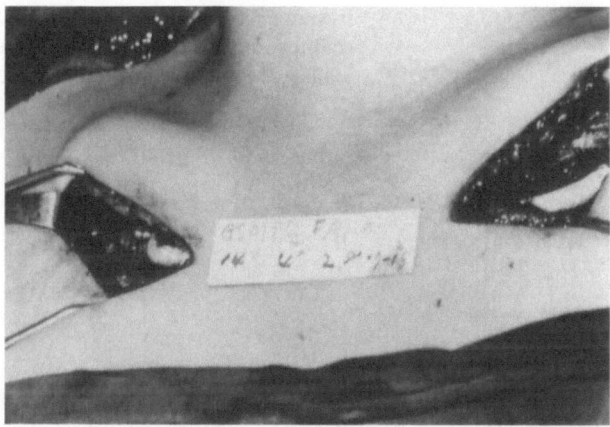

FIGURE 36.4. Operating view of successful axilloaxillary bypass.

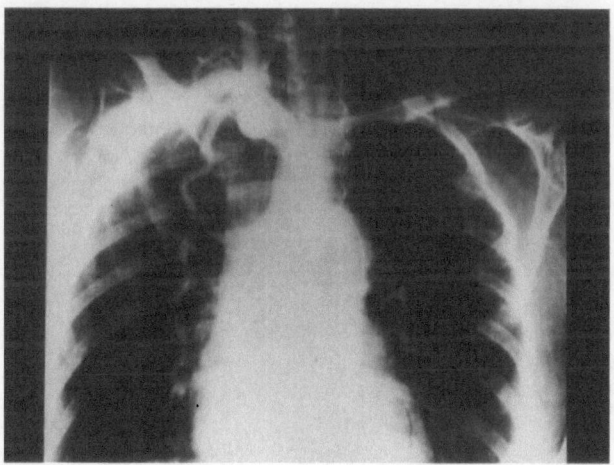

FIGURE 36.5. Arteriography of a type I patient showed occlusion of right and left subclavian, and left common carotid arteries.

4, endarterectomy with roof patch angioplasty using autogenous saphenous vein in 2, and right nephrectomy followed by aortoplasty in 1 case.

The surgical procedures for 2 cases of type IV were aneurysm resection with PTFE graft insertion for multiple aneurysms involving innominate and bilateral common carotid artery through median sternotomy (Figs. 36.10 and 36.11) and aneurysm repair by graft inclusion technique for saccular aneurysm of proximal thoracic aorta through left thoracotomy (Figs. 36.12–36.14).

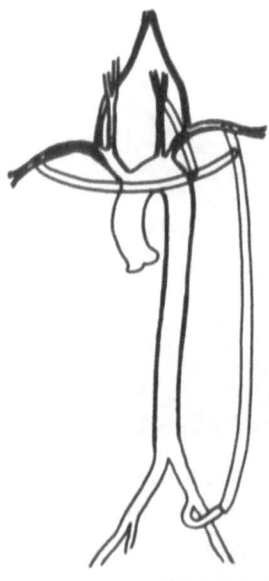

FIGURE 36.6. Schematic drawing of bypass procedures in this patient. Left internal iliac–axillary bypass was made to bring up blood.

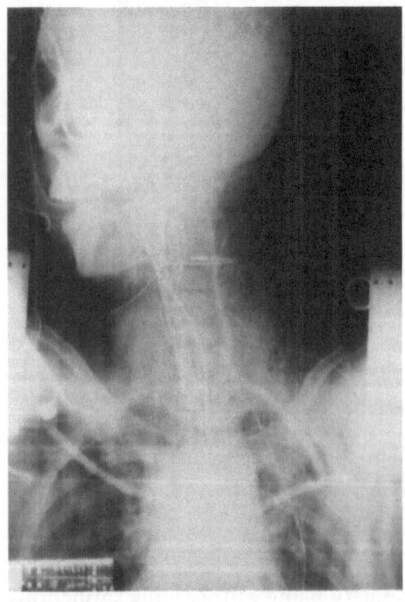

FIGURE 36.7. Intraoperative table arteriography showed good patency of all grafts. Dye was administered into left internal iliac artery.

Postoperative Results

Graft patency was confirmed by bedside Doppler examination. All patients were followed up continuously at 3-week intervals. Mean duration of time follow-up was 3.5 years.

All patients were given antiplatelet agents. Steroid therapy was given temporarily in cases of elevated ESR and worsened generalized malaise.

FIGURE 36.8. Arteriography of a type III patient showed diffuse irregular narrowing in midaorta, but visceral arteries were not involved.

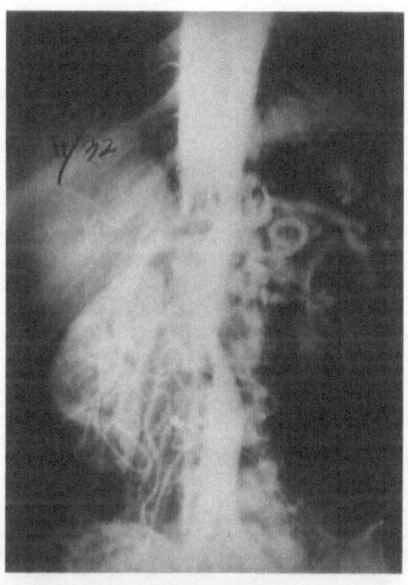

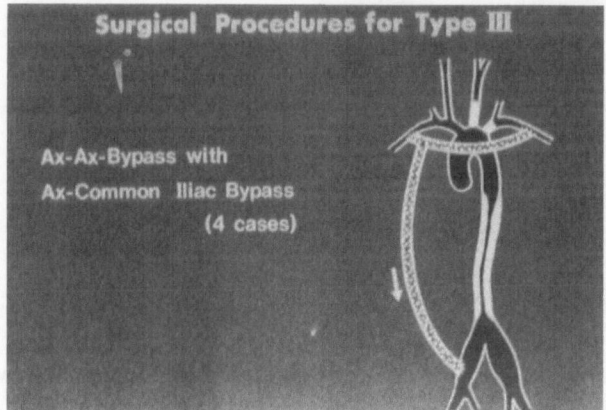

FIGURE 36.9. Schematic illustration of patient in Figure 36.8. Right axillary–common iliac artery bypass was made to bring down blood from upper to lower arterial system.

Restoration of radial pulses and brachial blood pressure and also improvement of arm and CNS ischemic symptoms were achieved in the majority of cases. In 5 cases, headache and dizziness persisted despite the patency of the grafts.

In 5 of 7 renovascular hypertension cases, blood pressure returned to normal; in 1 case it remained fluctuating, and 1 case required eventual nephrectomy after aortorenal bypass. Two patients with axillofemoral and 1 with axilloaxillary grafts experienced postoperative occlusion at 2, 5, and

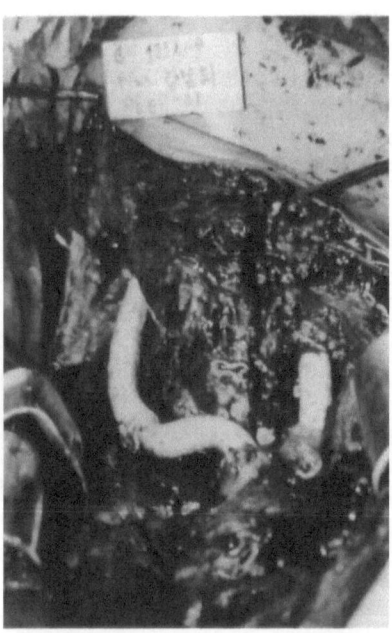

FIGURE 36.10. Arteriography of a type IV patient showed aneurysmal dilatation of innominate artery, right and left common carotid arteries.

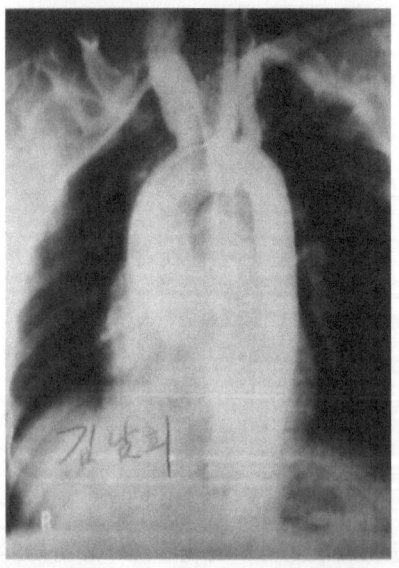

FIGURE 36.11. Operating view of patient shown in Figure 36.10. The innominate artery and the right and left common carotid arteries were replaced by PTFE graft. Intraluminal shunt was not used during cramping of the carotid artery because the stump pressure was over 90 mmHg.

6 months, respectively. Recanalization was restored by successful Fogarty thrombectomy and temporal heparinization except for 1 case, probably due to poor distal runoff.

A 22-year-old male patient whose common carotid and left subclavian artery were occluded visited the hospital because of recent stroke and left side hemiplegia. After a successful bypass procedure, his left lower extremity

FIGURE 36.12. Arteriography of a type IV patient showed saccular thoracic aneurysm just below ligament of ductus arteriosus.

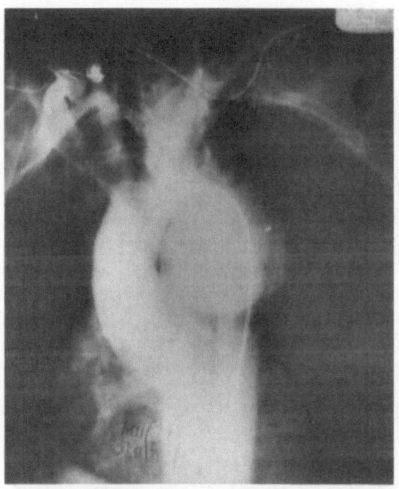

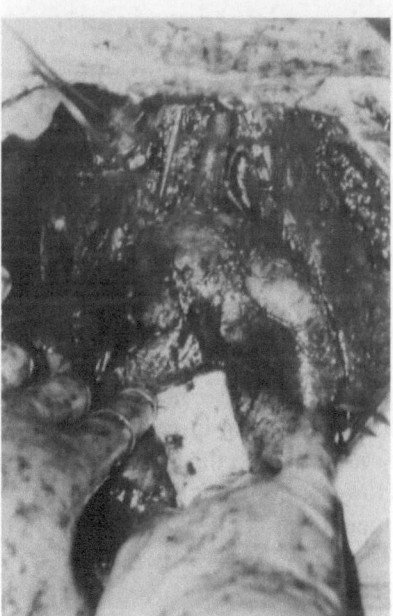

FIGURE 36.13. Operating view of patient shown in Figure 36.12 showed saccular thoracic aneurysm.

plegia recovered but his upper extremity plegia remained even though the graft was patent.

No anastomotic leakage or false aneurysms and no operative deaths were encountered in our cases.

Three patients died between 3 and $3\frac{1}{2}$ years following operation, although their grafts were found patent at their last hospital visit. The ages at death were 31, 26, and 52 years, and the duration of illness from initial disease to death was about 11, 6, and 4 years, respectively. Causes of death were noted

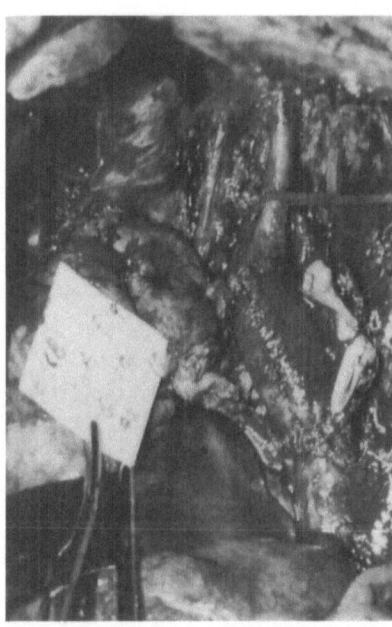

FIGURE 36.14. Successful aneurysmal repair was carried out by graft inclusion technique using Hemashield Dacron graft.

to be cerebral infarction. Perhaps a longer disease period is related to mortality.

Summary

In review of our 27 patients with Takayasu's arteritis who underwent various vascular bypass surgical procedures, we found that relatively simple extra-anatomic bypasses using PTFE were safe and effective measures which could bring functional improvement of preoperative disabling ischemic complications, although the underlying systemic disease cannot be treated surgically. However, longer follow-up than that reported here will be required to determine the ultimate effectiveness of our surgical procedures.

References

1. Ueno A, Awane Y, Wakabayashi A, Shimizu K. Case reports, successfully operated obliterative brachiocephalic arteritis (Takayasu) associated with the elongated coarctation. Japan Heart J 1967;8:538–544.
2. Lupi-Herrera E, Sanchez-Torres G, Marcushamer J. Takayasu's arteritis. Clinical study of 107 cases. Am Heart J 1977;93:94–103.
3. Takagi A, Tada Y, Sato O, Miyata T. Surgical treatment for Takayasu's arteritis. A long-term follow-up study. J Cardiovasc Surg 1989;30:553–558.
4. Shelhamer JH, Volkman DJ, Parrillo JE, Lawley TJ, Johnston MR, Fauci AS. Takayasu's arteritis and its therapy. Ann Intern Med 1985;103:121–126.

5. Yamamoto S, Nozawa T, Aoki H, Isobe Y. Femoro-internal carotid artery bypass for cerebral ischemia in Takayasu's arteritis. Arch Surg 1984;119:1426–1429.
6. Lagneau P, Michel JB, Vuong PN. Surgical treatment of Takaysu's disease. Ann Surg 1987;205:157–166.
7. Koh YB, Cho KW, Park CH, Lee YK. Bypass surgery of Takayasu's arteritis. J Korean Surg Soc 1988;34:493–503.
8. Song BJ, Kim EK, Kim SN, Koh YB, Lee YK. A clinical evaluation of Takayasu's arteritis. J Korean Surg Soc 1988;34:530–539.

37
Characteristic Angiographic Findings of Thromboangiitis Obliterans

CHOONG KI PARK, BUM GYU AHN, AND CHANG SIG CHOI

Representative diseases producing peripheral arterial occlusions in Korea are atherosclerosis obliterans (ASO) and thromboangiitis obliterans (TAO). However, the differential diagnosis becomes controversial on occasion. Tissue biopsy, we believe, should be taken in every equivocal case for an ultimate confirmation of the diagnosis. Clinically, however, this is not routine practice, and diagnosis still largely depends upon clinical information and angiographic findings. Although angiographic reading has its own limitation, usually the findings are typical enough to suggest the diagnosis of TAO, and we would like to review individual characteristics of angiographic findings.

Patients and Methods

Patients

Twenty-two patients who were admitted to Chunchon Sacred Heart Hospital between March 1986 and March 1992 with final diagnosis of TAO were enrolled in the study. All patients were male and under the age of 35 without a history of diabetes mellitus or hyperlipidemia. Three patients were in the second decade, 11 in the third delade, and 8 in the fourth decade.

A total of 36 angiographic studies were obtained from 22 patients. Follow-up angiography was performed in 12 patients: twice in 9 patients and 3 times in 3 patients. Thirty-two studies were femoral angiographies and 4 studies were brachial angiographies. The results were analyzed to show distribution and obstructive patterns of involved arteries, patterns of collateral circulation and distal runoff, changes of opacified arteries proximal to the occlusions, and patterns of venous drainage.

Methods

Angiography was performed by the Seldinger method. The femoral artery was punctured by a Seldinger needle, the guide wire was introduced through the needle into the femoral artery, and the guide wire was replaced by a 7 Fr pigtail catheter. The tip of the catheter was placed in the distal abdominal aorta, and 30–50 mL of water-soluble contrast medium (Rayvist 300 or Ultravist 370) was injected by an automatic injector for 6–10 seconds. The filming sequence depended on flow and station.

Results

Distribution of Involved Vessels

A total of 62 arteries were involved. The posterior tibial, anterior tibial, and peroneal arteries were commonly involved. All medium-sized arteries were involved (Table 37.1). Several veins were also found to be involved, but most veins were opacified in the early phase proximal to the lesions.

TABLE 37.1. Distribution of involved arteries.

Sites (artery)	Right	Left
Hypogastric a.		1
Deep femoral a.		1
Superficial femoral a.	3	3
Popliteal a.	3	3
Femoropopliteal a.	1	
Anterior tibial a.	6	6
Posterior tibial a.	7	9
Peroneal a.	4	4
Radial a.	3	3
Ulnar a.	2	2
Interosseous a.	1	
Total	30	32

TABLE 37.2. Obstructive patterns ($n = 62$).

Sites	
Nonbifurcation	52
Bifurcation	10
Occlusion	
Segmental	22
Nonsegmental	40
Margins	
Tapering	29
Round or beak	32
Flat	1

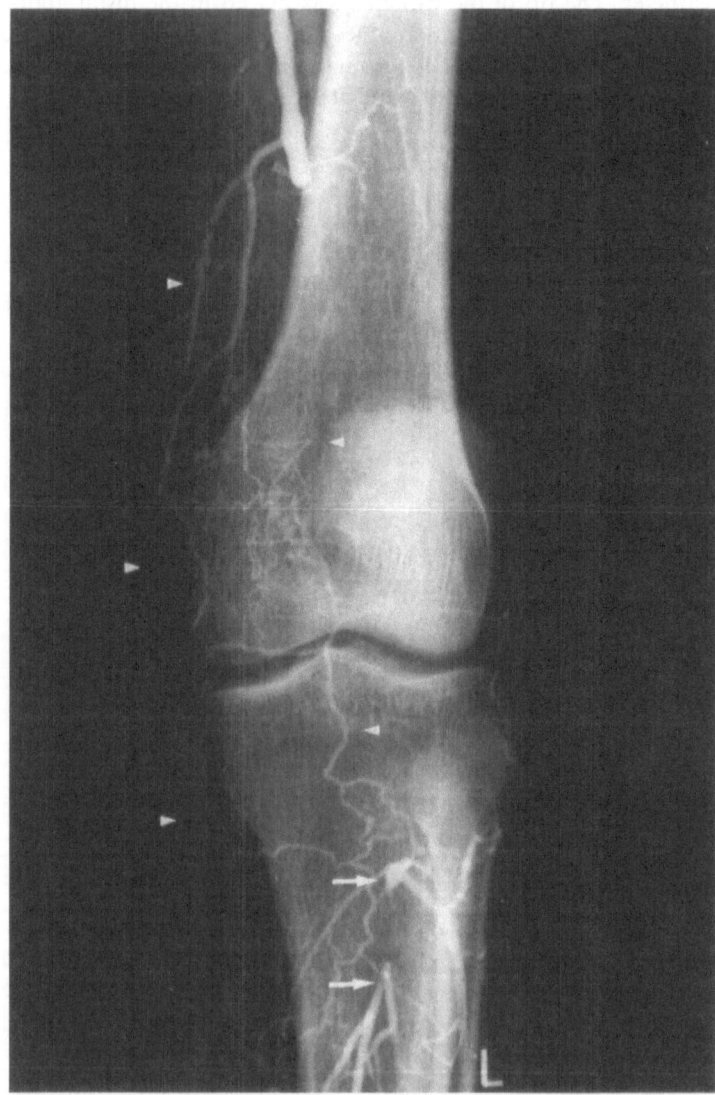

FIGURE 37.1. Image of typical thromboangiitis obliterans. Mulitple segmental occlusions are demonstrated at the distal femoral and popliteal arteries and femoropopliteal trunk. Indirect collaterals (arrowheads) and runoff vessels (arrows) are opacified at the anterior tibial, posterior tibial, and peroneal arteries.

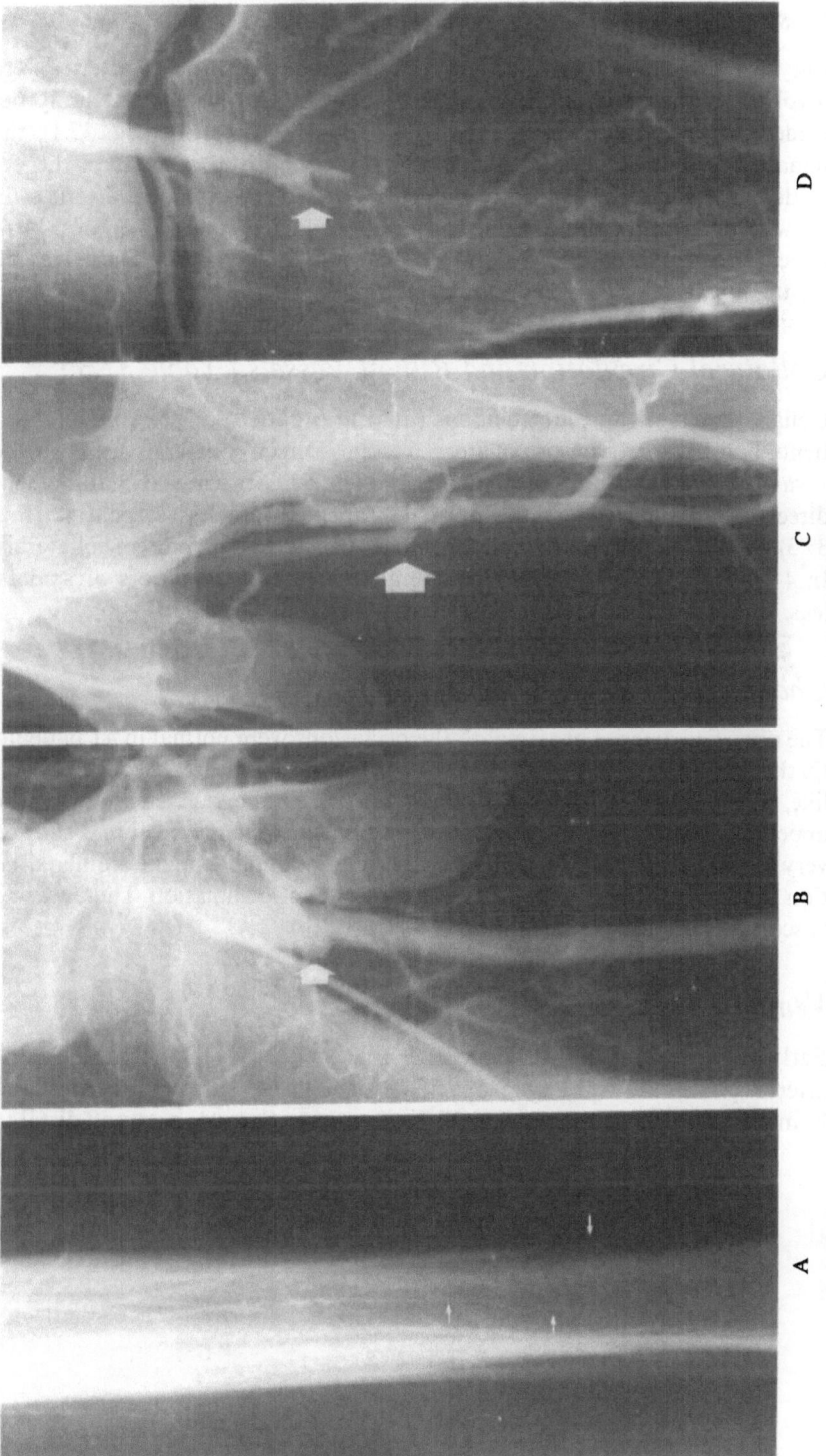

A   B   C   D

FIGURE 37.2. Various patterns of occlusion (arrows). Four different angiograms demonstrate (a) tapering of lower leg vessels, (b) round occlusion of the deep femoral artery, (c) bird beak appearance of the occluded superficial femoral artery, and (d) flat type occlusion of the popliteal artery.

Obstructive Patterns of Involved Arteries (Table 37.2)

Fifty-two arteries were involved at nonbifurcation sites, and 10 arteries were involved at the bifurcation site. Twenty-two arteries were segmentally occluded, including one case of multisegmental involvement (Fig. 37.1); the remaining 40 arteries were totally occluded. The distal margins of the occluded arteries were smoothly defined. Among 62 occluded arteries, 29 showed tapering of the opacified arteries, 32 had a rounded or bird-beak appearance, and one artery showed a flat margin (Fig. 37.2). There was no rat-tail appearance or round filling defect.

Collateral Circulation and Runoff Vessels (Table 37.3)

Collateral vessels were not demonstrated in 5 patients. The remaining patients had various type of collateral vessels. Direct collaterals through the vasa vasorum were more serpentine, producing a corkscrew appearance. Indirect collaterals through the normal branches were less serpentine (Fig. 37.3). Seventeen patients had direct collaterals and 15 had indirect collaterals. In 4 of 17 patients, corkscrew collaterals appeared as treeroots or spiders' legs. Runoff vessels were demonstrated in 8 patients (Fig. 37.1)

Changes of Inflow Arteries (Table 37.4)

The opacified arteries proximal to the occlusions were normal in 41 patients. Of the remaining 21 arteries, 12 were corrugated in appearance, 5 were wavelike, and 4 showed diffuse narrowing (Fig. 37.4). The corrugated and wavelike appearances and the diffuse narrowing were nearly symmetrical and showed very constant intervals. These findings are clear enough to make a differentiation from the atheromatous plaque and poststenotic dilatation. There was no vascular redundancy of the inflow arteries.

Venous Drainage (Table 37.5)

Early venous drainage was clearly seen in 6 patients (Fig. 37.4D). On the arterial phase, the veins were opacified through the surrounding muscular branches. These patients showed relatively poor collaterals or runoff distal to

TABLE 37.3. Collateral and runoff vessels ($n = 22$).

No collateral vessels	5
Collaterals	17
Direct (corkscrew appearance)	17
Tree roots or spiders' legs	4
Indirect	15

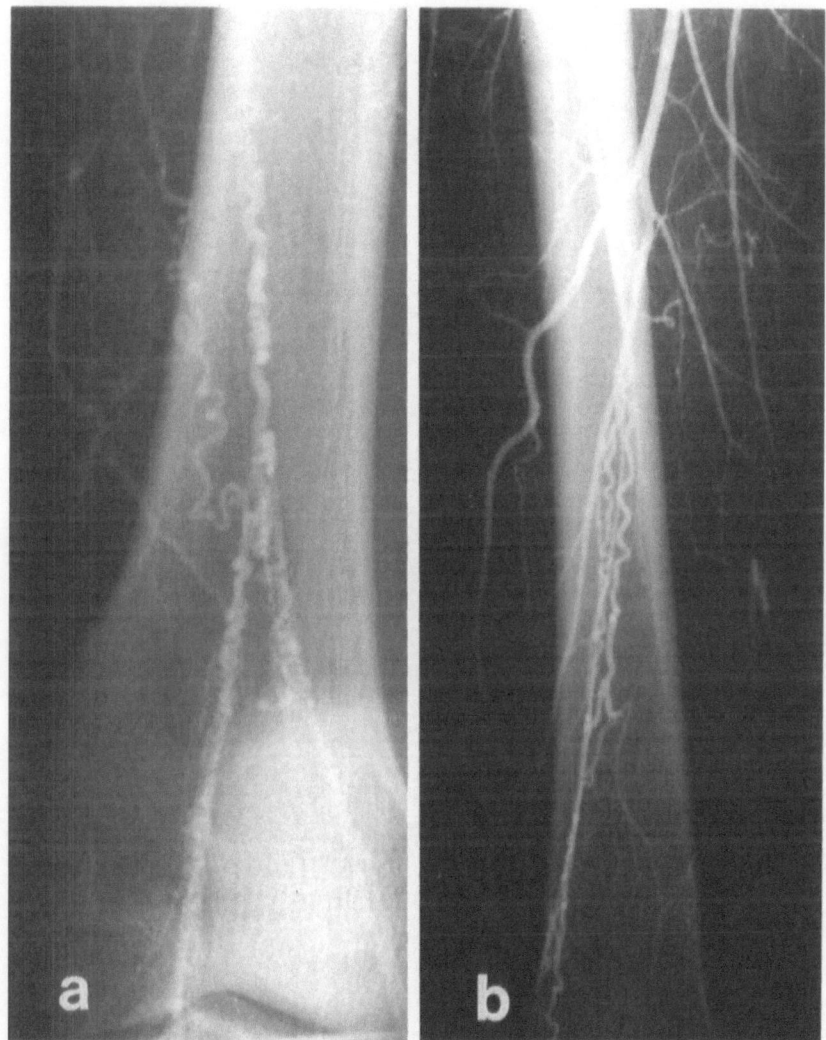

FIGURE 37.3. Collateral vessels. Two angiographic studies demonstrate tree-root or spider's leg appearances which originated from direct (a) and indirect (b) collaterals.

TABLE 37.4. Changes of inflow arteries ($n = 62$).

Normal	41
Abnormal	21
Corrugated appearance	12
Wave appearance	5
Diffuse narrowing	4
Atheromatous plaque	0
Poststenotic dilatation	0

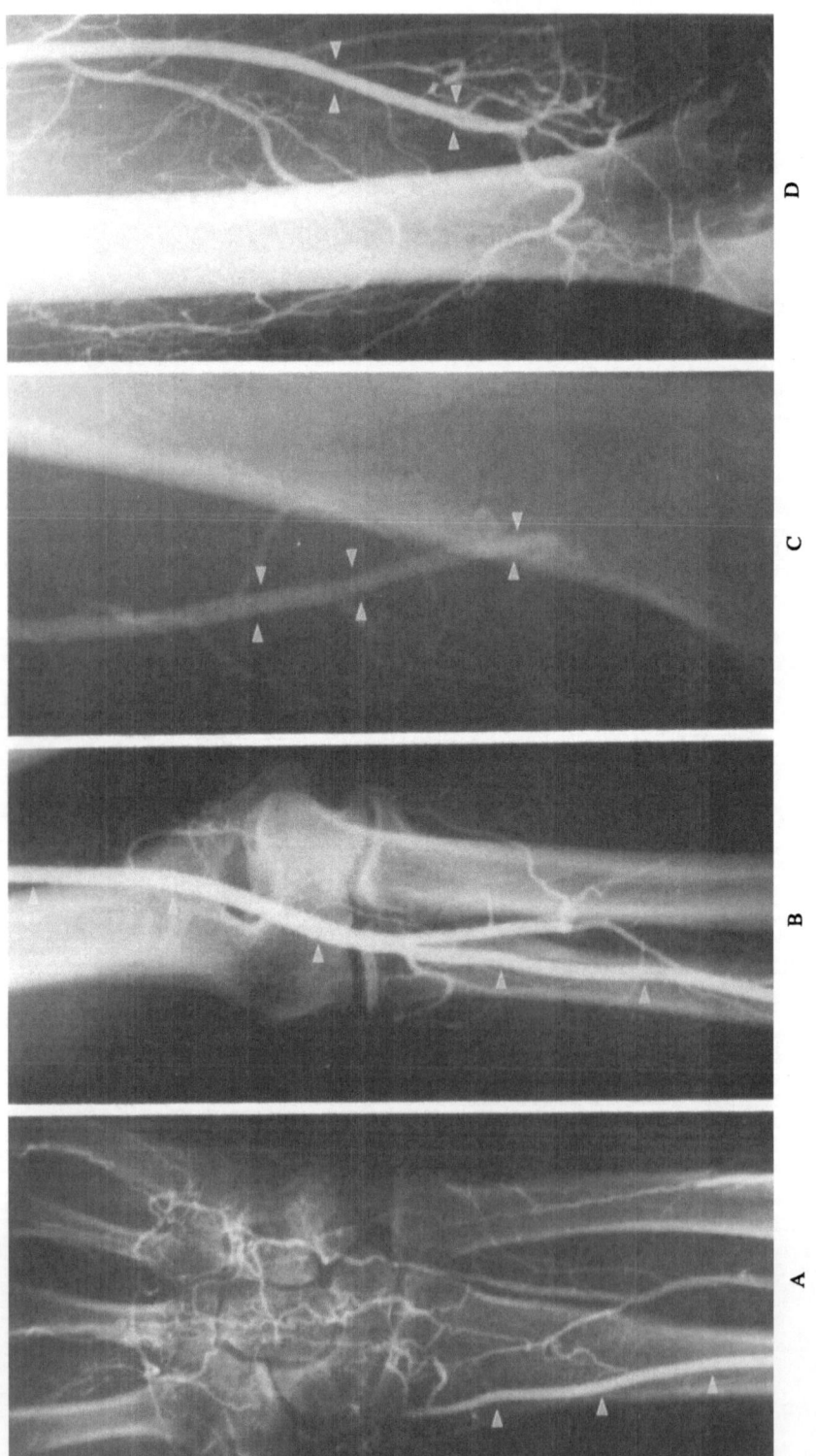

FIGURE 37.4. Changes of inflow arteries (arrowheads). Four different angiograms show (a) normal inflow artery, (b) corrugated appearance, (c) wave appearance, (d) diffuse narrowing.

TABLE 37.5. Venous drainage (*n* = 22).

Early venous drainage	6
Irregular venous pooling	5

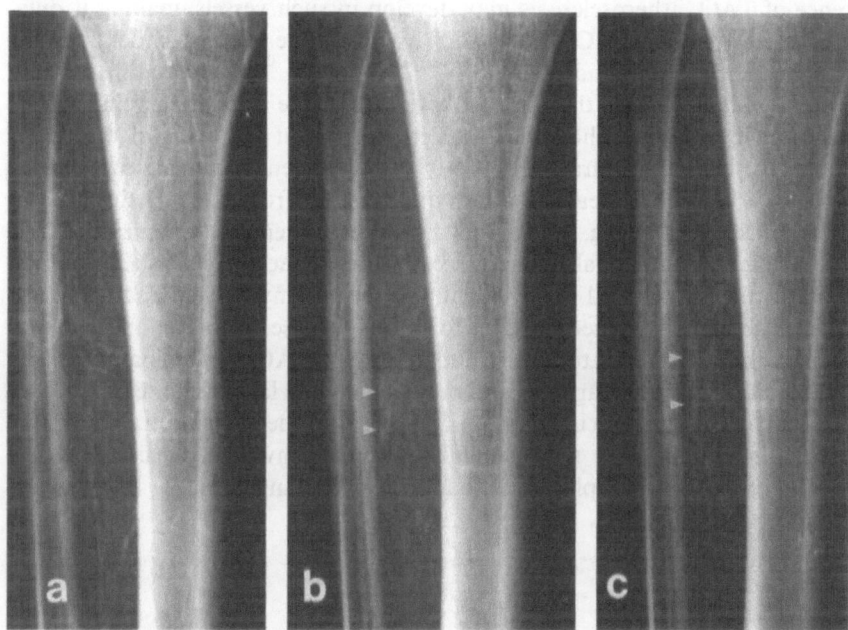

FIGURE 37.5. Venous involvement proved by angiography. Serial angiograms demonstrate (a) irregular opacification of the peroneal artery on late arterial phase, and then (b, c) irregular pooling of contrast media in the peroneal vein even on delayed venous phase (arrowheads).

the occlusions. Pooling of contrast medium in the draining veins was also detected in 5 out of 6 patients (Fig. 37.5).

Follow-up Studies

On follow-up angiography in 12 patients, the occlusions were gradually extended whether on not they received sympathectomy or sympathectomy with bypass graft.

Discussion

TAO is a distinct entity, but the other causes of peripheral vascular disease such as atherosclerosis and thromboembolism should be excluded before a definite diagnosis is made. It is now a well-known fact that TAO is a peripheral vascular occlusive disease that occurs almost exclusively in young men who are smokers. In many patients TAO affects the arms as well as the legs. It demonstrates a close relationship of remission and relapse to cessation or resumption of smoking and it manifests as excruciating pain. Usually there is no atherosclerosis in the vessels having TAO. But over the years of recurrence of TAO, atherosclerosis may develop in such vessels, making it difficult to differentiate TAO from ASO.[1] Therefore we selected patients under the age of 35 for this study.

Histopathologically, the acute involvement of the artery and vein is characterized by polymorphonuclear cell infiltration of all layers of the vessel wall, together with mural thrombosis of the lumen. Small microabscesses within the thrombus create a pattern quite distinct from the pure thrombosis of atherosclerosis[2] (Fig. 37.6). The thrombus undergoes organization and recanalization, and small microabscesses are replaced by fibrosing granulomas. After the arterial involvement, the accompanying vein and nerve are often secondarily affected, leading to fibrous encasement. The affected segment of the vessel tends to be firm and indurated. TAO predominantly affects the medium and small arteries and occasionally the larger arteries.

Whenever diagnostic uncertainty remains after the evaluation of the clinical findings or prior to treatment planning, it is invariably decided by the results of the angiographic examination.[3-6] The angiographic findings are

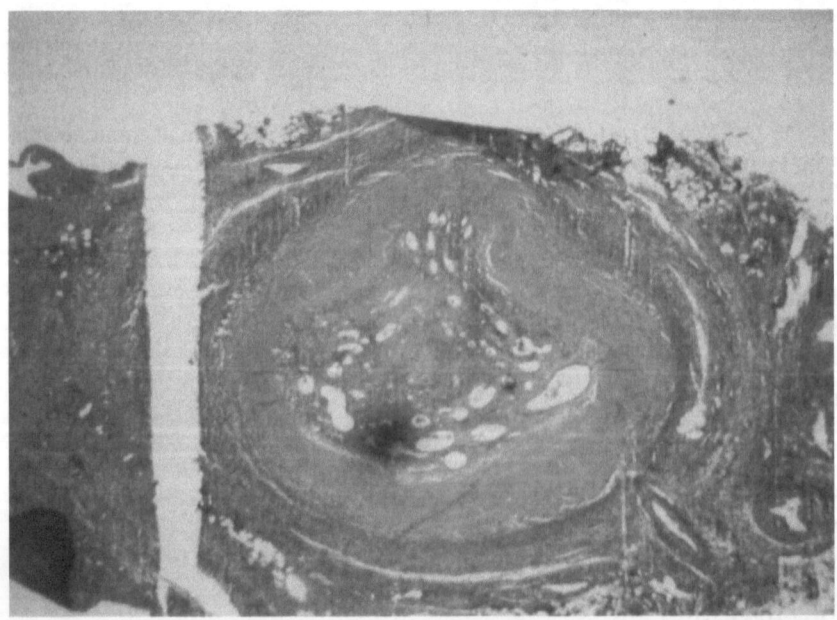

FIGURE 37.6. Histopathologic photograph. Small microabscesses are demonstrated within the thrombus and polymorphonuclear cell infiltration at all layers of vessel wall.

already established, but still not enough to guide treatment. The individual angiographic finding of TAO must represent a specific pathologic process.

The obstructive patterns of the involved arteries probably suggest the age of thrombus formation as well as differentiating among other peripheral vascular occlusive diseases. TAO usually involves the nonbifurcation site, whereas atherosclerosis usually involves the bifurcation site. Segmental involvement is almost characteristic of TAO. A tapered margin of the occluded artery suggests acute involvement which is not filled by thrombus. Regardless of etiology, the ultimate responses to the occlusion are thrombosis and collateral circulation. A flat margin of the opacified artery suggests a fresh thrombus, and a round margin toward the occlusion means an old thrombus, because the advanced cases have more concave margins. If the thrombus is fresh, it can be resolved by anticoagulant therapy. If the margin is convex, it should be differentiated from embolism.

Evaluation of collateral circulation and runoff vessels is necessary for bypass grafting. In acute involvement, the affected vessels are very scanty, and unfortunately there are no collaterals. Indirect collaterals can be developed in any peripheral arterial occlusive disease. However, direct collaterals are characteristic in TAO. McKusick et al[8] say that the direct collaterals of corkscrew appearance are the result of the engorged vase vasorum, but Rivera[9] insists that the collaterals result from recanalization of the thrombus. The corkscrew collaterals along with the branches of the original vessels can have a characteristic appearance like that of tree roots or spiders' legs.

Changes of inflow arteries usually shows a distinct differentiation between TAO and ASO. The inflow arteries are usually normal in TAO. But in one-third, the involved vessels demonstrate fine characteristic signs of corrugated and wave appearance and diffuse narrowing. The reasons for this wave appearance are still unknown. Several authors report that the wave is caused by hyperplastic endometria,[10] structual changes of the arterial wall that remains even after sympathectomy,[11] local spasm,[12] or discordant pulses between normal and occlusion.[13] These phenomena are not found in ASO and reveal atheromatous plaque and tortuous redundancy at inflow arteries.

Early venous opacification is a direct result of vascular occlusion and shortage of blood flow via surrounding muscular branches. Opacification of the peripheral vessels interferes with early venous drainage. Irregular pooling of contrast media in the draining veins is strongly suggestive of venous invasion.

In conclusion, TAO is an apparently distinctive disease characterized by progressive and segmental occlusion in small to medium-sized arteries with several characteristic signs.

References

1. Arteriosclerosis. In: *Pathologic Basis of Disease*, 2nd ed. Robbins SL, Cotran RS, eds. Philadelphia: WB Saunders, 1979, pp. 598–613.

2. Thromboangiitis obliterans (Buerger's disease). In: *Pathologic Basis of Disease*, 2nd ed. Robbins SL, Cotran RS, eds. Philadelphia: WB Saunders, 1979, pp. 617–618.

3. Oh KS, Suh HJ, Kim SS, Huh JD, Joh YD. Digital subtraction angiography in occlusive disease of the lower extremity. J Korean Radiol Soc 1990;26:1144–1149.

4. An BY, Cha SJ, Kim JH, Cha IH, Suh WH. Serial femoral arteriography in Buerger's disease. J Korean Radiol Soc 1985;21:318–322.

5. Cho WY, Suh JS, Park CY: Buerger's disease. J Korean Radiol Soc 1986;22:238–244.

6. Kang HS, Kim JW, Han MC. Arteriography in thromboangiitis obliterans. J Korean Radiol Soc 1979;15:95–100.

7. Brewer ML, Kinnison ML, Perler BA, White RI. Blue toe syndrome: Treatment with anticoagulants and percutaneous transluminal angioplasty. Radiology 1988; 166:31–36.

8. McKusick VA, Harris VS, Ottesen OE, et al. Buerger's disease. JAMA 1962;181: 5–12.

9. Rivera R. Roentgenographic diagnosis of Buerger's disease. J Cardvasc Surg 1973;14:40–46.

10. Shionoya S, Ban J, Nakata G, et al. Involvement of the iliac artery in Buerger's disease. J Cardiovasc Surg 1978;19:69–76.

11. Szilagyl DE, DeRusso FJ, Elliot JP. Thromboangiitis obliterans clinico-pathological correlations. Arch Surg 1964;88:824–835.

12. Wickbom I, Bartley O. Arterial spasm in peripheral arteriography using the catheter method. Acta Radiol 1957;47:433–447.

13. Leher H. The physiology of arteriographic arterial waves. Radiology 1967;89: 11–19.

XIII
Congenital Vascular Defects

38
Surgical Treatment of Congenital Vascular Defects

STEFAN BELOV

Introduction

The primary defect in vascular formation, which is the result of disturbances in embryonic development, is designated as *vitium vasorum congenitum* or congenital vascular defect. The term includes the congenital organic diseases of the vascular system that cause hemodynamic disturbances.

As Lamy and Bourde[1] indicated in 1957, the treatment of vascular malformations deviates from the framework of the generally accepted operative methods in vascular surgery. These authors pay attention to the fact that the appearance of abundant hemorrhages, endangering the patient's life during the operation, menaces every one of the surgeon's movements. Moreover, according to Fontaine,[2] he is constantly placed between Charybdis and Scylla, i.e., between excessive radicalness, which portends a postoperative severe ischemia, and excessive caution, which portends a relapse. Therefore, the old therapeutic conception recommends predominantly conservative treatment, most frequently elastic bandages, limited vascular surgery in the form of removal of small and well-localized arteriovenous malformations and of additional phlebectasias, and symptomatic operative procedures.

The modern causal and multidisciplinary treatment of congenital vascular defects, which Malan and Puglionisi[3,4] established in 1964 and 1965, included the classic methods for removing the diffuse vascular malformations with or without vascular reconstruction, operations for reduction of arteriovenous shunts, and combined multidisciplinary therapy. In the recent past, new surgical techniques for treatment of the "conventionally inoperable forms" of vascular defects were added to the active treatment.

The therapeutic strategy, surgical tactics, and operative techniques that we created over the course of many years were applied in 1,809 cases of congenital vascular defects by vascular surgeons in six different countries and were reported at the 15th World Congress of the International Union of Angiology in Rome in 1989.[5] They are based on a prolonged and thorough study of the anatomopathology of vascular malformations, on the disturbances in hemodynamics and tissue metabolism which they have caused, and on the pathogenesis of the clinical picture. The logic of their argumentation was confirmed by the good postoperative results.[5]

Therapeutic Strategy

The therapeutic strategy we propose includes the following principles.[6]

Active Treatment in Childhood

The ages between 5 and 12 years are the most convenient. Cases with complications (abundant hemorrhage, cardial overloading, and severe tissue ischemia) are indicated for urgent operation. In determining the time of treatment, it is necessary to consider a) the normal development of the vascular system after birth, b) the evolution of the vascular malformation, c) the clinical period of disease (compensated, subcompensated, and decompensated), and d) the period of the child's growth. This factor is important for correcting discrepancies in the length of the lower limbs in the postoperative period.

Treatment by Several Stages

Severe and diffuse forms of vascular malformation are operated in many stages. In cases of peripheral vascular defects causing congenital vascular-bone diseases with discrepancy in the length of the extremities, the first operation should be performed at the age indicated above. Periodic control of the patient's condition is necessary for many years.

Causal Treatment

Therapeutic methods must be in accordance with Hippocrates' principle *sublata causa tollitur morbus* (when the cause is removed, the illness is removed). They should combat the pathogenesis of the disease. The success of treatment depends on precise information about the morphology of the vascular malformation and the hemodynamics of each patient and on a sound knowledge of its impact on tissue metabolism.

Functional Radical Treatment

Since vascular malformations rarely allow the performance of an anatomically radical intervention, the aim is to have the operation functionally radical. This is sometimes very difficult, and the surgeon's personal experience is the greatest help for it.

Individual Treatment

This is a basic principle in which the surgical tactics established are implemented by means of a large number of variants in operative techniques, conforming to the polymorphism in congenital vascular pathology.

Combined Multidisciplinary Treatment

Since congenital vascular defects most frequently show polyangiopathies with great morphological variety, it is imperative in many forms of vascular malformation treatment to be multidisciplinary. In these cases vascular surgery is combined with other nonhemodynamic operations or with existing nonsurgical methods.

Surgical Tactics and Operative Techniques in Congenital Vascular Defects

The surgical tactics and operative techniques practiced by us in treatment of congenital vascular defects[6] are shown in Table 38.1.

TABLE 38.1. Surgical tactics and operative techniques in congenital vascular defects.

Surgical tactics	Operative techniques
Reconstructive operations (revascularization)	1. Resection of malformed segment of the vessel and reconstruction 2. Bypass operations 3. Patch-plastic 4. Membranotomy, membranectomy
Operations to remove the vascular defect (devascularization)	1. Resection of truncular dysplastic phlebectasias 2. Resection of deep truncular A-V communications 3. Resection of superficial truncular A-V communications together with efferent veins 4. Extirpation of extratruncular vascular malformations
Operations to reduce arteriovenous shunt (hemodynamic nonradical operations)	1. Arterial deafferentation 2. Skeletization of principal vessels: arteries and veins 3. Ligature by stages of 2 principal arteries distally from elbow, knee
Combined multidisciplinary treatment	1. Vascular surgery and nonhemodynamic operations 2. Vascular surgery and nonsurgical methods

Reconstructive Operations (Revascularization)

The percentage of reconstructive operations is significantly smaller than that of operations to remove the vascular defect. This is explained by the fact that vascular reconstruction can be applied predominantly in juxtacardial central defects and rarely in visceral defects and some peripheral arterial malformations (aneurysms of main arteries). The operative techniques for vascular reconstruction are: 1) resection or dilatation of a segment with vascular stenosis, or of a dysplastic arterial segment with arteriovenous communications and vascular suture, implantation of an autogenous venous graft, vascular prosthesis; 2) bypass operations; 3) patch-plastic; 4) membranotomy, resection of an obstructive membrane in the vascular lumen. The results of these operations are usually good, because of radical removal of the malformation and restitution of the integrity of the affected blood vessel.

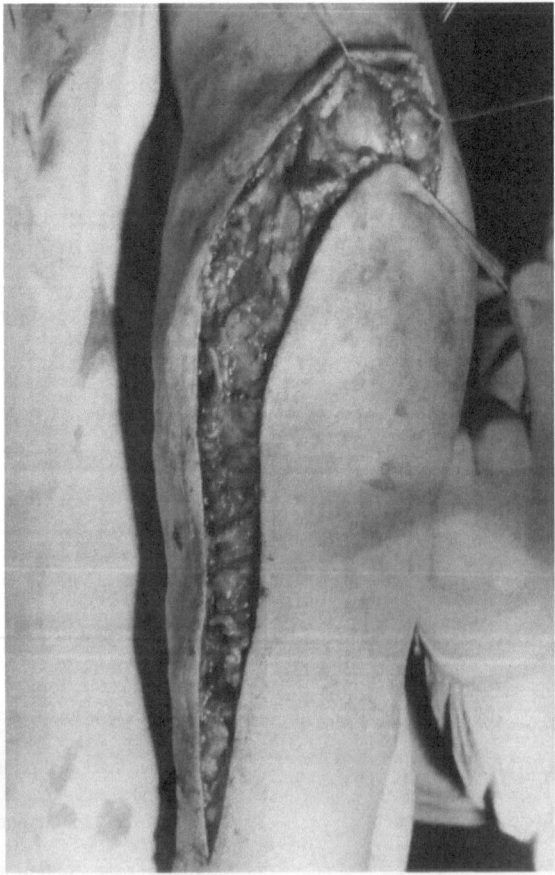

FIGURE 38.1. Surgical approach for resection of malformed phlebectasias in the calf.

Operations to Remove the Vascular Defects (Devascularization)

The operations to remove vascular defects are predominantly applied in the large number of peripheral vascular malformations. The following operative techniques are applied: 1) resection of the malformed phlebectasias and venous convolutions (Fig. 38.1); 2) resection of multiple deep truncular arteriovenous fistulae or aneurysms which connect main arteries and veins (Fig. 38.2); 3) resection of superficial truncular arteriovenous communications together with the efferent phlebectasias (Fig. 38.3); 4) extirpation of extratruncular venous or arteriovenous malformations (Fig. 38.4).

In cases where removal of the peripheral vascular defects is performed in the above-indicated years in childhood by several stages, functionally radical, successively and patiently, the normalization of hemodynamics and tissue metabolism in the extremities leads to correction of the length discrepancy of the lower limbs. These excellent postoperative results achieved by the active

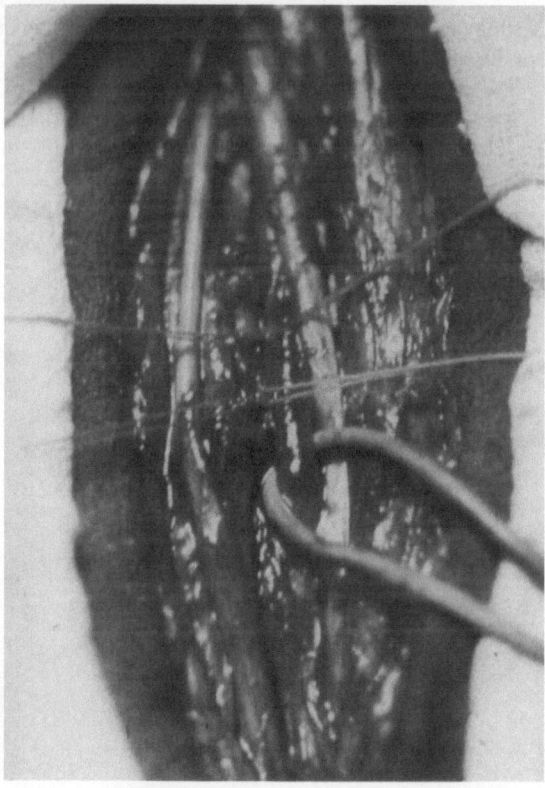

FIGURE 38.2. Resection of multiple deep truncular arteriovenous fistulae which connect the brachial artery and vein.

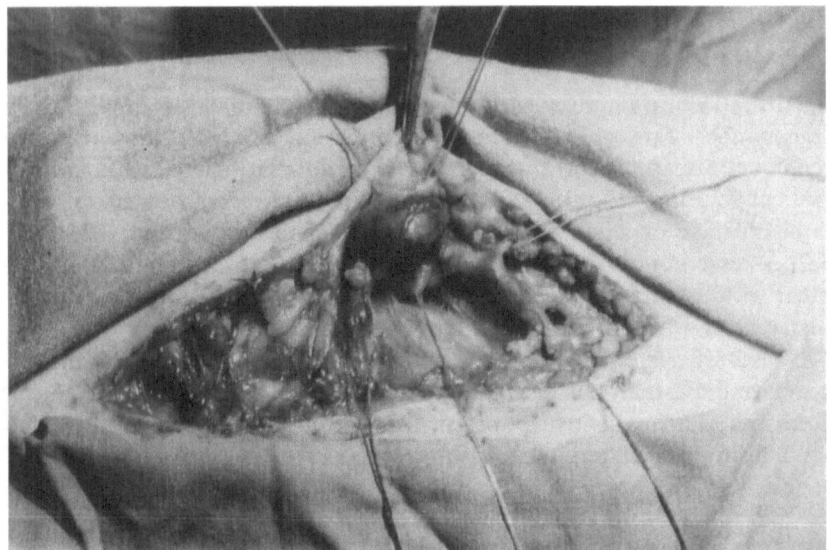

FIGURE 38.3. Resection of superficial truncular arteriovenous communications together with segment of the efferent phlebectasias in the thigh.

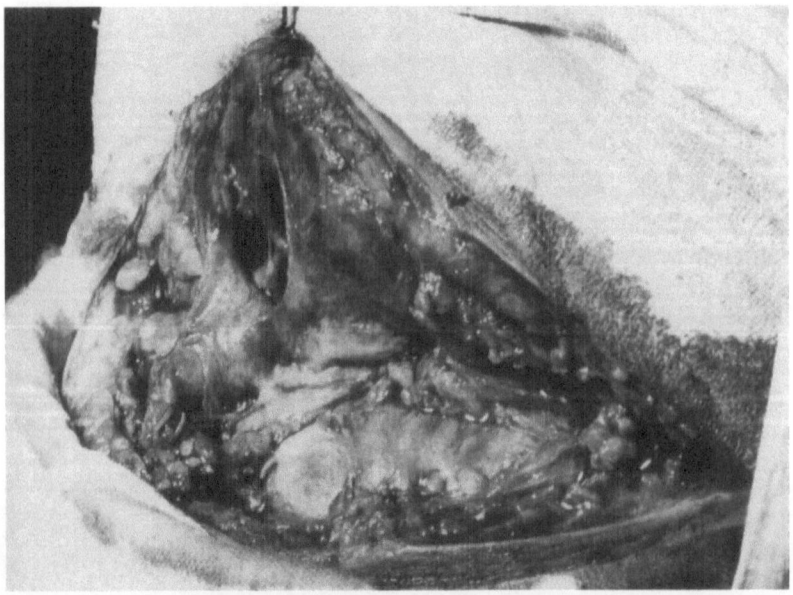

FIGURE 38.4. Extirpation of extratruncular venous malformation in the thoracic wall.

pathogenic approach in the treatment of vascular malformations have been published several times.[7-9]

Operations to Reduce Arteriovenous Shunt (Hemodynamic Nonradical Operations)

These are indicated in cases in which it is impossible to remove the vascular defect. These operative techniques are not radical surgery, but a reduction of the parasitic circulation is achieved. Operations to reduce arteriovenous shunts are: 1) arterial deafferentation (Malan's method),[10] consisting of isolating the principal artery of the limb and tying all the branches that supply the arteriovenous fistulae; 2) skeletization of principal vessels (arteries and veins) (Vollmar's method)[11]; 3) ligature or resection, by stages of two principal arteries distally from elbow, or knee (Vollmar's method).[12]

Experience has shown that the result of these operative techniques is a temporary reduction of the arteriovenous shunt. To achieve a better and more lasting effect, it is necessary to combine these operations with a partial resection of the fistular area or with additional desiccation by means of embolization.

Combined Treatment

Vascular Surgery and Nonhemodynamic Operations

Nonhemodynamic operations consist of the following:

Operations on the Lymphatic System

These are used for combined hemolymphatic malformations and include lymphovenous anastomoses, resection of malformed lymphangiectasias, and total superficial lymphangiectomy.[13]

Operations on the Bones

These are operations to stimulate bone growth, operations to arrest bone growth, and corrective lengthening or shortening osteotomies.[14,15] Indications for these operations are great discrepancy in length of lower limbs, impossibility of normalizing the hemodynamics by vascular operation, or finalizing the process of bone growth. In all these cases, however, the operations on the bones should be combined with operations to remove the vascular malformations or to reduce their hemodynamic activity.

Skin Plastics

Free and attached skin plastics can achieve postoperative success in correcting tissue defects.

Amputation of Extremities

This is the final method in treatment of vascular malformations. Primary amputation is indicated only when it is impossible to perform a vascular operation or desiccation by embolization of the fistular area. Amputation is indicated in cases in which, independently of treatment, the patients' condition has worsened because of severe dysfunction, considerable disfiguration, and complications endangering life.

Vascular Surgery and Nonsurgical Methods

These methods are laser therapy, cortisone therapy, sclerotherapy, and embolization.

In a number of severe cases, surgical methods are unable to manage treatment unaided and should be skilfully combined with existing nonsurgical methods of treatment, especially with embolization.[16,17] They may be performed before, during, or after operation. The indications are anatomically inaccessible and technically unresectable extratruncular infiltrating diffuse and multiple arteriovenous fistulae, as well as surgically nonextirpable infiltrating arteriovenous areas. Combined treatment has often considerably bettered the last postoperative results.

Surgical Techniques for Treatment of "Conventionally Inoperable Forms" of Congenital Vascular Defects

According to Vercellio et al.,[18] the concept "inoperable lesion" is still doubtful in the field of vascular malformations, is continuously evolving, and finally depends on the experience and skill of the vascular team. We fully support this concept, and therefore we will consider the anatomopathological forms of peripheral vascular defects, qualified according to the existing conventional criteria as inoperable, and the new surgical techniques for their treatment.

The first place among the conventionally inoperable cases is occupied by vascular malformations with deep venous reduction which cause congenital disturbed venous drainage. These are the cases with aplasia or hypoplasia of long segments in the deep veins of the extremities, in which vascular reconstruction is impossible. These patients are treated conservatively. Regretfully, elastic bandages do not improve but worsen the patients' condition because of increased venous stasis and ischemia in the extremities.

In the second place are the extratruncular forms that infiltrate the surrounding tissues and organs, destroying their structure and function. Dysplastic infiltrating vascular areas very often cannot be operatively dissected and resected with the existing conventional surgical techniques. In a number of cases, the character and localization of these vascular malformations do

not admit desiccation of arteriovenous communications through embolization, and these patients are considered incurable.

Because these congenital vascular defects cause significant dysfunction and
disfiguration and frequent complications, such as abundant hemorrhages in
shunting defects, new surgical techniques have been created to treat them.
These techniques are based on the logic of hemodynamic conditions and on
the morphological peculiarities of vascular malformations.

Skeletization of the Embryonal Vein

In a large number of patients with congenital angioosteohypertrophy, in
which aplasia of long, segments of the deep veins in the leg is found,
hemodynamic investigation and serial arteriography discover multiple small-
caliber arteriovenous fistulae flowing directly in the superficial embryonal
vein.

The literature is rich in cases in which arteriovenous communications are
found in venous decompensation, probably to assist the drainage of blood
from the affected part of the body by way of the intermediary satellite circulation.[1,19-22] When the hemodynamic activity of these communications sur-
passes the limits of compensation, the satellite circulation transforms into
pathologic parasitic circulation.

The pathogenetic connection between the decompensated venous reduction and the opening of short circuits was indisputably proved by the experiments of Soltesz,[21,22] who after ligature of the main venous trunks in young
animals obtained hypertrophy of the respective extremities with oxyhemo-
metric, arteriographic, and radiocirculographic proof of opened arteriovenous communications.

In 1968, the hemodynamic and pathogenic data suggested to us the idea of
removing the parasitic circulation and considerably reducing venostasis by
way of skeletization of the embryonal vein.[23]

The surgical technique consists in dissection and resection of all superficial
arteriovenous fistulae by numerous incisions along the vein (Fig. 38.5).[24] A
significant improvement of local hemodynamics is achieved, expressed in
decrease of unpleasant complaints and, in childhood, in considerable correction of the discrepancy in length of the lower limbs.

Operation to Divert the Venous Flow and
Restore Deep Venous Drainage

In many cases with congenital angioosteohypotrophy, phlebography reveals
hypoplasia of a long segment of the deep vein, while hemodynamic investigations show venous stasis and reduced circulation in the extremities. The com-
pensatory collateral superficial veins which communicated with the hypoplastic deep vein are also malformed, dilated, and tortuous and increase the
venous stasis.

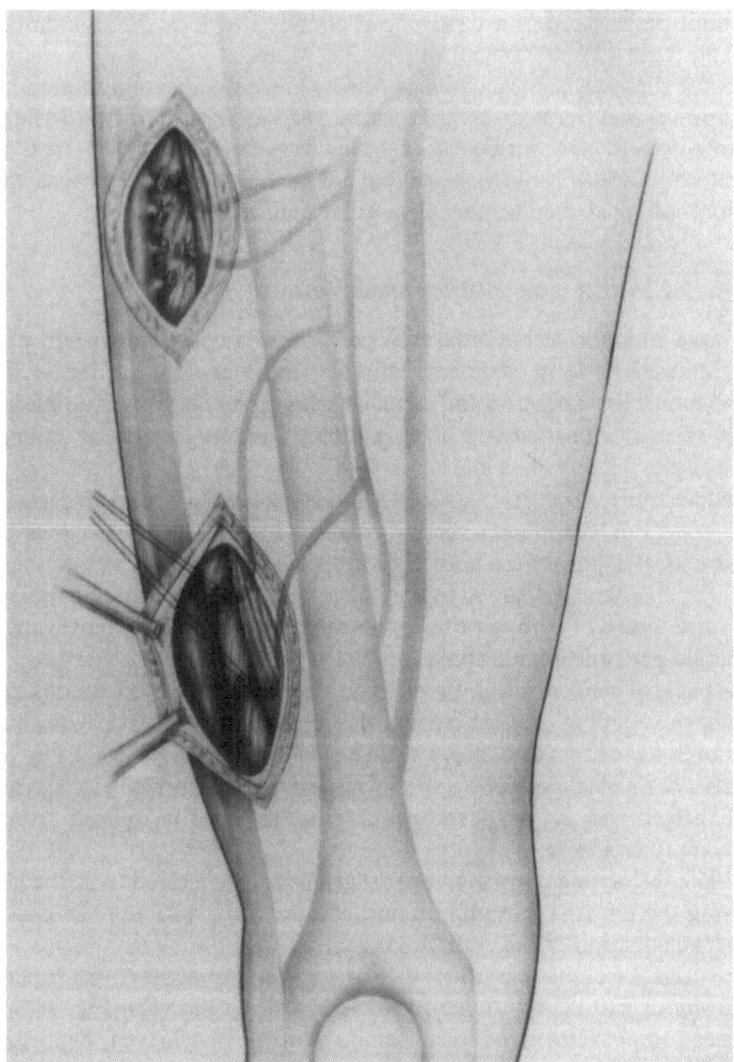

FIGURE 38.5. Skeletization of the embryonal vein. Dissection and resection of all superficial arteriovenous fistulae by numerous incisions along the vein (Reprinted with permission from Belov S. Surgical treatment of congenital predominantly venous defects. In: Belov S, Loose DA, Weber J (eds.). *Vascular Malformations*. Reinbek: Einhorn-Presse Verlag, 1989).

In 1978 these findings indicated to us a method of reducing venostasis by removal of one of the causes for the disturbed venous drainage, namely the phlebectasias, and by establishing the basic venous flow through its normal way, i.e., the principal deep vein, which dilates its lumen to normal size.[24, 25]

The surgical technique consists of careful resection, sometimes in several stages, of the highly dilated superficial veins (Fig. 38.6). A considerable reduc-

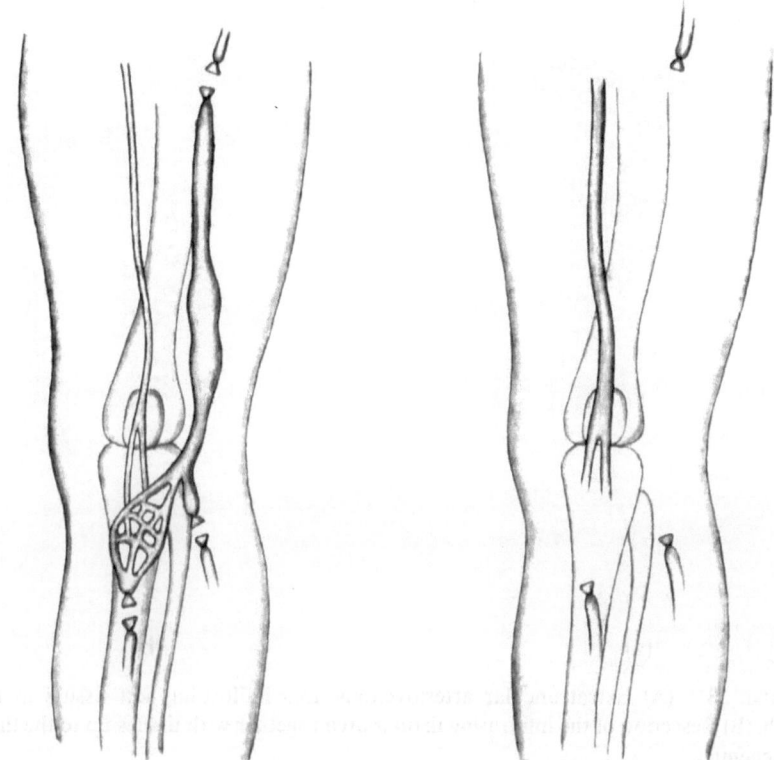

FIGURE 38.6. Operation to divert the venous flow. Resection of dilated superficial veins to divert the basic venous flow toward the principal deep vein. The hypoplastic vein is dilated consequently up to normal size and ensures good venous drainage.

tion of the venous stasis and improvement of the local hemodynamics are achieved.

Atypical Resection of Infiltrating Vascular Area Together with Tissues

The tendency for benign infiltrative growth of angiodysplasias in the surrounding tissues is specific for vascular malformations. We frequently observed the extratruncular infiltrating form in predominantly arteriovenous shunting defects and rarely in predominantly venous defects. Dissection of the malformed vascular areas in many cases is very difficult or impossible owing to hypoxic fibrosis of the soft tissues and fragility of the dysplastic vessels, and is always connected with abundant uncontrolled hemorrhage.

Practical experience in surgical removal of extratruncular dysplastic formations indicates the possibility of their resection together with tissues.[26,27]

Our surgical technique consists in step-by-step resection of the vascular

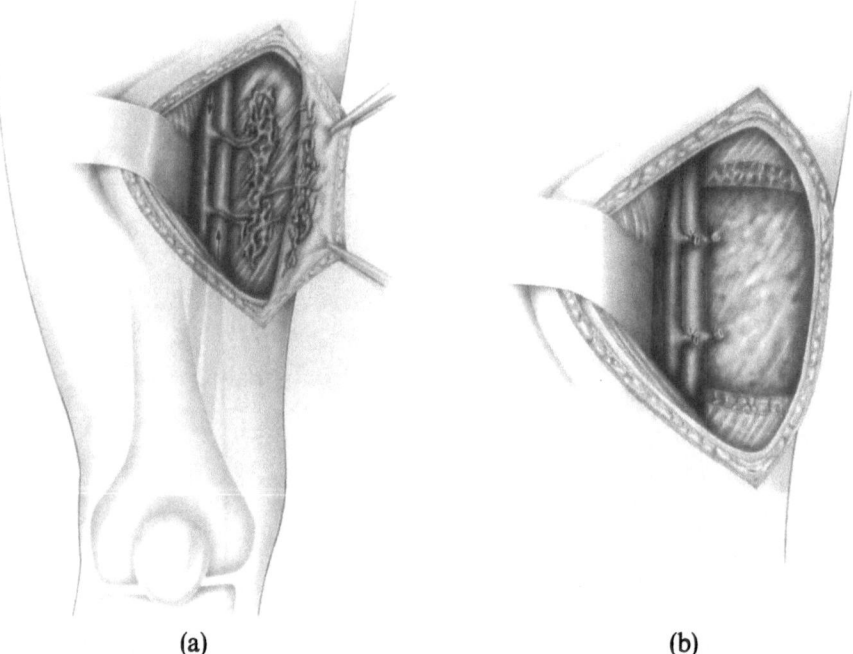

(a)   (b)

FIGURE 38.7. (A) Extratruncular arteriovenous area infiltrating soft tissues in the thigh. (B) Resection of the infiltrating fistular area together with tissues up to the limit of ischemia.

area together with tissues, using small hemostatic clamps and consecutive hemostasis of the bleeding surfaces (Fig. 38.7 A and B). The removal of vascular malformations by this technique must be performed up to the limit of ischemia, dysfunction, and disfiguration, retaining the principle "as radical as possible and as conservative as necessary."

In radically nonresectable infiltrating venous or arteriovenous areas, a segmental resection of the extratruncular vascular malformation is performed.[28] Our surgical technique consists of partial resection of the dysplastic area using atraumatic Satinsky vascular clamps and a continuing hemostatic suture according to Blalock (Fig. 38.8).

These surgical techniques make operative intervention possible in cases of extratruncular infiltrating vascular defects which were formerly qualified as inoperable, and improve significantly the form and function of the affected part of the body.

Summary

The efforts of many excellent specialists working today in different countries and our experience in diagnosis and treatment of congenital vascular defects over more than 30 years have shown that the belief that there is no hope for

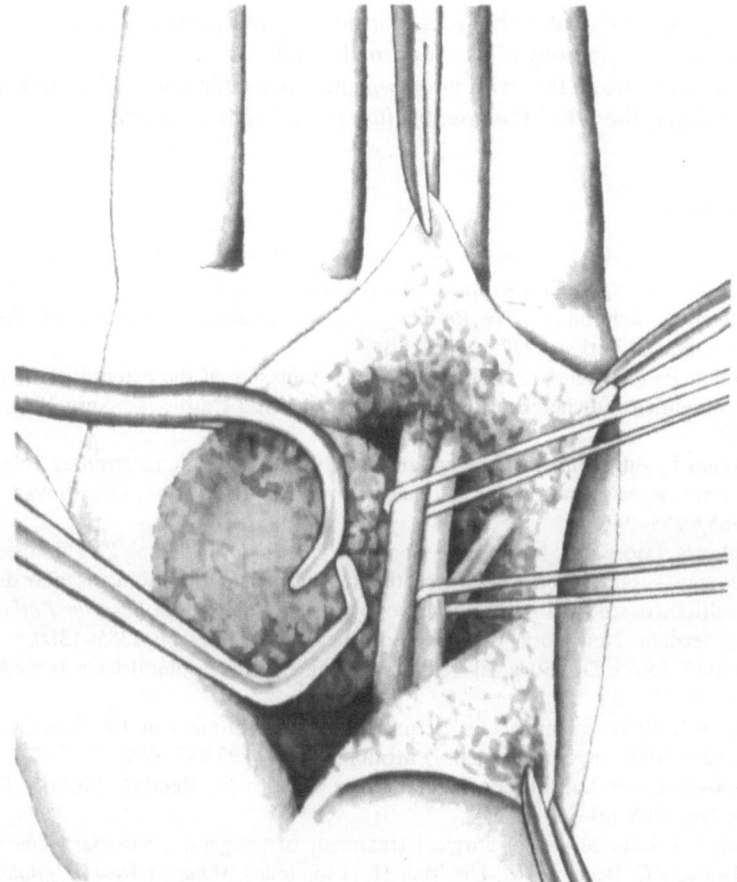

FIGURE 38.8. Partial resection of radically nonresectable infiltrating arteriovenous area in the hand.

therapy of vascular malformations is false. The simple old practice "elastic bandages—arterial ligatures—removing limited single arteriovenous fistulae —amputation" must be abandoned.

Modern treatment of congenital vascular defects should be early, active, and causal. It should conform to the above-mentioned therapeutic strategy and surgical tactics, but the operative technique must be individual for each patient and in accordance with the polymorphism of the congenital vascular pathology.

In a great number of cases with severe combined vascular defects, treatment is multidisciplinary. Vascular surgery should be combined with other nonhemodynamic operations and with existing nonsurgical methods.

The operative treatment of vascular malformations goes beyond the bounds of generally accepted surgical methods. It is often unconventional in applying new surgical techniques, considering the peculiarities in hemodynamics and morphology of vascular malformations.

Experience shows that with good will, indispensable knowledge, and surgical creativity, the art of the possible (*ars possibilis*) is probable.

References

1. Lamy J, Bourde C. *Urgenes vasculaires des membres*. Paris: Masson, 1957.
2. Fontaine R. Spezielle therapeutische Aspekte gewisser arteriovenöser Missbildungen. In: Schobinger RA: *Periphere Angiodysplasien*. Bern–Stuttgart–Vienna: Hans Huber Verlag, 1977, pp. 197–206.
3. Malan E, Puglionisi A. Congenital angiodysplasias of the extremities. (Note I: Generalities and classification; venous dysplasias). J Cardiovasc Surg 1964;5:87–130.
4. Malan E, Puglionisi A. Congential angiodysplasias of the extremities. (Note II: Arterial, arterial and venous, and haemolymphatic dysplasias). J Cardiovasc Surg 1965;6:255–345.
5. Belov S, Loose DA, Mattassi R, Spatenka J, Tasnadi G, Wang Z. Therapeutical strategy, surgical tactics and operative techniques in congenital vascular defects (multicentre study). In: Strano A, Novo S (eds.). *Advances in Vascular Pathology*. Amsterdam–New York–Oxford: Excerpta Medica, 1989, pp. 1355–1360.
6. Belov S, Loose DA. Surgical treatment of congenital vascular defects. Inter Angio 1990;9:175–182.
7. Belov S. Spätergebnisse der chirurgischen Behandlung von 100 Kranken mit kongenitalen Angiodysplasien. Zentralbl Chir 1974;99:935–945.
8. Belov S, Loose DA, Müller E. *Angeborene Gefässfehler*. Reinbek: Einhorn-Presse Verlag, 1985, pp. 73–86.
9. Belov S. Late results of surgical treatment of congenital vascular defects. In: Maurer PC, Becker HM, Heidrich H, et al., (eds.). *What Is New in Angiology?* Munich–Bern–Vienna: W Zuckschwerdt Verlag, 1989, pp. 249–250.
10. Malan E. *Vascular Malformations (Angiodysplasias)*. Milan: Carlo Erba Foundation, 1974, pp. 104–107.
11. Vollmar J, Vogt K. Angiodysplasie und Skelettsystem. Chirurg 1976;47:205–213.
12. Vollmar J. Die Chirurgie kongenitaler arteriovenöser Fisteln der Gliedmassen. In: Vollmar JF, Nobbe FP (eds.). *Arteriovenöse Fisterln–Dilatierende Arteriopathien (Aneurysman)*. Stuttgart: Thieme, 1976, pp. 66–76.
13. Servelle M. La lymphangiectomie superficielle totale. Rev Chir (Pairs) 1947;66: 294.
14. Wettstein P, Hackenbruch W. Die Epiphysiodese. Therapeutische Umschau 1975;32:317–318.
15. Noesberger B, Fernandez D. Technik der Verkürzungs- und Verlängerungsosteotomie an der unteren Extrimität. Therapeutische Umschau 1975;32:119–128.
16. Loose DA. The combined surgical therapy in congenital AV-shunting malformations. In Belov S, Loose DA, Weber J (eds.). *Vascular Malformations*. Reinbek: Einhorn-Press Verlag, 1989, pp. 213–225.
17. Loose DA, Weber J. Indications and tactics for a combined treatment of congenital vascular defects. In: Balas P (ed.). *Progress in Angiology 1991*. Turin: Edizioni Minerva Medica, 1992, pp. 373–378.

18. Vercellio G, Coletti M, Agrifoglio G. Our experience in the treatment of congenital AV-shunting malformations of the limbs. In: Belov S, Loose DA, Weber J (eds.). *Vascular Malformations*. Reinbek: Einhorn-Presse Verlag, 1989, pp. 206–210.

19. Jouve A, Bourdoncle E, Bourde C. Fistules artério-veineuses congénitales des membres et syndrome de Klippel-Trenaunay. Sem Hop (Paris) 1952;28:2674.

20. Rudofsky G, Brosig H-J, Ehinger W, Vogt K, Nobbe F, Vollmar J. Klinische und hämodynamische Untersuchungsbefunde beim Gliedmassenriesenwuchs (Typ Klippel-Trenaunay, Typ FP Weber). In: Vollmar J, Nobbe F (eds.). *Arteriovenöse Fisteln-Dilatierende Arteriopathien (Aneurysmen)*. Stuttgart: Thieme, 1976, pp. 82–86.

21. Soltesz L. Contributions of clinical and experimental studies of the hypertrophy of the extremities in congenital arteriovenous fistulae. J Cardiovasc Surg 1965, p. 260.

22. Solti F, Soltesz L, Ungvari G, Szlavi L, Gloviczki P. Limb circulation after deep venous thrombosis. Acta Chirurg Acad Scient Hung 1982;23:145–152.

23. Belov S. Congenital agenesia of the deep veins of the lower extremities: Surgical treatment. J Cardiovasc Surg 1972;13:594–598.

24. Belov S. Surgical treatment of congenital predominantly venous defects. In: Belov S, Loose DA, Weber J (eds.). *Vascular Malformations*. Reinbek: Einhorn-Presse Verlag, 1989, pp. 158–162.

25. Belov S. *Vascular Malformations—Diagnosis and Surgical Treatment*. Sofia: Medicina i Fizkultura, 1982, pp. 100–102.

26. Belov S. Chirurgische Behandlung der kongenitalen Angiodysplasien. Zentralbl Chir 1967;92:1595–1602.

27. Belov S. Surgical treatment of congenital predominantly arteriovenous shunting defects. In: Belov S, Loose DA, Weber J (eds.). *Vascular Malformations*. Reinbek: Einhorn-Presse Verlag, 1989, pp. 229–234.

28. Belov S. Operative-technical peculiarities in operations of congenital vascular defects. In: Balas P (ed.). *Progress in Angiology 1991*. Turin: Edizioni Minerva Medica, 1992, pp. 379–382.

XIV
Femoral Popliteal Artery Disease

39
Clinical Review of 49 Cases of Lower Limb Ischemic Disease

BYUNG JUN SO AND KWON MOOK CHAE

Lower limb ischemia due to various causes has been increasingly treated by surgical and medical methods. Forty-nine patients with lower limb ischemic disease, who were treated from July 1, 1981, to December 31, 1991, in our clinic, were studied retrospectively to determine the causes and clinical characteristics. The incidence of lower limb ischemic disease was as follows: atherosclerotic occlusion, 23 cases (46.9%); Buerger's disease, 15 cases (30.6%); thromboembolism, 11 cases (22.4%). The predominant ages were the sixth and seventh decades in atherosclerotic occlusion and thromboembolism, and the fourth and fifth decades in Buerger's disease. The most common symptom of atherosclerotic occlusion was intermittent claudication (56.5%); of Buerger's disease, rest pain (100%); and of thromboembolism, acute pain and coldness (100%). On angiogram, the most common sites of occlusion were the aortoiliac segment (52.1%) in atherosclerotic occlusion, infrapopliteal multiple lesions (85%) in Buerger's disease, and the femoral artery (63.6%) in thromboembolism. The associated diseases were hypertension (34.8%), diabetes mellitus (30.4%), and cardiac disease (21.7%) in atherosclerotic occlusion; and cardiac disease (72.7%) and cerebrovascular accident (27.2%) in thromboembolism.

Lower limb ischemic disease can be caused by the various occlusive processes of the infrarenal arterial system, such as chronic occlusive disease, acute occlusive disease, aneurysm, arteriovenous fistula, and vasomotor disturbance. Among the lesions of chronic occlusion, atherosclerotic disease is the most common in modern Western society, and it is well known that Buerger's disease is more prevalent in the Middle and Far East than in Europe and the United States.[1,2] Arterial thromboembolism is the main cause of acute arterial occlusive disease. A thorough understanding of the arterial obliterative process and its natural history is essential for the proper selection of candidates for appropriate surgical procedures to achieve limb revascularization.[3,4]

We have been concerned about the prevalent causes and clinical characteristics of lower limb ischemic disease in our province. Therefore, 49 patients with lower limb ischemic disease who were treated in our clinic from July 1, 1981, to December 31, 1991, were studied retrospectively.

Materials and Methods

During the period from July 1, 1981, to December 31, 1991, 49 patients with lower limb ischemic disease were admitted and treated in our clinic. For evaluation of clinical characteristics, the hospital records and outpatient charts of all patients were reviewed. The patients were classified into three groups on the basis of the angiographic and clinical findings: group I ($n = 23$, 46.9%), atherosclerotic disease; group II ($n = 15$, 30.6%), Buerger's disease; group III ($n = 11$, 22.4%), thromboembolism.

Our angiographic findings in group I were variable. However, in terms of location and extent of the atherosclerotic process, they were classified into three basal patterns: 1) aortoiliac, 2) femoropopliteal, and 3) tibioperoneal lesions. Group II showed multiple segmental occlusion of distal extremity arteries, primarily of the foot and calf. The arterial wall proximal to the occlusion was usually normal, and extensive collateral vessels developed. The angiographic findings of group III were abrupt occlusion of uniform caliber vessel, and showed superior convex meniscus and unopacified filling defect in cases of partially occluding emboli.

Clinical manifestations of group I varied with their location and extent, and included claudication, rest pain, and ulcer/gangrene. Our clinical criteria for the diagnosis of group II (Buerger's disease) were: 1) heavy smoker, 2) onset before the age of 50 years, 3) infrapopliteal arterial occlusions, 4) history of superficial phlebitis, and 5) absence of atherosclerotic risk factors other than smoking. Sudden onset of pain was universal in patients of group III. Numbness, paralysis, coldness, pallor, and pulse loss were present in most cases.

Results

General characteristics of group I patients are shown in Table 39.1. The mean age was 61.8 years, ranging from 43 to 79 years. The most common presenting complaint was claudication ($n = 13$); others were rest pain ($n = 10$) and ulcer/gangrene ($n = 3$). Thirty percent were diabetic. Thirty-four percent gave a history of hypertension, and 22% had known coronary artery disease. A history of smoking was obtained in 30%. The angiographic findings of this group were classifed into three groups: aortoiliac lesion ($n = 12$), femoropopliteal lesion ($n = 9$), and lesion below knee joint ($n = 2$). Disabling claudication ($n = 11$) and rest pain ($n = 5$) were the indications for the operation in 16 procedures in 16 patients. Reconstructive procedures included aortofemoral bypass ($n = 10$), femoro-posterior tibial bypass ($n = 4$), and axillofemoral bypass ($n = 2$). There were no immediate postoperative deaths, and mean graft patency rate was 2.5 years (range 5 months to 6 years).

Table 39.2 lists the general characteristics of group II patients. The mean age was 38.3 years, ranging from 22 to 55 years. The presenting complaints

TABLE 39.1. Characteristics of 23 patients with atherosclerotic disease.

Sex ratio (M : F)	21 : 2
Mean age (years)	61.6 (43–79)
Presenting complaints	
Claudication	13
Rest pain	10
Ulcer/gangrene	3
Predisposing factors	
Hypertension	8 (34.8%)
Diabetes mellitus	7 (30.4%)
Cardiac disease	5 (21.7%)
Transient ischemic attacks	1
Hyperlipidemia	2
Smoking	7
Site of occlusion	
Aortoiliac	12
Femoropopliteal	9
Below knee	2
Treatment	
Bypass operation	16
Sympathectomy	1
Conservative Tx	6

TABLE 39.2. Characteristics of 15 patients with Buerger's disease.

Sex ratio (M : F)	14 : 1
Mean age (years)	38.8 (22–49)
Presenting complaints	
Rest pain	15
Coldness	9
Ulcer/gangrene	10
Predisposing factors	
Smoking	14
Treatment	
Lumbar sympathectomy only	5
Amputation only	1
Lumbar sympathectomy + amputation	8
Bypass	1

were rest pain in 15, coldness in 9, and ulcer/gangrene in 10. The incidence of smoking history was 93%, and other risk factors were not noticed. All the patients received conservative treatment consisting of abstinence from cigarettes and vasodiators such as nifedipine and prostaglandin E, (PGE$_1$). But we could not attain a successful result. Twelve of the 15 patients were given lumbar sympathectomy as an additional procedure, and subsequent amputation was needed in 8 patients due to dry gangrene and uncontrollable pain.

TABLE 39.3. Characteristics of 11 patients with thromboembolism.

Sex ratio (M : F)	9 : 2
Mean age (years)	59.5 (21–75)
Presenting complaints	
Acute pain	11
Coldness	11
Paresthesia	3
Edema	2
Paralysis	1
Underlying diseases	
Cardiac disease	8
Atherosclerosis	1
Transient ischemic attacks	3
Site of occlusion	
Abdominal aorta	1
Iliac	3
Femoral	7
Popliteal	2
Treatment	
Thrombolytic agent	2
Embolectomy	7
Embolectomy with bypass	2

The clinical details of the patients in group III are shown in Table 39.3. The mean age was 59.5 years, ranging from 21 to 75 years. All complained of acute pain and coldness. Other presenting complaints were paresthesia in 3, edema in 2, and paralysis in 1. Seventy-three percent gave a history of cardiac disease; 9% had atherosclerotic disease without heart disease; 27% of the patients were smokers. The most common site of occlusion was the femoral artery ($n = 7$); less common sites were the iliac artery ($n = 3$) and the popliteal artery ($n = 2$). The main modalities of treatment were embolectomy only ($n = 7$), embolectomy with bypass ($n = 2$), and thrombolytic agents only ($n = 2$). The results of embolectomy with Forgaty catheter were excellent in 7, without later recurrence. Two of 11 patients were given embolectomy with bypass due to combined segmental stenotic lesions. In 2 patients, thrombolytic agents were employed for the treatment of the occlusion, which was judged to be a spontaneous local thrombosis.

Discussion

Atherosclerosis is the underlying cause of chronic limb ischemia in the vast majority of patients. From a clinicopathologic point of view, atherosclerotic processes may be responsible for several ischemic diseases by way of complicated lesions, such as acute thrombosis, ischemic occlusive disease, or aneurysm.[5] During the past 10 years, we have experienced 8 aneurysmal diseases, but their main problem were not ischemic symptoms. Therefore, we did not include the cases in this analysis, and acute thrombotic occlusion was classified in group III. The symptoms of the chronic occlusive process are claudication, rest pain, and ulcer/gangrene. Claudication is the single most important symptom of arterial occlusive disease. It consists of three essential features: 1) the pain is always experienced in a functional muscle unit; 2) it is reproducibly precipitated by a consistent amount of exercise; 3) it is promptly relieved by merely stopping exercise.[6] In our group, claudication also was the most common symptom ($n = 13$, 56.5%). Some of the more common initiating factors of the atherosclerosis are tobacco, diabetes, radiation, hypertension, hyperlipidemia, and direct arterial injury.[7] The incidence of smoking history in our group was 34.8%. The occlusive process of the femoropopliteal segment is the most common lesion of the lower extremities. Its preponderance, exclusive of its combination with other arterial lesions, has been documented by several statistical surveys, with incidence ranging from 47[8] to 65.4%.[9] Our studies showed that the aortoiliac segment was the most common site of chronic obliterative atherosclerosis ($n = 12$, 57.1%). A variety of reconstructive procedures are available to the surgeon: prosthetic bypass grafting and endarterectomy may be feasible. Extraanatomic procedures are reserved for high-risk patients unable to tolerate conventional anatomic reconstruction. We performed 16 reconstructive procedures which included aortofemoral bypass ($n = 10$), femoro-posterior tibial bypass ($n = 4$), and axillofemoral bypass ($n = 2$).

Thromboangiitis obliterans was originally described by Leo Buerger in 1908 and become firmly established, along with atherosclerosis, as one of the two major causes of peripheral arterial occlusive disease.[10] Thromboangiitis obliterans typically occurs in heavy smokers. The disease begins in young adult life, usually between 20 and 35 years of age. Although Buerger's disease affects all races, it is more prevalent in the Middle and Far East than in Europe and United States.[1,10] The Mayo Clinic reported an incidence of 97.5 cases per 100,000 patients in 1950, 48.6 in 1955, 18.8 in 1965, and 11.6 in 1969.[11] Park et al.[12] of Yonsei University College of Medicine reported an incidence of 9.5% of 1,620 patients with peripheral ischemic disease, and Park et al.[13] of Hanyang University College of Medicine reported an incidence 44.8% of 116 patients. Shigehiko et al.[14] reported a 15.9% rate. Our results showed a higher incidence, 30.6% of 49 patients.

The specific cause of Buerger's disease is not known. Secondary etiologic factors that have a positive effect on the disease include age, sex, race, hereditary factor [human lymphocyte antigen (HLA)], occupation, and smoking. HLA analysis in patients with Buerger's disease showed a higher frequency of Aw 24, Bw 40, Bw54, Cw 1, and DR 2 antigens and a lower frequency of DR 9 and DR w 52 compared with those in normal individuals.[15] However, the significance of these immunologic findings remains to be explained. In the Far East, the majority of patients have been outdoor workers, suggesting a relation with socioeconomic conditions, work environment, or both. Tobacco smoking, whether it is a direct etiologic factor or only a strongly contributory one, plays a pivotal role in disease development and progression. The incidence of smoking history of our patients was 93%. The major presenting symptoms are paresthesia, coldness, cyanosis, gangrene or ulcer, claudication, rest pain, and thrombophlebitis. At the author's institution, the presenting complaints were rest pain ($n = 15$, 100%), coldness ($n = 9$), and ulcer/gangrene ($n = 10$). The only way to arrest the disease is abstinence from smoking. Any therapeutic procedure not accompanied by a cessation of smoking cannot achieve a successful result. No specific medication has found wide acceptance, although anticoagulants, dextran, phenylbutazone, pyridinol-carbamate, inositol niacinate, and steroids have all been recommended. More recently, prostaglandin therapy (PGA_1)[16] and defibrotide[17] have been advocated, as well as agents to prevent platelet aggregation. In cases of poor spontaneous healing potential, sympathectomy or arterial reconstruction should be considered. When gangrene occurs, amputation at the lowest possible level is indicated. At the authors' institution, all patients have received conservative treatment. Lumbar sympathectomy was performed in 12 of 15 patients with Buerger's disease. The result of sympathectomy was not satisfactory and subsequent amputation was needed in 8 patients.

Acute arterial obstruction constitutes a true surgical emergency, and the importance of early operative intervention has been stressed by all investigators of the problem. The relative incidence of acute thrombosis vs. arterial embolism is not always easy to establish, especially in elderly patients with combined cardiopathy and peripheral arteriosclerosis. As a result, all episodes of acute arterial obstruction, regardless of orgin and etiology, are often classified as "acute arterial occlusions."[3,4] The onset is sudden and characterized by severe pain, paresthesia, and numbness in the toes and foot. The heart is the source of embolism in 80% to 90% of the published cases.[3,18,19] Acute occlusion may also be of thrombotic origin, prompted by chronic degenerative atherosclerotic disease of the periphery. The etiologic factors in our patients were cardiac disease in 8, advanced atherosclerotic disease in 1, and unknown origin in 2. The natural clinical course of a peripheral arterial embolism depends upon the location of the occlusion, the degree of completeness of the luminal obliteration, the extent of secondary thrombosis, and the degree of spontaneous restoration of the collateral circulation. Among these, secondary thrombosis is one of the most important local factors. The majority of surgically treatable emboli lodge in the lower extremities, usually at bifurcations. The incidence of impaction is highest in the femoral arterial bed, with frequent occurrence in the iliac, aortic, and popliteal areas as well. Our results were as follows: 63.6% in the femoral artery, 27.2% in the iliac artery, and 18.1% in the popliteal artery. Since the introduction of the balloon catheter, the technique of embolectomy has been simplified. Thrombolytic agents such as streptokinase, urokinase, tissue plasminogen activator

(TPA), and prourokinase have been employed for the treatment of actue arterial occlusion. If acute thrombotic occlusion is suggested after adequate arteriographic evaluation of the arterial tree has been performed, a decision must be made as to whether revascularization is feasible. A thrombectomy is rarely, if ever, useful in acute arterial occlusion. A bypass is necessary in the majority of cases, provided a runoff is delineated by an adequate arteriogram. Neverthless, thrombectomy alone was reported to provide good results in 53% of cases by Planell[20] and 65% of cases by Enjabert et al.[21] Raithel, using a ring-stripper together with a Fogarty catheter, was able to facilitate the pullout of the occluding thrombus with the involved arterial intima.[22] At the authors' institution, embolectomy was performed in 7 cases, and embolectomy with bypass in 2 cases. Thrombolytic agents were employed in 2 cases. All of them achieved limb salvage, and immediate postoperative death was absent.

In summary, 49 patients with lower limb ischemic disease were treated in our clinic during the last 10 years. The most common cause of lower limb ischemic disease was atherosclerotic occlusion (46.9%), and the second most common cause was Buerger's disease. These results correspond to the relatively high incidence of Buerger's disease in Asia. The majority of our patients achieved good results, except for those with Buerger's disease. However, we think that further outstanding diagnostic and therapeutic options for management of arterial occlusive disease will be needed for our clinic to approach more peripheral occlusive disease.

References

1. Mckusik VA, Harris WS. Buerger syndrome in Orient. Bull Johns Hopkins Hosp 1961;109:242.
2. Wessler S, Ming SC, Gurewich V, Freiman DG. A critical evaluation of the thromboangiitis obliterans. N Engl J Med 1960;262:1149.
3. Blaisdell GS, Steele M, Allen RE. Management of lower extremity arterial ischemia due to embolism and thrombosis. Surgery 1978;84:822.
4. Cambria RP, Abbott WM. Acute arterial thrombosis of the lower extremity. Its natural history contrasted with arterial embolism. Arch Surg 1984;111:784.
5. Haimovici H. *Vascular Surgery, Principles and Techniques.* 3rd ed. Norwalk, CT: Appleton & Lange, 1989, p. 184.
6. Rutherford RB. *Vascular Surgery.* 3rd ed. *Vol. 1.* Philadelphia: WB Saunders, 1989, p. 207.
7. Cohen JR. Vascular surgery for the house officer. Baltimore: Williams & Wilkins, 1986, p. 20.
8. Humphries AW, deWolfe VG, et al. Evaluation of the natural history and the results of the treatment in occlusive arteriosclerosis involving the lower extremities. In: Wesolowski SA, Dennis C (eds.). *Fundamentals of Vascular Grafting.* New York: McGraw-Hill, 1963, p. 423.
9. Fontaine R, Kieny R, et al. Long term results of restorative arterial surgery in obstructive disease of the arteries. J Cardiovasc Surg 1964;5:463.

10. Wessler S. Buerger's disease revisited. Surg Clin North Am 1969;49:703.
11. Juergens L. Thromboangiitis obliterans (Buerger's disease. TAO) Japanese Ministry of Health and Welfare, 1970;18–19: pp. 3–17.
12. Park TY, Choi HY, Kim CK. Clinicostatistical analysis of Buerger's disease. J Korean Surg Soc 1981;23:19.
13. Park DY, Kwak JY. Statistical study of peripheral arterial disease. J Korean Surg Soc 1987;3:19.
14. Shigehiko S, Ichiro B, Yukifumi N, Matsumi N, Matsubara J, Hirai M, Hiroshi M, Seichi K. Vascular reconstruction in Buerger's disease. Br J Surg 1981;63:841.
15. Numano F, Sasazuki T, Koyama T, et al. HLA in Buerger's disease. Exp Clin Immunogenet 1986;3:195.
16. Shionoya S. What is Buerger's disease? World J Surg 1983;7:544.
17. Ulution ON. Clinical effectiveness of defibrotide in vaso-occlusive disorders and its mode of actions. Semin Thromb Hemost 1988;14 (Suppl): 58.
18. Haimovici H. Peripheral embolism. A study of 330 unselected cases of embolism of the extremities. Angiology 1950;1:20.
19. Warren R, Linton RR. The treatment of arterial embolism. N Engl J Med 1948; 238:421.
20. Planell ES. Emergency thrombectomy in the treatment of acute arterial thrombosis. J Cardiovasc Surg (Special Issue: 11th World Congress, International Cardiovascular Society, Barcelona, Sept. 1973)
21. Enjalbert A, Gedeon A, Puel P, et al. Emergency thrombectomy in acute arterial obliterations: Experience with 204 operated cases. J Cardiovasc Surg (Special Issue: 11th World Congress, International Cardiovascular Society, Barcelona, Sept. 1973)
22. Raithel E. Ein neuartiger katheter—stripper zue Behandlung der akuten Gliemassenischaemie. Chirug 1973;44:434.

40
Current Status of the Surgical Treatment of Chronic Arterial Occlusive Disease in Japan

Yoshio Mishima

Summary

1. The number of patients who underwent operation has increased greatly, especially in the last 10 years.
2. Patients over 75 years old have also increased in the past 5 years. The main indication in the younger age group is intermittent claudication, whereas arterial reconstruction is mainly performed for limb salvage in the higher age group.
3. The long-term patency rate of aortoiliac reconstruction was 85.2% in all cases; however, it was 94.6% for the last 10 years.
4. The cumulative patency rate of femoropopliteotibial reconstruction in 135 cases was 85.6% after 1 year, 76.7% after 2 years, and 53.2% after 5 years. The patency rate in the above-knee region using polytetrafluoroethylene (PTFE) graft was 87.7% after 1 year, 80% after 2 years, and 63.3% after 5 years. On the other hand, the long-term patency rate in the below-knee region became remarkably lower after 4 years when PTFE was used.
5. Fortunately, we have encountered few cases with concomitant occlusive disease of the carotid, coronary, or renal arteries; however, we think that these associated atherosclerotic lesions will be a very important problem in the near future.

Clinical, hemodynamic, and angiographic findings provide the basis for the criteria in selecting patients with occlusive arterial disease for reconstructive surgery. Based on these criteria, three major indications are generally considered, according to Fontaine's classification. The indication for stage II is essentially for functional improvement and possibly also for prophylaxis against further progression of disease. The indications for stages III and IV are for limb salvage.

The causes for delay or avoidance of conventional aortoiliac vascular surgery are the presence of peritonitis, active inflammatory bowel disease, or sources of contamination, such as temporary colostomy or draining sinuses involving the abdomen. A routine systematic evaluation of all the vital organs is essential in all patients being considered for arterial surgery: cardio-vascular status, cerebral history with special reference to carotid arteries, renal function, especially in diabetic patients, chest films, blood pressure determinations over a period of several days, blood chemistry, and lipid profile.

Historically, the introduction of endarterectomy by J. Cid dos Santos in 1947 and the bypass graft technique by Kunlin in 1948 marked the beginnings of methods for direct revascularization of the lower extremity. Of the two procedures, the bypass has gained wider acceptance and has largely superseded the former, as attested to by the vast worldwide literature on this subject.

During the late 1970s, we adopted the use of the synthetic bypass graft in preference to endarterectomy in the aortoiliac segment. However, if there is a short, localized occlusive process involving the common iliac artery and extending slightly into the bifurcation, endarterectomy may be chosen. In my opinion, a synthetic graft should be used even in the latter circumstances, particularly if the vessels are hypoplastic or if there is extensive calcification of the vessels.

In those patients with severe organic disease that is not amenable to improvement, there is the option of employing extraanatomic bypasses, such as axillofemoral or femorofemoral grafts, with significantly less risk to the patients. Although hemodynamic noninvasive studies suggest that the amount of blood flow provided by these procedures is not as great as that with aortic grafts, they are very appropriate in high-risk patients where relatively short-term benefits are reasonable because of advanced organic disease.

The lack of an autologous vein of adequate length and the necessity of bypass grafting to the distal popliteal or the infrapopliteal branches has led to the use of either a composite or a sequential graft. The sequential technique consists of a single graft with multiple anastomoses for the purpose of reducing resistance and increasing flow. The sequential bypass has been reported to improve distal perfusion in markedly ischemic limbs, leading to patency rates of 76% at 1 year and 31% at 8 years. When occlusion of the distal bypass occurs with continued patency of the proximal segment, it is usually due to poor distal runoff. It is reasonable to attempt this technique in well-selected cases.

During the past few years, there has been an increasing use of balloon dilatation (percutaneous transluminal angioplasty) in selected patients. In our institution, balloon angioplasty was performed in 36 limbs of 33 patients. The mean age was 68 years. It was mainly performed in the iliac segment with an initial success rate of 72%. In this area this procedure is almost always feasible, if the guidewire can be inserted beyond the stenotic portion, from our experience.

Patients who are ideally suited for angioplasty are those with focal stenosis of the iliac and common femoral arteries. Patients with diffuse disease are more likely to benefit from surgical reconstruction. More recent experience shows that intraarterial low-dose urokinase can be used in patients with recent iliac and femoral artery occlusions (less than about 8 months duration) to provide thrombolysis, followed by balloon angioplasty. In patients with unilateral iliofemoral artery occlusion and stenosis of the contralateral iliac artery who are not candidates for either vascular reconstruction or thrombolytic therapy, balloon angioplasty can be used in conjunction with a less invasive surgical procedure. In such patients, balloon angioplasty of the stenotic iliac artery with subsequent femorofemoral crossover bypass graft may provide an alternative vascular reconstructive procedure. In addition, postoperative stenoses after aortoiliac and aortobifemoral bypass grafts can also be managed successfully with balloon angioplasty.

The occlusive patterns and the age distribution of the patients suffering from chronic arterial occlusive disease in Japan are somewhat characteristic and are different from those in the United States and European countries. Presumably, atherosclerosis is the main cause of chronic arterial occlusion in

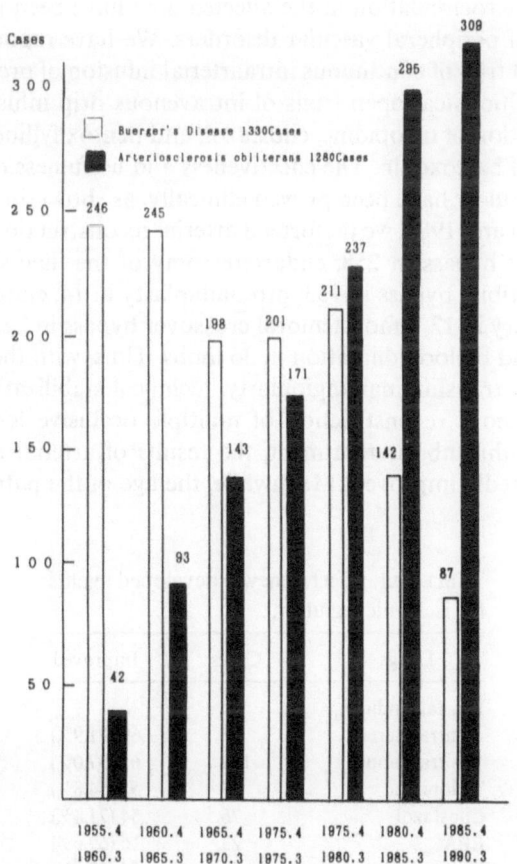

FIGURE 40.1. Chronological change of chronic arterial occlusive diseases in Japan, 1955–1990.

the Western countries, whereas Buerger's disease or its related pathology was the main cause until recently in the Orient, including Japan. During the past 10 years, however, the typical cases of Buerger's disease have decreased in number, and arteriosclerosis obliterans has greatly increased in Japan, as a result of progress in diagnostic procedures, the Europeanization of life styles, and dietary habits after World War II, as shown in Figure 40.1. The nature and that pattern of chronic arterial occlusion in Japan will also more and more resemble those observed in the Western countries from the pathophysiological point of view. Suspicion of chronic arterial occlusion is the signal for complete abstinence from smoking and the institution of a variety of other supportive measures, although none of them is specific.

Until recently, the so-called vasodilating substances have been prescibed mainly for patients suffering from chronic arterial occlusive diseases. In recent years, however, the study of platelet function and of hemorheology has progressed greatly both experimentally and clinically. Consequently, agents that improve microcirculation in the affected area have been introduced for the treatment of peripheral vascular disorders. We have reported a double-blind controlled trial of continuous intraarterial infusion of prostaglandin E_1 (PGE,) and multiclinical open trials of intravenous drip infusion of PGE_1, oral administration of ticlopidine, cilostazol, and pentoxifylline, and intravenous infusion of batroxobin. The effectiveness and usefulness of these agents for ischemic leg ulcer have been proved clinically, as shown in Table 40.1.

Between 1970 and 1989, we performed arterial reconstruction in 460 limbs: aortoiliofemoral bypass in 258, endarterectomy of the iliac segment in 32, femoropopliteotibial bypass in 153, profundaplasty in 14, endarterectomy of the femoral artery in 12, femorofemoral crossover bypass in 22, axillofemoral bypass in 16, and balloon dilatation in 36 limbs. Thus, with the introduction of percutaneous transluminal angioplasty, technical stabilization of outflow plasty, simultaneous reconstruction of multiple occlusive lesions, and the progress of antithrombotic treatment, the results of arterial reconstruction have been markedly improved. Meanwhile, the age of the patients undergo-

TABLE 40.1. Effect of newly developed agents for ischemic leg ulcer.

Drugs	Cases	Improved
Prostaglandin E_1		
Intraarterial	96	69 (71.9%)
Intravenous	114	65 (57.0%)
Ticlopidine	93	51 (54.8%)
Cilostazol	76	54 (71.4%)
EPA	23	16 (69.6%)
Pentoxifylline	41	24 (58.5%)
Batroxobin	85	57 (67.1%)
Argatroban	50	29 (58.0%)

ing arterial reconstructive surgery has increased. The number of patients who have undergone arterial reconstruction has increased greatly, especially during the last 10 years. Also, the frequency of both reconstruction for femoropopliteotibial segment occlusions and simultaneous reconstruction for multiple segmental occlusions increased in the 1980s.

The number of patients more than 75 years old has tended to increase in the last 5 years. The mean age of the patients has also gradually increased. The main indication in the younger age group is intermittent claudication, whereas arterial reconstruction is mainly performed for limb salvage in the higher age group. In the latter group, arterial reconstruction was performed only for cases with the symptoms of Fontaine's stage IV until 1979; however, it is now also performed for patients with stages II and III, reflecting the need of patients to improve the quality of daily life.

The long-term patency rate of aortoiliac reconstruction was 85.2% in all cases; however, it was 94.6% in the last 10 years. Thus, the long-term patency rate increased from 72.4% to 94.6% during the last 20 years. This result is though to be almost satisfactory. This improvement of the long-term patency rate is a result of the simultaneous performance of outflow plasty and multiple reconstructions. Regarding the cumulative patency rates of femoropopliteotibial reconstruction in 135 cases, the patency rate was 85.6% after 1 year, 76.7% after 2 years, and 53.2% after 5 years. This result is far from satisfactory. Because to date we have preferred to use the polytetrafluoroethylene (PTFE) graft in femoropopliteotibial reconstruction, the PTFE graft may play a significant role in the low patency rate in the long term. In the cases with femoropopliteotibial reconstruction using the PTFE graft, the

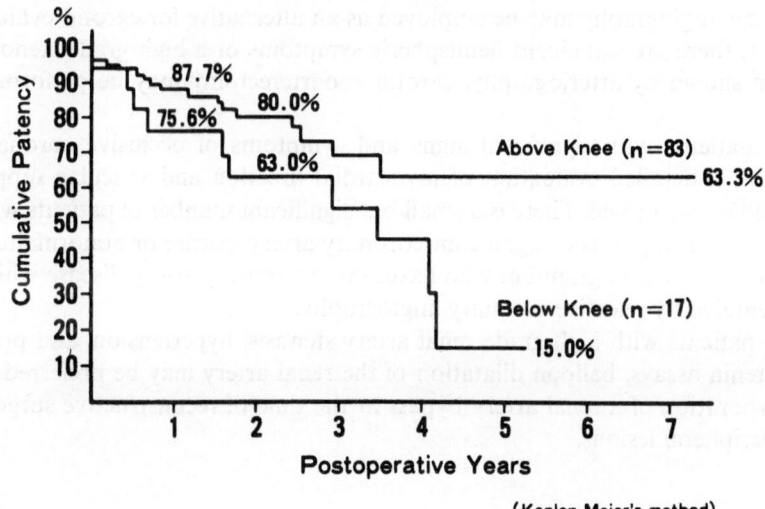

(Kaplan Meier's method)

Figure 40.2. Late results of femorodistal bypass using PTFE graft.

patency rate in the above-knee region was 87.7 after 1 year, 80% after 2 years, and 63.3% after 5 years. This result is a little less than the long-term patency rate of the autovein graft; however, it is almost as satisfactory as the rate using artificial vessels. On the other hand, the long-term patency rate in the below-knee region decreased remarkably after 4 years (Fig. 40.2). The clinical use of the PTFE graft, particularly in limb salvage situations, has resulted in early and late patency rates comparable to those achieved with autogenous saphenous veins in the femoropopliteal region. The durability of patency after implantation has been ascertained by several statistical studies in recent years. Experience with the PTFE, including our own experience, has shown that in the above-knee location, patency rates and durability differ little from those of an autogenous vein. Although long-term experience equivalent to the 15- to 20-year experience with the saphenous vein grafts is not available, recent 5- to 6-year results are encouraging. However, its use in the infrapopliteal leg arteries remains less acceptable, thus leaving the autogenous vein the graft of choice.

To date, there have been many heated discussions in congresses of surgery, vascular surgery, and neurosurgery about concomitant occlusive lesions of the visceral arteries. Fortunately, we have encountered few cases with concomitant occlusive disease of the carotid, coronary, or renal arteries; however, we believe that these associated atherosclerotic lesions will be a very important problem in the near future. In patients who also have carotid bruit or a history of transient ischemic attacks, or stroke, suitable noninvasive assessement and even selective arteriography should be performed prior to making the final decision regarding peripheral arterial reconstruction. Carotid arteriography may be coupled with aortofemoral studies, provided that the amount of contrast medium used is reasonable. Intravenous digital subtraction angiography may be employed as an alternative for carotid evaluation. If there are significant hemispheric symptoms or a high-grade stenotic lesion shown by arteriography, carotid endarterectomy may be performed first.

In patients with significant signs and symptoms of occlusive coronary disease, a detailed evaluation of myocardial function and vascular supply should be performed. There is a small but significant number of patients who exhibit no symptoms of significant coronary artery disease or abnormalities of the electrocardiogram but who have severe coronary artery disease which is identified by selective coronary angiography.

In patients with high-grade renal artery stenosis, hypertension, and positive renin assays, balloon dilatation of the renal artery may be preferred to incorporation of a renal artery bypass at the time of reconstructive surgery for peripheral lesions.

41
Long-Term Results of Arterial Bypass in the Femoropopliteal Region

SOHEI SUZUKI, MASAYUKI SHIMIZU, MASAHIKO TANAKA,
SHINJI NOMURA, AND HISAAKI KOIE

Introduction

The region of the superficial femoral and popliteal arteries is the most common area for an arterial obstruction in the lower extremities. The classical operative method for the problem using the reversed autogenous saphenous vein is considered established to a certain degree. However, the long-term results are not yet satisfactory, most likely due to problems other than operative technique.

Recently, methods such as the utilization of in situ saphenous vein, sequential bypass, new substitutional grafts and others, and adjuvant therapy such as antiplatelet and antilipemic drugs and prostaglandins have been employed.

In the present study, we review our clinical experience over the past 15 years with bypass operation in the femoropopliteal region and describe the in situ saphenous vein bypass performed in our institute.

Materials and Methods

From February 1977 to February 1992, 161 bypass operations for chronic arterial obstructions in the femoropopliteal region were performed in 128 patients, 4 of whom were females. The ages ranged from 28 to 79 years, with a mean of 60.7 ± 11.0 years. The population included 105 patients with arteriosclerosis obliterans (ASO) and 23 patients with thromboangiitis obliterans (TAO: Buerger's disease). The ages of ASO patients ranged from 43 to 79 years with a mean of 64.2 ± 7.6 years; the ages of TAO patients ranged from 28 to 65 years with a mean of 44.7 ± 10.4 years. Preoperative associated risk factors included diabetes mellitus in 27 patients (21.1%), hyperlipemia in 25 patients (19.5%), hypertension in 63 patients (49.2%), apparent symptomatic myocardial ischemia in 16 patients (12.5%), and cerebrovascular disease in 8 patients (6.3%). Indications for surgery were intermittent claudication in

60.9% of the patients, ischemic rest pain in 22.7%, and nonhealing ulcer or gangrene in 16.4%.

Femoropopliteal bypasses with above-knee anastomosis were performed in 112 limbs and with below-knee anastomosis in 49 limbs. Autogenous saphenous vein grafts were used in 109 procedures, which included 58 reversed veins and 51 in situ veins. The in situ vein bypass was performed in our clinic for the first time in 1981. Of the 58 reversed saphenous veins used, 29 were in above-knee bypass while the remaining 29 were below-knee. As for the in situ saphenous vein, 38 were used in above-knee bypass and 13 were used in below-knee bypass.

Our operative method of in situ saphenous vein bypass is as follows. For the patients who are expected to have an in situ bypass operation, a venography is performed prior to the operation to assess the anatomy of the saphenous vein, i.e., its course, length, caliber, and branches. The saphenous vein is exposed along its entire course in the appropriate region, except for the knee-crossing area, with care to minimize the trauma by manipulation. The vein is unroofed and visualized directly, and all branches detected are ligated. Loose fatty and connective tissue around the vein should not be dissected to excess. The proximal and distal portions of the vein are dissected and mobilized in proper length for anastomosis. After intravenous administration of 0.8–1.0 mg/kg of heparin, the vein is divided proximally and distally, and a valvulotome or valve cutter is introduced intraluminally to make the venous valves incompetent. The vein is gently perfused with a salt balanced solution which contains heparin and papaverin, to dilate, to be sure of adequate size, to look for leakage, and to avoid vasospasm. When the fluid is infused easily, even though some segment of the vein is occluded proximally with a digital compression, there must be an arteriovenous (A-V) fistula. The proximal anastomosis is performed with 5–0 monofilament continuous sutures with three anchor stitches to the toe and the heel; the distal anastomosis in above-knee bypass is usually done in the same fashion, and in below-knee bypass with 6–0 interrupted sutures. After completion of the anastomosis, an angiography is performed to check stenosis concerning operative procedure or residual A-V fistula. Reversed saphenous vein bypass is done in a standard fashion.

When the autogenous saphenous vein is unsuitable as a graft due to previous phlebitis, its short length, or small caliber, other substitutional grafts are employed. Expanded polytetrafluoroethylene (EPTFE) vascular grafts have been used in 44 femoropopliteal bypasses since 1979. Modified human umbilical vein grafts were used in 4 cases, and externally suported Dacron grafts (EXS) in 3. A composite graft with EPTFE and saphenous vein was used in one case.

The patients are treated preoperatively and postoperatively for 3 weeks with prostaglandin E_1 (PGE_1) or Lipo-PGE_1,[1] which is stable PGE_1 incorporated in lipid microspheres, and postoperative medication of antiplatelet drugs (aspirin, dipiridamole, or ticlopidine) is continued. Urokinase is usually used for several days after operation, but heparin or warfarin is not used. Most of the patients are followed once every 2 weeks as a rule. Patency is assessed clinically by symptoms or physical examination, including use of Doppler ultrasound and calculation of ankle–brachial pressure index, When evidence of deterioration is observed, an arteriography is performed. Cumulative graft patency rates were calculated utilizing the life table analysis, and statistical significance was determined by the log rank test.

Results

There were three deaths within 30 days from myocardial infarction and one each from acute renal failure and acute respiratory insufficiency. The overall patency rate was 64% at 15 years. There was no significant difference between ASO and TAO, in early and late patency rate for all grafts, as shown in Figure 41.1. Figure 41.2 shows the patency rates for the two types of grafts, the autogenous saphenous vein and EPTFE. Seventeen of 44 EPTFE grafts failed within the first year. The patency rate for overall autogenous saphenous vein was 77% at 8 years and 54% for EPTFE, and the 13-year patency rate for saphenous vein remained at 77%, whereas EPTFE decreased to 33%.

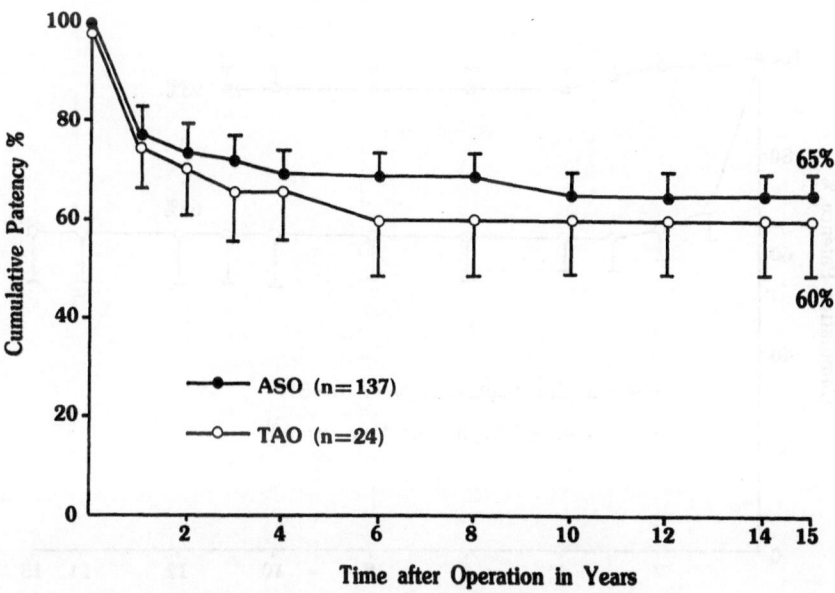

FIGURE 41.1. Cumulative patency rates for femoropopliteal bypasses of patients with arteriosclerosis obliterans (ASO) and thromboangiitis obliterans (TAO). The standard error of each point is shown. There is no statistically significant difference by the log rank test.

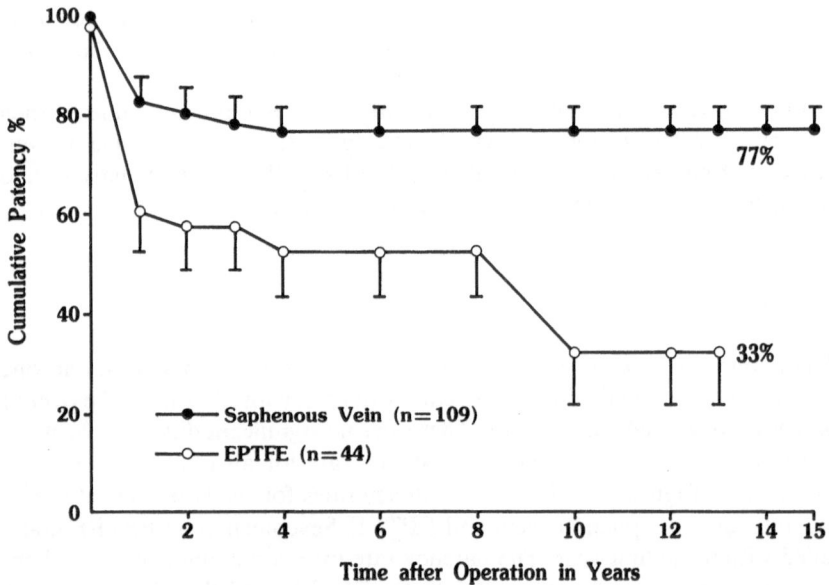

FIGURE 41.2. Cumulative patency rates for saphenous vein and EPTFE femoropopliteal bypasses. The standard error of each point is shown. The differences between the groups are statistically significant ($p < 0.001$).

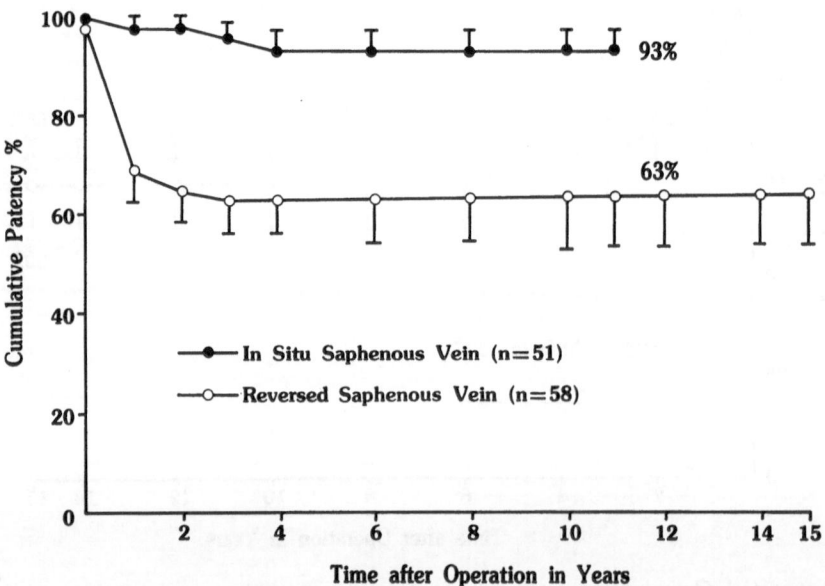

FIGURE 41.3. Cumulative patency rates for in situ saphenous and reversed saphenous vein femoropopliteal bypass. The standard error of each point is shown. The differences between the groups are statistically significant ($p < 0.005$).

As seen, the difference in patency rates between the groups was statistically significant ($p < 0.001$) (Fig. 41.2).

The 109 saphenous veins that were utilized included 58 reversed and 51 in situ saphenous veins. Eighteen of 21 graft failures in the reversed-vein group occurred within the first year. The 11-year patency rate for in situ saphenous vein was 93%, compared with 63% for reversed saphenous vein (Fig. 41.3); the difference is statistically significant ($p < 0.005$). Cumulative patency rates in above-knee femoropopliteal bypass for three kinds of grafts are shown in Figure 41.4. Reversed saphenous vein in above-knee bypass had a cumulative patency rate of 65%, and EPTFE had patency rates of 58% at 8 years and 35% at 13 years. There was no significant difference between the groups. However, the patency rate of 94% for in situ saphenous vein at 11 years was significantly greater than both the 65% patency rate for reversed saphenous vein ($p < 0.005$) and the 35% rate for EPTFE ($p < 0.001$) (Fig. 41.4). In below-knee femoropopliteal bypass, in situ grafts tended to have a higher patency rate than reversed-vein grafts, but no statistically significant difference was found between these two types of grafts (Fig. 41.5).

Six sequential bypasses to the infrapopliteal arteries were performed in 6 patients. Two of them failed, one at 6 months and the other at 5 years. One

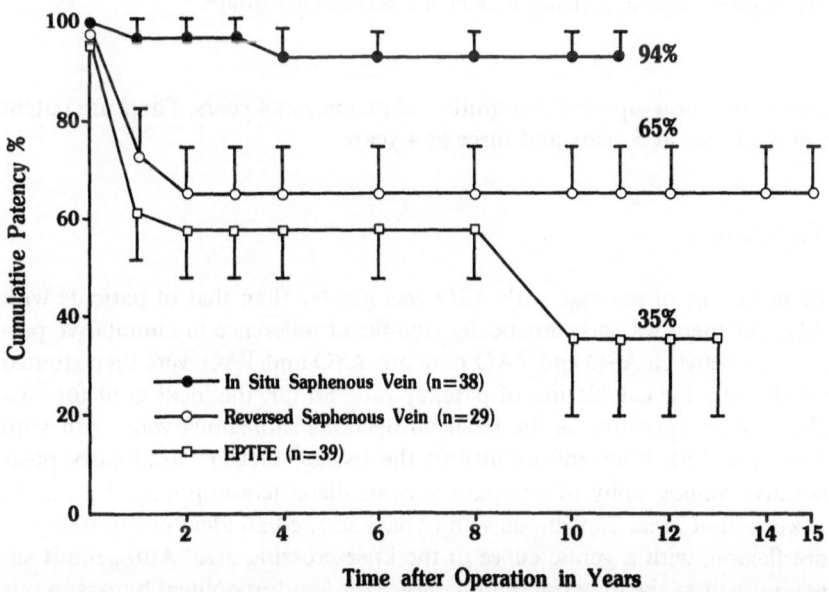

FIGURE 41.4. Cumulative patency rates for above-knee femoropopliteal bypasses in three kinds of grafts. The standard error of each point is shown. There is no significant difference between the reversed-vain bypass and the EPTFE bypass, whereas the patency rates for in situ saphenous vein are significantly higher than those for reversed vein ($p < 0.005$) and for EPTFE ($p < 0.001$).

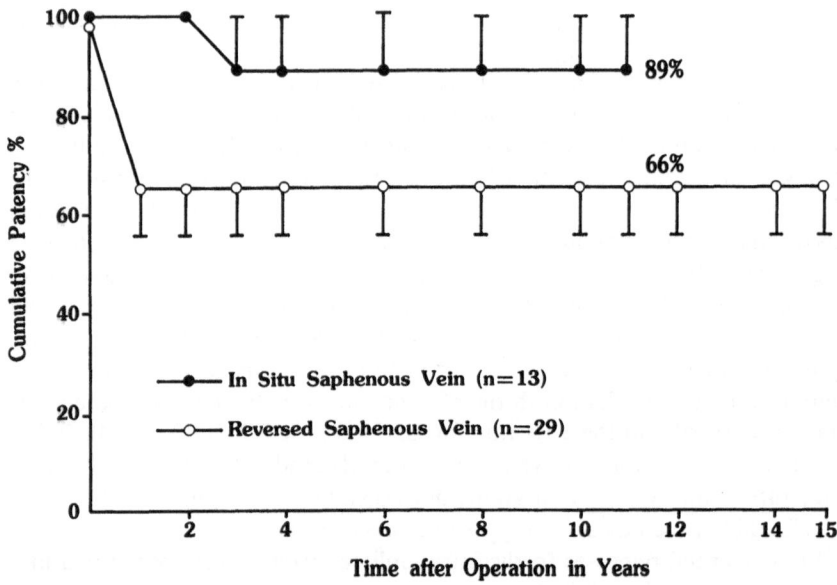

FIGURE 41.5. Cumulative patency rates for below-knee femoropopliteal bypasses with in situ saphenous vein and reversed vein. The standard error of each point is shown. There is no statistically significant difference between the groups.

was lost to follow-up after recognition of patency at 4 years. Three are patent at present, one at 5 years and three at 4 years.

Discussion

The mean age of patients with ASO was greater than that of patients with TAO, but there was no statistically significant difference in cumulative patency rate between ASO and TAO patients. ASO and TAO were then studied cumulatively for calculation of patency rate. So far, the ideal graft for vascular bypass operation is the fresh autogenous saphenous vein, with vital vascular endothelium and affinity to the tissue.[2] Geiger[3] used early postoperative angiography to compare various distal femoropopliteal grafts in the knee joint area. Saphenous vein bypass showed an ideal position during knee flexion, with a gentle curve in the knee-crossing area. Autogenous saphenous vein is the material of first choice for femoropopliteal bypass in our institute.

When the autogenous saphenous vein is absent or unavailable, EPTFE is used as the second choice. A ring-supported EPTFE is adopted in the case in which a reconstruction crossing the knee joint is required. The patency rate for EPTFE femoropopliteal bypass was 58% at 3 years and 54% at 5 to 8 years, and was close to the other reports.[4-6] In several reports,[5,7] the early patency rate for EPTFE was close to that of vein graft and later became worse than that of vein graft. In our study, early EPTFE graft failures within the first year were not few. The overall cumulative patency rate for autogenous saphenous vein graft was significantly better than for EPTFE.

In above-knee bypass, there was no significant difference between patency rates for reversed-vein bypass and EPTFE, while the patency rate for in situ vein bypass was better than that for both reversed-vein bypass and EPTFE. The long-term patency rate of the in situ saphenous vein was the most satisfactory in above-knee bypasses. In below-knee bypasses, the 11-year patency rate for in situ saphenous vein was 89%, as opposed to 66% for reversed vein. Though there was no significant difference between them, we believe that the in situ saphenous vein is superior for below-knee femoropopliteal bypass. Further experience and investigations are required.

In our experience, most graft failures in reversed saphenous vein and EPTFE occurred within the first year, although the reason for this is unclear. It seems important to prevent early occlusion for good long-term patency. Occasionally, the patients requiring below-knee bypass had poor runoff vessels. In such cases, the patency would be affected by a trivial technical matter or an incidental occlusive disease of inflow, such as in the common iliac artery or the common femoral artery. When there is coexistence of proximal occlusive disease, more recently, we have performed percutaneous transluminal balloon or laser angioplasty prior to the bypass operation if possible, or simultaneous bypass operation such as aortoiliac, aortofemoral, or iliofemoral bypass with femoropopliteal bypass. Sequential bypass seemed worthwhile in cases with poor distal runoff. Although these cases were few in number, the results were fairly good.

We consider an in situ saphenous vein to be the best conduit for femoropopliteal bypass at present because of many advantages: the adequacy of caliber in distal anastomosis, the tapered shape that permits blood to flow smoothly, and preservation of the vasa vasorum that supply blood to the endothelial surface. Nevertheless, there are some problems as well. We generally perform the proximal anastomosis of the femoropopliteal bypass to the common femoral artery. Occasionally, the proximal portion of the graft is too short to be anastomosed to the required position. In such cases, we try to dissect the saphenous vein to a further extent at the proximal side. We applied a branch of the saphenous vein to the proximal anastomosis in one case. When the common femoral artery cannot be used as a proximal anastomosis, the superficial femoral artery is selected, with endarterectomy if required. The method of producing valvular incompetence is also important. We utilize three types of valve cutter and valvulotome as the case may be. Residual A-V fistula is the controversial problem. The residual A-V fistula may cause bypass failure or thrombophlebitis.[8-10] To detect residual fistula, intraoperative or postoperative Doppler ultrasound is utilized.[10-13] This method is very attractive but has not been applied yet in our clinic. During the operation, we expose the saphenous vein along its entire length so that it can all be seen, a procedure followed by other authors.[12,13] It is easy to detect branches in comparison with preoperative venography. Flushing the vein with heparinized fluid, as mentioned above, is useful to look for branches, and an intraoperative angiography after completion of anastomosis is reliable. When any residual branch is detected, it can easily be ligated. We consider that even though the exterior part of the saphenous vein is dissected, the vein is buried in the fatty tissue, so disruption of the blood flow to the vasa vasorum is minimal. Besides, insertion and manipulation of the valvulotome or valve cutter can be done safely under direct vision without injury to the endothelial surface, as the surgeon can look through the instrument to verity the position of the top and the direction of the instrument. We have experienced no cases of residual A-V fistula.

Preoperative and postoperative administration of antiplatelet drugs and prostaglandin E_1 is considered very effective. Considerable hemorrhagic tendencies or excess bleeding caused by the drugs are not seen. Low-grade elevation of transaminase by ticropidine was found in a few patients, but they improved after change of drugs.

The results of this study suggest that the in situ autogenous saphenous vein graft is the most useful for a femoropopliteal bypass. When the saphenous vein is not suitable as an in situ graft, the vein is used as a reversed-vein bypass. If the autogenous saphenous vein is not available, we would employ EPTFE graft. Nevertheless, there is another problem. Patients with ASO frequently have other coexistent arterial occlusive diseases. In recent coronary bypass operations, the internal mammary artery and the gastroepiploic artery have been used for the graft instead of the saphenous vein. However, repeat coronary bypass operations have increased. Furthermore, patients, who have undergone femoropopliteal bypass on occasion have suffered from further peripheral arterial occlusive disease. In such circumstances, the autogenous saphenous veins would be necessary at the second operation. EPTFE or other substitutional graft should be applied in above-knee bypass if possible. Meticulous surgical technique and further efforts are required to obtain good results not only in the autogenous saphenous vein bypass, but also in the substitutional graft bypass.

Bibliography

1. Mizushima Y, Yanagawa A, Hoshi K. Prostaglandin E_1 is more effective, when incorporated in lipid microspheres, for treatment of peripheral vascular disease in man. J Pharm Pharmacol 1983;35:666–667.
2. Wright CB, Hobson RW II, Giordano JM. et al. Acute femoral venous occlusion (Management by segmental venous replacement in the dog). J Cardiovasc Surg 1977;18:523–529.
3. Geiger G, Hoevels J, Storz L, et al. Vascular grafts in below-knee femoropopliteal bypass. A comparative study. J Cardiovasc Surg 1984;25:523–529.

4. Veith FJ, Gupta S, Daly V. Management of early and late thrombosis of expanded polytetrafluoroethylene (PTFE) femoropopliteal bypass grafts: Favorable prognosis with appropriated reoperation. Surgery 1980;87:581–587.
5. Ascer E, Veith FJ, Gupta SK, et al. Six year experience with expanded polytetrafluoroethylene arterial grafts for limb salvage. J Cardiovasc Surg 1985;26:468–472.
6. Johnson WC, Squires JW. Axillo-femoral (PTFE) and infrainguinal revascularization (PTFE and umbilical vein). J Cardiovasc Surg 1991;32:344–349.
7. Veith FJ, Gupta SK, Ascer E, et al. Six-year prospective multicenter randomized comparison of autologous saphenous vein and expanded polytetrafluoroethylene grafts in infrainguinal arterial reconstructions. J Vasc Surg 1986;3:104–114.
8. Dundas P. The in situ vein bypass. J Cardiovasc Surg 1970;11:450–453.
9. Shearman CP, Gannon MX, Gwynn BR, et al. A clinical method for the detection of arteriovenous fistulas during in situ great saphenous vein bypass. J Vasc Surg 1986;4:578–581.
10. Chang BB, Leopold PW, Kupinski AM, et al. In situ bypass hemodynamics. The effect of residual A-V fistulae. J Cardiovasc Surg 1989;30:843–847.
11. Strayhorn EC, Abott WM, Brewster DC. Doppler identification of in situ vein graft arteriovenous fistulas. Surg Gynec Obstet 1985;160:562–564.
12. Strayhorn EC, Wohlgemuth S, Deuer M, et al. Early experience utilizing the in situ saphenous vein technique in 54 patients. J Cardiovasc Surg 1988;29:161–165.
13. Wengerter KR, Veith FJ, Gupta SK, et al. Prospective randomized multicenter comparison of in situ and reversed vein infrapopliteal bypasses. J Vasc Surg 1991;13:189–199.

42
Reevaluation of Effectiveness of Low-Dose Warfarin as Antithrombotic Therapy After Vascular Reconstruction

Joonghee Kang, Masato Sakon, and Jun-ichi Kambayashi

Introduction

As the hypercoagulable state is known to persist after vascular reconstruction, various regimens of antithrombotic therapy with warfarin and/or anti-platelet agents have been examined in our vascular service and elsewhere.[1,2] Recently, some hemostatic examinations (so-called molecular markers) have been developed, and their usefulness in predicting hemostatic condition in vivo has been reported. Thrombin–antithrombin III complex (TAT), one such molecular marker, is considered to reflect in vivo thrombin generation, and therefore it appears to be an useful tool in the prediction of graft occlusion.[3] In this study, we attempted to evaluate the effectiveness of low-dose warfarin administration by serial determination of TAT (normal range, less than 5 ng/ml). We also measured the plasma level of fibrin degradation product (D/D) (D-dimer) as a marker of in vivo hyperfibrinolysis (normal range, less than 0.5 μg/ml).[4]

Patients and Methods

Twenty-nine patients who underwent vascular reconstruction at our vascular service from 1989 to 1992 were studied. All patients in this study suffered from severe arteriosclerosis and poor runoff. Table 42.1 shows the profile of the patients. Twenty-five patients received low-dose warfarin (2.6 $\pm$ 1.1 mg/day), and the remaining 4 patients had no warfarin. We serially measured the plasma levels of TAT to evaluate the postoperative state of hypercoagulability. Surgical procedures are also shown. One of the patients on warfarin with aorto femoral bypass was implanted with aorta-left-femoral bypass, and the others were implanted with aorto bifemoral bypass grafts. Warfarin was given for at least 3 days before TAT measurement. TAT was measured by the EIA method, and D-dimer was measured by enzyme-linked immunosorlent assay (ELISA). Other conventional hemostatic examinations were also performed.

TABLE 42.1. Profile of cases.

Cases on warfarin	
No. of cases	$n = 25$ (M = 23, F = 2)
Age (years)	65.0 ± 8.8 (50–80)
Dose of warfarin	2.6 ± 1.1 (0.5–4.5) mg/day
Administration	5.5 ± 3.9 (3–12) days after surgery
Cases without warfarin	
No. of cases	$n = 4$ (M = 2, F = 2)
Age (years)	65.3 ± 4.6 (56–68)
Surgical procedures	
Cases on warfarin	
PTFE graft	Aortofemoral bypass (7)
	Axillofemoral bypass (4)
	Femorofemoral bypass (6)
	Femoropopliteal bypass (1)
Autogenous saphenous vein	Femoropopliteal (7)
Cases without warfarin	
PTFE graft	Aortofemoral bypass (4)

PTFE, Polytetrafluoroethylene.

Results

In patients without warfarin, the plasma level of TAT was elevated to 19.2 ± 6.0 ng/ml (mean $\pm$ SD) on postoperative day. 7 and remained high even 4 weeks after surgery (Fig. 42.1). These data indicate that the hypercoagulable state persists for more than 1 month after vascular reconstruction. On the other hand, regardless of the early administration of low-dose warfarin, TAT was significantly elevated (12.3 ± 9.3 ng/ml, mean $\pm$ SD) within 1 month, and there was no significant correlation between TAT and prothrombin time (PT) (Fig. 42.2). In this period, PT value was kept at $50.7 \pm 15.3\%$. Furthermore, there was no difference in the value of TAT between patients with different surgical procedures. In 2 patients who suffered from early graft

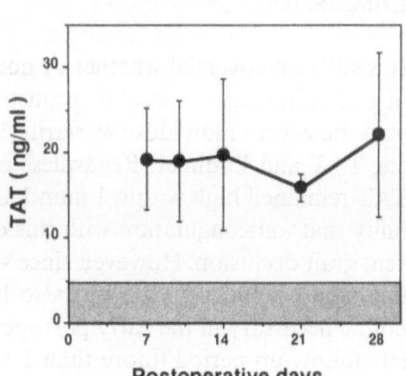

FIGURE 42.1. Changes of TAT after vascular reconstruction (cases without warfarin).

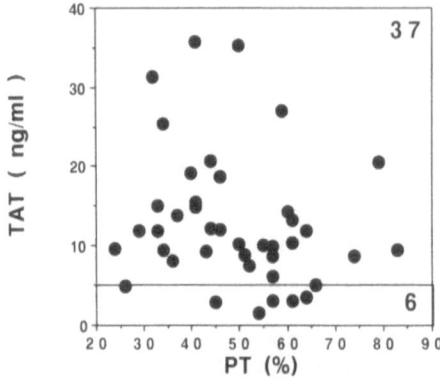

FIGURE 42.2 Relationship between TAT and PT in cases with warfarin administration (within 1 month after surgery).

occlusion, an apparent elevation of TAT preceded the clinical manifestations of graft failure, including decrease of ankle–arm pressure. The clinical course of one patient is shown in Figure 42.3. TAT value was 6.5 ng/ml on postoperative day 1 and 9.4 ng/ml on postoperative day 2. TAT then increased up to 24.6 ng/ml on postoperative day 13, but there was no clinical manifestation of graft failure in this period. We confirmed graft occlusion using duplex scan on postoperative day 14. We performed thrombectomy on postoperative day 16. The elevation of TAT was followed by the increase of D-dimer, a molecular marker of secondary fibrinolysis. These data indicate that TAT is a powerful tool for prediction of early graft failure. On the other hand, the values of TAT were well correlated with those of PT, when examined more than 1 month after surgery (Fig. 42.4). In cases with PT less than 55%, TAT value was normal in 85% of all determinations, while in cases with PT more than 65%, 70% of TAT determinations exhibited a marked increase. The relationship between TAT and D-dimer is shown in Figure 42.5. These molecular markers were well correlated with each other ($R^2 = 0.688$).

Discussion

It is still controversial whether or not warfarin is essential for the prevention of graft failure after vascular reconstruction.[5] In the present study, we evaluated the effect of low-dose warfarin (1–5 mg/day) using two molecular markers, TAT and D-dimer. Regardless of warfarin therapy, the plasma level of TAT remained high within 1 month after surgery. These data raise the possibility that anticoagulation with this dosage of warfarin is insufficient to prevent graft occlusion. However, since surgical stress generally induces not only the hypercoagulable state but also hyperfibrinolysis,[6] anticoagulation may not be necessary in the early postoperative period. On the other hand, in the late follow-up period (more than 1 month after surgery), low-dose warfarin administration (1–5 mg/day) to lower the PT value below 55% was found to

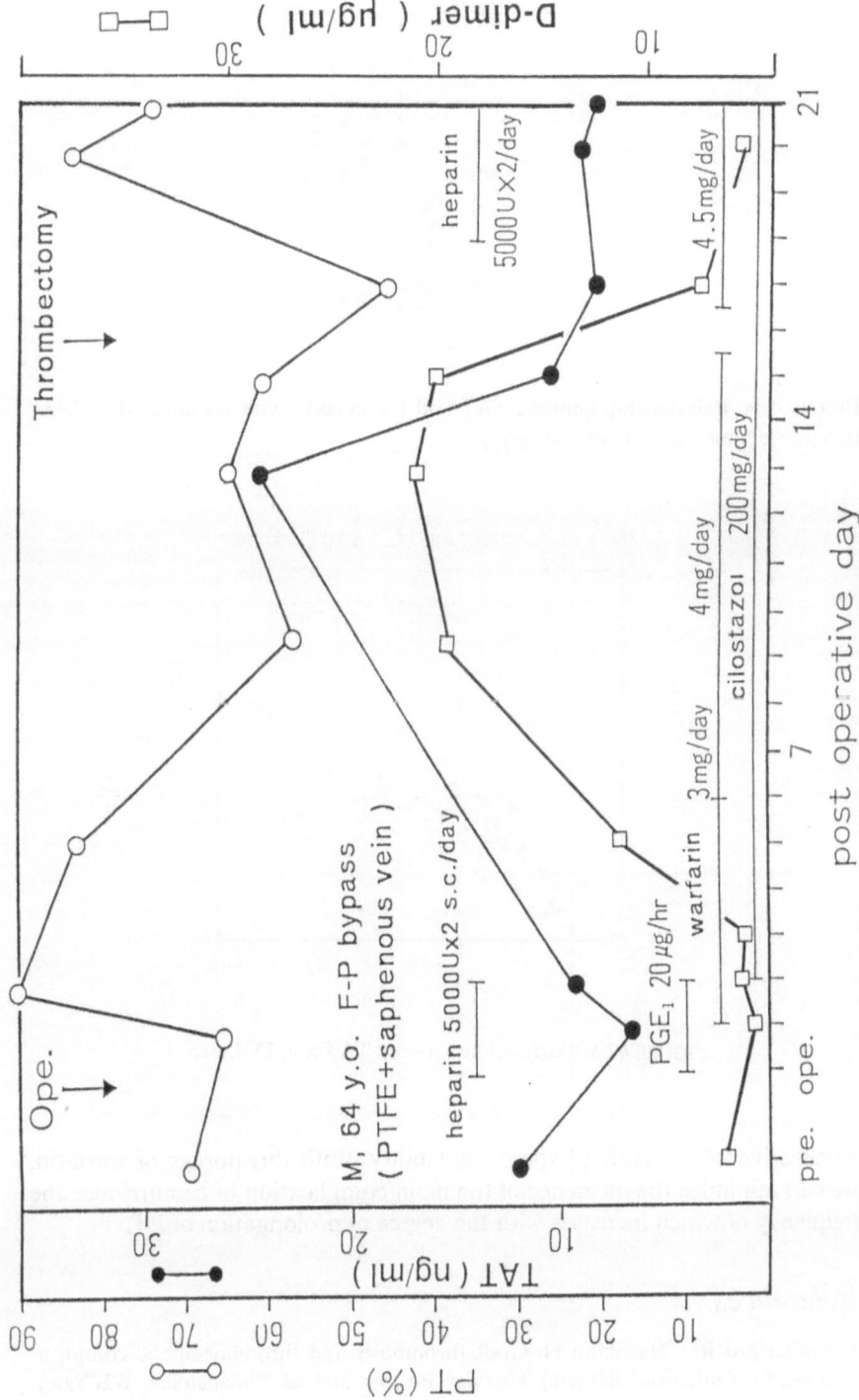

FIGURE 42.3. Clinical course of patient who suffered from early graft failure.

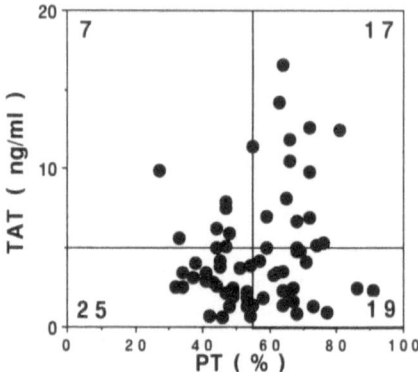

FIGURE 42.4. Relationship between TAT and PT in cases with warfarin administration (more than 1 month after surgery).

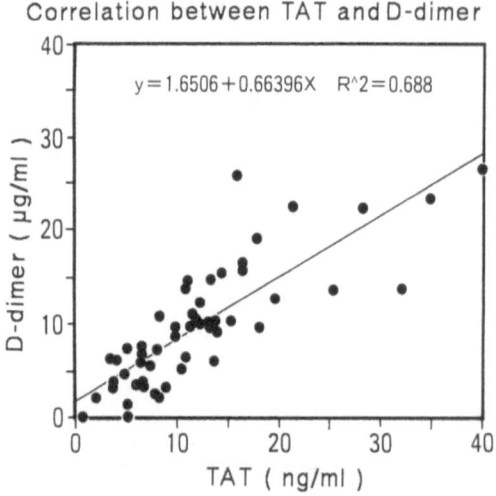

FIGURE 42.5. Correlation between TAT and D-dimer.

be effective in preventing hypercoagulability. With this dosage of warfarin, we can minimize the incidence of the main complication of hemorrhage, the frequency of which increases with the degree of prolongation of PT.

References

1. Rutherford RB, Nishikimi N. Graft thrombosis and thromboembolic complications. In: Rutherford RB (ed.). *Vascular Surgery*. 3nd ed. Philadelphia: WB Saunders, 1989, pp. 487–491.

2. Kapsch DN, Silver D. Anticoagulants (heparin, warfarin). In: Wilson SE, Veith FJ, Hobson RW, Williams RA (eds.). *Vascular Surgery (Principles and Practice)*. New York: McGraw-Hill, 1987, pp. 231–240.
3. Pelzer H, Schwarz A, Heimburger N. Determination of human thrombin-antithrombin III complex in plasma with an enzyme-linked immunosorbent assay. Thrombos Haemostasis 1988;59:101–106.
4. Elms MJ, Bunce FIH, Bundesen PG, Rylatt DB, Webber AJ, Masci PP, Whiteker AN. Rapid detection of cross-linked fibrin degradation products in plasma using monoclonal antibody coated latex particles. Am J Clin Pathol 1986;85:360–364.
5. Kang J, Kambayashi J, Sakon M, Tsujinaka T, Mori T. Postoperative changes in hemostasis analyzed by the serial determination of fibrinopeptides and D-dimer. Jpn J Surg 1989;19:262–268.
6. Rosenthal D, Mittenthal MJ, Ruben DM, Jones DH, Estes JW, Stanton PE, Lamis PA. The effects of aspirin, dipyridamole and warfarin in femorodistal reconstruction. Am Surg 1987;53:477–481.

43
Percutaneous Transluminal Angioplasty and Segmentally Enclosed Thrombolysis for Femoropopliteal Occlusions

Bo Jørgensen and Jørn Dalsgaard Nielsen

Introduction

The method of transluminal arterial recanalization envisioned by Dotter and Judkins in 1964[1] and the balloon-tipped double-lumen angioplasty catheter introduced by Grüntzig and Hopff 10 years later[2] founded the field of endovascular surgery. Percutaneous transluminal angioplasty (PTA) has become a leading endovascular technique for treatment of obliterative lower limb arteriosclerosis, and is replacing endovascular bypass surgery due to acceptable clinical results, low mortality and morbidity, and low cost of treatment.[3] The outcome of PTA for femoropopliteal arterial occlusions is, however, not entirely satisfactory due to failed recanalization or reocclusion, preventing these procedures from competing with surgical bypass.

Deep arterial wall injuries intrinsic to PTA[4,5] produce subendothelial collagen exposure and tissue factor release, leading to local platelet activation, thrombin formation, and mural thrombosis.[6] High plasma concentrations of β-thromboglobulin and fibrinopeptide A (FPA) indicative of intravascular fibrin formation can be prevented during femoropopliteal PTA by conventional administration of a heparin bolus injection.[7,8] The reduction of markers of platelet activation and thrombin activity in peripheral blood by heparin, however, does not preclude arterial reocclusion shortly after balloon angioplasty procedures.

Identification of factors determining the technical competence and clinical outcome of PTA is important for placement of balloon angioplasty among other interventional vascular procedures, including surgery, and may provide further improvements of endovascular techniques. This chapter describes a novel thrombolytic procedure applied in high-risk patients for prevention of early rethrombosis following femoropopliteal PTA.

Femoropopliteal Occlusions: A Risk Factor in PTA

Reports on femoropopliteal PTA specifically dealing with occlusions are infrequent.[9] Most studies include a minority of occlusions and present the results together with that of stenoses.[10] We evaluated the outcome of femoropopliteal PTA selectively for 70 occlusions and 58 stenoses in consecutive aspirin-and heparin-treated patients with respect to severity of the vascular disease, tibial runoff, and length and type of obstruction, factors that have been reported to influence long-term results.[11] Noninvasive measurements of ankle–brachial systolic blood pressure index (ABI) at short intervals were used for patency assessment in technically successful PTA procedures. Our findings indicated that the type of obstruction is a major determinant of early vascular patency in femoropopliteal PTA (Table 43.1).[12] Hemodynamic and clinical signs of early rethrombosis occasionally found following PTA for stenoses presented regularly for occlusions ranging in length from 1 to 27 cm, opposing the recommendation of PTA for femoropopliteal occlusions less than 10 cm.[13] A significant difference in long-term patency between occlusions and stenoses was attributable to early events, the later restenosis rate being indifferent. Inferior results of PTA for femoropopliteal occlusions compared with stenoses were subsequently reported by others.[14]

The risk of sudden relapse due to early rethrombosis following balloon angioplasty is increased by organized thrombus in the vascular obstruction.[15] Fibrin-bound thrombin with preserved procoagulant activity is released from the clot by balloon compression,[16] and thrombus residues produce a highly thrombogenic surface on the vessel wall. These factors

TABLE 43.1. Outcome of technically successful femoropopliteal PTA for 70 occlusions and 58 stenoses evaluated according to various pretreatment subsets.

Subset	Hemodynamic success	Clinical success
Claudication	28/37 (76%)	18/37 (49%)
Ischemia	60/91 (66%)	49/91 (54%)
	$p = 0.39$	$p = 0.74$
Good runoff	50/68 (74%)	40/68 (59%)
Poor runoff	38/60 (63%)	27/60 (45%)
	$p = 0.29$	$p = 0.17$
Length ≤ 5 cm	56/74 (76%)	39/74 (53%)
Length > 5 cm	32/54 (59%)	28/54 (52%)
	$p = 0.07$	$p = 0.93$
Stenosis	49/58 (84%)	37/58 (64%)
Occlusion	39/70 (56%)	30/70 (43%)
	$p < 0.01$	$p < 0.03$
Total	88/128 (69%)	67/128 (52%)

Hemodynamic success was >0.15 ABI increase 24 hours after PTA, whereas clinical success was at least one Fontaine stage improvement at the latest clinical examination before any vascular surgery. The observation period was 16 (1–60) months (mean and range).[12] *Ischemia* refers to patients with rest pain or gangrene. Tibial runoff in 2 or 3 patient arteries was considered good, otherwise poor.

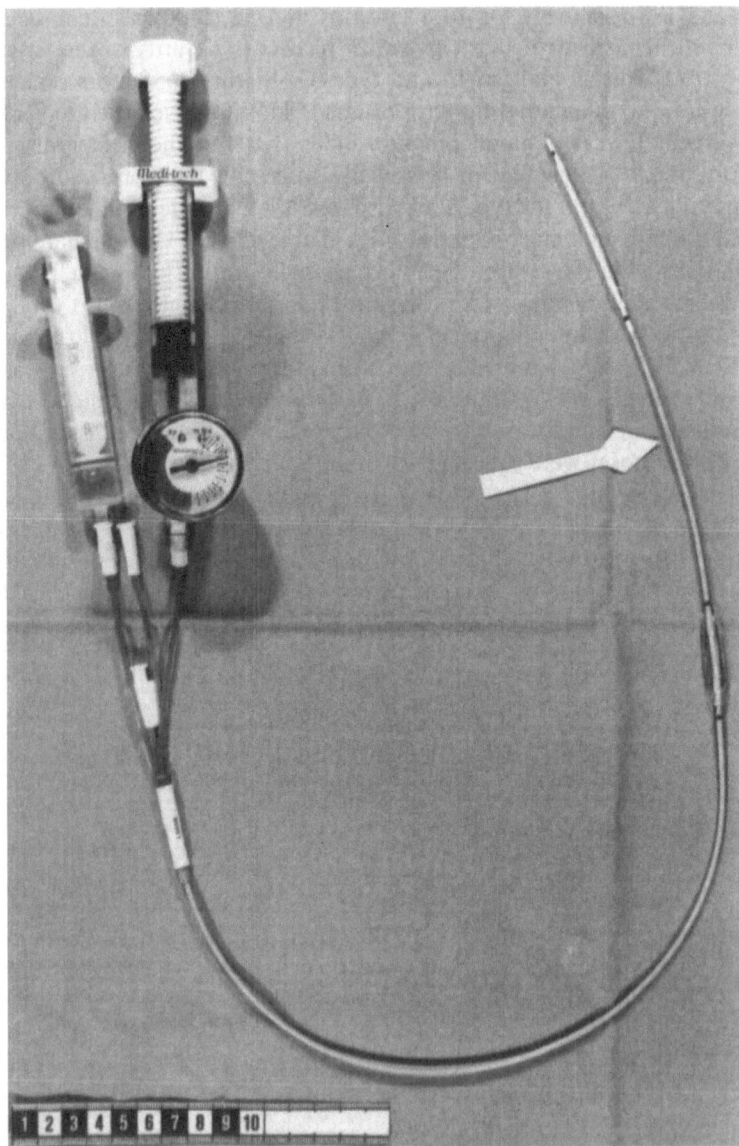

FIGURE 43.1. The double balloon catheter used for segmentally enclosed thrombolysis. The distal balloon is inflated with a high-pressure device for dilatation purposes. The proximal balloon inflated with a syringe is used during enclosed thrombolysis. There is one connection for each of the balloons, one for the central lumen, and one for the sideport centered between the balloons (arrow).[19]

may, together with the deep vessel wall injury, explain the prevalence of early rethrombosis following PTA for femoropopliteal occlusions.

Segmentally Enclosed Thrombolysis

With the aim of improving early vascular patency by dissolving residual thrombus, preventing subsequent thrombus formation at dilated sites, and at the same time avoiding bleeding complications induced by systemic infusion of fibrinolytic agents,[17] a double balloon catheter (Fig. 43.1) was used to enclose recombinant tissue plasminogen activator (TPA) and heparin in dilated arterial segments for a short period of time immediately after PTA.[18] High efficacy and rapidity of segmentally enclosed thrombolysis (SET) was facilitated by the preceding use of PTA to disintegrate the occluding thrombus, and by enclosing higher concentrations of TPA and heparin than can be obtained systemically without causing hemorrhage.

In a pilot study on 34 patients,[19] in whom the severity of their vascular disease and length of occlusions was comparable with our previous series,[12] PTA was performed with the distal balloon of the double balloon catheter. Arterial access was obtained via the popliteal artery in selected cases of proximal superficial femoral artery obstruction or obesity.[20] Immediately after PTA, the double balloon catheter was advanced as appropriate to isolate the dilated arterial segment by simultaneous inflation of both balloons (Fig. 43.2B). Small dosages of TPA (5 mg) and heparin (1,000 IU) dissolved in high concentrations of 1 mg/ml and 200 IU/ml, respectively, were injected through the sideport and enclosed for 30 minutes. The catheter was then withdrawn for a completion angiogram (Fig. 43.2C) and removed. Attempts to aspirate remains of TPA and heparin from secluded arterial segments before catheter removal ceased when SET proved not to cause depletion of coagulation factors. Additional heparin was administered during and after the procedures.[19] Patency was evaluated by ABI measurements. Assessment of hemostatic and fibrinolytic parameters included fibrinogen, cross-linked fibrin degradation products (D-dimer), α-2-antiplasmin, FPA, and TPA antigen. We employed a method of intraarterial, translesional FPA measurement to estimate the thrombotic response to PTA, and the antithrombin effect of SET (Table 43.2).[21]

Results

Early rethrombosis occurred in three (9%) patients following subintimal dissection or intimal flap formation. One-year cumulative patency including all procedures was 80% (Fig. 43.3).[19] The effect of SET on hemostasis and fibrinolysis is shown in Table 43.2. Fibrinogen was reduced by 18% 6 hours after SET, and there was a transient 13% reduction in α-2-antiplasmin. Fibrin

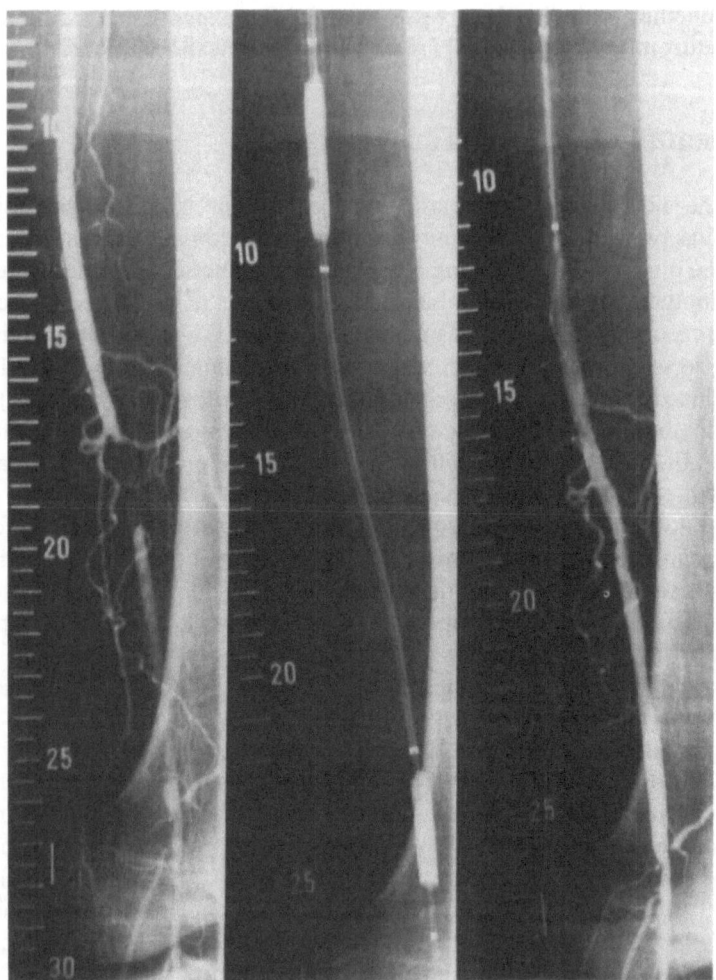

FIGURE 43.2. Left: A 2-cm superficial femoral artery occlusion with adjacent thrombus before recanalization. Middle: Following recanalization and dilatation, the double balloon catheter is situated with a balloon at each end of the relevant arterial segment. Segmentally enclosed thrombolysis is ongoing. Right: Completion angiogram after segmentally enclosed thrombolysis. The tip of the double balloon catheter is at the upper end of the angiogram.[19]

degradation was indicated by the D-dimer increase, which correlated with the length of occlusions and not with the inter-balloon distance. A 50-fold thrombin activity increase measured in the vicinity of dilated sites immediately after PTA was eliminated immediately after SET (Fig. 43.4).[21]

Leakage of TPA to the general circulation was prominent during SET. However, the average TPA concentration retained in secluded arterial

TABLE 43.2. Hemostatic and fibrinolytic parameters before and after segmentally enclosed thrombolysis.[19,21]

	Fibrinogen (g/L)[1]	D-dimer (ng/ml)[1]	α-2-AP (% normal)[1]	FPA (ng/ml)[2]
Before	5.0 ± 0.4	785 ± 118	102 ± 5	21.5 ± 4.4
+30 min	4.7 ± 0.4	15,755 ± 7,570[c]	89 ± 5[b]	24.0 ± 170.5
+2 hours	4.7 ± 0.5	5,737 ± 1,604[b]	103 ± 6	28.0 ± 6.1
+6 hours	4.1 ± 0.5[a]	3,238 ± 1,129[a]	105 ± 6	42.3 ± 277.4

Values are mean ± SE[1] or median ± SE.[2] Levels of significance compared with values before SET: [a] $p < 0.05$; [b] $p < 0.0005$; [c] $p < 0.00005$. D-dimer, Cross-linked fibrin degradation products. α-2-AP, α-2-Antiplasmin. FPA, Fibrinopeptide A.

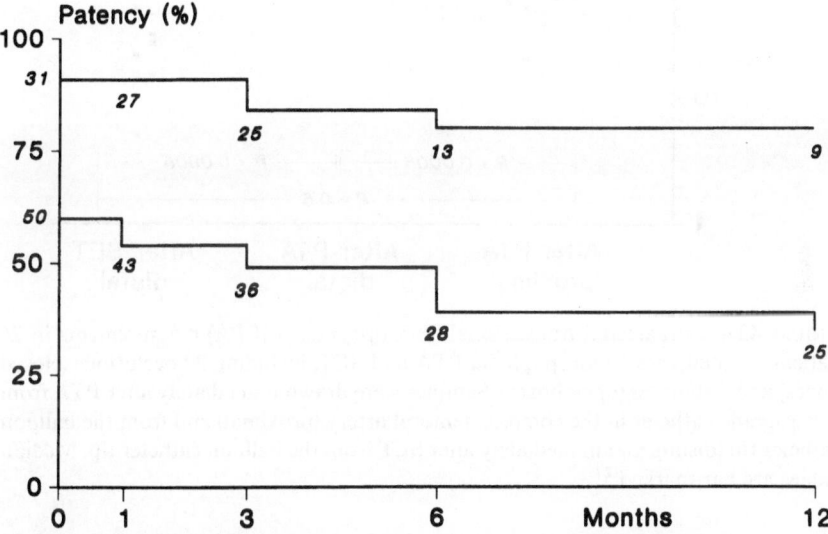

FIGURE 43.3. One-year cumulative patency in 34 PTA and SET (upper curve) compared with all technically successful PTA for femoropopliteal occlusions performed before the introduction of SET (lower curve). Patency was significantly ($p < 0.001$) improved by SET, providing a marked reduction in early rethrombosis rate. The origin of the curves corresponds to patency on the day after the treatment. Inset values are number of patients at risk at the beginning of each interval.[19]

segments was about 30,000 ng/ml or 20 times higher than steady-state concentrations obtained during systemic infusion.[22] The TPA concentration in peripheral blood was 2% of contemporary inter-balloon concentration, and 10% of steady-state concentration obtained during systemic infusion. We determined a 6 times longer plasma elimination rate of TPA after SET termination[23] than that reported in other human studies on TPA pharmacokinetics.[24]

The overall complication rate was higher when heparin was administered

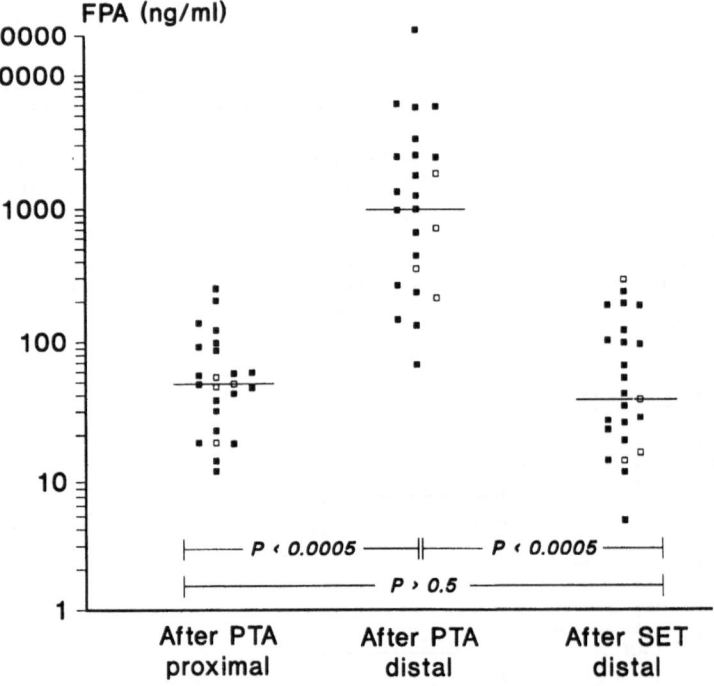

FIGURE 43.4. Intraarterial translesional fibrinopeptide A (FPA) measurements in 24 patients treated with femoropopliteal PTA and SET, including 20 occlusions (closed boxes) and 4 stenoses (open boxes). Samples were drawn immediately after PTA from a retrograde catheter in the common femoral artery (proximal) and from the balloon catheter tip (distal), and immediately after SET from the balloon catheter tip. Median values are bar-marked.[21]

TABLE 43.3. Complications.

Complication	Intravenous heparin ($n = 11$)	Subcutaneous heparin ($n = 23$)	Total
Puncture site hemorrhage	1	1	2
Hemathemesis	1	0	1
Calf hematoma	1	0	1
Puncture site hematoma	2	3	5
Microembolization	3	1	4
Total	8 (73%)	5 (22%)	13 (38%)

Complications were more frequent when using intravenous than subcutaneous heparin treatment during 24 hours following segmentally enclosed thrombolysis ($p < 0.02$).[19] Intravenous heparin regimen: 1,000 IU per hour. Subcutaneous heparin regimen: 3 times 5,000 IU.

intravenously rather than subcutaneously subsequently to SET (Table 43.3). Double balloon catheter seclusion did not cause peripheral circulatory arrest but decreased lower leg subcutaneous blood flow rate by an average of 42%.[19]

Discussion

Patency rates of 52%–80% within a few weeks, and 32%–57% after 1 year, have been reported following PTA for femoropopliteal occlusions.[9,12,14] Introducing SET as an adjunctive therapy, we obtained 80% 1-year patency due to a marked 75% reduction in early rethrombosis rate compared with previous results.[19] In our hands, SET produced midterm patency of PTA for femoropopliteal occlusions comparable with that of short stenoses.[25] Long-term and randomized studies on this novel thrombolytic procedure in PTA are required to confirm results.

We demonstrated for the first time that PTA in the vicinity of dilated sites produces a vast thrombin activity, which is not expressed in peripheral blood.[21] These findings, which may be due to the 2- to 3-minute half-life of FPA in plasma,[26] indicate that assessment of thrombin activity by FPA and the effect on thrombin activity of anti-thrombin regimens in endovascular surgery should rely on direct intraarterial measurements. Elimination of local thrombin activity by TPA and heparin briefly enclosed in dilated segments after PTA illustrates the effect of SET to restore anticoagulant properties in the freshly injured arterial wall, and to reduce the risk of early thrombotic reocclusion. Whereas high dosages of heparin may fail to control a paradoxical thrombin activity causing thrombotic occlusion after systemic thrombolytic therapy,[27] SET provided a method to suppress thrombin activity, indicating its potent anti-thrombin action.[21]

Accumulation of TPA during systemic infusion leads to significant amounts of circulating free plasmin, as indicated by marked reductions in fibrinogen and α-2-antiplasmin coinciding with a risk of hemorrhage.[22,28] Depletion of these factors is related not only to the dosage of TPA but also to the duration of infusion.[22,28] Short-term, segmentally enclosed application of small amounts of TPA caused peak values in peripheral blood comparable with TPA concentrations found during systemic infusion, but of short duration. The minimal reductions in fibrinogen and α-2-antiplasmin were clinically irrelevant and indicated the safety of SET, causing a small and transient systemic load of free plasmin.

Although the total rate of puncture site complications was somewhat higher than the 6% reported following conventional PTA,[29] none coincided with consumption of coagulation factors induced by SET. The risk of hemorrhage during intravenous heparin treatment after thrombolytic therapy has also been recognized by others.[22]

The average inter-balloon TPA concentration obtained by SET was about

100 times higher than contemporary systemic concentration, although less than 5% of injected TPA was retained.[23] Binding properties of TPA to sub-endothelial tissues, including fibroblasts[30] exposed to the vessel lumen by the deep injury enforced by PTA, may be an important mechanism for the long TPA half-life. In effect, SET may result from a dual action of TPA and heparin applied in high concentrations. Dissolution of thrombus and fibrin mesh for subsequent washout of fibrin-bound thrombin and activated platelets is provided by the action of TPA, and inhibition of local platelet activation and thrombus formation is provided by heparin.[31] Long-lasting fibrinolytic activity obtained by TPA accumulated in the injured vessel wall also counteracts thrombus formation at dilated sites.

Residual stenoses uncovered in most patients following intraarterial thrombolytic therapy for femoropopliteal occlusions are often corrected with PTA to secure patency.[22,28] We reversed the strategy and combined recanal-ization, dilatation, and thrombolysis in a procedure that is fast and requires no more staff, patient monitoring, or repeat arteriography than conventional PTA. Short-term target application of high TPA and heparin concentrations in relevant arterial segments by SET provides a safe and highly potent thrombolytic and anti-thrombotic procedure, which may allow treatment of vascular occlusions otherwise remote to interventional therapy, and opens the prospect of segmental treatment of vessels with a variety of pharmacolog-ical compounds.

Acknowledgments. The research presented in this chapter was financially supported by Kathrine & Vigo Skovgaards Fond, Therese Marie Hansen, født Beers, Fond, and the Danish Medical Research Council (Grants no. 12-9178 and 12-9845).

References

1. Dotter CT, Judkins MP. Transluminal treatment of arteriosclerotic obstruction. Description of a new technic and a preliminary report of its application. Circula-tion 1964;30:654–670.
2. Grüntzig A, Hopff H. Perkutane rekanalisation chronischer arterieller versch-lüsse mit einem neuen dilatationskatheter. Modifikation der Dotter-technik. Dtsch Med Wochenschr 1974;99:2502–2505.
3. Fletcher JP, Little JM, Kershaw LZ. The changing pattern of vascular surgery: The effect of percutaneous transluminal angioplasty. Aust N Z J Surg 1987;57: 221–224.
4. Kinney TB, Chin AK, Rurik GW, Finn JC, Shoor PM, Hayden WG, Fogarty TJ. Transluminal angioplasty: A mechanical-pathophysiological correlation of its physical mechanism. Radiology 1984;153:85–89.
5. Lyon RT, Zarins CK, LU CT, Yang CF, Glagov S. Vessel, plaque, and lumen morphology after transluminal balloon angioplasty. Quantitative study in dis-tended human arteries. Arteriosclerosis 1987;7:306–314.

6. Chesebro JH, Zoldhelyi P, Badimon L, Fuster V. Role of thrombin in arterial thrombosis: Implications for therapy. Thromb Haemost 1991;66:1–5.
7. Blättler W, Foullon N, Cappius G, Roth FJ. Platelet activation at the time of percutaneous transluminal angioplasty. In: Dotter CT. Grüntzig AR, Schoop W, Zeitler E (eds.) *Percutaneous Transluminal Angioplasty. Technique, Early and Late Results.* Berlin: Springer-Verlag, 1983, pp. 91–94.
8. Blättler W, Cappius G, Haeberli A, Foullon N, Roth FJ. Thrombinemia during percutaneous transluminal angioplasty of chronic femoral artery occlusions. VASA 1986;15:379–386.
9. Martin EC, Fankuchen EI, Karlson KB, Dolgin C, Collins RH, Voorhees AB, Casarella WJ. Angioplasty for femoral artery occlusions: Comparison with surgery. AJR 1981;137:915–919.
10. Tegtmeyer CJ. Percutaneous transluminal angioplasty. Curr Probl Diagn Radiol 1987;16:75–139.
11. Morin JF, Johnston KW, Wasserman L, Andrews D. Factors that determine the long-term results of percutaneous transluminal dilatation for peripheral arterial occlusive disease. J Vasc Surg 1986;4:68–72.
12. Jørgensen B, Meisner S, Holstein P, Tønnesen KH. Early rethrombosis in femoropopliteal occlusions treated with percutaneous transluminal angioplasty. Eur J Vasc Surg 1990;4:149–152.
13. Zeitler E, Richter EI. Roth FJ, Schoop W. Results of percutaneous transluminal angioplasty. Radiology 1983;146:57–60.
14. Johnston KW. Femoral and popliteal arteries: Reanalysis of results of balloon angioplasty. Radiology 1992;183:767–771.
15. Mabin TA, Holmes DR, Smith HC, Vlietstra RE, Bove AA, Reeder GS, Chesebro JH, Bresnahan JF, Orszulak TA. Intracoronary thrombus: Role in coronary occlusion complicating percutaneous transluminal coronary angioplasty. J Am Coll Cardiol 1985;5:198–202.
16. Francis CW, Markham RE, Barlow GH, Florack TM, Dobrzynski DM, Marder VJ. Thrombin activity of fibrin thrombi and soluble plasmic derivatives. J lab Clin Med 1983;102:220–230.
17. Ricotta JJ, Green RM, DeWeese JA. Use and limitations of thrombolytic therapy in the treatment of peripheral arterial ischemia: Results of a multi-institutional questionnaire. J Vasc Surg 1987;6:45–50.
18. Jørgensen B, Tønnesen KH, Bülow J, Nielsen JD, Jørgensen M, Holstein P, Andersen E. Femoral artery recanalisation with percutaneous angioplasty and segmentally enclosed plasminogen activator. Lancet 1989;1:1006–1008.
19. Jørgensen B, Tønnesen KH, Nielsen JD, Holstein P, Bülow J, Jørgensen M, Andersen E. Segmentally enclosed thrombolysis in percutaneous transluminal angioplasty for femoropopliteal occlusions: A report from a pilot study. Cardiovasc Intervent Radiol 1991;14:293–298.
20. Tønnesen KH, Sager P, Karle A, Henriksen L, Jørgensen B. Percutaneous transluminal angioplasty of the superficial femoral artery by retrograde catheterization via the popliteal artery. Cardiovasc Intervent Radiol 1988;11:127–131.
21. Jørgensen B, Nielsen JD. Intra-arterial thrombin activity produced by percutaneous transluminal angioplasty eliminated by segmentally enclosed thrombolysis. Eur J Vasc Surg 1992;6:153–157.
22. Graor RA, Risius B, Lucas FV, Young JR, Ruschhaupt WF, Beven EG, Grossbard EB. Thrombolysis with recombinant human tissue-type plasminogen acti-

vator in patients with peripheral artery and bypass graft occlusions. Circulation 1986;74:115–120.

23. Jørgensen B, Nielsen JD. Long half-life of tissue-type plasminogen activator after segmentally enclosed thrombolysis. Lancet 1991;337:795–796.

24. Tanswell P, Seifried E, Su PC, Feuerer W, Rijken DC. Pharmacokinetics and systemic effects of tissue-type plasminogen activator in normal subjects. Clin Pharmacol Ther 1989;46:155–162.

25. Jørgensen B, Tønnesen KH, Holstein P. Late hemodynamic failure following percutaneous transluminal angioplasty for long and multifocal femoropopliteal stenoses. Cardiovasc Intervent Radiol 1991;14:290–292.

26. Nossel HL, Yudelman I, Canfield RE, Butler VP, Spanondis K, Wilner GD, Qureshi GD. Measurement of fibrinopeptide A in human blood. J Clin Invest 1974;54:43–53.

27. Eisenberg PR, Sherman L, Rich M, Schwartz D, Schechtman K, Geltman EM, Sobel BE, Jaffe AS. Importance of continued activation of thrombin reflected by fibrinopeptide A to the efficacy of thrombolysis. J Am Coll Cardiol 1986;7:1255–1262.

28. Earnshaw JJ, Westby JC, Gregson RH, Makin GS, Hopkinson BR. Local thrombolytic therapy of acute peripheral arterial ischaemia with tissue plasminogen activator: A dose-ranging study. Br J Surg 1988;75:1196–1200.

29. Gardiner GA, Meyerovitz MF, Stokes KR, Clouse ME, Harrington DP, Bettmann MA. Complications of transluminal angioplasty. Radiology 1986;159:201–208.

30. Reilly TM, Whitfield MD, Taylor DS, Timmermans PB. Binding of tissue plasminogen activator to cultured human fibroblasts. Thromb Haemost 1989;61:454–458.

31. Heras M, Chesebro JH, Penny WJ, Bailey KR, Lam JY, Holmes DR, Reeder GS, Badimon L, Fuster V. Importance of adequate heparin dosage in arterial angioplasty in a porcine model. Circulation 1988;78:654–660.

44
Results of Surgical Treatment of Multivessel Disease of Lower Limb

ROY VARGESE, A.N. KOSENCOV, AND YURY V. BELOV

Introduction

A combination of lesions in two or more sites occurs in about 5.7% of patients presenting with lower limb ischemia.[1] Numerous improvements in patient selection and arterial reconstructive techniques have contributed to the current excellent results of direct aortic surgery for aneurysmal or occlusive disease.[2] The diffuse nature of atherosclerotic disease presents unique problems in the long-term management of these patients in large parts of the world where the facilities are less than ideal for follow-up and secondary management. For these reasons, in these patients, despite the available technology and technique, amputation has been the mode of treatment. At the National Research Center for Surgery we operated on patients with multilevel disease in whom one-level reconstruction was not deemed adequate, and the long-term results were analyzed to determine whether revascularization in this subgroup of patients was worthwhile.

Patient Population

From 1986 to 1991 we treated 1,835 patients presenting with lower limb chronic critical ischemia. One hundred eighty patients were offered two-level reconstructions in the aortoiliac (AI) and femoropopliteal (FP) zones and below. One hundred patients had the reconstructions in one sitting, and 80 patients had them within the same period of hospitalization. The latter group consisted of patients who had proximal revascularization and who on postoperative examination did not have relief, therefore the distal reconstruction was done.

The mean age of the patients was 56. All were male and all were smokers. The number of patients with associated diseases was: diabetes, 15; chronic cholecystitis, 4; chronic obstructive pulmonary disease, 5; malignancy, 5; renal disease, 4; essential hypertension, 12; total 50 (36%).

The number of patients with symptomatic vascular lesions in other regions was: coronary, 21; brachiocephalic, 18; renal, 7; total 46 (25.5%).

Criteria for Patient Selection

The indications for simultaneous proximal reconstructions were:

1. Hemodynamically significant occlusion the AI zone more than 10 cm in length combined with occlusion of the superficial femoral artery, associated with occlusive changes in the profunda femoris.
2. Poor outflow (less than 120 mL/min) after proximal aortofemoral (AF) reconstruction, and the profunda was angiographically normal.
3. Associated arteritic changes (common in patients of Central Asian origin).
4. Extensive disease of the popliteal trifurcation. No patient was refused revascularization when the alternative was amputation.

The indications for operation were: rest pain, 68; nonhealing ulcer, 76; toe gangrene, 36.

Operation

The operation was carried out under general anesthesia by two teams each consisting of a surgeon and an assistant. In 28 patients 6-mm polytetrafluoroethylene (PTFE) grafts were used due to nonavailability of the autogenous saphenous vein, and in 6 patients a combination of vein and PTFE was used due to inadequacy of the vein. The median operating time was 260 minutes. Thirty-three patients had the distal anastomosis at or below the tibial artery. No patients had in situ vein grafts. The average length of the bypass in the FP segment was 46 ± 3cm.

Results

There were 6 (3.2%) deaths in the 30-day period all from myocardial infarction. Two other patients with myocardial infarction were managed successfully. One patient had pulmonary insufficiency and was managed successfully. Eight patients had thrombosis in the veins, and 5 were reoperated successfully. Seven patients had infections, and 5 were managed successfully. Eight (4.4%) patients had amputations all at the above-knee level. The mean hospital stay was 22 days. The immediate rise in ankle–brachial index (ABI) was 0.31 ± 0.05 to 0.55 ± 0.03 after AF reconstruction. and after total reconstruction in the FP-tibial zone it rose to 0.89 ± 0.67.

Long-term follow-up was done by primary care physicians, with strict instructions to refer patients back immediately in case of symptom recurrence, thrombosis, or any other disability. Twelve (6.6%) patients came back for secondary procedures due to thrombosis in the FP zone. The maximum period of follow-up available was 53 months.

The results were analyzed by log rank tests. The long-term patency was

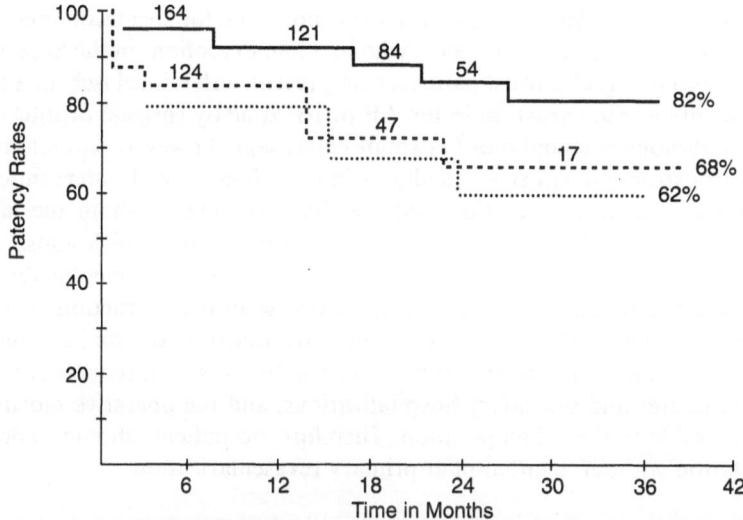

FIGURE 44.1. Cumulative life table patency rates. Top line, AF zone patency; Bottom line, FP zone patency; Middle line, Limb salvage.

82% in the AF zone and 62% in the FP zone. The overallrate of limb salvage was 68%. (Fig. 44.1).

Discussion

This study was primarily done to learn the effectiveness of surgical reconstruction in patients with multilevel disease in a setting where facilities for secondary care are not optimal, a situation not uncommon in large parts of the world. It is of particular importance to detect failing grafts, which, if reoperated before thrombosis, yield good results.[3] The 68% limb salvage rate compares favorably with published data of above 70% from developed nations.[4]. The operative mortality of 3.2% also compares well with the operative mortality for amputations in the literature.[5] The study also compares well with a recent study on concomitant revascularization.[6] The group of 80 patients consisted of our early patients who had interval revascularization because we were developing experience at that time in radical treatment (hence we subjected them to interval revascularization) and those patients in whom we thought that a proximal procedure would suffice but had outflow problems. The fact that these patients had ischemic problems after proximal reconstruction points out the practical utility of the criteria used by us for revascularization. It is possible that a small percentage of patients may have had overcorrection, but this is a small price to pay when the facilities are limited and the pressure on beds and specialists is high. In this series, active and expert care to detect failing grafts was not done for socioeconomic and geographic reasons. All the patients who had reinterventions in the long term had thrombosed grafts. Most patients who present with critical ischemia may require only a reconstruction in the AF or FP zone by surgical or interventional radiological techniques.[7] A small percentage, however, requires two-level reconstruction, either surgically or in combination with interventional radiological techniques. In this study we had patients in whom the latter technique was not deemed optimal because of the nature of the lesions.

This study shows, in conclusion, that in severe multisegmental disease of the arteries of the lower limb, surgical two-level reconstructions can be carried out safely with comparable results irrespective of optimal secondary facilities for follow-up. Concomitant reconstruction is safe, it reduces secondary procedures and secondary hospitalizations, and the operative mortality is comparable to that of amputation. Therefore, no patients should undergo amputation without an attempt at primary revascularization.

References

1. Aston No, Lea M, Thomas ML Burnand KG. The distribution of atherosclerosis in the lower limbs. Eur J Vasc Surg 1992;6:73–77.
2. Brewster DC. Surgery of late aortic graft occlusion. In: Bergan JJ, Yao JST (eds.). *Aortic Surgery*. Philadelphia: WB Saunders, 1989.
3. Second European Consensus Document on Chronic Critical Leg Ischemia. Vol. 6. Supplement A. p. 17, 1992.
4. Myers KA, Scott DF, Devine TJ. In: Greenhalgh R (ed.). *Indications in Vascular Surgery*. Philadelphia: WB Saunders, 1989, p. 226.
5. Hodson RW, Lynch TG Jamil Z, et al. Results of revascularisation and amputation in severe lower extremity ischemia: A five year clinical experience. J Vasc Surg 1985;2:174–182.
6. Harris PL, Cave Bigley DJ, McSweeney L. Aortofemoral bypass and the role of concommittant femorodistal reconstruction. Br Surg 1985;22:317.
7. Samson RH, Scher LA, Veith FJ. Combined segment arterial disease. Surgery 1985;97:35–39.

45
Late Complications Following Surgery for Popliteal Artery Entrapment Syndrome

TAKEHISA IWAI, SHOJI SATO, YOSHINORI INOUE, NORIAKI TAKIGUCHI, AND MITSUO ENDO

Introduction

Popliteal artery entrapment syndrome (PAES) is recognized as becoming symptomatic in relatively younger age groups, demonstrating popliteal arterial occlusive changes.[1] In our country by 1985, 40 surgical cases had been reported in the literature.[2]

The surgical principle includes arterial reconstruction using venous graft for the arterial occlusion, and when there are no occlusive changes in latent cases, resection of the abnormal muscle or resection of the artery with reanastomosis in the anatomically correct position.[3] The majority of the cases in the world literature have been reported as having an uneventful course postoperatively. Additionally, comparatively few graft thromboses have been reported.[4-7]

This syndrome is caused not only by the abnormal positioning of the vessels or musculature, but also by imbalance of the muscle belly. Therefore, late complications should be considered from the normal muscle arrangement and its relation to the new graft.[8,9]

We report two such cases which showed late complications 4 and 8 years after surgery, respectively.

Materials and Case Reports

Since 1975, 17 limbs and 13 cases of PAES have been treated surgically. The male-to-female ratio was 10:3 and the age ranged from 7 to 57 years with a mean age of 28.8. Surgical treatment included autosaphenous vein replacement in 12 limbs, and thromboendarterectomy (TEA) in one limb in the arterial occlusive group. Arterial reanastomoses in the anatomically correct position were performed in three limbs and tendon resection followed by reanastomosis in one limb in the latent PAES group. In these cases, two late complications were encountered.

Case 1

A 26-year-old male. The first surgery showed a rotated popliteal artery me-
dially surrounded by the medial head of the gastrocnemius muscle, and classified as Delaney type 3. The occluded popliteal artery was replaced with a
graft from the patient's contralateral saphenous vein. Intraoperatively the
medial head of the gastrocnemius muscle and the semimembranosus muscle
were found to be remarkably huge in size. Four years later the patient was
readmitted to our university hospital complaining of intractable popliteal
fossa pain on walking. Angiography revealed an aneurysmal change of the

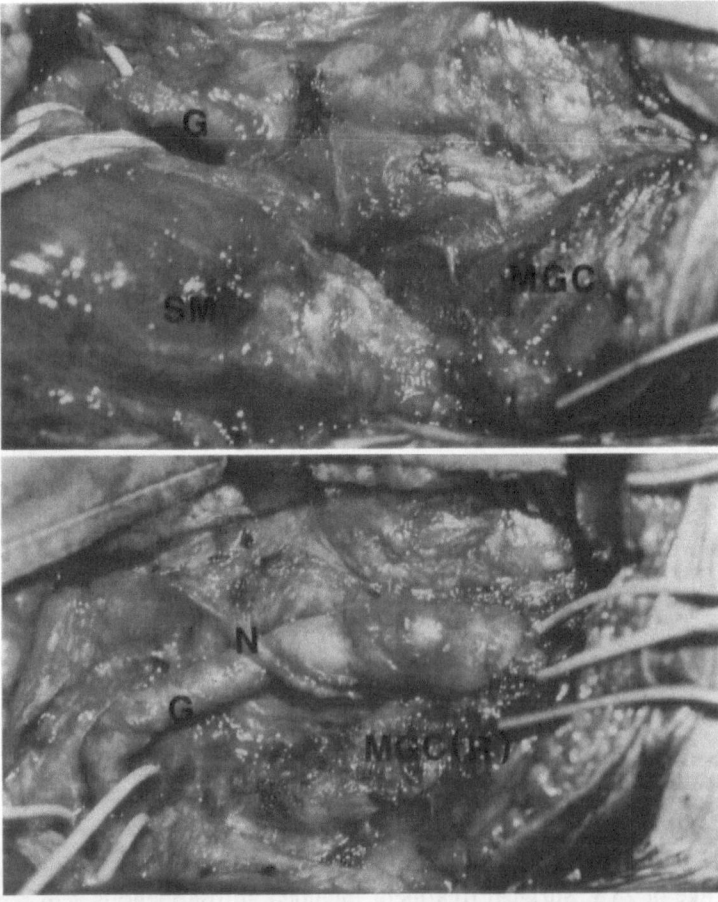

FIGURE 45.1. *Case 1.* A huge semimembranosus muscle (SM) and a big muscle belly of
the medial head of the gastrocnemius muscle (MGC) (above) G, Initial graft. Medial
view of the right leg in prone position. An aneurysmal change in the distal graft and
adhered nerve (N) (below). Left side is cephalic.

lower half of the vein graft. On modification surgery, the nerve to the medial head of the gastrocnemius muscle was found to have adhered to the graft, and this had compressed the middle part of the graft. The aneurysmal change was considered a result of the entrapment by the nerve. The operation was performed with transfer of the nerve downward to the new saphenous vein graft on the posterior approach. The abnormally large medial head of the muscle was also partially resected (Fig. 45.1). Additionally, to prevent further abnormal compression by the rest of the muscle, the graft was surrounded by Dacron mesh. For years after this procedure, the patient is free from any complaints (Fig. 45.2).

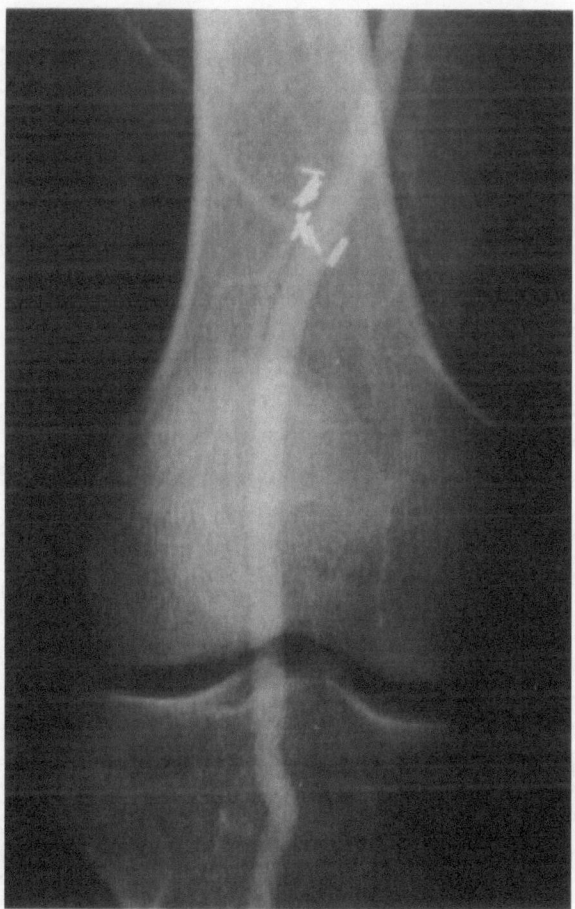

FIGURE 45.2. *Case 1.* Postoperative angiography showing good patency without any symptoms.

Case 2

A 24-year-old male. Initial surgery showed right popliteal artery occlusion, of Delaney type 2 classification, with intermittent claudication. The saphenous vein replacement was performed along the anatomical route. The intraoperative view showed a significantly large lateral head of the gastrocnemius muscle; however, it was left without any treatment. Eight years later, the patient visited us complaining of recurrent intermittent claudication. Angiography showed the graft was occluded, and he agreed to undergo surgical reconstruction again. Careful exposure in the popliteal fossa revealed the normally positioned graft which was apparently entrapped by the huge lateral head of the gastrocnemius muscle (Fig. 45.3). The new saphenous vein graft was then

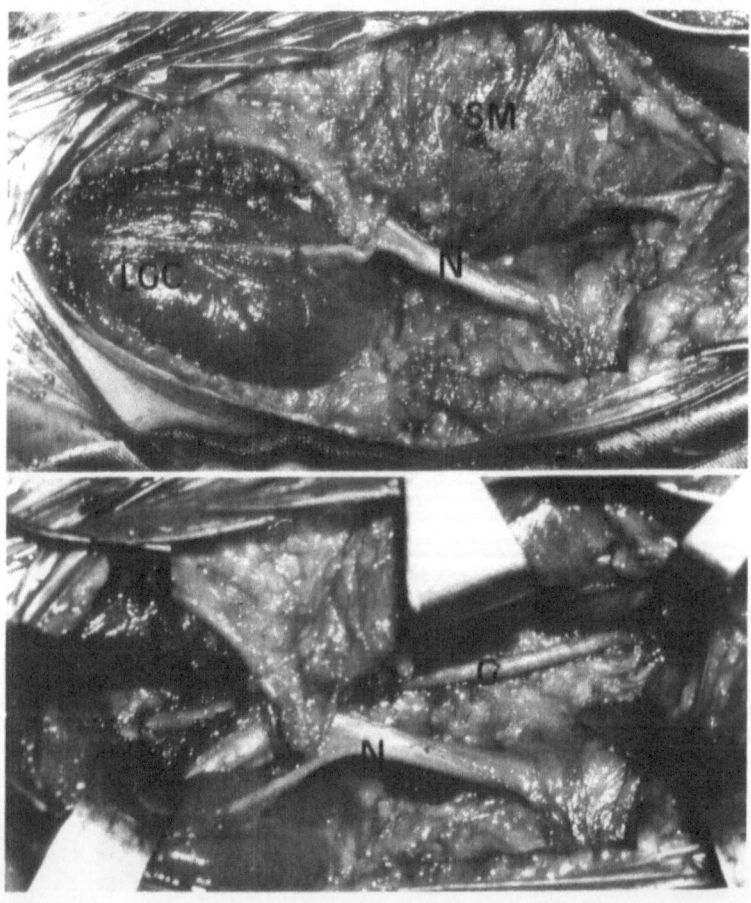

FIGURE 45.3. *Case 2.* A huge lateral head of the gastrocnemius muscle (LGC) and well-developed semimembranosus muscle (SM) (above). Lateral view of the right leg. Tibial nerve (N) and new saphenous vein graft (G) (below). Right side is cephalic.

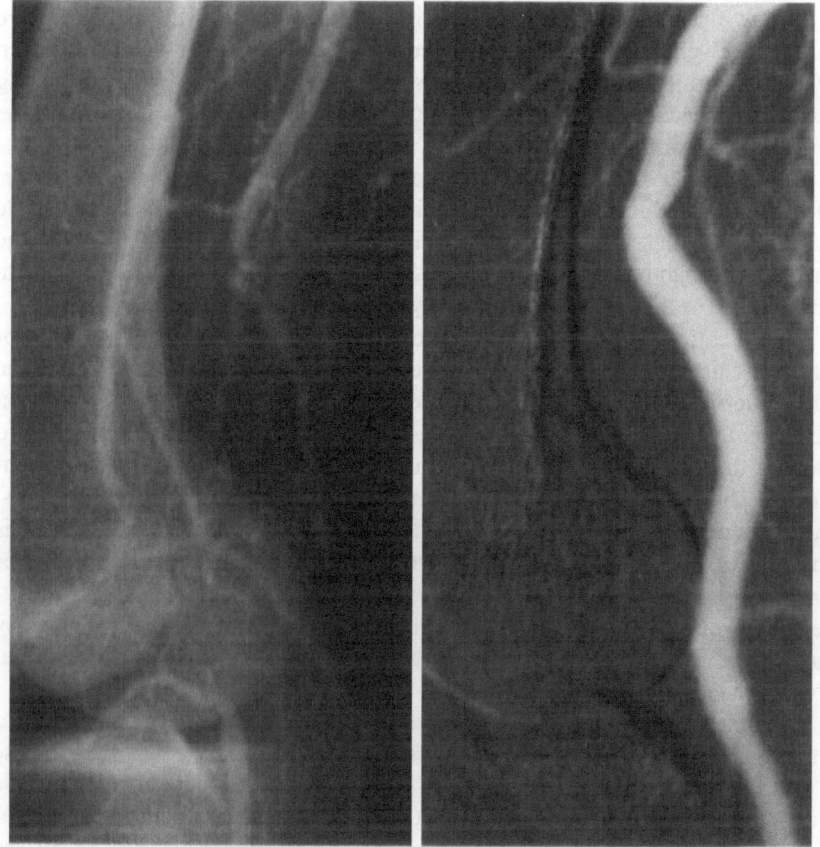

FIGURE 45.4. *Case 4.* Preoperative (left) and postoperative (right) angiography.

anastomosed, and the lateral head of the muscle was partially resected. Two years following the new procedure, the patient is well and able to walk without any problems (Fig. 45.4).

Discussion

More than 210 cases of PAES had been surgically treated in the world by 1986,[6] and more than 40 cases had been reported in Japan by 1985.[2] Possibly by now there are 50–60 cases in Japan. However, the reported follow-up period in Japan was not so long,[6] and long-term angiographic changes were not so clearly demonstrated up to the present. In addition to the surgical point of view, many patients who present with mild symptoms are treated conservatively, and in that latter group many patients might not even be diagnosed as having PAES throughout their lives.[8]

Follow-up care is less well established because most of the patients were young, the vein autograft was short enough for a thorough check, and even when the graft was occluded after surgery, with the exception of young athletes or occupational walkers, the average patient might not notice the chronic occlusion.

Reported cases that demonstrated early occlusion or aneurysmal changes after venous replacement are limited in number.[4-7] These included possible intimal hyperplasia[6] related to the vein itself, or misdiagnosis caused by the medial approach to the popliteal fossa.[4] From our collective review, late complications of PAES are very rarely seen in the literature.

Classification of PAES has been proposed by several authors.[4,10-13] Popular classifications are based on the relationship between the artery and the muscle alone. These classifications look easy to understand; however, when abnormally-sized or separated muscles are included, it is really impossible to classify the PAES accurately. We would therefore like to pay special attention to the muscular anomalies. Concerning the surgical procedure, most authors advocate placing the graft in the anatomically correct position. This therapeutic theory is somewhat incorrect when abnormal muscle structures are present. Our two cases were suggestive of this fact. Usually a short-segment venous replacement is safe and expected to have a long patency rate when 2 or 3 years have passed without any technical error or intimal hyperplasia.

Though a long patency was expected in our two cases, a large medial head of the gastrocnemius muscle and the semitendinosus muscle was seen in case 1 and a huge lateral head in case 2. In case 1, the nerve located on the middle part of the graft played a very important role in causing aneurysmal dilatation, which may have been accelerated by the stronger compression of the abnormally large muscle medial head. He is now completely symptom-free after 4 years. This clearly showed that correction of the popliteal anatomical route by the resection of part of the muscle and transposition of the nerve was the reasonable procedure. Case 2, on the other hand, demonstrated the vein as being reentrapped by the huge lateral head of the gastrocnemius muscle, even though the graft was placed in the correct route.

In our total experience with PAES of 17 cases, we can include cases where even with a normal course of the popliteal artery, the artery was occluded only by the huge muscle structure itself. Those cases included a huge medial head of the gastrocnemius muscle, and a long abductor muscle and semi-membranosus muscle. From this fact, late complications could be prevented by reestablishing the anatomically correct route as appropriately as possible. The main point is that the anatomical position is not always safe enough for a new graft. Our successful cases suggest that resection of the abnormally-formed muscle worked very well.

From the standpoint of surgery in PAES in which anomalous muscle is present, we therefore recommend the following principles for successful surgical treatment.

Preoperative definitive diagnosis is really essential when considering avoiding the medial approach or other procedures like percutaneous transluminal angioplasty (PTA). Surgery should be via the posterior approach to obtain a good view of the complete muscular orientation. Autosaphenous vein is harvested from the contralateral thigh and should be preserved in 4°C normal saline solution during the change of the patient's position from supine to prone, so that the vein is kept in a biologically fresh condition, and early complications such as intimal hyperplasia are prevented.

Finally, the graft route should be carefully reconstructed to partially remove the muscle or transfer the nerve. When the muscle belly is too heavy, we advocate resecting the tendinous part of the muscle completely. This treatment completely reduces contraction of the new graft by the muscle.

Summary

Two late complications in PAES surgery were reported. To avoid such complications, the graft route should be carefully reconstructed by resection of abnormally-sized muscle or by the transfer of the nerve.

Acknowledgment. The authors would like to thank Miss Kumi Masugi for her assistance.

References

1. Biemans RGM, van Bockel JH. Popliteal artery entrapment syndrome. Surg Gynecol Obstet 1977;144:604–609.
2. Matsuwaka R, Ohnishi K, Hata I, et al. Popliteal entrapment syndrome; Report of two cases and study of 40 cases in Japan. J Clin Surg 1985;40:1421–1426 (in Japanese).
3. Iwai T, Konno S, Soga K, et al. Diagnostic and pathological considerations in the popliteal artery entrapment syndrome. J Cardiovasc Surg 1983;24:243–249.
4. Kusaba A, Kiyose T, Moriyama M, et al. Popliteal artery entrapment syndrome. Cardioangiology 1977;1:81–93 (in Japanese).
5. Sakurai T, Yamada I, Ohta T, et al. Report of 3 cases of the popliteal artery entrapment syndrome—A review of the Japanese literature and differential diagnosis of the occlusive disease of the kid-popliteal artery. J Jpn Soc Clin Surg 1985;47:82–90.
6. Cavallaro A, Di Marzo L, Gallo P, et al. Popliteal artery entrapment. Analysis of the literature and report of personal experience. Vasc Surg 1986;20:404–423.
7. Darling RC, Buckley CJ, Abbott WM, et al. Intermittent claudication in young athletes: Popliteal artery entrapment syndrome. J Trauma 1974;14:543–553.
8. Bouhoutsos J, Daskalakis E. Muscular abnormalities affecting the popliteal vessels. Br J Surg 1981;68:501–506.
9. Bouhoutsos J. Popliteal artery entrapment syndrome: Report of 29 cases. Vasc Surg 1980;14:365–374.

10. Schurmann G, Mattfeldt T, Hofmann W, et al. The popliteal artery entrapment syndrome: Presentation, morphology and surgical treatment of 13 cases. Eur J Vasc Surg 1990;4:223–231.
11. Insua JA, Young JR, Humphries AW. Popliteal artery entrapment syndrome. Arch Surg 1970;101:771–775.
12. Delaney TA, Conzalez LL. Occlusion of popliteal artery due to muscular entrapment. Surgery 1971;69:97–101.
13. Rich NM, Collins GJ, Jr, McDonald PT, et al. Popliteal vascular entrapment. Its increasing interest. Arch Surg 1979;114:1377–1384.

XV
Tibial Peroneal Occlusive Disease

46
Tibial Revascularization Under Transmicroscopic Technique

MASAYASU YOKOKAWA, MASAKI TOMIKAWA, TAKESHI UEYAMA, AND
KEIICHI YAMAMOTO

Introduction

Bypass grafting to tibial arteries has extended our ability to revascularize severely ischemic lower extremities with threat of amputation. The evolution of vascular surgical knowledge and techniques has contributed to the success of these procedures.

Although the initial results in several recent reports seemed to be satisfying, the long-term patency has not been well discussed. Tibial arteries with diameters as small as 2.0 mm or less cause unsatisfactory results. Magnification of the operative field is considered a primitive technique for performing accurate operative procedure for such small-caliber arteries.[1] For this reason, we use the transmicroscopic technique of vascular surgery for performing accurate anastomosis in the region of tibial arteries.

We have obtained good results in long-term patency. Our experience and results of bypass grafting to the tibial artery with microscopic technique are reported. The transmicroscopic technical point for long-term patency is discussed.

Patients and Methods

Thirty-two tibial artery bypasses with transmicroscopic techncique were performed in 27 consecutive patients from June 1984 to December 1991. Twenty-three patients had arteriosclerosis obliterans, and 4 patients had thromboangiitis obliterans. Patients ranged from 37 to 78 years old, with a mean age of 62 years. Twenty-five were men and 2 were women.

Twenty bypasses were performed for limb-threatening ischemia, in which 7 (24.1%) presented tissue necrosis and 13 (44.8%) presented rest pain. Nine bypasses were performed for disabling claudication. Twenty-seven bypasses were primary and two were secondary in these operations.

The risk factors observed were hypertension (33.3%), prior history of stroke (14.8%), angina pectoris (3.7%), previous myocardial infarction (11.1%), diabetes mellitus (33.3%), and chronic renal failure (3.7%).

Angiographic Assessment

All patients were examined with conventional aortic lower extremity angiography preoperatively. Special attention was paid to the outflow tracts. Runoff was graded into three categories as follows. The presence of either three patent crural vessels or two patent vessels plus an intact pedal arch was classified as "good" runoff. The presence of two patent vessels without an intact arch or one vessel with an intact pedal arch was "fair." Any other runoff situation was "poor."

Transmicroscopic Technique

An ipsilateral autogenous greater saphenous vein was used in most instances. The reversed saphenous vein was used in 27 patients, the in situ saphenous vein in 3, and composite vein-to-vein graft in 2. The proximal anastomosis was placed on the common femoral artery in 13 patients, the superficial femoral in 2, the above-knee popliteal in 15, and the below-knee popliteal in 2. These anastomoses were performed without the microscope.

On the other hand, all the distal anastomoses were performed under transmicroscopic technique. We used the microscope provided by Zeiss (type: OPMi 7), which enabled magnification of the operative field by 5 to 10 times in all cases. A 7–0 or 8–0 polypropylene suture was used for distal end-to-side anastomosis. Continuous suture was performed in recipient vessels larger than 1.5 mm in diameter. However, interrupted 8–0 suture was chosen for smaller vessels. The distal anastomosis was made at the proximal portion of the tibial artery in 14 instances; of these, the tibioperoneal truncus was selected in 6, the anterior tibial artery in 1, the posterior tibial artery in 5, and the peroneal artery in 2. The distal portion of the tibial artery was used in 18 instances; of these, the posterior tibial artery was selected in 16 and the peroneal artery in 2. The bypass graft was passed along the medial border when the anastomosis was placed on the posterior tibial or peroneal arteries. The lateral border was selected in case of the anterior tibial artery.

Combined revascularization was performed in 8 patients at the same time. Iliofemoral bypass was performed in 2 patients and femoropopliteal bypass in 6. Three patients, in the presence of multiple occlusive disease, were revascularized by femoro-popliteal-tibial sequential bypass with autogenous greater saphenous vein graft.

Cumulative patency rates were calculated using the Kaplan-Meier method.

Results

The preoperative angiographically assessed condition of the tibial arteries affected the patency rate when runoff was poor or fair. Five instances were judged "poor" runoff. Two of these were occluded in the early postoperative

TABLE 46.1. Preoperative angiographic findings and graft failures.

| Runoff | | Graft failure | | |
Grade	No. of cases	Early graft failure	Late graft failure	Rate of failure (%)
Good	11	0	0	0
Fair	13	1	2	3/13 (20%)
Poor	5	2	1	3/5 (60%)
Total	29	3	3	6/29 (20.7%)

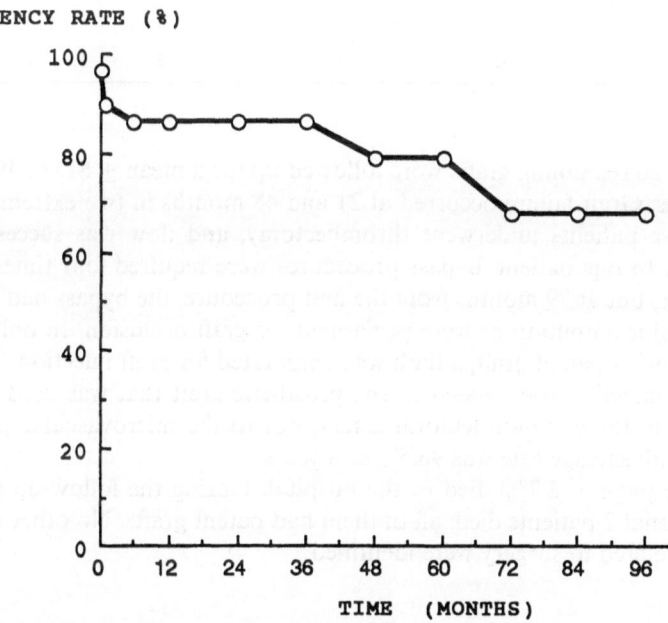

FIGURE 46.1 Graft patency calculated by Kaplan-Meier method.

period, and one of these in the late phase. Thirteen were judged "fair" runoff. One of these was occluded in the early postoperative period, and 2 of these in the late phase. Eleven were judged "good" runoff. No graft failures were identified throughout the follow-up period in the good runoff series (Table 46.1).

The cumulative patency rate was 86.2% at 1 year, 79.0% at 5 years, and 67.7% at 8 years (Fig. 46.1). The primary patency of the 14 grafts in which the distal anastomosis was placed proximal to the tibial artery was 85.7% at 1 year, 71.4% at 5 years, and 71.4% at 8 years. The patency rate of the 18 grafts that were placed distal to the tibial artery was 93.3% at 1 year, 93.3% at 5 years, and 46.7% at 8 years. No significant difference was observed in the primary graft patency of these two groups (Table 46.2).

Three (9.4%) graft failures occurred during the hospitalization period.

TABLE 46.2. Site of distal anastomosis and graft failures.

Anastomosis at the tibial artery		Graft failure		
Site	No. of cases	Early graft failure	Late graft failure	Rate of failure (%)
Proximal				
Truncus	6	1		1/6 (16.7%)
Anterior tibial	1			0
Posterior tibial	5	1		1/5 (20%)
Peroneal	2		1	1/2 (50%)
Distal				
Posterior tibial	16	1	1	2/16 (12.5%)
Peroneal	2		1	1/2 (50%)
Total	32	3	3	6/32 (18.8%)

The 26 remaining grafts were followed up for a mean $\pm$ SD of 49.5 $\pm$ 26.7 months. Graft failure occurred at 21 and 48 months in two extremities. One of these patients underwent thrombectomy, and flow was successfully restored. In one patient, bypass procedures were required four times for limb salvage, but at 79 months from the first procedure, the bypass had occluded. No major amputations were performed for graft occlusion. In only one patient with a patent graft, a limb was amputated for graft infection. The cause of the infection was related to the prosthetic graft that was used for patch plasty in the common femoral artery, not to the microvascular procedure. The limb salvage rate was 96.5% at 8 years.

One patient (3.7%) died in the hospital. During the follow-up period an additional 2 patients died; all of them had patent grafts. No other complications related to surgery were identified

Discussion

Femorotibial bypass under transmicroscopic technique could save severely ischemic limbs with low hospital mortality and good long-term patency. However, the transmicroscopic technique has been considered a complicated and time-consuming surgical procedure. The field under the standard operative loupe would be sufficient in vascular anastomosis to the tibial artery. However, in most cases of arteriosclerosis obliterans, the outer diameter of the tibial artery is smaller than 2.0 mm, gradually decreasing to as small as 1.5 mm at the distal portion of the tibial artery. The advantage of microscopic surgery is fine observation, because the magnificantion level is changeable, as needed. In anastomosis for small-caliber vessels such as the tibial artery, magnification by 10 times under the microscope is important to observe the characteristics of the intima of the recipient artery. Subsequently, the procedure is performed by transmicroscopic technique under 5 times magnification, which provides much higher accuracy for suturing than the operative loupe.[1,2] High magnification prevents intraoperative technical error or unexpected injury. The patency rates of the tibial bypasses with microvascular technique reported in this paper were better than any other results reported recently.

The controversy still remains regarding the utility of distal arterial bypass for limb salvage.[3] Using the microsurgical technique, no significant difference in the patency rate was found between distal tibial bypass grafting and proximal tibial bypass grafting. When tibial bypass graft is performed for threatening ischemic limb, the most distal of the arteries that is disease-free and continues with the pedal circulation is preferred as the site of anastomosis.[4,5] When a suitable autogenous saphenous vein is available, selecting the most distal portion for the anastomosis is expected to improve the clinical symptoms and limb salvage rate effectively.

No graft failure was found in "good" runoff series. However, occlusion of the bypass graft occurred in 60% of "poor" runoff and 20% of "fair" runoff series. This confirms the earlier reports that graft failure is affected by the poor runoff of the tibial artery.[2,6] There was no major amputation due to graft failure. A failed tibial bypass graft does not preclude salvage of the limb and does not predispose to subsequent amputation.[7] We recommend trying to revascularize the tibial artery under transmicroscopic technique, even if the runoff is judged "poor" preoperatively.

The prerequisite for tibial bypass grafting is the availability of suitable bypass materials. When autogenous vein is not available, human umbilical vein, prosthetic graft, or composite graft can be used in order to avoid amputation.[8,9] However, many reports show the superiority of autogenous saphenous vein grafts compared with composite grafts or prosthetic grafts.[6,10] Good results have been recently reported by use of in situ technique.[4,11] On the other hand, Taylor et al.[12] described the superiority of the reversed-vein graft for patency, vein utilization, and limb salvage. He argued that the recently improved figures for patency and limb salvage after tibial bypass grafting reflect overall improvement in perioperative and intraoperative care, and not the use of in situ technique. Wengerter et al.[13] reported the influence of vein diameter on graft patency. Vein grafts less than 3.0 mm in diameter, either reversed or in situ, have poor patency. We consider that grafts other than autogenous saphenous vein should never be used in the primary operation for tibial bypass grafting. We prefer the use of reversed-vein grafts, because it is simple technique providing good utilization of the autogenous vein. All three bypass grafts with in situ technique were patent. The relative superiority of reversed and in situ grafts was not determined.

The microsurigcal technique for performing vascular anastomosis is still a primitive method to complete the accurate anastomosis. Of course, microsurgical technique can be combined with other vascular techniques to improve the operative result. By extending the use of microsurgical technique, the patency rate of tibial artery bypass grafting will be improved.

References

1. Tomikawa M, Ueyama T, Yokokawa M, et al. Tibial artery revascularization utilizing microscopic vascular technique. Vasc Surg 1990;24:475–481.
2. Klamer TW, Lambert GE, Richardson JD, et al. Utility of inframalleolar arterial bypass grafting. J Vasc Surg 1990;11:164–170.
3. Harrington EB, Harrington ME, Schanzer H, et al. The dorsalis pedis bypass— Moderate success in difficult situation. J Vasc Surg 1992;15:409–416.
4. Shah DM, Darling RC, Chang BB, et al. Is long vein bypass from groin to ankle a durable procedure? An analysis of a ten-year experience. J Vasc Surg 1992;15: 402–408.
5. Andros G, Harris RW, Salles-Cunha SX, et al. Lateral plantar artery bypass grafting: Defining the limits of foot revascularization. J Vasc Surg 1989;10:511– 521.
6. Sipponen J, Ala-Kulju K, Kentonen P, et al. Femorotibial bypass grafting for lower limb ischaemia. Int Angiol 1989;8:65–69.
7. Bloom RJ, Stevick A. Amputation level and distal bypass salvage of the limb. Surg Gynecol Obstet 1988;166:1–5
8. Feinberg RL, Winter RP, Wheeler JR, et al. The use of composite grafts in femorocrural bypasses performed for limb salvage: A review of 108 consecutive cases and comparison with 57 in situ saphenous vein bypasses. J Vasc Surg 1990; 12:257–263.
9. Londrey GL, Ramsey DE, Hodgson KJ, et al. Infrapopliteal bypass fro severe ischemia: Comparison of autogenous vein, composite, and prosthetic grafts. J Vasc Surg 1991;13:631–636.
10. Chang JB. Femoropoliteal and femorotibial arterial bypasses for limb salvage. Vasc Surg 1981;15:240–257.
11. Leather RP, Shah DM, Karmody AM. Infrapopliteal arterial bypass for limb salvage: Increased patency and utilization of the saphenous vein used "in situ". Surgery 1981;90:1000–1008.
12. Taylar LM, Edwards JM, Porter JM, et al. Reversed vein bypass to infrapopliteal arteries. Ann Surg 1987;205:90–97.
13. Wengerter KR, Veith FJ, Gupta SK, et al. Influence of vein size (diameter) on infrapopliteal reversed vein graft patency. J Vasc Surg 1990;11:525–531.

47
Clinical Review of Adjunctive Arteriovenous Fistula with Tibial and Peroneal Reconstruction for Extensive Occlusive Arterial Disease of Lower Extremity

Yong Bok Koh, Cho Hyun Park, Jong Man Won, and Chang Joon Ahn

Introduction

The ischemic extremity secondary to occlusive arterial disease has been managed by bypass graft, thromboendarterectomy, or sympathectomy. A new revascularization procedure for end-stage occlusive arterial lesions of the lower extremity is desirable since lumbar sympathectomy may yield poor results.

In recent years, operative procedures for limb salvage have extended more distally, and femorotibial or peroneal bypass is now increasingly common.

Vascular reconstruction to the tibial and peroneal arteries will yield good patency rates with improvement of ischemic symptoms if the runoff is good, including an intact pedal arch. However, with poor runoff, bypass has been discouraging due to inability to maintain adequate graft flow.

An arteriovenous fistula at the site of the distal anastomosis could overcome this problem by increasing graft flow velocity and by allowing much of the blood entering the graft to bypass the foot, thereby permitting continued graft patency. Dardik et al.[1] have been leading proponents of the use of an adjunctive arteriovenous fistula to improve graft patency.

This report presents the results of the effects of an adjunctive arteriovenous fistula in femorodistal bypass grafting.

Materials and Method

During the 6-year period from 1985 through 1991, 40 patients underwent adjunctive arteriovenous fistula with tibial and peroneal reconstruction for extensive occlusive arterial disease of the lower extremity.

The causes of occlusive arterial disease included arteriosclerosis obliterans (ASO) in 24 patients (60%) and thromboangiitis obliterans (TAO) in 16 patients (40%). Ages ranged from 26 to 76 years. Twelve of 24 patients (50%)

with ASO had diabetes mellitus; 28 patients had had one or more previous revascularization procedures; 21 of 24 patients (88%) with ASO had one or more of the risk factors, including previous myocardial ischemia, hypertension, chronic obstructive pulmonary disease, and renal insufficiency.

All patients were threatened with imminent limb loss due to end-stage arterial occlusive disease. The indications for surgery were rest pain in all patients, distal gangrene in 20, and nonhealing ulcer in 13 patients. Preoperative arteriography was performed in all cases (Fig. 47.1). In cases with poor

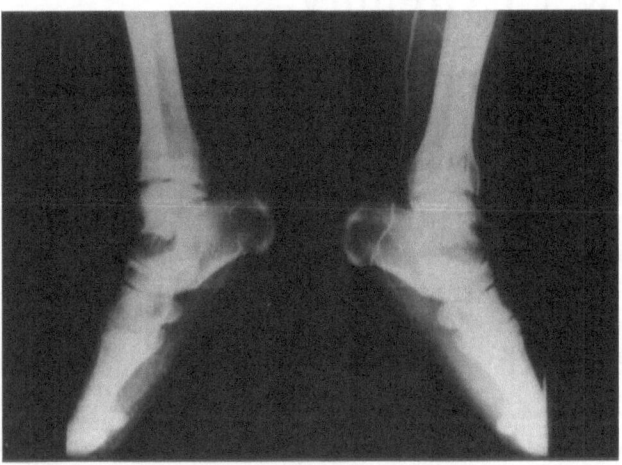

FIGURE 47.1. Preoperative arteriography showing nonvisualization of runoff vessels with absent pedal arch of right lower extremity.

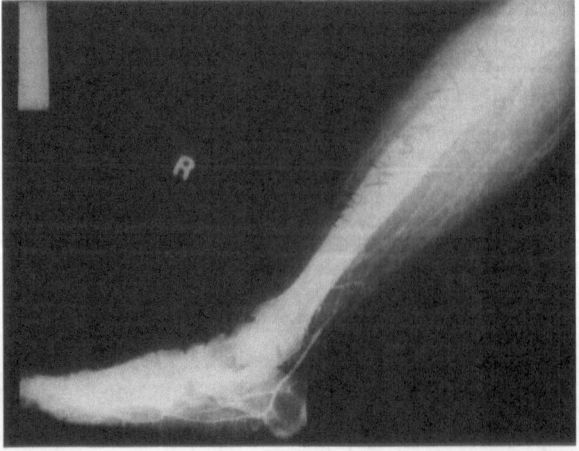

FIGURE 47.2. Intraoperative arteriography demonstrating posterior tibial artery with multifocal areas of stenosis.

runoff or nonvisualization in preoperative routine arteriography, operative maneuvers such as sounding, fluid injection, and intraoperative table arteriography were performed (Fig. 47.2). The operative technique for adjunctive arteriovenous fistula formation in distal anastomosis was similar to that reported by Dardik et al.[1] (Fig. 47.3). Proximal anastomosis was done on the common femoral artery in 32 cases (80%) and the superficial femoral artery in 8 cases (20%). Reversed autogenous saphenous vein graft was used in 12 patients (30%), in situ autogenous saphenous vein graft in 6 patients (15%),

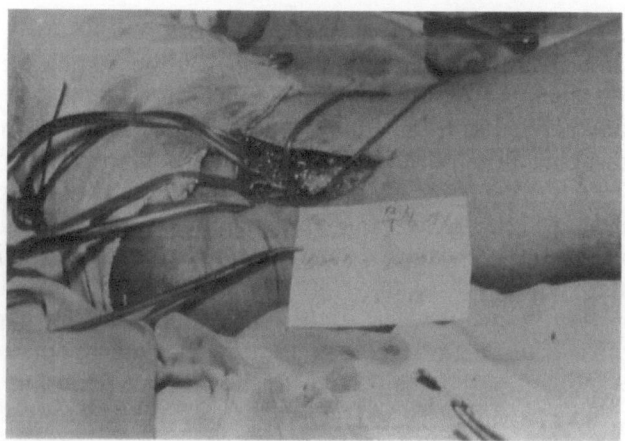

FIGURE 47.3. Photogram of operative field creating arteriovenous fistula at the site of the distal anastomosis at the malleolus level.

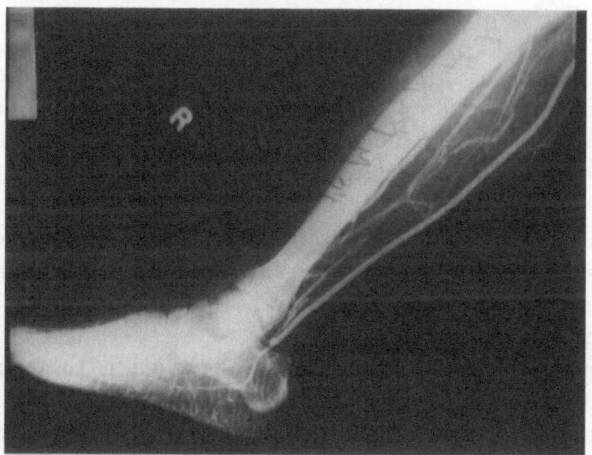

FIGURE 47.4. Intraoperative arteriography showing femoral posterior tibial bypass with adjunctive arteriovenous fistula. Excellent venous network is well demonstrated.

and polytetrafluoroethylene (PTFE) graft in 22 patients (55%). Twenty-six (65%) bypasses were performed to the posterior tibial artery and 10 (25%) to the anterior tibial artery; 4 (10%) were performed to the peroneal artery.

After completion of reconstruction, operative arteriography was performed (Fig. 47.4). Postoperative observations consisted of graft patency, reversal of ischemic symptoms and signs, and healing of lesions by physical examination, Doppler ultrasound, and postoperative arteriography.

Results

During the immediate postoperative period, no deaths or significant morbidity occurred. Patent grafts were characterized by a soft pulse, a palpable thrill, and an audible bruit. Functional grafts resulted in reversal of the ischemic signs and symptoms and healing of ulcers. Thirty-six (90%) of 40 bypass grafts were patent postoperatively, and amelioration of rest pain with healing of ischemic lesions was achieved in 34 patients (85%). In 2 patients, the grafts and fistulas remained patent postoperatively, but persistent ischemic symptoms necessitated above-knee amputation. Graft thrombectomy was performed in 3 patients whose grafts occluded immediately after reconstruction with eventual below-knee amputations. One other patient required above-knee amputation because of postoperative graft occlusion within 1 month. Another 4 patients who had undergone successful reconstruction also required amputation during 2 to 9 months of follow-up period. Ancillary toe and transmetatarsal amputations were performed in 10 due to preexisting gangrene without uneventful wound healing.

Discussion

Since Dean and Read[2] first described the concept of using an arteriovenous fistula to improve graft flow and patency in a canine model, the use of an arteriovenous fistula to maintain flow in prosthetic grafts in small artery and venous reconstructive surgery has been studied predominantly in the laboratory.[3-6]

Although initial results were unsatisfactory, an arteriovenous fistula for treating arterial insufficiency has been investigated extensively, and certain types of arteriovenous fistulas were shown to maintain viability of ischemic extremities in experimental animals.[7-9]

The rationale for the use of an arteriovenous fistula in the treatment of the ischemic extremity is twofold.[1,8] first, an arteriovenous fistula is a potent stimulus for the formation of collateral vessels about the fistula. Second, the fistula establishes retrograde arterial blood flow in the distal venous limb of the fistula.

In 1966, Blaisdell et al.[10] reported the use of a "Y" fistula to maintain the patency of a prosthetic graft used in reconstruction of small arteries in 4 cases but noted subsequent failure in 3 of them. However, various types of reconstructions have been developed and have achieved relatively good patency rates.

Dardik et al.[1] reported 13 cases of composite side-to-side arteriovenous fistula with simultaneous distal end-to-side anastomosis of bypass to fistula in tibial and peroneal reconstruction.

The indication for adjunctive arteriovenous fistula was inadequate runoff and pedal arch in all 13 patients, calcification in 9, multifocal stenosis in 3, small caliber of the crural artery in 4, and previous surgery in 9. In a population undergoing limb salvage with multiple failed reconstructions, they achieved a 1-year patency rate of 39% and a limb salvage rate of 52%. They suggested that an adjunctive arteriovenous fistula can maintain patency in a femoro tibial or peroneal bypass graft while preserving flow into the markedly diseased distal circulation.

Kusaba et al.[11] also reported 57% graft patency rate in 63 cases of end-stage occlusive arterial disease of the lower extremity with use of the "A-V shunt procedure."

The most critical factor in maintaining a patent graft in instances of inadequate runoff is the ability to shunt an adequate volume from the arterial circuit into the low-resistance venous circuit.[1] Stagnation and eventual thrombosis can be prevented with creation of an arteriovenous fistula. Thus distal arteriovenous fistulas provide improved patency rates by the augmentation of graft flow.

An arteriovenous fistula may cause an increase in blood volume and cardiac output. This did not occur in this series, presumably because fistulas were constructed to small veins with an average diameter of less than 2 mm. Schenk et al.[12] reported that fistulas placed in medium-sized vessels are well tolerated if they are less than 1 cm in diameter and carry less than 20% of the cardiac output.

Development of venous hypertension and edema is another theoretical objection in the construction of an arteriovenous fistula. We observed transient edema of the lower leg in nearly all patients. Supportive measures such as leg elevation and/or wearing an elastic stocking could adequately control the progression of edema. Leg edema was usually not evident 2 to 3 weeks postoperatively.

The steal phenomenon has not been demonstrated in this series. The authors reduced the diameter of the vein used in construction of the arteriovenous fistula when the lumen was large enough to produce suspected steal of blood from the distal arterial bed.

The patients in this series were all threatened with imminent loss of limb due to end-stage arterial occlusive disease. Conventional bypasses were considered likely to fail because of the probability of graft occlusion. Although long-term results are essential in order to elucidate the role of adjunctive arteriovenous fistulas in these desperate cases of vascular reconstruction, the early patency rate is excellent.

These results demonstrate that an arteriovenous fistula at distal anastomosis of a long femorotibial or peroneal bypass is of benefit when blood flow through the graft is limited with poor runoff.

References

1. Ibrahim IM, Sussman B, Dardik I, Kahn M, Israel M, Kenny M, Dardik H. Adjunctive arteriovenous fistula with tibial and peroneal reconstruction for limb salvage. Am J Surg 1980;140:246.
2. Dean RE, Read RC. The influence of increased blood flow on thrombosis in prosthetic grafts. Surgery 1964;55:581.
3. Blaisdell FW, Lim RC, Hall RD, Thomas AN. Reconstruction of small arteries with an arteriovenous fistula. Arch Surg 1966;92:206.
4. Steinman C, Alpert J, Haimovici H. Inferior vena cava bypass grafts: An experimental evaluation of a temporary arteriovenous fistula on their long term patency. Arch Surg 1966;93:747.
5. Hobson RW, Wright CB. Peripheral side-to-side arteriovenous fistula. Hemodynamics and application in venous reconstruction. Am J Surg 1973;126:411.
6. Wilson SE, Johauer A, Stone RT, Stanley TM. Patency of biologic and prosthetic inferior vena cava grafts with distal limb fistula. Arch Surg 1978;113:1174.
7. Root HD, Cruz HB. Effects of arteriovenous fistula on the devascularized limb. JAMA 1965;191:645.
8. Matolo NM, Cohen SE, Wolfman EF, Jr. Use of an arteriovenous fistula for treatment of the severely ischemic extremity. Ann Surg 1976;184:622.
9. Johansen K, Bernstein EF. Revascularization of the ischemic canine hindlimb by arteriovenous reversal. Ann Surg 1979;190:243.
10. Blaisdell FW, Lim RC, Hall AD, Thomas AN. Revascularization of severely ischemic extremities with an arteriovenous fistula. Am J Surg 1966;112:166.
11. Kusaba A, Inokuchi K, Furuyama M, Okadome K. A new revascularization procedure for extensive arterial occlusions of lower extremity. A-V shunt procedure. J Cardiovasc Surg 1982;23:99.
12. Schenk WG, Martin JW, Leslie MB, Partin AB. The regional hemodynamics of chronic experimental arteriovenous fistulae. Surg Gynecol Obstet 1960;110:44.

XVI
Acute Arterial Occlusion

48
Results of Treatment of Acute Arterial Occlusion

Takashi Komiyama, Hiroshi Shigematsu, Hiroshi Yasuhara, and Tetsuichiro Muto

Introduction

Despite recent advances in vascular surgery, acute arterial occlusions still cause death and the loss of limbs. Over the past 15 years, we have treated 176 patients who suffered from acute arterial occlusions. The purpose of this report is to present the results of treatment of these cases.

Patients and Methods

One hundred seventy-six patients who suffered from acute arterial occlusions required treatment, including conservative therapy, in our department of the University of Tokyo Hospital. Of these 176 patients, 160 had their cases documented and reviewed during the 15-year-period from January 1977 to May 1992. Their average age was 63.2 years (range 10–87). One hundred thirty-four were male and 26 were female.

The primary treatments were classified as reconstruction, conservative therapy, or limb amputation. The reconstruction group (R) included patients who had bypass reconstruction, thrombectomy, embolectomy, thromboendarterectomy (TEA), and profundaplasty. The conservative therapy group (C) included patients who had anticoagulation therapy with heparin and warfarin, thrombolytic therapy with urokinase, and other drug therapy with prostaglandin E_1. The results are classified as limb salvage, limb amputation, or death.

Results

Gender, Age, and Cause of Occlusion

There are two causes of acute arterial occlusion: acute thrombosis and arterial embolism. The two conditions were differentiated primarily on the basis of arteriography, operative findings, and pathological data. Since there were wide differences between the therapeutic and prognostic aspects of these two conditions, they must be addressed separately.

Of 160 patients who were treated for acute arterial occlusion, 50 suffered from embolism and 110 suffered from thrombosis. Among the 110 patients with thrombosis, 99 were men and 11 were women. They ranged in age from 10 to 87 years, with a mean of 60.8. The cases of thrombosis in our series were due to atherosclerotic obstruction (43%), graft occlusion (24%), traumatic arterial injuries (18%), various aneurysms (9%), and other causes (6%).

In contrast, the average age of the 50 patients in the embolism group of 35 men and 15 women was 68.0 (range 46 to 82), which is significantly higher than that in the thrombosis group (Mann–Whitney U test, $p < 0.05$). Embolisms were due to cardiogenic origins (78%), atherosclerotic debris (12%), mural thrombi in aneurysms (7%), and other causes (3%).

Site of Occlusion

The sites of occlusion in thrombosis and embolism also differed (Fig. 48.1). While only 5% of the thromboses occurred in the upper extremities, 21% of the embolisms occurred in these areas. Occlusion of the aorta occurred in 14% of the thrombosis cases but in only 3% of the embolism cases. Occlusion of the iliac arteries occurred in 23% of the thrombosis cases but in only 18% of the embolism cases. In the lower extremities, thrombosis tended to occur in more proximal sites than embolism.

Ankle–Brachial Pressure Index

The preoperative ankle–brachial pressure index (ABI) was measured in 16 patients with thrombosis and in 10 with embolism. The average preoperative

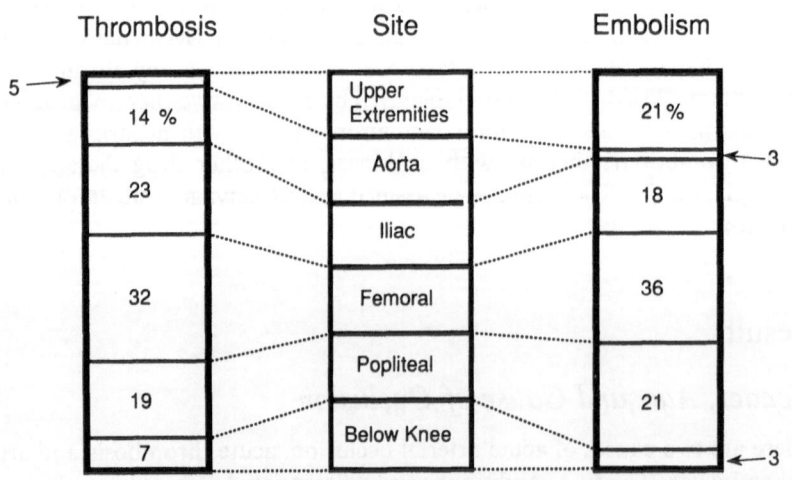

FIGURE 48.1. Sites of occlusion in thrombosis and embolism.

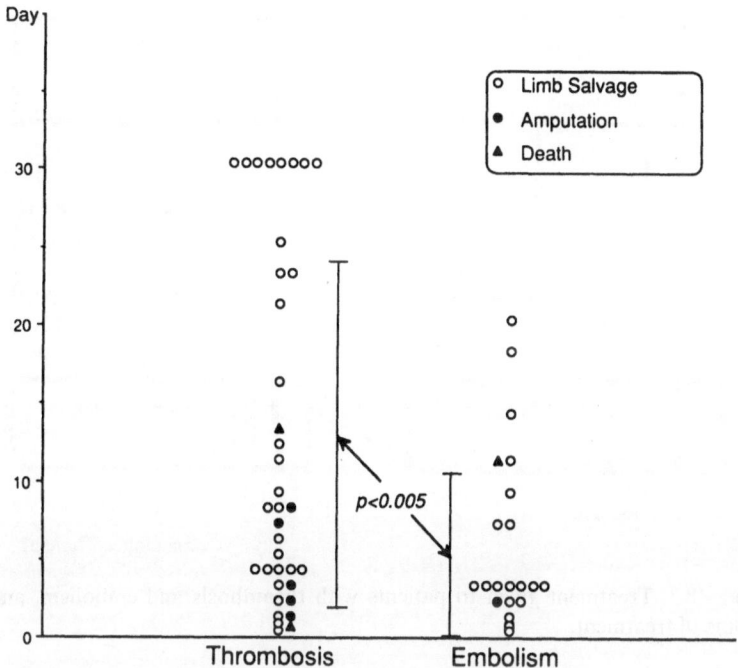

FIGURE 48.2. Duration from the onset of symptoms to treatment in patients with thrombosis and embolism, and the outcome of treatment.

ABIs of the two groups (0.36 ± 0.31 in the thrombosis cases vs. 0.32 ± 0.17 in the embolism cases) were not significantly different.

Duration Prior to Treatment

It is well known that early treatment of acute arterial occlusion leads to a good prognosis. Figure 48.2 shows the duration from the onset of symptoms to the beginning of treatment in both groups. Patients with thrombosis (12.6 days) received treatment significantly later than those with embolism (4.8 days) (Mann-Whitney U test, $p < 0.005$).

Types of Treatment

Figure 48.3 shows the treatments and the results in these patients. Arterial reconstructions were performed in 70% of the patients in both groups. However, there were differences between the reconstructive procedures used in the thrombosis and the embolism groups. Bypass reconstructions were performed in 39 (51%) of 77 cases with thrombosis. On the other hand, while only 4 (11%) of 35 cases with embolism received bypass operations, 29 (83%) patients received a simple embolectomy. In the thrombosis group, limbs were successfully salvaged in 66 (79%) of 77 R patients and in 14 (70%) of 20 C

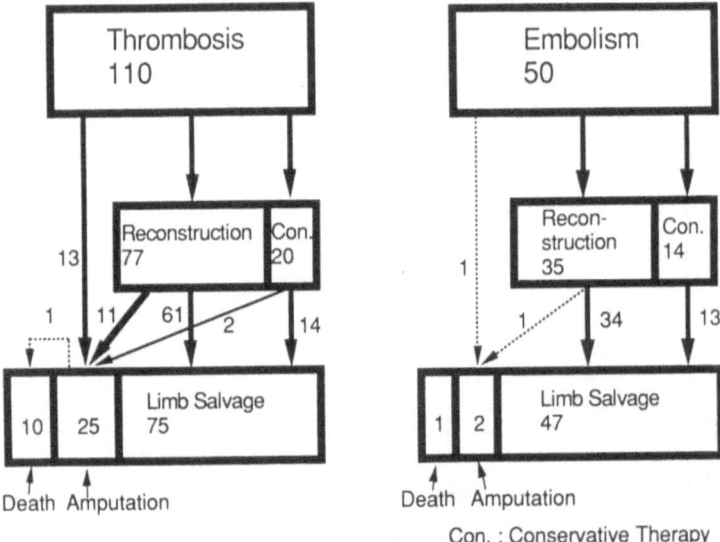

FIGURE 48.3. Treatment given to patients with thrombosis and embolism, and the outcome of treatment.

patients. A total of 75 (68%) of 110 patients with thrombosis ultimately received successful treatment. In the embolism group, the limbs of 34 (97%) of 35 R patients and of 13 (93%) of 14 C patients were salvaged. A total of 47 (94%) of 50 patients with embolism ultimately received successful treatment.

Amputation

Limb amputation was the primary treatment in 13 patients (12%) of the thrombosis group and in 1 patient (2%) of the embolism group. In the thrombosis group, limb amputation was performed in 11 of 77 R cases and in 2 of 20 C cases. One of these 13 patients lost his life. Ultimately 25 (23%) of 110 patients with thrombosis had a successful limb amputation. In contrast, limb amputations were performed in only 2 (4%) of 50 patients with embolism: in 1 patient who underwent limb amputation after reconstruction and in another patient who underwent limb amputation as a primary treatment.

Mortality and Causes of Death

Ultimately, 11 patients (10 with thrombosis and 1 with embolism) lost their lives. The overall mortality rate from acute arterial occlusions was 6.9%, which reflects mortality rates of 9.1% in patients with thrombosis and 2% in patients with embolism. The 10 patients with thrombosis died of metabolic complications after revascularization, so-called myonephropathic metabolic syndrome (MNMS) (5 cases), myocardial infarction (3 cases, including 2 after arterial reconstruction and 1 after limb amputation), and other causes (3 cases, including 1 after arterial reconstruction and 2 after conservative therapy). The patient in the embolism group who died suffered from multiple organ embolism (so-called shower embolism) after thromboembolectomy. MNMS caused death in 5 (45%) of the fatal cases (3.1% of the total 160 cases).

Discussion

Despite the fact that it is important to differentiate between thrombosis and embolism to determine a proper course of treatment, it is often difficult to assess them accurately, especially in patients who require emergency treatment. In this study, the incidence of thrombosis in acute arterial occlusions was 70%, which is higher than the 30% to 63% reported by other studies.[1,2] Although the reason for this discrepancy is not clear, it may be due to the increasing incidence of acute thrombosis as the cause of atherosclerotic occlusive diseases.[3-6] From this point of view, it should be noted that the number of patients who suffered from embolisms in atherosclerotic lesions was about one-fifth of the total number of patients with embolisms. In our study, preoperative ABI was not an adequate indicator of the severity of acute arterial occlusion. Although there are many parameters that show the severity of ischemia in the lower extremities, it is still difficult to decide upon the most appropriate treatment for each patient. A differential diagnosis cannot be made without taking a careful history and physical examination. The sudden onset of symptoms, a history of cardiac diseases, a prior embolic episode, and the absence of a history of claudication and atrophy in the contralateral limb may indicate the likelihood of embolism. Angiography can also be extremely useful in differentiating between thrombosis and embolism.

There was a tendency for the duration from the onset of symptoms to treatment to be slightly longer in our study than in other reports.[7,8] This difference may be due to our policy of performing the delayed reconstruction even in the patients with critical but reversible ischemia who have been treated conservatively more than a week after onset in other institutes. Various reasons have been suggested to explain why patients with thrombosis waited longer to receive treatment than those with embolism.[9,10] The main reason involved differences in the development of collateral arteries. Since patients who suffered from embolism felt more severe pain than those who suffered from thrombosis, they may have sought treatment sooner.

Bypass reconstructions were performed in 51% of the patients with thrombosis, whereas 83% of the patients with embolism were treated with a simple embolectomy. This is the same tendency observed in other institutions after the invention of the Fogarty balloon catheter.[11] The delayed embolectomy has gradually been recognized to be effective in patients who present more than a week after the embolic episode with reversible ischemic extremities.[11]

This study confirmed the validity of this therapy, although the detrimental metabolic disorders caused by revascularization could not be ignored.

In this study, limb salvage was achieved in 76% of the patients who suffered from acute arterial occlusions, with an overall mortality rate of 6.9%. The rate of limb salvage was higher with embolism (94%) than with thrombosis (68%), while the mortality rate was lower in embolism (2%) than in thrombosis (9.1%). Although different reports involve different patient populations, types of diseases, and sites of occlusions, limb salvage may be achieved in 50% to 70% of patients with acute arterial occlusions, with mortality rates ranging from 10% to 30%.[3] Although our results might compare favorably to other reports, especially with regard to patients with embolism, several patients who suffered from thrombosis lost their limbs or their lives. MNMS caused half of the deaths in this study. In addition, the mortality rate due to MNMS was 3.1% of the total cases and 4.5% of the 112 patients who received reconstructive operations. The clinical course of this syndrome may be affected not only by the duration of the occlusions but also by the extent, the level, and the type of arterial occlusion.

Conclusion

Acute arterial occlusions can be caused by either thrombosis or embolism. Our results suggest the importance of an accurate diagnosis because of the different treatments and the prognoses of these two conditions.

References

1. Haimovici H. Acute arterial thrombosis. In: *Vascular Surgery*. Norwalk, CT: Appleton & Lange, 1989, pp. 354–360.
2. Hirose M, Matsumoto K. The complications and their treatments of the reconstructive operations to patients with acute arterial occlusion. Geka 1984;46:1493–1498.
3. Ozaki S, et al. Investigation of the cases of acute arterial thrombosis of lower extremities. J Jpn Surg Soc 1987;88:205–210.
4. Furuta G, et al. Acute arterial thrombosis. Cardioangiology 1981;10:409–418 (Japanese).
5. Tawes RL, Jr, et al. Arterial thromboembolism. Arch. Surg 1985;120:595–599.
6. Sakaguchi S, et al. Problems in treatments of arterial thrombosis. J Jpn Coll Angiol 1980;20:75–79 (Japanese).
7. Kondo J, Matsumoto A. Treatments and results of acute arterial occlusion. Geka 1984;46:1499–1506 (Japanese).
8. Hoshino S. Ischemia by acute arterial occlusion and limb salvage. Geka 1991;53:357–363.
9. Hollier LH. Acute Arterial Occlusion. Cardiovasc Dis 1982;13:49–57.
10. Shigematsu H, Morioka Y. Acute arterial occlusion and limb salvage. Operation 1988;42:9–17 (Japanese).
11. Brewster DC, et al. Arterial thromboembolism. In: *Vascular Surgery*. Philadelphia: WB Saunders, 1989, pp. 548–564.

XVII
Amputation

49
Should Chemical Sympathectomy Precede Below-Knee Amputation?

Leonid Lantsberg and Mark Goldman

Introduction

Amputation continues to present a challenge for surgeons, especially in the choice of amputation level. Preservation of the knee joint increases the likelihood of successful rehabilitation, but unfortunately a more distal amputation exposes the patient to an increased risk of wound breakdown, which varies from 10% to 50% in most series.[1]

Lumbar sympathectomy still holds a place as an attempt at limb preservation in the treatment of ischemia of the lower limb, especially when a patient is considered unsuitable for direct arterial reconstruction.[2]

We have explored the possibility of an alternative use of chemical lumbar sympathectomy to preserve the knee joint in patients already condemned to major amputation.

Materials and Methods

We studied 21 consecutive patients suffering from severe ischemia of the lower extremities, which had led to gangrene or rest pain of the foot.

The median age was 73 years (range 33–87). Ten patients were suffering from diabetes mellitus. When amputation was indicated by the clinical condition of the patient, the skin flaps for proposed long posterior flap (Burgess type) were drawn prior to operation. The cutaneous microcirculation was assessed at the distal limit of the anterior flap by laser Doppler flowmetry (LDF).

The LDF unit used in the study (model periflux PF2, Perimed, Sweden) emitted a monochromatic helium-neon laser beam that was conducted to the skin by flexible fibro-optic probe. The Doppler shift detected by sensitive photodetector is related in a linear fashion to the mean velocity of red blood cells within skin capillaries.

Measurements were obtained with the patient in the supine position with the measuring head in contact with the skin, heated to 42°C, to ensure vasodilation during the recording. The measurements obtained reflected an average over a semicircle of skin approximately 1 mm in radius. The LDF monitor was set at a gain frequency of 10 kHz, and values were expressed in millivolts (mV).

The level of amputation was chosen at operation by traditional clinical criteria, attempting to preserve maximum limb length. Below-knee (BK) amputations were performed with a posterior flap technique (Burgess), and above-knee (AK) procedures with equal anterior and posterior flaps.

To examine the effect of chemical lumbar sympathectomy (CLS), 21 additional patients with severe limb ischemia had LDF measurements at the same BK site, utilizing the above-described method. There were 11 men and 10 women with a median age of 75 (39–88 years). Patients underwent CLS using an injection of 8 ml of phenol under x-ray control. Trophic changes of their limbs were an indication for sympathetic ablation in 14 patients, 3 complained of rest pain, and 1 had claudication. Two patients were suffering from vasospastic disorders and 1 had Buerger's disease.

One week after sympathectomy an identical repeat examination of the leg was undertaken.

Results

Fifteen patients (from the "amputation" study) underwent BK and 6 AK amputation, all of which healed by primary intention. The median LDF values obtained on the anterior skin flaps in the BK group were 42 mV (range 20–85) (Fig. 49.1). In the group of patients that were selected by clinical judgment for primary AK amputation statistical significance was noted at the 1% level (Wilcoxon unpaired samples test) in LDF values on BK flaps; the median flow on anterior flaps was as low as 11 mV (9–20).

Twenty of our 21 patients (from the "sympathectomy" study) reported improvements of limb condition or relief of symptoms after sympathectomy. LDF values rose significantly from 26 mV (10–75) to 50 mV (10–100) ($p < 0.001$). In particular, 7 patients had initial LDF levels below 20 mV, and in 5 chemical sympathectomy produced elevation to the level commensurate with BK stump healing.

Discussion

In our retrospective study,[3] chemical lumbar sympathectomy appears to be appropriate for patients with critical ischemia in whom alternative reconstruction procedures cannot be utilized.

We therefore assessed sympathectomy by measuring skin blood flow before and after the procedure using LDF and transcutaneous oxygen tension

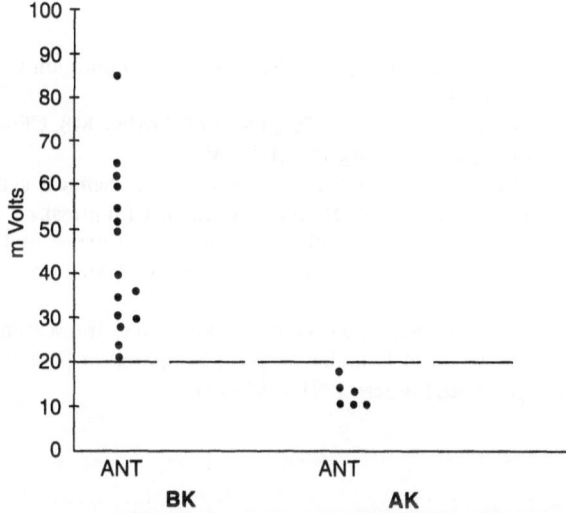

FIGURE 49.1. Laser Doppler flowmetry values obtained from BK flaps greater than or equal to 20 mV were associated with primary BK stump healing. Patients selected for AK amputation had LDF values less than 20 mV.

(TCpO$_2$) techniques. Our results have shown that sympathetic ablation of the leg increased skin blood flow and skin oxygenation at the foot and below the knee.[4]

Improved circulation of the foot after sympathectomy is presumably the mechanism whereby our patients gained clinical relief of symptoms, but it is important to note that our measurements cannot indicate the contribution of pain relief and control of infection that may also follow sympathectomy.

Assessment of skin flap perfusion by LDF appears to be a useful and simple objective test in patients undergoing amputation.[5]

The results of this study showed that preoperative LDF values of less than 20 mV in the BK flap are correlated with failure to heal at the BK level. All BK patients in our series had cutaneous LDF values greater than or equal to 20 mV, and none of them failed to heal. By contrast, in all AK amputees skin LDF values at BK levels were less than 20 mV.

In practical terms, our findings may have important implications for patients faced with inevitable amputation due to foot gangrene. Though such patients would not normally be considered for chemical sympathectomy, our study suggests that better results might be achieved in some patients following amputation, or a lower level of amputation might be possible if this procedure was performed preoperatively. We think that chemical lumbar sympathectomy can improve BK skin blood flow and may enhance primary wound healing.

References

1. Barnes RW, Thornhill B, Nix L, et al. Prediction of amputation wound healing. Arch Surg 1981;116:80–83.
2. Collins GS, Rich NM, Glagett CP, Salander SM, Spebar MS. Clinical results of lumber sympathectomy. Am Surg 1981;1:31–35.
3. Lantsberg L, Goldman M, Hibbert R, Khoda J. Is chemical sympathectomy worthwhile in the ischemic leg? J Bloodless Med Surg (in press).
4. Lantsberg L, Goldman M. Low limb sympathectomy assessed by laser Doppler blood flow and transcutaneous oxygen measurements. J Med Eng Technol 1990; 14:182–183.
5. Lantsberg L, Goldman M. Laser Doppler flowmetry, transcutaneous oxygen tension measurements and Doppler pressure compared in patients undergoing amputation. Eur J Vasc Surgery 1991;5:195–197.

XVIII
Vascular Grafts

50
Increased Resistance to Staphylococcal Graft Infection by Rifampicin Impregnation of Gelatin-Sealed Dacron

JOHN P. FLETCHER, J. AVRAMOVIC, J. KENNY, AND F. SARDELIC

Introduction

A vascular prosthetic graft is susceptible of becoming infected from contamination at the time of graft insertion, at a subsequent reoperation, or from seeding onto the graft during an episode of bacteremia, either early or late after graft insertion. Infection of a vascular prosthesis is associated with significant morbidity and mortality, with reported incidences ranging from 0.25% to 6%.[1-5] At our institution, similar to the experience of others, a 3.4% incidence of prosthetic vascular graft infection was caused by *Staphylococcus aureus* in two-thirds of cases, with *Staphylococcus epidermidis* being responsible for the majority of the remainder.[5]

Our vascular graft of choice for aortic reconstruction has been a gelatin-sealed knitted Dacron graft (Gelsoft, Vascutek, Scotland). The gelatin seal of this graft has an affinity for rifampicin, which is incorporated by a process of ionic binding to carboxyl groups of succinylated gelatin. In vitro studies have shown retention of rifampicin activity for up to 4 days[6] and in vivo studies for at least 2 days.[7] Rifampicin has very strong antistaphylococcal activity and is not a commonly used antibiotic in clinical practice, making it an attractive prophylactic agent for this use.

The efficacy of rifampicin impregnation of gelatin-sealed Dacron in reducing vascular graft infection has been studied in a sheep carotid artery model, and this chapter summarizes our experimental work.

Materials and Methods

An animal model was used in which a 2-cm length by 5-mm diameter interposition graft was placed in sheep carotid artery and inoculated before wound closure with 10^8 colony forming units (cfu) of *Staphylococcus aureus*. This concentration of organisms had been shown to cause infection in all prosthetic grafts if no systemic or local antibiotic was used.[8]

Animal operations were approved by the Animal Care and Ethics Committee and were performed under general anesthesia. The *Staphylococcus aureus* inoculum was prepared from human blood culture isolate. After recovery, the sheep were returned to grazing for 3 weeks and then anesthetized again for harvesting of the vascular graft and determination of the presence or absence of graft infection.[9]

Four groups of animals were studied, with one to four subgroups in each group. Group 1 received untreated grafts, with polytetrafluoroethylene (PTFE) to subgroup 1a, knitted unsealed Dacron to subgroup 1b, and gelatin sealed Dacron to subgroup 1c. Group 2 received a gelatin-sealed Dacron graft with perioperative intravenous antibiotic (cefoxitin). Group 3 had the wound irrigated with rifampicin saline solution (1 mg/ml) after graft insertion prior to wound closure; subgroup 3a received PTFE, subgroup 3b knitted unsealed Dacron, and subgroup 3c gelatin-sealed Dacron. Group 4 received a graft which had been soaked in rifampicin saline solution (1 mg/ml at 37°C for 15 minutes) prior to insertion; subgroup 4a received PTFE, subgroup 4b knitted unsealed Dacron, subgroup 4c gelatin-sealed Dacron, and subgroup 4d gelatin-sealed Dacron with perioperative intravenous antibiotic (cefoxitin).

Results

The results are summarized in Table 50.1. All untreated grafts in group 1 became infected. Use of perioperative intravenous antibiotic in group 2 reduced the graft infection rate to 75%. Irrigation of the wound with rifampicin saline solution in group 3 reduced the infection rate to 27%. Soaking of the

TABLE 50.1. Summary of results for each group of sheep.

Group	Total no. grafts	No. infected
Group 1: Untreated grafts		
1a: PTFE	10	10
1b: unsealed Dacron	10	10
1c: gelatin-sealed Dacron	10	10
Group 2: Intravenous antibiotic		
2a: gelatin-sealed Dacron with cefoxitin	8	6
Group 3: Wound irrigation with rifampicin		
3a. PTFE	10	3
3b: unsealed Dacron	10	2
3c: gelatin-sealed Dacron	10	3
Group 4: Rifampicin graft soaking		
4a: PTFE	10	8
4b: unsealed Dacron	10	6
4c: gelatin-sealed Dacron	10	1
4d: gelatin-sealed Dacron with cefoxitin	10	2

graft in rifampicin saline solution prior to insertion in group 4 further reduced the graft infection rate to 15% in gelatin-sealed Dacron grafts, but the infection rate in PTFE grafts remained high at 80%.

When graft infection occurred, phage typing was used to confirm that the infecting organism was identical to the inoculating organism. The infecting organism was also tested for rifampicin sensitivity, and there was no evidence of development of resistance to rifampicin.

The reduction in graft infection with intravenous antibiotic was significant (chi-square 3.69, $p = 0.05$). The reduction in graft infection was highly significant both for rifampicin wound irrigation (chi-square 31.65 $p < 0.001$) and for rifampicin impregnation of gelatin-sealed grafts (chi-square 34.94, $p < 0.001$). There was a significant difference between rifampicin soaking of gelatin-sealed Dacron and unsealed (Dacron and PTFE) grafts (chi-square 10.23, $p = 0.001$).

Discussion

Vascular graft infection is a serious complication of vascular surgery, with a high mortality and amputation rate. It is believed that most infections occur at the time of graft insertion,[2,10] and vascular surgeons are mindful of strict aseptic technique. Perioperative intravenous antibiotics are used routinely.[11] Bonding of an antibiotic to a vascular graft has been shown experimentally to be an effective additional prophylactic measure to further reduce the risk of graft infection.[12-16] However, this process has been limited by the complex preparation required for chemical bonding to the graft and by the rapid elution of antibiotic from the graft when it is passively incorporated.[17]

Rifampicin impregnation of gelatin-sealed Dacron is readily accomplished by soaking the graft for 15 minutes in warm saline (37°C) to which is added rifampicin to achieve a concentration of 1 mg/ml. The simplicity of this process makes it readily applicable to clinical practice. Rifampicin has a wide spectrum of activity against Gram-positive bacteria, especially staphylococci,[18] as well as Gram-negative organisms. In our experience and that of others, *Staphylococcus aureus* and *Staphylococcus epidermidis* have been the main pathogens responsible for vascular graft infection.[3,5] Rifampicin has been associated with the rapid emergence of resistance, but this has been in situations where the site of infection has a heavy bacterial population and when rifampicin is used as a single agent for prolonged periods.[19-21] The load of organisms likely to be encountered when used for prophylaxis in vascular surgery should be small, and rifampicin has been shown to be effective in eliminating small inocula of staphylococci.[22] In clinical practice, with this application of graft impregnation the rifampicin will be used as a once-only dose in conjunction with perioperative intravenous antibiotics, usually a cephalosporin. The use of rifampicin in combination with another antibiotic appears to limit the emergence of bacterial resistance.[7,21] Of particular note is that in our experimental work we have not encountered rifampicin resistance when impregnated grafts have become infected.

Wound irrigation alone with rifampicin was associated with a significant reduction in graft infection in our animal studies. However, there was a further reduction in infection rate with rifampicin graft impregnation, and there was a significant difference between gelatin-sealed Dacron grafts and unsealed grafts (Dacron and PTFE) soaked in rifampicin. It is likely that wound irrigation will lead to some graft impregnation when a gelatin-sealed Dacron graft is used, but soaking of the graft will give a more certain impregnation.

Rifampicin has been a very well tolerated antibiotic, but adverse effects encountered have been gastrointestinal upset, a "flu-like" syndrome, renal impairment, thrombocytopenia, and hepatic dysfunction.[7] The risk of adverse effects should be minimal with rifampicin graft impregnation because of the very small systemic absorption, estimated to be no more than 20 mg.[7]

On the basis of our experimental work, we have undertaken initial clinical trials of the use of rifampicin-impregnated gelatin-sealed Dacron grafts in patients having aortic reconstructive surgery, and this has confirmed that this method is readily adaptable to routine clinical practice.

A clinical study to demonstrate a significant difference in the incidence of vascular graft infection would require large numbers of patients. As there does not appear to be a significant difference in long-term results of prosthetic femoropopliteal bypass between Dacron and PTFE,[23] we have commenced a multicenter study in which patients having an infrainguinal prosthetic vascular graft are randomized to receive either a gelatin-sealed Dacron graft or a PTFE graft, with or without rifampicin impregnation.

In conclusion, rifampicin impregnation of gelatin-sealed Dacron vascular grafts has been shown experimentally to be effective in reducing the incidence of graft infection after a bacterial challenge of *Staphylococcus aureus*. Initial clinical trials have confirmed its application to routine clinical practice in aortic surgery, and an ongoing randomized, prospective trial for infrainguinal reconstruction has commenced.

References

1. Goldstone J, Moore WS. Infection in vascular prostheses: Clinical manifestations and surgical management. Am J Surg 1974;128:225–233.
2. Liekweg WG, Greenfield LJ. Vascular prosthetic infections: Collected experience and results of treatment. Surgery 1977;81:335–342.
3. Blunt TJ. Synthetic vascular graft infections. Surgery 1983;93:733–746.
4. Reilly LM, Altman H, Lusby RJ, Kersh RA, Ehrenfeld WK, Stoney RJ. Late results following surgical management of vascular graft infection. J Vasc Surg 1984;1:36–44.
5. Fletcher JP, Dryden M, Sorrell TC. Infection of vascular prostheses. Aust NZ J Surg 1991;61:432–435.
6. Ashton TR, Cunningham JD, Paton D, Maini R. Antibiotic loading of vascular

grafts. Proceedings of the 16th Annual Meeting of the Society for Biomaterials, Charleston, South Carolina, 1990, p. 235.

7. Goeau-Brissonniere O, Leport C, Bacourt F, Lebrault C, Comte R, Pechere J-C. Prevention of vascular graft infection by rifampin bonding to a gelatin-sealed Dacron graft. Ann Vasc Surg 1991;5:408–412.

8. Fletcher JP, Dryden M, Munro R, Xu JH, Hehir MD. Establishment of a vascular graft infection model in the sheep carotid artery. Aust NZ J Surg 1990;60:801–803.

9. Avramovic Jr, Fletcher JP. Rifampicin impregnation of a protein-sealed Dacron graft: An infection-resistant prosthetic vascular graft. Aust NZ J Surg 1991;61:436–440.

10. Szylagyi DE, Smith RF, Elliott JP, et al. Infection in arterial reconstruction with synthetic grafts. Ann Surg 1972;176:321–333.

11. Kaiser AB, Clayson KR, Mulherin JL, et al. Antibiotic prophylaxis in vascular surgery. Ann Surg 1978;188:283–289.

12. McDougal EG, Burnham SJ, Johnson G. Rifampicin protection against experimental graft sepsis. J Vasc Surg 1986;4:5–7.

13. Moore WS, Chvapil M, Seiffert G, Keown K. Development of an infection-resistant vascular prosthesis. Arch Surg 1981;116:1403–1407.

14. Shue WB, Worosilo SC, Donetz AP, Trooskin SZ, Harvey RA, Creco RS. Prevention of vascular prosthetic infection with an antibiotic-bonded Dacron graft. J Vasc Surg 1988;8:600–605.

15. Clark RE, Magraf HW. Antibacterial vascular grafts with improved thromboresistance. Arch Surg 1974;109:150–162.

16. Krag LE, Solhcim K. Antibiotic binding polytetrafluoroethylene via glucosaminoglycan-keratin luminal coating. Surgery 1986;100:629–634.

17. Powell TW, Burnham SJ, Johnson G. A passive system using rifampicin to create an infection-resistant vascular prosthesis. Surgery 1983;94:765–769.

18. Thornsberry C, Hill BC, Swenson JM, et al. Rifampicin: Spectrum of antibacterial activity. Rev Infect Dis 1983; 5 (Suppl 3):S412–S419.

19. Acar F, Goldstein FW, Duval J. Use of rifampicin for the treatment of serious staphylococcal and Gram-negative infections. Rev Infect Dis 1983;51 (Suppl 3):S502–S507.

20. Kunin CM, Brandt O, Wood HG. Bacteriologic studies of rifampicin: A new semi-synthetic antibiotic. J Infect Dis 1969;119:132–138.

21. Sande SA. The use of rifampicin in the treatment of non-tuberculous infections: An overview. Rev Infect Dis 1983;5 (Suppl 3):S399–S411.

22. Mandell GL, Vent KT. Killing of intraleucocytic *Staphylococcus aureus* by rifampicin: In vitro and in vivo studies. J Infect Dis 1972;125:486–489.

23. Rosenthal D, Evans RD, McKinsey J, Seagraves A, Lamis PA, Clark MD, Daniel WW. Prosthetic above-knee femoropopliteal bypass for intermittent claudication. J Cardiovasc Surg 1990;31:462–468.

51
Involvement of Growth Factors in Pseudointimal Hyperplasia, Analyzed by Synthetic Somatostatin Analogues

Jun-ichi Kambayashi, Suguru Shibuya, and Makoto Watase

Introduction

Pseudointimal hyperplasia (PH) is known as a major etiologic factor for late graft failure. Nevertheless, studies of the histology and pathogenesis of PH have been very limited, in contrast to those on intimal hyperplasia (IH), which is associated with stenosis or occlusion of native artery or vein grafts. During our experimental studies on venous prostheses,[1-3] it was observed that the lumen of polytetrafluoroethylene (PTFE) interposed in rabbit inferior vena cana (IVC) was markedly narrowed by PH within 4 weeks after grafting, regardless of the complete lining of luminal surface with endothelial cells. Ultrastructural studies on this PH by electron microscopy revealed that PH is mainly caused by proliferation of fibroblasts rather than smooth muscle cells, which are known as dominant proliferative cells in IH. When the same graft was interposed in the abdominal aorta of rabbits, histologically identical PH formation was observed but the process was much slower than in the venous system. These findings indicate the animal model to be ideal to study pathogenesis of PH in a relatively short period.

As the first step to elucidate the pathogenesis, attempts were made to study a possible involvement of growth factors in PH. Although a variety of growth factors, such as growth hormone (GH), insulin-like growth factor (IGF), fibroblast growth factor (FGF), epidermal growth factor (EGF), and platelet-derived growth factor (PDGF), have been implicated in IH,[4-7] little is known about the involvement of any growth factor in PH. To investigate this problem, the effect of somatostatin analogues was examined, employing the above-mentioned animal model.

Materials and Methods

Animal Experiments

Twelve Japanese albino rabbits weighing 2.2 to 2.5 kg were used; they were fed a standard diet for at least 1 week before use. The animals were anesthetized by intravenous administration of sodium pentobarbiturate (30 mg/kg), and an additional dose was given to prevent the rabbits from suffering further discomfort. Through a midline laparotomy, the IVC was gently exposed from the renal veins to the iliac bifurcation. After an intravenous bolus injection of heparin (50 U/kg), two small atraumatic clamps were placed on the IVC just below the renal veins and above the bifurcation. A 1-cm segment of IVC was resected and replaced by a 3-cm-long PTFE graft (3 mm internal diameter, 0.32 mm wall thickness, 30 μm internodal distance, kindly supplied by Japan Gore-Tex, Tokyo). The anastomoses were carefully created in end-to-end fashion by a running suture with 7–0 polypropylene. After completion of the anastomosis, the clamps were removed and the venous circulation was restored. After immediate patency was confirmed, the abdomen was closed in one layer and an aminoglycoside antibiotic (amikacin, 100 mg) was intramuscularly given to prevent graft infection. The rabbits were then kept in a cage with a standard diet. After 4 weeks, under the same anesthesia as described above, the patency was examined and the graft was harvested with a portion of host veins after perfusing thoroughly under constant pressure with heparinized saline.

Determination of the Intraluminal Deposit and Histological Examination

The harvested specimen was divided longitudinally into three sections: one quarter for light microscopy (LM), one half for scanning electron microscopy (SEM), and one quarter for future analysis by transmission electron microscopy (TEM). For LM, the specimens were fixed in 10% buffered formaldehyde solution, embedded in paraffin, sectioned, and stained with hematoxylin-eosin. For SEM, the longitudinal halves of the harvested grafts were fixed in 2.5% glutaraldehyde for 12 hours and then rinsed in Millonig buffer for 2 hours, followed by postfixing in 1% osmium tetroxide for an hour. They were then dehydrated in graded ethanol series (50–100%), after which they were dried in a critical point drying system. Before mounting for SEM, dehydrated specimens were weighed and the dried weight of the intraluminal deposit was estimated by subtracting the weight of the unused PTFE graft from that of the dried whole specimen.

Administration of Somatostatin Analogues

Twelve rabbits were equally divided into 3 groups: group 1 (control group), no drug was given; group 2, daily subcutaneous injection of angiopeptin at a dose of 20 μg/kg for 4 weeks from the day of grafting; group 3, daily subcutaneous injection of sandostatin at a dose of 20 μg/kg. Angiopeptin is a synthetic octapeptide somatostatin analogue (Ala-Cys-Tyr-Trp-Lys-Vsl-Cys-Thr) and was purchased from Sigma Chemicals (St. Louis). Sandostatin is also an octapeptide somatostatin analogue (Phe-Cys-Phe-Trp-Lys-Thr-Cys-Thr) and was kindly donated by Sandoz Pharma AG (Basel). Both peptides were dissolved in sterile water for injection. The direct effect of these agents on rabbit platelets was examined by means of platelet aggregation and secretion.

Results

Patency and Dry Weight of the Intraluminal Deposit

All the rabbits survived for 4 weeks after grafting, when the abdomen was reopened and the graft was harvested. No apparent hematoma or infection was noted in the abdominal cavity. All the grafts except for one from a rabbit in the sandostatin group were found to be patent, as summarized in Table 51.1. The mean dry weight of the intraluminal deposit as an indicator of the degree of PH is also summarized in Table 51.1. There was a significant reduction in the weight of group 2 rabbits receiving angiopeptin in comparison with that of control rabbits. Administration of sandostatin, however, was not effective in reducing the weight. The platelet activation either by ADP or thrombin was not influenced by even a high dose of both analogues (data not shown).

Light Microscopic Findings

Longitudinal sections at anastomotic sites and midportions of the harvested grafts were subjected to light microscopic examination to study the thickness of PH and to estimate composition of PH. As reported previously,[3] in this particular model the PH of the midportion was thicker than that of the anastomotic site. Furthermore, the variation of thickness was far less in the midportion than in the anastomotic sites. A representative light micrograph of the midportion from each group is shown in Figure 51.1. Apparently, the thickness of PH in group 2 is thinner than that of group 1 or group 3, which is well correlated with the results of the dry weight mentioned above. It was difficult to identify cell species composing the PH by LM, but the general components were not significantly different among the three groups. Comparing these micrographs, it is found that the difference in the thickness of

TABLE 51.1. Patency and dry weight of the intraluminal deposit.

Group	Patency (4 weeks)	Dry weight of intraluminal deposit (mg per 3-cm graft)
1. No drug	4/4	40 ± 8 (mean $\pm$ SD)
2. Angiopeptin	4/4	26 ± 3*
3. Sandostatin	3/4	40 ± 2

* Significantly lower ($p < 0.05$) than groups 1 and 3.

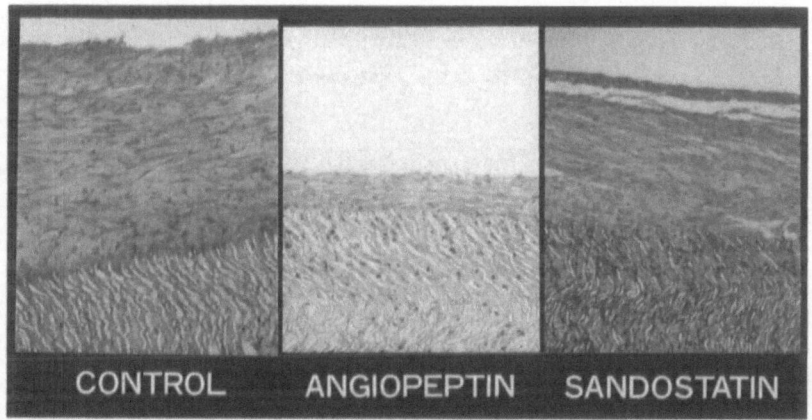

FIGURE 51.1 Light micrographs of longitudinal section of midportion of the grafts harvested from each group. Sections were stained with hematoxylin–eosin. Original magnification is × 50.

TABLE 51.2. Lining of the luminal surface with endothelial cells, based on the findings of SEM.

	Endothelial cell coverage		
Group	Cranial	Middle	Caudal
1. No drug	+ + +	+ +	+ + +
2. Angiopeptin	+ + +	+ +	+ + +
3. Sandostatin	+ + +	+ + +	+ + +

Luminal surface moderately (+ +) or thoroughly (+ + +) covered with mature endothelial cells.

PH is likely due to the difference in the number of spindle cells near the inside surface of the grafts.

Endothelial Cell Lining Observed by Scanning Electron Microscopy

The lining of the intraluminal surface with endothelial-like cells, which have been identified as endothelial cells by TEM[3] was evaluated by SEM and the results are summarized in Table 51.2. In all groups, the luminal surface near the cranial or caudal anastomotic sites was fully covered with endothelial cells. As shown in figure 51.2, the luminal surface of the midportion of the graft from group 1 or 2 was not fully covered with matured endothelial cells, while that from group 3 was fully covered with the flattened matured endothelial cells.

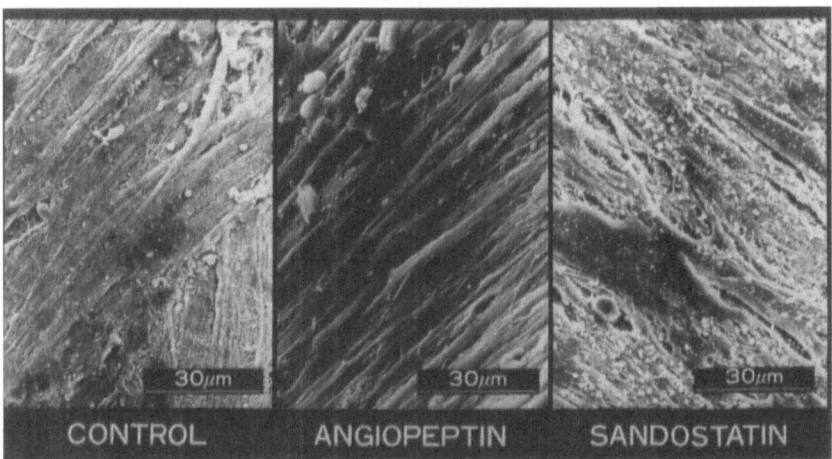

FIGURE 51.2. Scanning electron micrographs of the luminal surface of the midportion of the harvested grafts from each group.

Discussion

Pseudointimal hyperplasia (PH) is defined as intimal thickening of synthetic vascular prostheses,[8] but occasionally this condition has been erroneously called intimal hyperplasia (IH), which is thickening of damaged native vessels or autogenous vein grafts. Because IH has been known to be an important etiologic factor in various disease conditions such as atherosclerosis, restenosis after angioplasty, stenosis of vein grafts, and transplantation-related atherosclerosis, the pathogenesis and the pharmacological control of intimal hyperplasia have been extensively investigated in recent years.[9] At present, it is generally accepted that proliferation and/or migration of smooth muscle cells is the most important etiologic factor for IH and that the proliferation is mediated by certain growth factors, as mentioned earlier. On the contrary, studies on the pathogenesis of PH are very limited and the process is poorly understood, although PH is a major etiologic factor for late occlusion of synthetic vascular prostheses, especially in venous reconstruction.[1,2] We have extensively studied the process and the composition of PH by ultrastructural analysis with TEM, and we have determined that the proliferation of fibroblasts is the main contributing factor in PH.[3] The fibroblasts may be transformed via myofibroblasts into smooth muscle cells.[3]

As probes to elucidate the involvement of growth factors in PH, two kinds of somatostatin analogues, angiopeptin[10] and sandostatin,[11] were employed in the present study. As the half-lives of these octapeptide analogues are significantly longer than that of the original tetradecapeptide somatostatin, it has been shown that daily subcutaneous injection of the analogues in the dose employed in the present study is sufficient to exert a pharmacological effect in laboratory animals.[12] In the present study, angiopeptin apparently suppressed PH without affecting the endothelial lining of the luminal surface. The inhibitory effect of angiopeptin or even any other somatostatin analogues has never been reported before, though it has been shown to inhibit IH due to balloon injury,[13] IH in autogenous vein grafts,[12] and transplantation-associated IH.[14] As it inhibited in vitro proliferation of tumor cells[15] and in vitro thymidine uptake by arterial tissues,[16] the effect of angiopeptin has been considered a direct rather than an indirect action via somatostatin. The direct antiproliferative effect of angiopeptin may be due to interference with receptors for certain growth factors or to intracellular signal transduction after receptor–agonist coupling. The present histological findings suggested that the suppression of PH by angiopeptin is likely due to the inhibition of fibroblast proliferation, although no direct evidence is available at present. As angiopeptin as well as sandostatin exhibited no significant effect on platelet activation which may release PDGF, the suppression of PH by angiopeptin is not mediated by inhibiting a release of PDGF. In contrast, PH was not suppressed at all by another analogue, sandostatin, but this was not surprising because the inhibitory spectrum is apparently different between the two octapeptides. Sandostatin was originally designed to inhibit specifically GH release without affecting the release of insulin or glucagon.[11] Thus, the present observation with sandostatin indicated that GH is not involved in PH. Studies on the direct antiproliferative effect of sandostatin are very limited. Recently, Bensaid et al.[17] reported that sandostatin at a very low dose suppressed FGF-induced rat pancreatic cancer cell proliferation and that this is possibly due to interference with FGF receptors. This finding may rule out positive participation of FGF in the occurrence of PH. There was a slight effect by sandostatin on the extent and the maturity of the endothelial cell lining in the midportion of the grafts. However, there are not enough data to explain the above findings. In conclusion, the findings of the present study clearly demonstrated that growth factor is involved in PH and angiopeptin is a useful tool to analyze the pathogenesis of PH in the future.

References

1. Itoh T, Kambayashi J, Tsujinaka T, Sakon M, Ohshiro T, Mori T. Pathogenesis of early thrombus formation in experimental vein graft. Thrombos Res 1989;53: 357–365.
2. Itoh T, Shiba E, Kambayashi J, Watase M, Kawasaki T, Sakon M, Mori T. Pathogenesis of late thrombus formation in experimental vein grafts. Eur J Vasc Surg 1990;4:625–631.
3. Watase M, Kambayashi J, Itoh T, et al. Ultrastructural analysis of pseudo-intimal hyperplasia of polytetrafluoroethylene prostheses implanted into the venous and arterial systems. Eur J Vasc Surg 1992;6:371–380.
4. Astora S, Foegh M, Conte JV, Cai BR, Ramwell PW. Inhibition of tritium-thymidine incorporation by angiopeptin in the aorta of rabbits after balloon angioplasty. Transplant 1989;21:3695–3696.

5. Cerek B, Fishbein MC, Forrester JS, et al. Induction of insulin-like growth factor messenger RNA in rat aorta after balloon denudation. Circ Res 1990;66:1755–1760.

6. Powell JS, Clozel JP, Muller RKM, et al. Inhibition of angiotensin-converting enzyme prevents myointimal proliferation after vascular injury. Science 1989;245:186–188.

7. Linder V, Lappi DA, Baird, A. et al. Role of basic fibroblast growth factor in vascular lesion formation. Circ Res 1991;68:106–113.

8. Sottiurai VS, Batson RC. Role of myofibroblasts in pseudointima formation. Surgery 1983;94:792–801.

9. Clowes AW, Reidy MA. Prevention of stenosis after vascular reconstruction: Pharmacological control of intimal hyperplasia—A review. J Vasc Surg 1991;13:885–891.

10. Lundergan C, Foegh ML, Vargas R, et al. Inhibition of myointimal proliferation of the rat carotid artery by the peptides, angiopeptini and BIM 23034. Atherosclerosis 1989;80:49–55.

11. Bauer W, Briner U, Doepfner W, et al. SMS 201–995; A very potent and selective octapeptide analogue of somatostatin with prolonged action. Life Sci 1982;31:1133–1140.

12. Calcagno D, Conte JV, Howell MH, et al. Peptide inhibition of neointimal hyperplasia in vein grafts. J Vasc Surg 1991;4:475–479.

13. Conte JV, Foegh ML, Calcagno RB, et al. Peptide inhibition of myointimal proliferation following angioplasty in rabbits. Transplant Proc 1989;21:3686–3688.

14. Foegh ML, Khirabadi BS, Chambers E, et al. Inhibition of coronary artery transplant atherosclerosis in rabbits with angiopeptin, an octapeptide. Atherosclerosis 1989;78:229–236.

15. Taylor JE, Bodgen A, Moreau J-P, et al. In vitro and in vivo inhibition of human small cell lung carcinoma (NCI-H69) growth by somatostatin analogue. Biochem Biophys Res Commun 1988;153:81–86.

16. Vargas R, Bormes GW, Wroblewska B, et al. Angiopeptin inhibits thymidine incorporation in rat carotid artery in vitro. Transplant Proc 1989;21:3702–3704.

17. Besaid M, Tahiri-Jouti N, Cambillau C, et al. Basic fibroblast growth factor induces proliferation of a rat pancreatic cancer cell line. Inhibition by somatostatin. Int J Cancer 1992;50:796–799.

52
Experimental Evaluation of a New Compliant Biological Arterial Substitute

Armin Welz, G. Murrmann, S. Grenzner, R. Triefenbach, and M. Beyer

Introduction

Autologous vessels are the grafts of choice for small arterial grafting. This is especially true with myocardial revascularization. However, due to the increasing number of reoperations and the extension of the indication to the elderly, we have to deal with some patients in whom we may encounter problems harvesting sufficient autologous materials.[1-3] For these cases, a reliable small-diameter arterial graft would be needed.

In the development of new arterial prostheses, most emphasis has been placed on blood compatibility and thrombogenicity. Only a few studies have evaluated the physical characteristics of grafts and arteries.

It is well known that there are three major functions of arteries besides pure blood flow transmission. These are energy transmission, pulse smoothing, and impedance matching.[4-6] They all depend on the elastic behavior of the arterial wall.

The radial compliance C, calculated through the formula

$$C = \frac{\Delta C}{C \Delta P} \times 100\% \tag{1}$$

D = diameter
p = blood pressure

describes the elastic property of the wall of arteries.

The study was done to investigate the compliance of a dialdehyde starch-preserved bovine internal mammary artery (BIMA; Bioflow^R graft, Biovascular, St. Paul, Minnesota) and its changes during graft healing.

Materials and Methods

Experimental Model

The canine femoral artery was used as a model. Twenty small mongrel dogs (mean body weight 20 kg, range 16–27 kg) had the femoral artery of one side

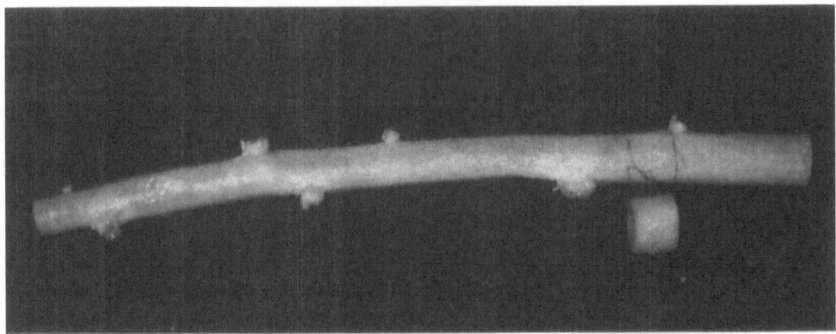

FIGURE 52.1. Dialdehyde starch-preserved BIMA ready for an experimental implantation. The graft is shown together with the cross section of a removed proximal segment.

replaced with the BIMA (Fig. 52.1). For comparison, the opposite side was implanted with a polytetrafluoroethylene (PTFE) graft. The length of all grafts was 7 cm, the diameter 4 mm. The study comprised 2 groups for a 3-month (group I, $n = 10$) and 6-month follow-up (group II, $n = 10$).

Patency was assessed daily by the transcutaneous ultrasound Doppler technique. Suspected graft occlusion was confirmed by angiography. All grafts were harvested at the end of the scheduled follow-up period or immediately after the diagnosis of graft failure.

All animals received humane care, and the experimental protocol satisfied the requirements of the Federal Republic of Germany law for the prevention of cruelty to animals.[7]

Compliance Measurements

To calculate the compliance C (see formula 1), the determination of the small changes in diameter of the vessels during the pulse cycle is crucial. To do this, we developed a new device with implantable sensors based on the physical induction phenomena.

An alternating current, generated at a primary coil, induces an alternating voltage at a secondary coil according to formulas 2 and 3.

$$\Phi' \text{ (flow of induction)} = \frac{1}{c} L_{1,2} I_1 \tag{2}$$

$$E \text{ (electromotive force)} = -\frac{1}{c} \frac{d\Phi'}{dt} \tag{3}$$

I_1 = current at the primary coil
C = electrical constant
$L_{1,2}$ = coefficient of induction

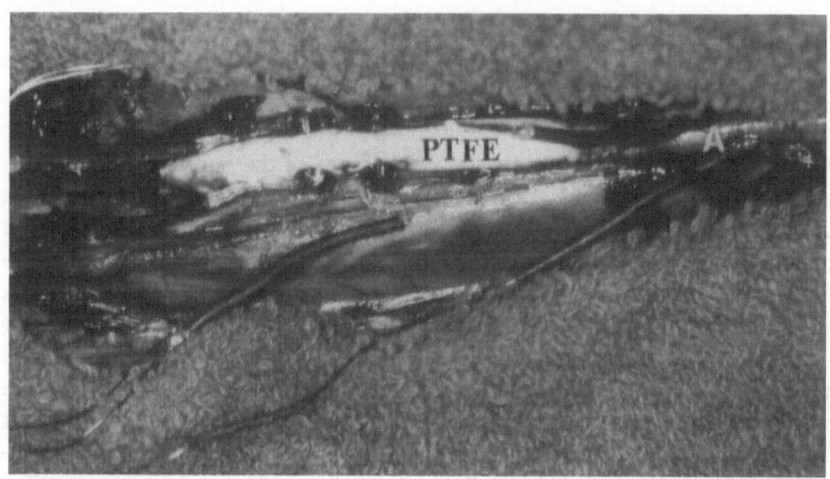

FIGURE 52.2. Implantable device for the measurement of radial compliance. Two sensors are implanted in the PTFE graft (PTFE), one in the femoral artery (A).

The coefficient of induction $L_{1,2}$ depends on, among other factors, the distance between the two coils. This device has been described in detail earlier.[7]

At least two sensors were implanted to one leg of the experimental animals (Fig. 52.2). Each sensor consisted of two small coils ($0.5 \times 1.5 \times 2.5$ mm) which had to be sutured to the vessel wall exactly opposite to each other. One sensor was implanted in the femoral artery 2 cm upstream to the proximal anastomosis, the other in the graft. All sensors of one side were attached to one electrical connector which could be covered subcutaneously.

To determine the arterial blood pressure, a permanent indwelling catheter was introduced into the femoral artery through a side branch.

Compliance measurements were carried out at implantation and after 1, 3, and 6 months.

Graft Healing

To study the healing characteristics, all grafts were fixed with 2% glutaraldehyde. Cross sections of the midgraft area and longitudinal sections of the anastomosis were stained using hematoxylin-eosin (H-E), Elastica van Gieson, and Alcian-periodic-acid-Schiff (PAS) techniques for light microscopy.

Statistics

All results are expressed as mean and standard error of the mean. To confirm statistical significance ($p < 0.05$), Student's t-test was used.

Results

Compliance

Immediately after implantation, the compliance of the native femoral artery adjacent to the proximal anastomosis was $0.06 \pm 0.0025\%$ mm Hg^{-1}. This value went down to $0.041 \pm 0.007\%$ mm Hg^{-1} within 1 month ($p < 0.05$) and remained essentially constant thereafter (Table 52.1). At implantation the biograft (BIMA) also showed a well-preserved elasticity. The compliance was calculated to be $0.028 \pm 0.009\%$ mm Hg^{-1}. It peaked to $0.046 \pm 0.022\%$ mm Hg^{-1} ($p < 0.05$) during the early interval of graft healing. Besides this early rise, the compliance profile of the BIMA paralleled that of the native femoral artery. In particular, after 6 months the compliance of the biograft was 0.027 $\pm 0.005\%$ mm Hg^{-1}, which was well matched now to the compliance of the native arterial vessel ($0.039 \pm 0.01\%$ mm Hg^{-1}).

At implantation the PTFE graft was nearly stiff, revealing a compliance of only $0.008 \pm 0.005\%$ mm Hg^{-1} ($p < 0.05$). Because of its inelasticity and the high rate of graft occlusion, PTFE was not included in the long-term compliance study.

Graft Healing

With regard to the intimal, medial, and adventitial layer of the vessel, the description of the healing characteristics of the bovine graft will be divided into three sections.

Up to 6 months, no pseudoneointima formed in the functioning biograft. In all specimens examined, the luminal surface was made up of the smooth inner elastic membrane. Rarely, some proteinaceous materials were adherent. The original endothelial layer was removed by the processing technique.

If H-E-stained specimens were studied, the inner half of the muscular layer showed some decrease in density after 2 weeks. The Alcian PAS technique proved this to be due to the disappearance of interstitial mucopolysaccharides. After 3 months, the biograft specimens revealed a mononuclear and

TABLE 52.1. Long-term determination of the radial compliance.

Vessel	Compliance ($\%$ mm Hg^{-1})			
	At implantation $n = 10$	1 month $n = 5$	3 months $n = 5$	6 months $n = 5$
Femoral artery	$0.06 \pm 0.025^*$	$0.041 \pm 0.007^*$	0.043 ± 0.003	0.039 ± 0.013
BIMA	$0.028 \pm 0.009^*$	0.046 ± 0.022	0.027 ± 0.004	0.027 ± 0.005
PTFE	0.008 ± 0.005	—	—	—

$^* p < 0.05$

polymorphonuclear cellular infiltrate apparently invading the muscular layer from the luminal side. But this cellular infiltrate was always confined to the inner half of the medial layer. It never proceeded further during the following 3 months (Figure 52.3).

All biografts retained an intact adventitial layer with strong bundles of collagen. This was never penetrated by host tissue. An outer capsule made up of fibroblasts and newly synthesized collagen was formed within 3 months.

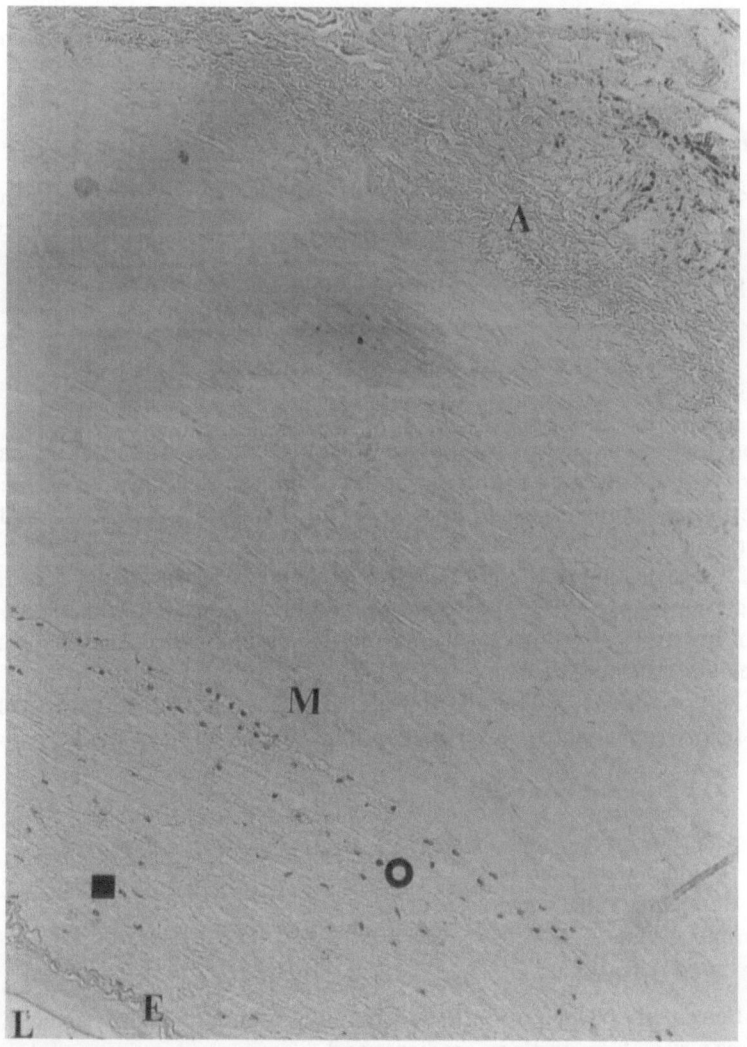

FIGURE 52.3. Cross section of a patent BIMA, implanted for 6 months. L, Luminal surface; E, inner elastic membrane; M, medial layer; A, adventitial layer; ○, mononuclear cell; ■, polymorphonuclear cell.

TABLE 52.2. Patency rate of the dialdehyde starch-preserved BIMA and PTFE grafts (4 mm, 7 cm).

Graft	No. patent grafts	
	3 months ($n = 10$)	6 months ($n = 10$)
PTFE	6	2
BIMA	7	6

Up to 6 months, anastomotic neointimal hyperplasia was not seen with either graft.

Patency Rate

After 3 months, the patency rate of the 4-mm biograft did not differ from that of the PTFE prosthesis (group I). After 6 months, however, the patency rate of the biograft was clearly superior (Table 52.2). Six biografts and only two PTFE vessels out of 10 were still functioning (group II).

Discussion

Compliance remains a continuing problem when new arterial grafts have to be developed. Because of the pulsatility of the arterial flow, the elasticity of arterial substitutes is essential for an optimal transmission of flow and flow energy.

If a nonelastic graft is implanted into the arterial tree, some detrimental effects can be expected with regard to theoretical considerations. Some arise from the stiff segment itself, others from the junction where the elastic artery meets the stiff substitute.

The equation of Moens Korteweg defines the relationship between the elastic properties of the vessel wall and the velocity of the pulse wave v.

$$v_p = \sqrt{\frac{Eh}{2r\rho}} \tag{4}$$

E = Young's elastic modulus
h = thickness of the vessel wall
r = inner radius
ρ = blood density

The velocity of the pulse wave increases in a noncompliant segment. This causes a rise of the pressure gradients and a faster acceleration and deceleration of the inert blood during the pulse cycle. Thus energy is wasted due to the need to overcome viscous resistance and fluid inertia. Furthermore, the shear stress between blood and the luminal surface is accentuated. Platelets exposed to high shear stress are believed to release mitogenic factors.[8-10] In addition, shear stress and turbulent flow can be responsible for graft vibrations. The result may be neointimal formation and hyperplasia. This is especially true with PTFE grafts.[11-13] In part due to its compliance, the BIMA showed no neointima or pseudoneointima development.

At implantation, the compliance of the femoral artery was calculated to be $0.06 \pm 0.025\%$ mm Hg^{-1}. This result was in accordance with the data reported in previous publications which ranged from 0.059 to 0.12% mm Hg^{-1}.[14-16] The BIMA displayed half the compliance of the native femoral artery. However, the value of $0.028 \pm 0.008\%$ mm Hg^{-1} was superior compared to the stiff PTFE. Our results did not differ from values found with other biological grafts. The compliance of the vein grafts ranged from 0.027 to 0.048% mm Hg^{-1}, and that of the umbilical vien from 0.037 to 0.049% mm Hg^{-1}.[16-18]

Several authors found different compliance profiles during graft healing.[6,14,19] However, long-term studies using implantable sensors are lacking.[15,19-23] Our results arising from compliance measurements without graft dissection established the clear impact of the collagenous outer capsule surrounding the graft and the adjacent artery on the elastic properties of the vessels. Healing reduced the compliance of both the graft and the native femoral artery. However, the decline was greater in the primarily more elastic native artery, resulting in comparable compliance values of the BIMA and the femoral artery after 6 months. The initial increase in compliance of the biograft paralleled the early loss of basic interstitial mucopolysaccharides displayed by histological examinations.

Wall stability is always a major concern with biografts.[24-6] A decreased stability of the graft followed by aneurysm formation or at least graft rupture may be the result of biodegradation and collagen breakdown.

When a cellular invasion into the fixed muscular layer of the BIMA was first observed after 3 months beginning biodegradation was suspected. But this invasion did not proceed beyond the inner half of the medial layer of the graft. We think this to be due to the dependency of the invading cells on the limited oxygen diffusion capacity from the luminal side. Host tissue was never seen to penetrate the adventitial layer and thus start collagen breakdown. This is in accordance with a constant collagen content of the biograft as we reported earlier. In addition, the slight decrease in compliance of a biograft has been reported to be a strong indicator of retained graft stability.[27]

In comparison to PTFE, the dialdehyde starch-preserved BIMA showed no diameter-reducing neointimal formation. This may be due to the retained elasticity and the lack of any porosity of the biograft. It ultimately translated into the clearly superior long-term patency rate of the biological graft compared to PTFE.

Conclusions

The development of arterial grafts has been focused on the thrombogenicity of the inner surface. A complete neointimal inner lining including an endothelial cell layer is believed to be the most important factor to obtain a nonthrombogenic graft. However, any degree of neointima reduces the inner diameter, thus increasing the viscous fluid resistance, which correlates to $1/r^4$ according to the law of Poiseuille. This is especially true with small-diameter grafts. In an 8-mm graft, a 0.5-mm-thick neointima increases the resistance by 30% as compared to 200% in a 4-mm arterial substitute. Additionally, until now there has been no reliable method of controlling the growth of the neointimal tissue.

With regard to these theoretical considerations, we hypothesize the small-diameter graft of choice to be an elastic nonthrombogenic tube with "nothing" growing inside. In the experimental situation, the dialdehyde starch-preserved BIMA revealed some of these desired properties. It showed favorable results regarding wall stability, compliance, and healing. In accordance with these basic parameters, its patency rate was superior to that of PTFE.

References

1. Szilagyi DE. Some controversial topics in vascular surgery. Am J Surg 1969;118: 406.
2. Li Calzi LR, Stansel HC, Jr. Failure of autogenous reversed saphenous vein femoropopliteal grafting: Pathophysiology and prevention. Surgery 1982;91:352.
3. Szilagyi DE, Elliott JP, Hogemen JH, et al. Biologic fate of autologous vein implant as arterial substitutes. Ann Surg 1973;178:232.
4. Hales S. Statistical essays: Containing Haemostatics 1773. History Of Medicine Series. Vol 22. Library of New York Academy of Medicine. New York: Hafner Publishing, 1964.
5. Cox RH. Blood flow and pressure propagation in the canine femoral artery. J Biomech 1970;3:131.
6. Kidson IG. The effect of wall mechanical properties on patency of arterial grafts. Ann R Coll Surg Engl 1983;65:24–29.
7. Welz A, Triefenbach R, Murrmann G, Grenzner S, Hammer C. Experimental evaluation of the dialdehyde starch preserved bovine internal mammary artery as a small diameter arterial substitute. Cardiac Surg 1992;7:163.
8. Baumgartner HR. Platelet and fibrin deposition on subendothelium opposite dependence on blood shear rate (Abstract). Thromb Haemost 1977;38:133.
9. Brown CH, Leverett LB, Lewis CW. Morphological, biochemical and functional changes in human platelets subjected to shear stress. J Lab Clin Med 1975;86:462.
10. LoGerfo FW, Sonscrant T, Teel T, Dewey CJ. Boundary layer separation in models of side to side arterial anastomose. Arch Surg 1979;114:1369.
11. Caron SN, Hunter G, French S, Lord P, Wong HN. Occurrence of occlusive intimal changes in an expanded polytetrafluoroethylene graft. J Cardiovasc Surg 1980;21:503.

12. Satturai VS, Yao JST, Flinn WR, Batson RC. Intimal hyperplasia and neointima. An ultrastructural analysis of thrombosed grafts. Surgery 1983;93:809.
13. Bergeur R, Higgins RF, Reddy DJ. Intimal hyperplasia: An experimental study. Arch Surg 1980;115:332.
14. White R, Klein SR, Shors EC. Preservation of compliance in a small diameter microporous silicone rubber vascular prosthesis. J Cardiovasc Surg 1987;28:485.
15. Baird RN, Kidson IG, L'Italien GJ, Abbott WM. Dynamic compliance of arterial grafts. Lancet 1976;2:948.
16. Kidson IG, Abbott WM. Low compliance and arterial graft occlusion. Circulation 1978;58 (suppl I): I-1.
17. Kinely CE, Marble AE. Compliance: A continuing problem with vascular grafts. J Cardiovasc Surg 1989;21:163.
18. Walden R, L'Italien GI, Megermann I, Abbott WM. Matched elastic properties and successful arterial grafting. Arch Surg 1980;115:1166.
19. Schmitz Rixen T, Megermann J, Andersen JM, Warnod DF, L'Italien GI, Erasmi H, Horsch S, Abbott WM. Longterm study of a compliant biological vascular graft. Eur J Vasc Surg 1991;5:149.
20. Gow BS. An Electrical caliper for measurement of pulsatile arterial diameter changes in vivo. J Appl Physiol 1966;21:1122.
21. Mallos AI. An electrical caliper for continous measurement of relative displacement. J Appl Physiol 1962;17:131.
22. Hokanson DE, Mozersky DI, Summer DS, Strandness DE. A phase-locked echo tracking system for recording arterial diameter changes in vivo. J Appl Physiol 1972;32:728.
23. Megermann J, Harson IE, Warnod DF, L'Italien GI, Abbott WM. Noninvasive measurement of nonlinear arterial elasticity. Am J Physiol 1986;250:181.
24. Brayn T, Christensen O, Fossdal IE, et al. Early complications with a new bovine arterial graft (Solograft P). Acta Chir Scand 1986;152:263.
25. Dale WA, Lewis MR. Further experiences with bovine arterial grafts. Surgery 1976;80:711.
26. Halpert B, DeBakey ME, Jordan GL, et al. Fate of vascular homografts and prostheses of human aorta. Surg Gynecol Obstet 1960;111:659.
27. Hamilton G, Megermann J, L'Italien GI, Warnock DF, Schmitz-Rixen T, Brewster DC, Abbott WM. Prediction of aneurysm formation in vascular grafts of biologic origin. J Vasc Surg 1988;7:400.

XIX
Venous System

53
A New Valvuloplasty for Primary Deep Venous Insufficiency

Katsushi Akemoto and Takeshi Ueyama

Postphlebitic syndrome caused by venous obstruction or valvular destruction presents lower limb stasis syndrome. It results in skin pigmentation and ulceration of lower extremities. Conventional treatments, such as compression stockings, many kinds of massage therapies, or Linton's interruption of perforating veins have been done in this syndrome,[1] but those methods have not led to good results.

Primary nonobstructive deep venous incompetence was recognized by evaluation of descending phlebography, and it was classified by Kistner's grading system.[2] Then direct surgical approaches such as valvuloplasty,[3,4] vein transposition,[5] and valve transplantation[6] were able to prevent venous regurgitation in this disease.

The first valvuloplasty was performed by Kistner in 1968.[3,4] He reported that the pathological condition of valve incompetence is prolapse of the valves due to elongation of the cusp edge. The surgical procedure consisted of venotomy, and shortening the cusp by tucking suture at the point of valve commissure. However, this technique requires anticoagulant therapy both during and after the operation to prevent thrombus formation at the site of venotomy. Therefore, simultaneous use of this technique with stripping of saphenous vein is associated with danger of hematoma formation. Sometimes valves are injured during repair and then the superficial femoral vein must be ligated.

We also performed valvuloplasty by our new technique with good results. This paper reports our operative method and its benefits.

Materials and Methods

From December 1986 to December 1991, 5 patients were admitted to our institute for pigmentation, ulceration, and severe bursting pain of the lower legs (Table 53.1). There were 1 male and 4 females, with ages ranging from 39 to 63 years (mean 53.2). The duration of disease was very short except for case 1, and this disease tends to progress rapidly.

TABLE 53.1. Patient features.

Case no.	Age	Sex	Clinical features	Duration of disease
1	63	M	Ulceration Skin pigmentation Spontaneous bleeding	16 years
2	56	F	Ulceration Skin pigmentation	3 years
3	54	F	Skin pigmentation Bursting pain	6 months
4	39	F	Bursting pain Venous claudication	6 months
5	54	F	Ulceration Skin pigmentation	1 year

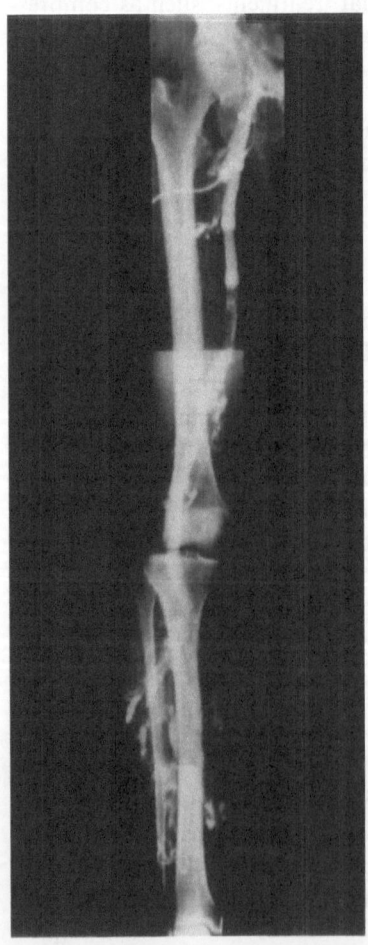

FIGURE 53.1. Preoperative descending phlebography. Massive reflux can be seen from common femoral vein toward the periphery.

Patient Evaluations

We do Doppler ultrasound directional examination and duplex scan in our
outpatients to exclude moderate or mild reflux of the deep vein. If severe
reflux sound is audible in the groin region, we do descending phlebography
by an alternative method such as direct puncture of the common femoral or
external iliac vein in the semistanding position (60 degrees) (Fig. 53.1). The
Valsalva maneuver is not used because of overestimation. The findings are
classified by the grading system proposed by Kistner.[2] Grades I and II reflux
are manifested by conventional compression therapy, and grades III and IV
reflux should be investigated for valvuloplasty. It is very important, however,
that if insufficiency of the saphenofemoral or saphenopopliteal junction is
detected and varicose veins of the saphenous system are remarkable, the
indication of valvuloplasty should be reevaluated after treatment and manifestation of superficial venous insufficiency, such as stripping of saphenous
veins or sclerotherapy of varicosis.

Operative Procedure

First, closer evaluation of preoperative descending phlebography is necessary
to determine the distance from the common femoral vein to the incompetent
valve. Next, under epidural anesthesia, we expose the target valve, which is

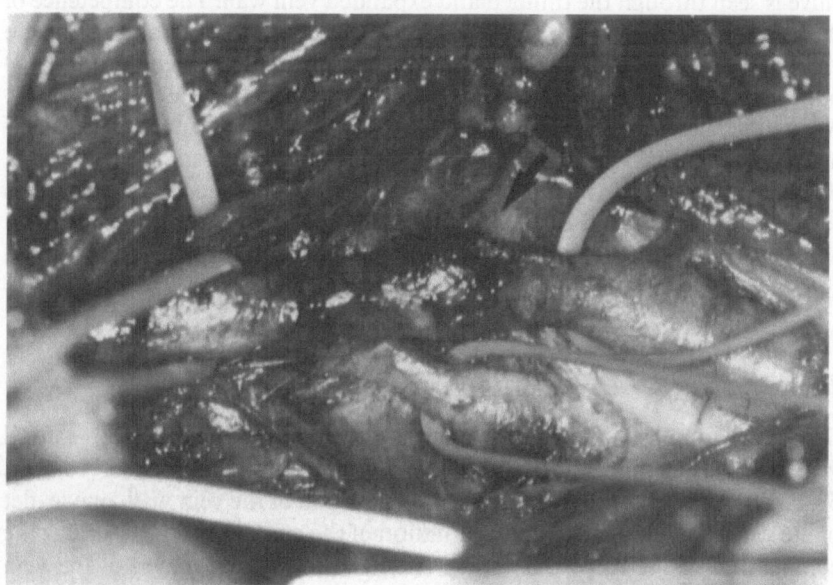

FIGURE 53.2. Intraoperative findings. Left side is cranial. Arrow; point of incompetent
valve.

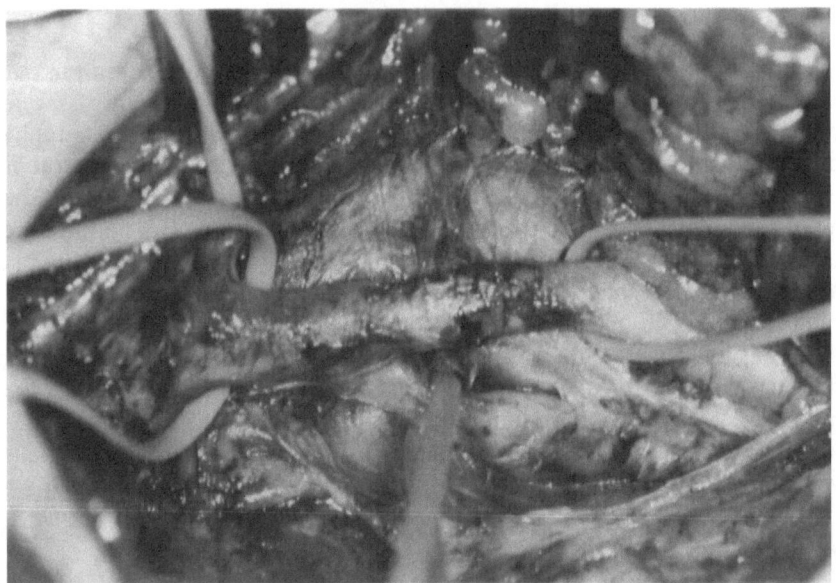

FIGURE 53.3. The incompetent vein was reefed.

the highest valve of the superficial femoral vein (Fig. 53.2). The insufficient valve is seen through the thinned and expanded vein wall. The competence of the valve is checked by the milking test from distal to cranial beyond the valve. The wall is then plicated with four to seven interrupted sutures (7–0 polypropylene) from the outside of the vein without venotomy (Fig. 53.3). After that, the valve should be checked for competence by the milking maneuver again. When insufficiency of the saphenous system exists, stripping of the greater saphenous vein and Linton's interruption of the perforating veins can be done at the end of the operation. No anticoagulation is performed either during or after the operation. Postoperative thrombosis is prevented simply by using elastic stockings and mechanical massage.

Intraoperative Angioscopic Findings

Before valvuloplasty, the angioscope was inserted from the common femoral vein, and the incompetent valve was directly intraluminally observed (Fig. 53.4). The valve was floppy with partial dilatation of the vein wall, one leaflet of the valve was elongated, and coaptation of the cusp was decreased. But the commissure of the valve was intact. After the plasty, the lumen of the vein had become narrow and one leaflet was reefed. Coaptation of the cusp had become perfect (Fig. 53.5).

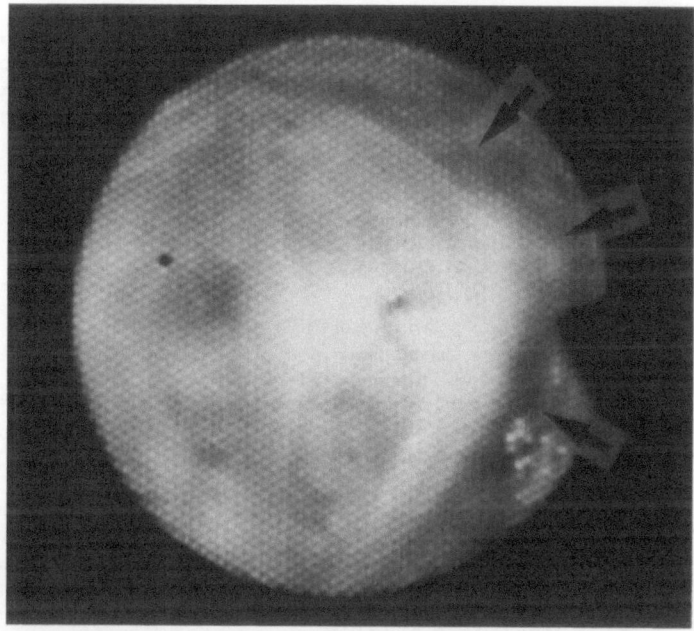

FIGURE 53.4. Angioscopic findings. One leaflet of right side is incompetent and valve commissure (arrow) is intact.

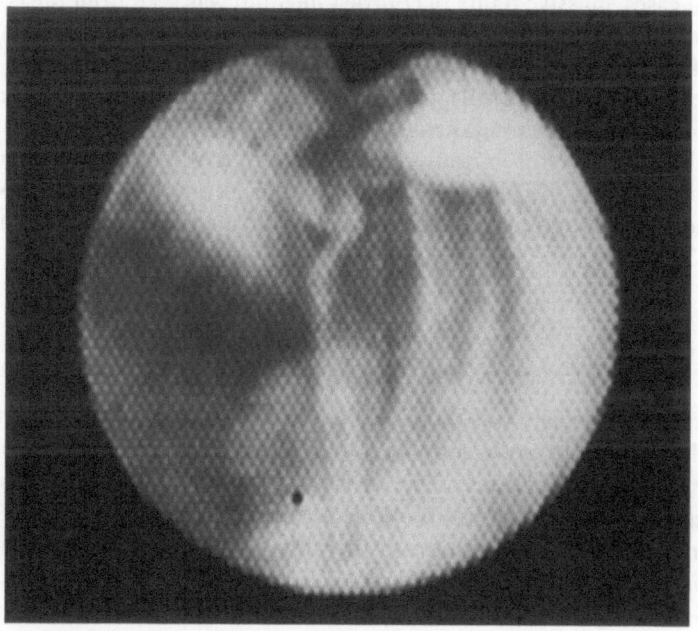

FIGURE 53.5. After plasty.

TABLE 53.2. Results of procedures.

Case no.	Grade of reflux[a]	Surgical procedure (Additional procedure)	Clinical result	Postoperative reflux
1	IV	Valvuloplasty Linton's method[b]	Excellent	
2	III	Valvuloplasty Linton's method Stripping of GSV[c]	Excellent	0
3	IV	Valvuloplasty	Excellent	0
4	III	Valvuloplasty Stripping of GSV	Excellent	0
5	IV	Valvuloplasty Stripping of GSV	Excellent	0

[a] Kistner's grading system.
[b] Subfascial interruption of the communicating veins.
[c] Greater saphenous vein.

Results

Five valve repairs were attempted. All of these 5 patients had primary non-obstructive deep venous insufficiency. There was no irregularity, stenosis, or occlusion of the deep femoral vein on preoperative ascending phlebography.

In all cases, massive reflux of contrast medium was seen from the common femoral vein to the distal site of the knee joint on descending phlebograms. The reflux grade was classified as grade 3 or 4 according to Kistner.

When incompetence of the greater saphenous vein was observed, stripping was done safely and simultaneously (Table 53.2).

In all cases, relief of various clinical symptoms was noted. Pigmentation and ulceration of the legs were healed within 3 months. On postoperative descending phlebography, all deep venous reflux had disappeared completely (Fig. 53.6).

Comments

The first valvuloplasty was reported by Kistner.[3] The important point of the procedure is tucking and shortening of the elongated valve cusps at the point of commissure. The sutures are made from the inside of the vein under longitudinal phlebotomy. The result of this operation is very wonderful.[7,8] However, at venotomy, the position of the anterior commissure of the valve is sometimes difficult to identify exactly,[7] and the risk of valve injury is a burden to the surgeon. Moreover, anticoagulation is necessary to avoid thrombosis at the site of venotomy. There is also a risk of hematoma formation after additional procedure. Therefore Kistner reported that stripping and

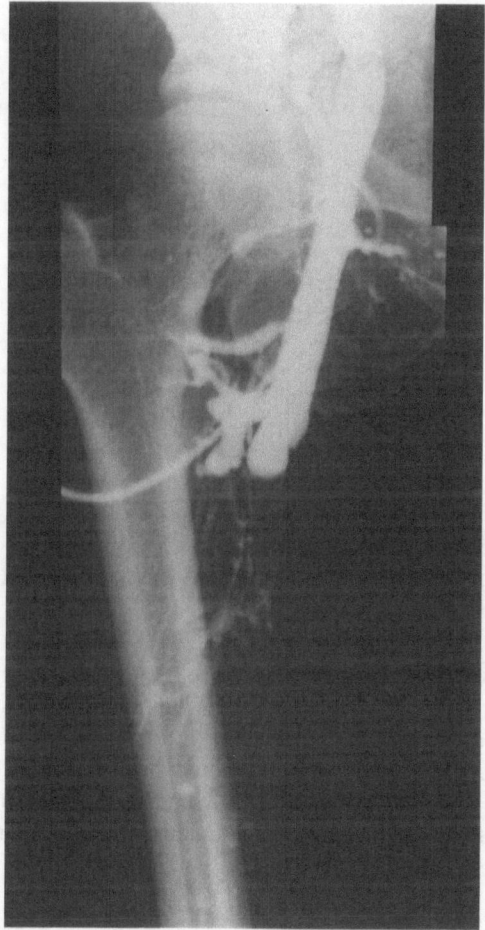

FIGURE 53.6. Postoperative phlebography. The reflux has disappeared completely.

subfascial interruption must be done first, and 3 days to 1 week later, femoral vein repair should be done under heparin sodium anticogulation. Anticoagulation is continued for a 2-month period.

In our technique (Fig. 53.7), neither phlebotomy nor anticoagulation is necessary. With only interrupted suture from the outside of the vein, the expanded vein wall is plicated, a leaflet of the valve is reefed, and coaptation of the cusp is increased. In patients 1 and 2, Linton's interruption was performed at the same time. So the question of which procedure is more effective to improve the clinical symptoms may arise. However, the latter three patients had only valvuloplasty; all three patients did well and their complaints disappeared immediately.

In conclusions: (1) This method is simple and reliable and could be done

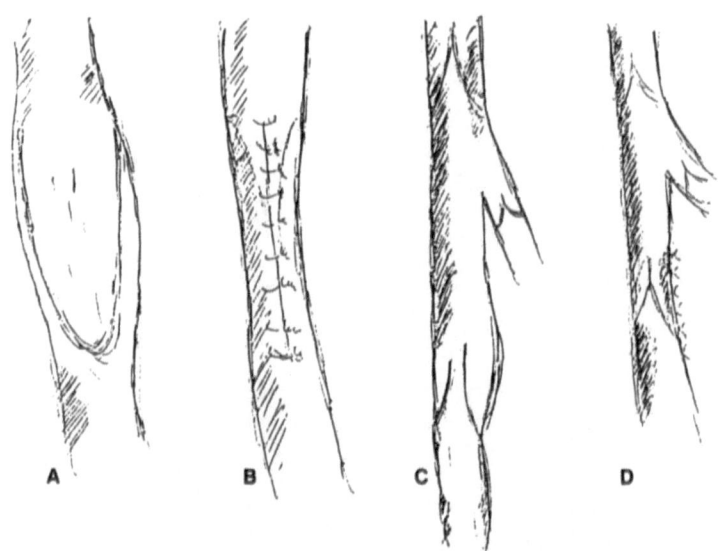

FIGURE 53.7. Scheme of the operation. A, B: Frontal view. C, D: Side view.

simultaneously with stripping of varicose veins. (2) No anticoagulant therapy was required during or after operation. (3) There were no postoperative complications, such as hematoma formation and thrombosis of the deep vein. (4) Postoperative thrombosis was prevented by using elastic stockings and HADOMER mechanical massage. Follow-up periods were 10 to 70 months, no recurrence was observed, and clinical results were excellent.

References

1. Linton R. The post-thrombotic ulceration of the lower extremity: Its etiology and surgical treatment. Ann Surg 1953;138:415–432.
2. Kistner RL, Ferris EB, Rndhawa G, et al. A method of performing descending venography. J Vasc Surg 1986;4:465–468.
3. Kistner RL, Surgical repair of a venous valve. Straub Clin Proc 1968;34:41–43.
4. Kistner RL. Surgical repair of the incompetent femoral vein valve. Arch Surg 1975;110:1336–1342.
5. Kistner RL, Sparkuhl MD. Surgery in acute and chronic venous disease. Surgery 1979;85:31–43.
6. Taheri SA, Lazar L, Elias S, et al. Surgical treatment of post-phlebitic syndrome with vein valve transplant. Am J Surg 1982;144:221–224.
7. Eriksson I, Almgren B, Nordgren L. Late results after venous valve repair. Inter Angio 1985;4:413–417.
8. Raju S, Fredericks R. Valve reconstruction procedures for nonobstructive venous insufficiency: Rationale, techniques, and results in 107 procedures with two- to eight-year follow-up. J Vasc Surg 1988;7:301–310.

54
Homolateral Long Saphenous Vein as a Valvulated Graft for Reflux Treatment of Deep Venous Postthrombotic Disease

J.M. Cardon, A. Joyeux, D. Noblet, M.M. Faye, and P. Bousquet

Surgery for deep venous reflux in postthrombotic disease is still an open field for research in vascular surgery. Many procedures have been proposed but are not always feasible nor effective. We review 15 patients who benefited from an original technique: the transplantation of the homolateral long saphenous vein.

Physiopathology

Deep Venous Reflux Is the Major Pathological Element

The evolution of deep venous phlebitis leads to a totally adhesive thrombus bridged by a quickly organizing collateral pathway; therefore, the obstructive syndrome disappears with its increase (Figs. 54.1a and 54.1b). Then, in a few years, there is a repermeation but with a valvular destruction inducing the reflux syndrome which is definitive and self increasing (Fig. 54.1c).

The reflux consequences are to induce a hyperpressure, which is the weight of a blood column from the heart to the ankle. That explains the forced opening of the perforating veins, swelling, dermatitis, pain, and ulcers. Experimental and clinical studies point out that if a single valve is interposed at the femoral or popliteal level, the pressure decreases sufficently at the ankle to alleviate the most serious symptoms.

The pathological association: obstruction-reflux (Fig 54.2) is frequent, particulary on the left side, where an obstruction syndrome often explains the remaining obstructive lesion on the iliac level associated with a femoropopliteal reflux. In these cases it is mandatory to preserve the collateral pathway arising from the saphenous junction.

Homolateral Long Saphenous Vein

The homolateral long saphenous vein (LSV) is the natural shunt for the leg in case of deep venous thrombosis. Immediately the flow becomes continuous and preserves the LSV from an extension of the thrombus inside the junction,

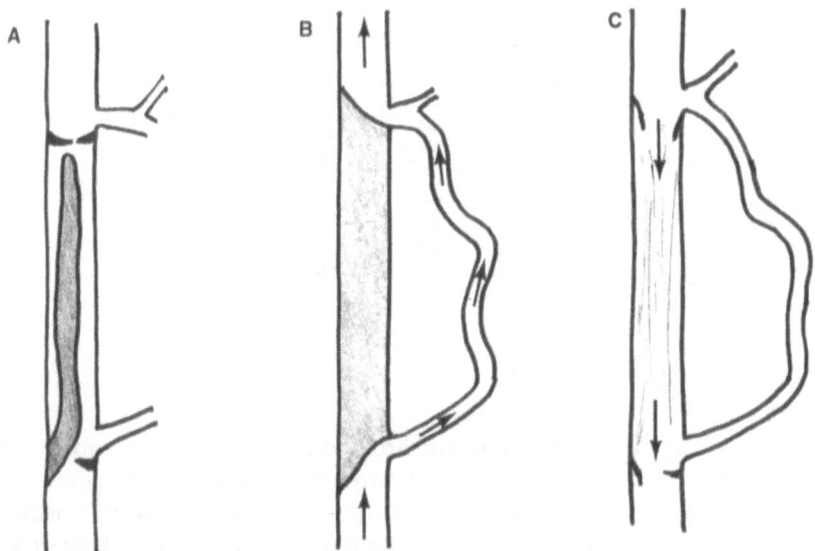

FIGURE 54.1. The long-term evolution of deep venous phlebitis. (a) Phlebitis. (b) Obstructive syndrome. (c) Reflux syndrome.

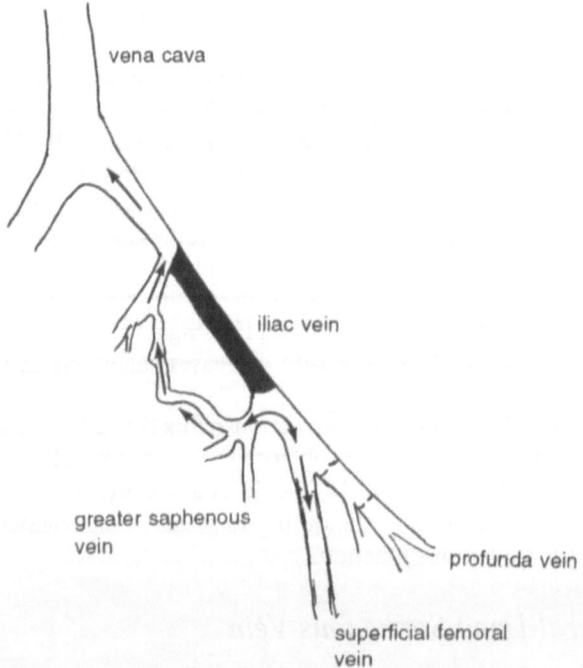

FIGURE 54.2. Pathologic association in postthrombotic disease. Obstruction of the iliac vein and reflux in the superficial femoral vein.

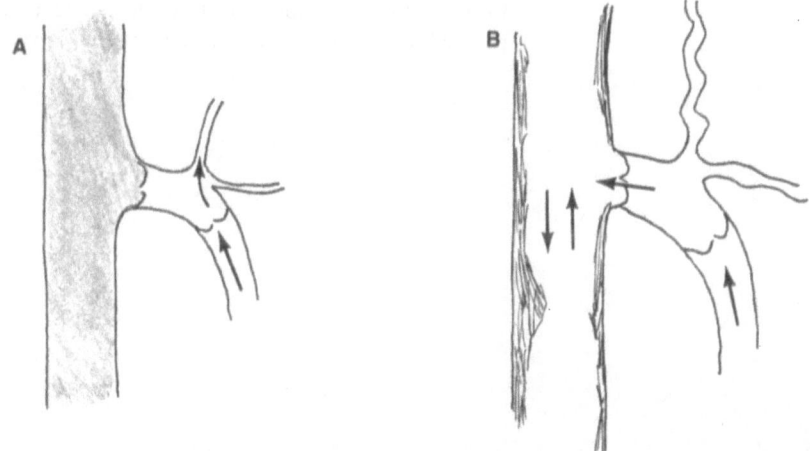

FIGURE 54.3. Preservation of a valvulated greater saphenous vein in spite of a deep venous reflux.

thus protecting its valves (Figs. 54.3a and 54.3b). On the other hand, the branches of the junction become the starting point of the pelvic collateral flow. In case of definitive iliac obstruction, this role remains essential.

Special conditions such as family history, pregnancy, hyperactivity, or postphebitic valvular destruction may make the LSV value incompetent. In these cases the LSV must not be used as a valvulated graft but must be destroyed to stop the reflux via the superficial veins. Fortunately, and especially in young patients, the LSV often remains competent and can be employed.

Surgical Techniques for Reflux Treatment Are Not Always Usable or Efficient

The transposition of the superficial femoral vein in the profunda vein (Fig. 54.4) is the best method, according to R.L. Kistner, giving good results at long-term follow-up, but it requires a good valvulation of the profunda, which is rather uncommon.

The transposition of an axillary valvulated vein graft (Fig. 54.5) gives good initial results but fails in the long term. The results are similar with external procedure and in the Psatakis procedure. Valvuloplasty can only be used if the valves are repairable, which is unusual.

For the use of the homolateral saphenous vein, several techniques have been described, but none is like ours, and the exact long-term results are unknown. Therefore we reviewed all patients since 1984 who benefited from our technique of homolateral transplantation of the LSV in case of post-

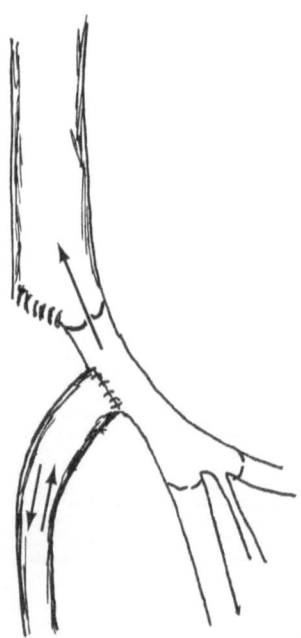

FIGURE 54.4. Transposition of an incompetent superficial femoral vein in a competent profunda vein.

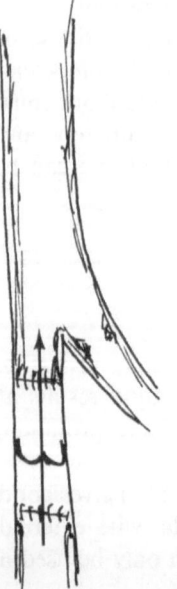

FIGURE 54.5. Transposition of an axillary vein.

thrombotic disease to establish the long-term outcome of patient and graft competence.

Methods

Patients

Only really handicapped patients (pain, ulcer) are operated on, and only if:
- A correct unsuccesful medical treatment with elastic compression has been observed;
- A correct unsuccesful surgical treatment of any leak from deep to superficial venous system has been corrected [small saphenous vein (SSV), perforating veins].

Screening

The screening of the patients includes;
- A color duplex scanning done in a standing position and with a Valsalva maneuver;
- An ascending phlebography to show obstructive and recanalized segments;
- A descending phlebography to assert the deep venous reflux. Only reflux in the calf vein (stage IV of Kistner) is proposed for surgery.

Operative Technique

- The anesthesia is epidural;
- The skin incision is vertical at the groin. The LSV and the deep venous veins are controlled;
- A stretch test at the deep femoral superficial vein confirms the deep venous reflux but shows that the LSV is competent (Fig. 54.6a);
- An end-to-side anastomosis is realized between the LSV and superficial femoral vein (Fig. 54.6b);
- This anastomosis is converted to an end-to-end one by a double ligation of the superficial femoral vein above the anastomosis (Fig. 54.6c);
- A new stretch test shows the competence of the graft. This technique is very simple: only one anastomosis; congruency of the anastomosis always matches; absolute respect of the collaterals from the junction.

Postoperative Management

- We elevate the foot end of the bed and give heparin for 48 hours; walking is then mandatory with elastic compression, which must be continued forever;

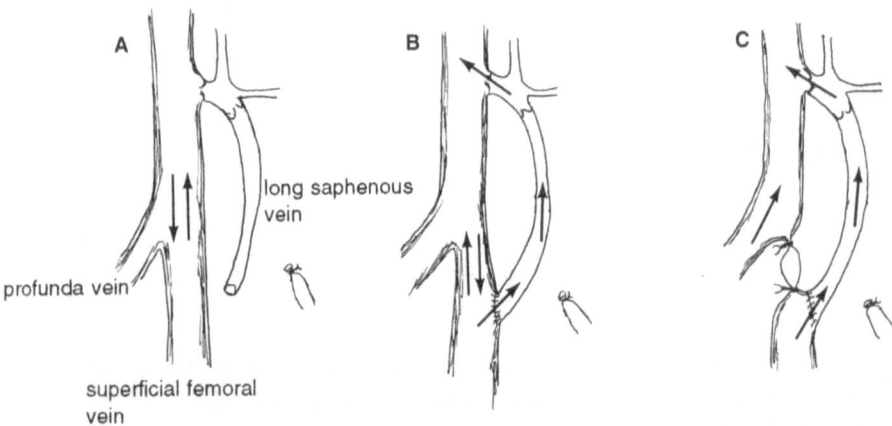

FIGURE 54.6. Homolateral long saphenous vein technique of transplantation.

• The control is realized by color dupex scanning and repeated every 6 months to confirm patency and competence of the graft and to screen any new active leak from the deep to the superficial system.

Results

From 1984 to 1991, 15 patients were operated on with this technique. There were 9 men and 6 women; the ages ranged from 25 to 76 (mean 56 years); the side was right in 7, left in 8. All had chronic pain that kept them from standing up without moving; 9 patients had a nonhealing ulcer; 8 had had previous treatment of the superficial venous system (small saphenous vein or perforators) without any improvement, all had a deep venous reflux, stage IV at descending phlebography.

Immediate Results

• No deaths or pulmonary embolism, no extensive deep venous thrombosis;
• At 3 months: all ulcers were cured. None complained of pain again, but nearly all had a persistent swelling as before the operation;
• The color duplex scan showed patency in 15/15 and competence in 15/15.

Long-Term Results (1–8 Years Mean 43 Months)

• Clinically: 11 have been definitively cured, and among them 5 had chronic ulcers: 4 had failures, all of which were recurrent ulcers;

• At the color duplex examination: 14 were patent; 1 thrombosed at 18 months after an orthopedic surgery. Of the 14 grafts at risk, 13 were competent at the end of the follow-up but 1 was incompetent.

Clinical Findings

Of the 9 recurrent ulcers, 5 were definitively and primarily cured: minimum follow-up was 17 months, maximum 44 months (mean 30 months); all had a competent and patent graft and no leak from deep to superficial venous system. The remaining 4 recurred: minimum follow-up was 12 months, maximum 47 months (mean 30 months); the color duplex scan showed that of these 4, 3 had a patent and competent graft but a huge reflux in the small saphenous vein. In these 3 patients the treatment of the new reflux in SSV cured the ulcer again with nonrecurrency. The fourth one had both an incompetent graft and a reflux in the SSV; in spite of adequate treatment the ulcer recurred again, but it was less painful and more easily controlled by medical care.

• Of the 6 patients with pain: 5 had a complete disappearance of pain and worked again in a standing position. The last one experienced new deep venous thrombosis 18 months later and had no further pain but complained of swelling.

• On swelling: the results are very poor in spite of elastic compression. All of the 15 patients have a mild ankle swelling in the evening. So we can conclude that there is no cosmetic indication in postthrombotic reflux.

Conclusions

• Perfect safety of the procedure;
• Effectiveness for pain;
• The primary efficacy in ulcer is 55% rises to 89% if a correct survey of the SSV and perforators is made;
• There is no cosmetic indication for this surgery. Only severely handicapped patients should be proposed for surgery.

Bibliography

Bergan JJ. Kistner RL. *Atlas of Venous Surgery*. Philadelphia: WB Saunders, 1992.

Raju S, Frederiks R. Valve reconstruction procedure for non obstructive venous insufficiency. Rationale, techniques and results on 107 procedures. J Vasc Surg 1988; 7:301–310.

Taheri, Pendergast DR, Lazar E. Vein valve transplantation. Am J Surg 1985;150: 201–202.

Ferris EB, Kistner RL. Femoral vein reconstruction in management of chronic venous insufficiency. Arch Surg 1982;117:1571–1579.

Kistner RL, Ferris EB, Randhawa G. A method of performing descending venography. J Vasc Surg 1986;4:646–468.

Nicolaides AN, Christopoulos DC. Methods of quantification of chronic venous insufficiency. In Bergan JJ, Yao ST (eds.). *Venous Disorders*. Philadelphia: WB Saunders, 1991, pp. 77–91.

Welkie JF, Comerota AJ, Kerr RP. The hemodynamics of venous ulceration. Ann Vasc Surg 1992;6:1–4.

55
Local Gas Analysis in Patients with Venous Ulcers

Živan V. Maksimović, Tomislav Jovanović, Slobodanka Dukić, and Siniša Jagodić

Introduction

Chronic postthrombotic states of the deep veins or damage to the superficial venous system leads to progressive incompetence of perforators (venae communicantes) manifesting as a pathological blood reflux from the deep into the surface system (calf pump failure). This leads to local metabolic, microcirculatory, and trophic changes which may be manifested in the form of a dermatosclerosis, the dying out of cells, and appearance of venous ulcerations.

There are three major theories attempting to explain the etiology of venous ulceration:

Stasis and hypoxia within the cutaneous microcirculation[1];
The opening of arteriovenous shunts[2] succeeded by hypoxia[3];
An interstitial diffusion blockade due to capillary permeability[4].

Examination of gas analyses of the venous blood in patients with venous ulcers was followed by contradictory results. Thus, Homans'[1] findings could not be confirmed on all occasions. Blalock[2] found that the venous blood oxygen content was at its peak if the estimates were performed while the patient was lying down, whereas the concentration of gas drastically dropped if the patient was standing up. The total blood flow and oxygen level is greater in the varicose veins and in the blood of patients with venous ulcers. Such results suggested that pathological arteriovenous shunts open up in venous ulcers, so that the blood bypasses the capillary bed,[5,6] thus being responsible for the escalation in the oxygen level of the venous blood in the ulcerating region.

Calf failure causes alteration of the local capillary network; dermal capillary loops tend to elongate and become tortuous,[7] with succeeding changes in the basement membrane, which becomes irregular and thickened. The basement membrane becomes more permeable, so that fibrinogen and other macromolecules escape into the pericapillary space, which causes an interstitial barrier, thus impeding gas exchange between the intercapillary and interstitial spaces.[4,8]

Despite all this, the enigma of oxygen concentration in the venous blood of patients suffering from venous ulcers still has not been solved, since it has been proven that in patients treated differently for venous ulcers, we can find both elevated and reduced oxygen tension values.[9] This chapter surveys gas analysis values in the venous blood of patients whose clinical and pathoanatomical venous ulcers have emerged in a variety of different forms.

Materials and Methods

Gas analysis was performed by a gas analyzer type ABL-2, Radiometer, Copenhagen. We took blood samples (approximately 2 ml) with a small-bore needle and heparinized syringe, drawing blood from a vein draining the venous ulceration. The control blood samples were taken under the same conditions from the adjoining healthy leg. Immediately upon obtaining the required amount of blood in the syringe, we squeezed out a small amount of blood while simultaneously jabbing the needle into a rubber stopper. This was done to prevent gas exchange between the blood samples and the atmosphere. We recorded the values of partial oxygen pressure (pO_2), partial carbon dioxide pressure (pCO_2), and acid-base status (pH), while the analyzer calculated the total carbon dioxide values (TCO_2), oxygen saturation (sO_2), and carbon dioxide concentration (HCO_3).

The examinations were carried out among two group of patients:

Group I: Patients with Doppler ultrasound and phlebographic results of regular, normal deep venous flows and damaged superficial veins and emerging unilateral surface venous ulcerations and subcutaneous varices (ulcers not caused by damage to deep veins).

Group II: Patients with Doppler ultrasound and phlebographic confirmation of postthrombotic venous stasis and visible deep and extensive unilateral venous ulcers (ulcers caused by damage to deep veins).

Results

Group I pO_2 values were considerably lower than those of the venous blood in the healthy leg. Group II showed considerably higher pO_2 values in relation to the venous blood drawn from the healthy leg (Table 55.1).

The sO_2 was also considerably lower in the blood samples taken from the ulcerating region than in the samples taken from the healthy leg. In group II we found surface values of sO_2 that were statistically more significant (Table 55.2). Similarly, as in the pO_2 case and during the estimation of sO_2, differences emerged in the mutually controlled samples that may be the effect of external factors or other various causes during the examinations of patients from groups I and II.

The pCO_2 of group I had significantly lower values in the venous blood

TABLE 55.1. Local pO_2 values (kPa) in patients with venous ulcers.

Group	Sample	No. of pts.	$\bar{X}$	SE	Significance
I	Ulcer	7	5.30	0.51	$t = 3.627$
	Control	7	6.97	1.11	$p < 0.01$
II	Ulcer	8	7.32	1.50	$t = 2.280$
	Control	8	5.60	1.53	$p < 0.05$

TABLE 55.2. Local sO_2 values (%) in patients with venous ulcers.

Group	Sample	No. of pts.	$\bar{X}$	SE	Significance
I	Ulcer	7	0.7507	0.0370	$t = 3.398$
	Control	7	0.8516	0.0693	$p < 0.01$
II	Ulcer	8	0.8272	0.1030	$t = 2.053$
	Control	8	0.6635	0.2006	$p < 0.05$

TABLE 55.3. Local pCO_2 values (kPa) in patients with venous ulcers.

Group	Sample	No. of pts.	$\bar{X}$	SE	Significance
I	Ulcer	7	6.21	0.48	$t = 2.537$
	Control	7	5.52	0.60	$p < 0.05$
II	Ulcer	8	5.83	0.77	$t = 1.440$
	Control	8	6.38	0.76	$p < 0.05$

taken from the ulceration region, whereas the lower values of pCO_2 in group II were not statistically significant (Table 55.3).

In group I HCO_3 values were higher in the venous blood in the ulceration region, whereas in group II the lower values were not statistically significant (Table 55.4). Similar ICO_2 values were also found (Table 55.5).

There were no statistically significant differences in pH (Table 55.6).

Conclusion

The results clearly show that there can be two different types of venous ulcers.[10]

Hypoxic ulcers are not caused by damage to deep veins. The anatomical and functional integrity of the deep system has not been damaged, but due to

TABLE 55.4. Local HCO_3 values (mmol/L) in patients with venous ulcers.

Group	Sample	No. of pts.	$\bar{X}$	SE	Significance
I	Ulcer	7	29.03	1.92	$t = 2.594$
	Control	7	26.74	1.33	$p < 0.05$
II	Ulcer	8	24.96	1.84	$t = 1.514$
	Control	8	26.51	2.20	$p < 0.05$

TABLE 55.5. Local TCO_2 values (kPa) in patients with venous ulcers.

Group	Sample	No. of pts.	$\bar{X}$	SE	Significance
I	Ulcer	7	30.13	1.95	$t = 3.154$
	Control	7	27.66	1.07	$p < 0.01$
II	Ulcer	8	26.26	1.99	$t = 1.782$
	Control	8	28.10	2.13	$p > 0.05$

TABLE 55.6. Local pH values in patients with venous ulcers.

Group	Sample	No. of pts.	$\bar{X}$	SE	Significance
I	Ulcer	7	7.407	0.043	$t = 1.292$
	Control	7	7.439	0.049	$p > 0.05$
II	Ulcer	8	7.375	0.038	$t = 0.831$
	Control	8	7.358	0.042	$p > 0.05$

the blood stasis caused by damaging to the non-deep superficial system, hypoxic and hypercapnial changes in the interstitial subcutaneous space have taken place, which can be manifested as varices and venous ulcers. Such ulcerations are shallow and limited, offering a good prognosis following surgical treatment and application of elastic bandaging.

Hyperoxic ulcers are caused by injury to deep veins. There is postthrombotic damage to the deep vein system with a subsequent progressive perforator incompetence as well as severe, chronic deep vein failure. Due to complex mechanisms (capillary exchange block, pericapillary morphological or metabolic block, etc.), there may consequently be a lack of exchange of gases and nutritive ingredients in the capillary segment. Thus, blood flowing into the venous level via the capillary level of circulation is practically without any capillary exchange. Such changes cause severe local nutritive alterations, bringing about intensive and extensive venous ulcerations which are resistant to therapeutic procedures.

The results and findings show there can be damage to capillary gas exchange in venous ulcers. The results also prove that other factors may be significant in the formation of venous ulcers, all of which could be of great importance for the treatment of patients with venous ulcers.

References

1. Homans J. The etiology and treatment of varicose ulcer of the leg. Surg Gynecol Obstet 1917;24:300.
2. Blalock A. Oxygen content of blood in patients with varicose veins. Arch Surg 1929;19:309.
3. Piulacks P, Vidal-Barraquer F. Pathogenic study of varicose veins. Angiology 1953;4:59.
4. Browse NL, Burnand KG. The cause of venous ulceration. Lancet 1982;2:243.
5. Holling HE, Beacher HK, Linton RR. Study of the tendency to oedema formation associated with incompetence of the valves of the communicating veins of the leg. Oxygen tension of the blood contained in varicose veins. J Clin Invest 1938; 17:555.
6. Fagrell B. Local microcirculation in chronic venous incompetence and leg ulcers. Vasc Surg 1979;13:217.
7. Fagrell B. Vital capillary microscopy. Scand J Clin Lab Invest (Suppl 133) 1973.
8. Burnand KG, Whimster I, Naidoo A, Browse NL. Pericapillary fibrin in the ulcer-bearing skin of the leg: The cause of lipodermatosclerosis and venous ulceration. Br Med J 1982;285:1071.
9. Stacey MC, Burnand KG, Layer GT, Pattison M. Transcutaneous oxygen tensions in assessing the treatment of healed venous ulcers. Br J Surg 1990;77:1050.
10. Maksimović Ž. Etiopatogeneza, klinika i operativno lečenje "Ulcus venosuma" donjih ekstremiteta. Ph.D. thesis, University Medical School, Belgrade, Yugoslavia, 1985.

56
Local Lactate and Pyruvate Values Prior to and Following a Shearing Operation for Venous Ulcers

Živan V. Maksimović, Veljko Djukić, Djordje Radak, and Tomislav Jovanović

Introduction

Venous ulcers manifest as loss of skin and subcutaneous tissues on the legs, usually localized on the lower legs around and above the medial malleolus, and caused by venous stasis.

Although there are differences in etiologic explanations, it is mostly accepted that postthrombotic disorders of deep veins of other lesions lead to incompetence of perforators (communicating veins) and consequently to pathologic blood reflux from the deep into the superficial veins. This leads to progressive impairment of microcirculation accompanied by proliferation of the capillaries, which become prolonged and twisted.[2] The endothelial cells become swollen and contain large vacuoles, and the basement membrane becomes irregular and thickened; these changes are manifested as lipodermatosclerosis, cell destruction, and ulcer development.[1-3]

Whatever the origin, severe deprivation of oxygen leads to a reduction in the tricarboxylic acid cycle and subsequently to glycolytic reduction of pyruvate to lactate. This develops into a severe form of acidosis, called lactic acidosis, which is associated with an increase in the lactate-pyruvate blood ratio, and lactate levels may rise as high as 25 mmol/L or higher.[4] Lactate in the presence of NAD^+ and lactate dehydrogenase (LDH), a hydrogen transfer enzyme, is oxidized to pyruvate:

$$Lactate + NAD^+ \xrightarrow{LDH} pyruvate + NADH + H^+$$

In severe shock and anoxia, LDH levels may be moderately elevated. There were no data available on the values of lactate and pyruvate in venous blood from venous ulceration sites, nor on possible changes of these values following static strain.

The treatment of patients with venous ulcers is aimed at interrupting the blood reflux in perforator veins. This could be temporarily achieved with special elastic bandages, which are regularly followed by ulcer recurrences. Surgical treatment of postthrombotic ulcerations, on the other hand, was followed by bad results and a high percentage of postoperative recurrences.

In the past three decades it was definitely concluded that surgical treatment consists of effective interruption of the pathological reflux through the incompetent perforating veins. This could be achieved with the following procedures:

Suprafascial (extrafascial) ligation of the medial communicating veins (Cockett's operation)[3];
Subfascial ligation and division of the medial communicating veins (Linton's[5] and Dodd's[6] operations);
Subfascial shearing (discission) perforators (Albanese's[7] Edwards',[8] or Petron and Pennin's[9] operations).

Extrafascial operations are difficult to perform in patients who have venous ulcerations with advanced lipodermatosclerosis. Therefore De Palma[10] suggested multiple incisions, although in such conditions there is a possibility of overlooking important incompetent perforators or their survival which later on increase and lead to recurrences. Also, in the direct subfascial approach to perforators, there is major surgical trauma due to surgical incisions through ulcerative surfaces, which is accompanied by necrosis and infections and which prolongs the postoperative course.

The subfascial shearing operation enables the approach to the pathological site from the healthy region by incision through healthy skin, subcutaneous tissue, and fascia outside the ulceration so that there is no possibility of increasing the intraoperative trauma. However, complications are possible with this method (hemorrhage, subfascial infection, or lesions of nerves or other subfascial structures). Nevertheless, this method offers favorable immediate and long-term results with tolerable complications if properly performed.

The aim of this report is to examine the regional lactate and pyruvate values before and after static strain. We also present immediate and long-term results of the shearing operation. Beside other parameters, we assessed the efficacy of this method by measuring the lactate and pyruvate values during the immediate postoperative period, and the findings were compared with the preoperative findings in patients with unilateral venous ulcers.

Materials and Methods

We studied a group of 96 patients (mean age 52.2 ± 6.3 years) with unilateral venous ulcers. The ulcerations had lasted on average 3.5 years (range 1–18 years, SE = 4.6 years) before surgery. During the period 1978–1982 we performed the so-called shearing operation as monotherapy or together with some other procedure (extirpation of varices, partial or complete stripping of vena saphena magna). The long-term results were analyzed in 1991 and 1992, and the average follow-up period was 10.1 years (range 12–14 years).

The sex distribution was almost equal, 49 female and 47 male patients, although the incidence of total venous diseases was twice as high in women for the given period. A positive family history was given by 62 patients (64.6%); a history of previous deep vein thrombosis by 77 (80.2%); a history of hormonal disorders or use of hormonal contraceptives by 44 (89.8%) women; a history of previous sclerosant therapy by 12 (12.5%); a history of previous trauma by 9 (9.4%); and a history of other associated diseases (hemorrhoids, lymphatic diseases, etc.) by 15 (15.6%).

Subfascial Shearing (Perforators Discission) Operation

A subfascial shearing operation was performed in all patients in the supine position with the affected leg elevated so that the lower leg was above the thoracic level, after the usual preparations and introduction of spinal epidural anesthesia. Incompetent perforators were localized by Doppler echography and marked. Phlebography was done in 21 patients with unclear status in order to discover the ulceration cause. Surgery is performed in the following way: a 6- to 10-cm-long incision is done above the ulceration on the medial side of the affected lower leg. The subcutaneous tissue and fascia are cut, and with the operator's finger the initial cleavage is done and a phlebotome is placed into it and passed all the way through the medial malleolus.[7-12] Immediately after the operation, after closure of fascia and skin with interrupted sutures, a stiff elastic bandage is placed. If there are indications, extirpation of varices or partial or complete stripping of vena saphena magna could be performed. To lower the occurrence of lesions of subfascial structures, we use the original modification of Edwards' phlebotome with a semispherical convexity at the "working part" of the phlebotome which bluntly separates subfascial structures (Fig. 56.1).

During the follow-up period we analyzed the incidence of symptoms and signs of venous stasis as well as signs of ulcer recurrences.

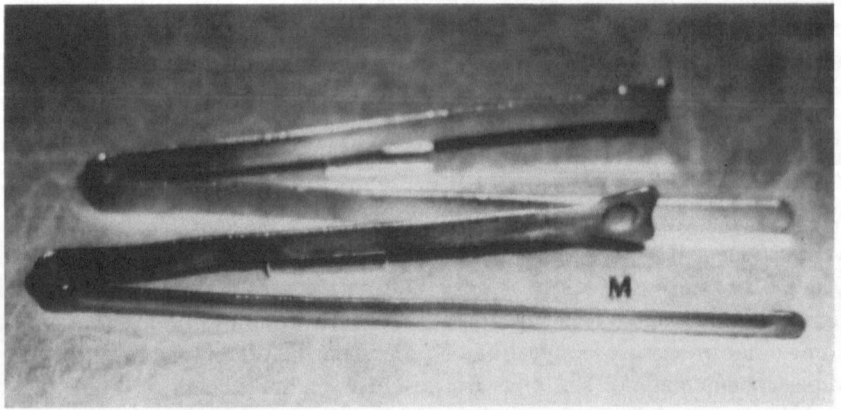

FIGURE 56.1. Edwards' phlebotome and modification of the working part (M).

Measurements of Regional Lactate and Pyruvate Values

Blood samples for lactate and pyruvate determination were taken from the vein draining the ulcerative region before and after static fatigue, in other words, by inactivating the venous pump with passive standing for 30 minutes. The control blood sample was taken under the same conditions from the other healthy leg. All samples were taken before meals, the day before surgery, and on the seventh day after the shearing operation. Lactate and pyruvate determination was done in 8 patients.

The Boehringer-Mannheim GmbH method[13] was used for determination of lactate levels; normal values in venous blood were 1.0–1.78 mmol/L.[14]

The level of pyruvate was measured using the Boehringer-Mannheim GmbH method[15] as well, and the normal values in venous blood were 41–67 μmol/L.[16]

Results and Discussion

The shearing operation was performed in all prospectively followed patients. In the majority of them (91 patients), extirpation of surrounding varices was performed before this operation, and partial or complete stripping of the vena saphena magna was performed in 50 patients, which was dictated by preoperative clinical, Doppler, and phlebographic findings.

Immediate postoperative complications were registered in 21 (21.9%) patients, which manifested as subcutaneous seromas (6 patients), local wound infection (4 patients), dermatitis (4 patients), subcutaneous hematomas (3 patients), edema of the wound and ulcer region (3 patients), and repeated thrombosis of distal deep veins (1 patients).

During the long-term postoperative course we followed 93 (96.9%); 3 patients did not respond to our calls. Satisfactory results were achieved (Table 56.1). Ulcer recurrences were found in only 7 patients, although 5 ulcers were registered at new sites (Table 56.1).

TABLE 56.1. Long-term results after shearing operation.

Finding	No.	%
Temporary mild pain	18	19.4
Constant pain at ulcer site	3	3.2
Heavy legs and leg edema	21	22.6
Itching, numbness, and paresthesia	31	33.3
Cramps of venous origin	9	9.7
Recurrent varices (various stages)	28	30.1
Persistent and developed hyperpigmentation	32	34.4
Ulcer recurrence and ulcer deterioration	2	2.2
New ulcers (at new sites)	5	5.4

Somewhat better results were reported by Simpson and Smeillie (3.9% of recurrences), but their long-term follow-up period was shorter (24 months).[11] However, during the long-term postoperative period over 10 years, the incidence of recurrences, varices, and other signs of ulceration was significant (Table 56.1). Other signs of venous stasis may also exist, as well as a significant incidence of neurological deficits, as a consequence of the subfascial shearing procedure (paresthesia and similar deficits). Those lesions rarely, according to the patients, have essential impact on their lives. Generally speaking, the shearing method of subfascial discission of the incompetent perforating vein is a reliable procedure for curing venous ulceration, and for that reason it is not clear why it is not applied more widely (Fig. 56.2).

Significantly lower venous blood values were found before static strain in the ulceration site, in contrast to values from blood taken from the healthy leg. Although the obtained concentrations are within normal ranges, such findings may indicate either decreased lactate production or its increased transformation into pyruvate (during rest). By excluding the venous pump during 30 minutes of passive standing, new conditions of venous stasis are created, which are manifested by significantly increased venous blood lactate values from the ulceration site (Table 56.2).

On the seventh postoperative day, venous blood lactate values from the ulceration site became normal, and static fatigue did not significantly affect the lactate blood concentration (Table 56.3).

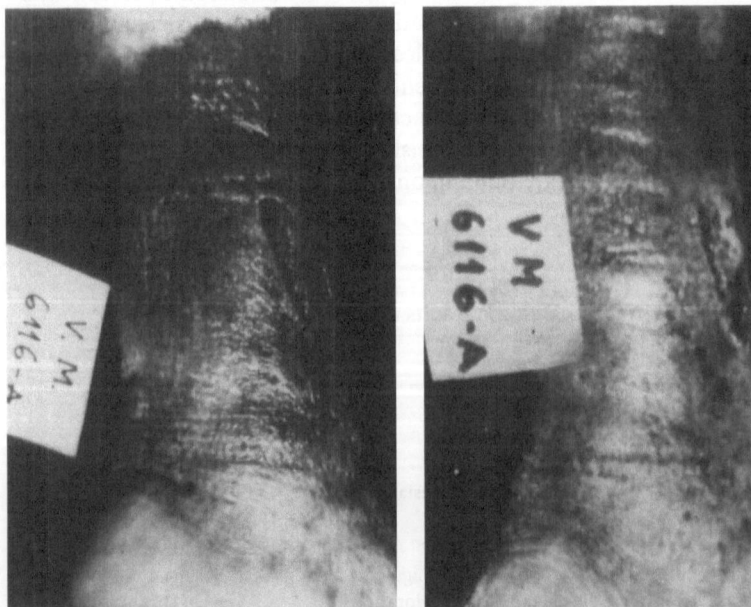

FIGURE 56.2. Postthrombotic leg ulcer (left) and healed ulcer on the seventh day after shearing operation (right).

TABLE 56.2. Preoperative local lactate values in venous blood before and after static fatigue.

Static fatigue	Sample	No.	X	SE	Significance
Before	Ulcer	8	0.59	0.19	t = 2.640
	Control	8	1.33	0.18	p < 0.05
After	Ulcer	8	1.86	0.26	t = 3.222
	Control	8	1.86	0.21	p < 0.01

TABLE 56.3. Postoperative local lactate values in venous blood before and after static fatigue.

Static fatigue	Sample	No.	X	SE	Significance
Before	Ulcer	8	1.41	0.14	t = 0.785
	Control	8	1.33	0.22	p < 0.05
After	Ulcer	8	1.56	0.10	t = 1.137
	Control	8	1.48	0.15	p > 0.05

TABLE 56.4. Preoperative local pyruvate values in venous blood before and after static fatigue.

Static fatigue	Sample	No.	X	SE	Significance
Before	Ulcer	8	63.63	6.09	t = 1.841
	Control	8	58.50	4.98	p > 0.05
After	Ulcer	8	78.87	5.30	t = 5.562
	Control	8	62.38	6.50	p < 0.05

TABLE 56.5. Postoperative local pyruvate values in venous blood before and after static fatigue.

Static fatigue	Sample	No.	X	SE	Significance
Before	Ulcer	8	60.43	4.16	t = 0.768
	Control	8	58.71	4.19	p < 0.05
After	Ulcer	8	67.00	5.60	t = 1.143
	Control	8	63.43	6.08	p > 0.05

Pyruvate values were higher in venous blood from the ulceration site, but the differences became significant only after 30 minutes of static strain (Table 56.4).

On the seventh day after the shearing operation, the concentration of pyruvate became normal and no statistically significant differences in venous blood of either region were found. Static fatigue also did not lead to significant increase of pyruvate concentration (Table 56.5).

Conclusion

Static fatigue (passive standing) for 30 minutes led to venous stasis and increased lactate and pyruvate blood values in the region of venous ulcers. This indicates that there were regional metabolic changes in the tricarboxylic acid cycle which may be responsible for the development of venous ulcerations.

The advantages of the shearing operation are: complete interruption of incompetent perforating veins, minimization of trauma by approaching the pathologic region from the healthy one, shorter duration of hospitalization, excellent immediate and reliable long-term cure of venous ulcers, and normalization of local lactate and pyruvate values before and after static fatigue.

References

1. Leu HJ. The prognostic significance of cutaneous and microvascular changes in venous leg ulcers. Vasc Dis 1965;2:77.
2. Corrigan TP, Kakkar VV. Early changes in the postphlebitic limb: Their clinical significance. Br J Surg 1973;60:808.
3. Cockett FB. The pathology and treatment of venous ulcers of the leg. Br J Surg 1955;43:260.
4. Tietz NW. *Fundamentals of Clinical Chemistry*. 3rd ed. Philadelphia: WB Saunders, 1987, p. 442.
5. Linton RR. The communicating veins of the lower leg and the operative technique for their ligation. Ann Surg 1938;107:582.
6. Dodd H. The diagnosis and ligation of incompetent perforating veins. Ann R Coll Surg Engl 1964;34:186.
7. Albanese AR. New instruments of varicose vein surgery. J Cardiovasc Surg 1965;6:65.
8. Edwards JM. Shearing operation for incompetent perforating veins. Br J Surg 1976;63:885.
9. Petrov ML, Pennin BA. Khirurgicheskoe lechenie pri posttrombophlebitischesko sindrome. Vest Khir 1976;116:48.
10. DePalma RG. Surgical therapy for venous stasis. Surgery 1974;76:910.
11. Simpson CJ, Smeillie GD. The phlebotome in the management of incompetent perforating veins and venous ulcer.
12. Maksimović ŽM. Etiopatogeneza, klinika i operativno lečenje "Ulcus venosuma" donjih ekstremitet. Ph. D. thesis, University Medical School, Belgrade, Yugoslavia, 1985.
13. Gutman I, Awhlefeld AW. In: Bargemeyer, HU (ed.). *Methoden der enzymatischen Analyse, 3. Auflage, Band II.* Weinheim: Verlag Chemie, 1974, S. 1510.
14. Laudahn G. Klin Wschr 1959;37:850.
15. Czok R, Lamprecht W. In: Bergmeyer HU (ed.). *Methoden der enzymatischen Analyse, 3. Auflage, Band II.* Weinheim: Verlag Chemie, 1974, S. 1491.
16. Landon J, et al. J Clin Pathol 1962;15:579.

57
Ablative Surgery Versus Sclerotherapy in the Treatment of Vein Disease

GEORGE M. ROBB

Introduction

Despite the many recent advances in reparative techniques in dealing with venous problems, ablative methods, whether by direct surgery or by compression sclerotherapy, remain the mainstay of current treatment protocols. The overall results in five thousand cases of venous insufficiency treated by one or both methods are reviewed. The findings would tend to suggest that although the sclerotherapy techniques are more acceptable to a larger number of patients, the results from surgery can be equally good, and of longer duration if modern techniques are used. In many cases the best results will be achieved by using a surgical approach initially and reserving sclerotherapy for problems with recurrent varicosities. However, in patients in whom there is no evidence of saphenofemoral incompetence or other perforator incompetence, sclerotheraphy alone will achieve satisfactory long-term results.

Surgical Techniques

Incisions

It has come to be realized by specialists in this field worldwide that the large incisions that were commonly employed for vein surgery a decade or so ago can no longer be justified in most cases. In the groin the incision has to be adequate to allow adequate exploration of the saphenofemoral junction. Except in the very obese, this means an incision in the 4- to 6-cm range. Furthermore, it is generally accepted that except in unusual circumstances the incision should be in the groin crease.

When stripping superficial varicosities, incisions about 3 mm in size are all that are required. The underlying vein is picked up with a hooking technique and exteriorized through the incision. Then, by continuous traction, as much of the vein as possible is exteriorized and then avulsed. No ties are necessary, and as many incisions are made as are necessary for complete stripping of the vein. The use of local anesthetic for this procedure is gaining popularity when treating short lengths of vein.

Procedures

Great Saphenous Stripping

Most centers recommend that stripping of the great saphenous vein be done when saphenofemoral incompetence has been demonstrated, but most are content with stripping out the vein in the thigh only—down to the level of about the knee joint—claiming that this is the basic minimal stripping that is necessary. This procedure is often referred to as "short stripping." Most authorities feel that simple ligation and division of the great saphenous is not adequate. Other workers in this field advocate sclerotherapy of the saphenofemoral junction, but this can make subsequent dissection more difficult in the event of failure of sclerotherapy, as will be the result in about 50% of cases so treated.

Small Saphenous and/or Gastrocnemius Vein Division

Stripping of the small spahenous vein may also be indicated occasionally. Some French workers have described indications for ligation and division of the gastrocnemius vein at its origin from the popliteal vein, and much has been written about the importance of adequate examination and treatment of veins issuing from the popliteal fossa.

Groin Exploration in Recurrent Varicose Veins

Under modern conditions, blind exploration of the saphenofemoral junction should seldom be necessary. In recurrent varicose veins, the presence of persistent reflux at the saphenofemoral junction can be readily confirmed or refuted by Doppler studies, especially with the use of the color Doppler. There should be no need then to advocate routine reexploration of the groin in all cases of vein recurrence, but only when such abnormal reflux has been demonstrated by Doppler or venogram. Indeed, as we achieve better results in initial exploration of the groin, the presence of persistent varices in this region is becoming less common in cases of recurrent varicose veins. A more fruitful field for exploration would be to look for an incompetent Hunter's canal perforator, or more commonly, incompetent perforating veins in the posterior compartment of the calf. However, these are often best dealt with by sclerotherapy, even if it might mean treatment every few years, because most patients find the scar necessitated by fasciotomy to be unacceptable. Whatever approach is chosen, it must not be forgotten that the related superficial varices must also be eradicated by one of the methods already described. Fasciotomy by endoscopy is also gradually taking a place in the methods to be considered.

Results of Review

In the series currently under review, treatment was mainly by surgery in the earlier years, and mainly by sclerotherapy in the later years. The cases reviewed were seen between 1976 and 1986. Ages ranged from 12 to 100 years, with a median age of 34. This period has seen a great reversal in the relative importance of sclerotherapy and surgery in the management of venous problems. Whereas in the 1970s it was usual to recommend surgery as the primary procedure and sclerotherapy mainly as a method of dealing with recurrences, a large number of patients are now encountered who request sclerotherapy as the primary approach in therapy. If there is no clinical or Doppler evidence of saphenofemoral incompetence or other significant perforator incompetence, there is ample experience now to give reasonable assurance to the patient that the immediate outcome will be satisfactory. The recurrence rate, however, is higher than with surgical removal. In such cases, multiple superficial avulsion through small incisions is an excellent primary procedure. On the other hand, sclerotherapy is a much simpler procedure initially, and repeat treatments for recurrence are well accepted so long as the possible need for this is explained to the patient at the outset. This is particularly true when one considers that sclerotherapy seldom entails any loss of work days.

Fifteen percent of patients in this review were initially seen for recurrent varices. These on the whole make rapid progress with sclerotherapy if there is no persistent saphenofemoral or perforator incompetence. Moreover, in such patients calf perforator incompetence is often readily dealt with by sclerotherapy. The main indications for surgery in these would be persistent incompetence at the saphenofemoral junction or failure of calf perforators to respond to sclerotherapy.

Patients selected for sclerotherapy had an average of three treatments over a period of 3 to 6 weeks and were then asked to attend for review in 3 months after completion of treatment. Treatment was continued until all significant varices were brought under control. When varices were very extensive, treatment was continued for a few months controlling the main sources of superficial venous hypertension. In such patients, the importance of annual or more frequent review and treatment was emphasized.

At 2 years postsclerotherapy the incidence of recurrence—including minimal recurrences—was 42%, but even those showing some recurrence nevertheless showed marked improvement in appearance as well as improvement in venous function, as evidenced by fewer problems with swelling, erythema, cellulitis, ulceration, etc. when compared with their initial presentation.

After surgery the patient was advised to report any small recurrences that might develop and have them treated. With surgery a recurrence rate of about 24% was found. These were usually treated by sclerotherapy. It should be borne in mind that the cases recommended for surgery as the primary treatment either had severe incompetence at the saphenofemoral junction or had very extensive varicose veins, often with advanced venous insufficiency.

In general, the more the superficial spread of varices has been allowed to extend, the more likely it is that recurrent or persistent varices will be a problem. Such cases also involve more discomfort with sclerotherapy. It is felt that a good case can be made for dealing with varicose veins at an early stage rather than leaving them to extend out of control, thus damaging perforators that are initially competent. In the few patients who are deemed unfit for surgery when it seems that surgery is the best choice, sclerotherapy alone can on occasion give amazingly good results. Sclerotherapy is also used in some centers as an adjunct to the treatment of varicose ulceration.

Reference

Hobb JT. The enigma of the gastrocnemius vein. Phlebology 1988;3:19–30.

58
Functional Evaluation of the Venocuff Sleeve in the Primary Great Saphenous Varicose Vein

Bo Yang Suh, Dong Kweon Suh, and Koing Bo Kwun

The conventional treatments for the primary saphenous varicose vein have been high ligation, stripping, and/or sclerotherapy. Therefore, the vein cannot be used as a substitutional graft vessel for either peripheral or coronary arteries. Moreover, high ligation frequently causes thrombophlebitis in the involved vein.[1] In 1988, Jessup et al.[2] reported the use of the Venocuff as a new surgical procedure in animal models. In 1988, Raju et al.[3] found that an addition of the Dacron sleeve following valvuloplasty on chronic venous insufficiency patients produced good results. Repair of venous valvular insufficiency with the use of the Venocuff sleeve allows recovery of valvular function and prevents backflow. It is simple and less invasive than other procedures.[4] We have utilized this technique for the past several years and found it to be very effective.

Materials and Methods

Eighteen patients with a primary great saphenous varicose vein were treated by application of Venocuff sleeves. They were 7 males and 6 females with an age range of 20 to 63 (mean 43 years). The average symptom duration was 4 years. The pre- and postoperative values of superficial venous pressure and venous refilling time using direct puncture method and photoplethysmography (PPG) were obtained from 13 patients and compared.

Measurement of Superficial Venous Pressure

The great saphenous vein was directly punctured at ankle level and connected to a 4-way channel monitor (Model SE-485 Monitor, Se-In Electric Company, An-Yang City, Korea). The superficial venous pressure was then measured and the venous refilling time was calculated with foot exercise.

PPG Test

The PPG monitor (VASOFLO®-2, Model 4600, Sonicaid Ltd. Chichester, England) was used. The photoelectric cell was applied at the skin just above

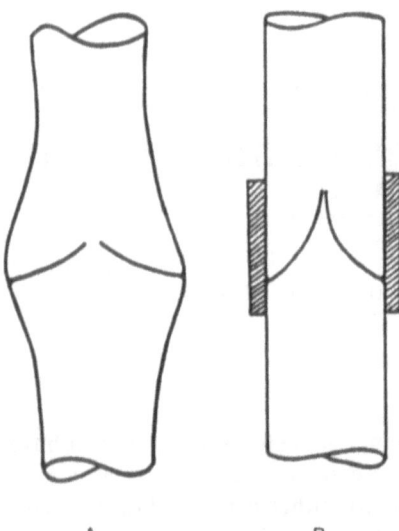

FIGURE 58.1. Cut surface of vein. (A) Valvular insufficiency. (B) Apposition of the insufficient valve after Venocuff application.

A   B

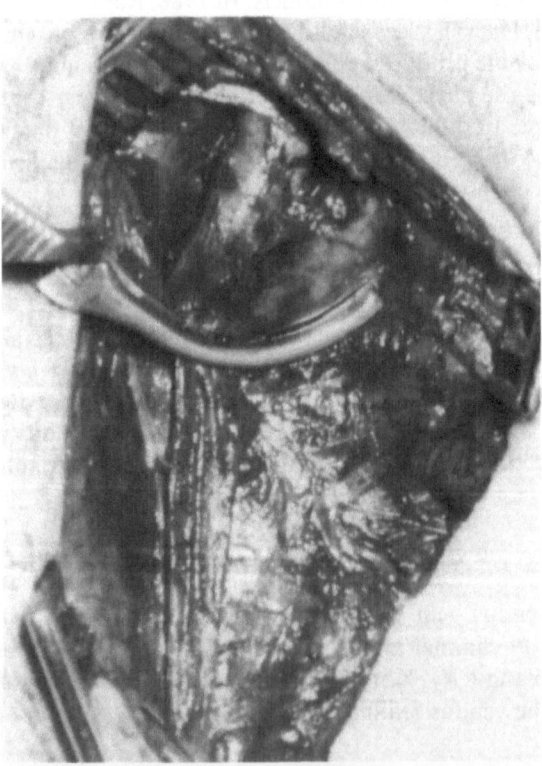

FIGURE 58.2. Saphenofemoral junction. Clamping proximal and distal part of the valve with vascular clamp prevented back flow.

the medial malleolus and then the venous refilling time was recorded with foot exercise.

The Venocuff material is usually either Dacron-reinforced silicone or polytetrafluoroethylene (PTFE; Goretex®). We used the Goretex cuff with an average width of 1.2–1.5 cm and diameter of 5–6 mm (Figs. 58.1 and 58.4).

The surgical procedure consisted of skin incision, exposure of the valve area of the saphenofemoral junction, checking for the presence or absence of backflow, and application of the Venocuff around the valvular site in order to reduce the circumference and to bring the valve cusp into apposition. After the valvular function was recovered, the absence of backflow was confirmed by the milking test or the clamp-release method using vascular clamps (Figs. 58.2–58.4).

All measurements were expressed by their mean value and standard deviation, and the statistical significance of the results was assessed by the paired Student's *t*-test.

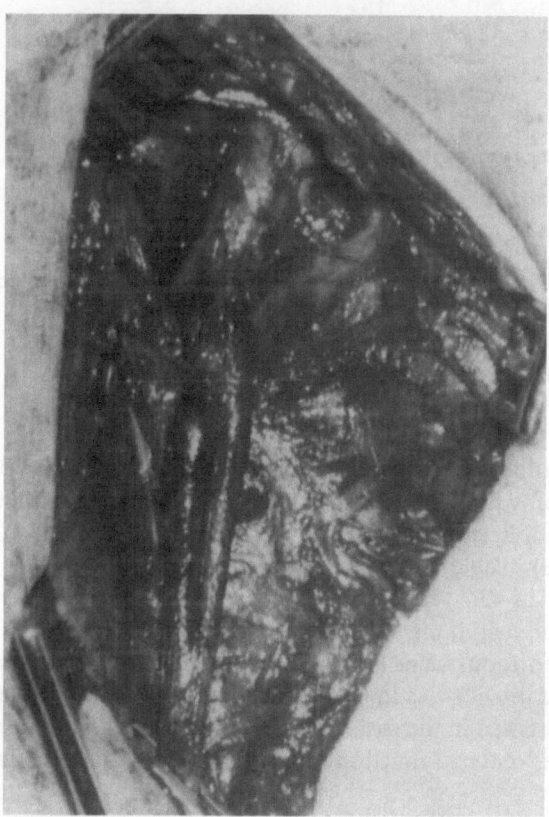

FIGURE 58.3. When the proximal vascular clamp was released, marked back flow was noted, which shows insufficient valvular function.

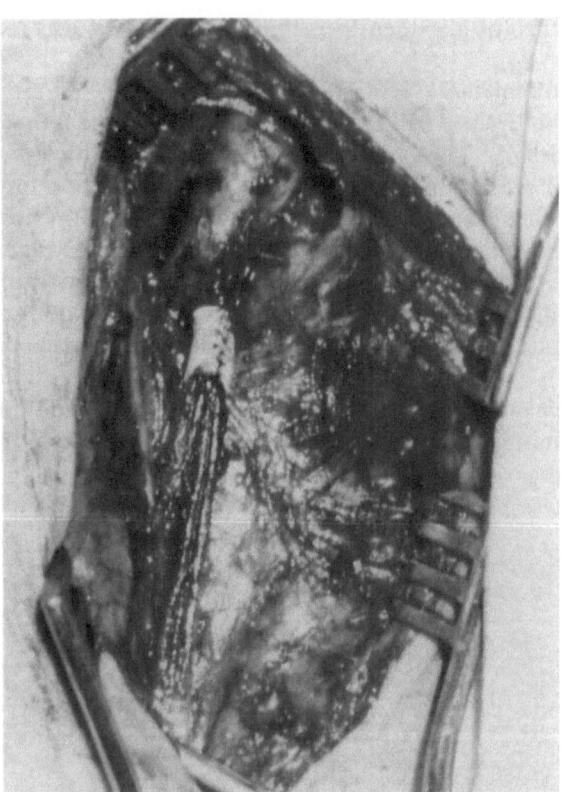

FIGURE 58.4. After Venocuff application, back flow was not noted, which shows recovery of valvular function.

Results

Among 18 patients who had been treated by this procedure, 13 patients who underwent full vascular laboratory examination before and after operations were analyzed. The average follow-up time was 13 months (postoperative 1–27 months) (Table 58.1). The male-to-female ratio was 7 to 6 and the average age was 43.2 years, with a range of 20–63 years (Table 58.2).

The clinical symptoms, including venous engorgement ($n = 12$), calf pain ($n = 3$), and tortuous veins ($n = 4$), were all improved after operation. However, swelling ($n = 2$) was improved in 1 out of 2 cases (Table 58.2). Recurrence was observed in the case of 1 patient, in which there was backflow due to the loss of Venocuff function and confirmed by the venous refilling time tests.

The mean venous refilling times measured by superficial venous punctures were 9.0 ± 1.5 seconds preoperatively and 20.5 ± 2.5 seconds postoperatively. The mean venous refilling times measured by PPG were 8.8 ± 1.1

TABLE 58.1. Venous pressure and photoplethysmography (PPG).

No. of patients	Follow-up duration (months)	Venous pressure refilling time (sec)		PPG refilling time (sec)	
		Pre-OP	Post-OP	Pre-OP	Post-OP
1	27	11	13	10	11
2	22	8	21	9	20
3	19	9	21	9	21
4	18	7	19	8	18
5	17	8	21	7	20
6	16	8	20	9	21
7	12	10	23	8	22
8	10	9	21	11	22
9	10	11	24	9	23
10	8	10	21	9	22
11	7	11	22	10	20
12	2	7	21	9	21
13	1	8	20	7	19
Mean ± SD	13.0 ± 7.7	9.0 ± 1.5	20.5 ± 2.6**	8.8 ± 1.1	20.0 ± 3.0**

** $P < 0.01$.

seconds preoperatively and 20.0 ± 3.0 seconds postoperatively ($p < 0.01$; Table 58.1; Figs. 58.5 and 58.6).

Discussion

Varicose veins can be classified into primary and secondary. The cause of secondary varicose veins is valvular insufficiency of either the deep vein or the perforating vein, or both. Secondary varicose veins can be partially treated by ligation of the perforating veins and/or stripping of the superficial veins.[5]

Primary great saphenous varicose veins are caused by valvular insufficiency of the saphenofemoral junction. The difference between primary and secondary varicose veins can be detected by the Trendelenburg test and the PPG test. The Trendelenburg test can detect valvular insufficiency of the saphenofemoral junction. The PPG test can detect valvular insufficiency of both the deep vein and the perforating vein (Figs. 58.5 and 58.6). To assess the competence of the saphenofemoral valve, the milking technique or the clamp-release test using vascular clamps was used at the operative field.

In most varicose veins, venous wall defects and venous distentions are observed, but valve cusps themselves are surprisingly well preserved.[6] Cotton[7] found macroscopically normal values in 123 of 156 valves examined. Edwards and Edwards[8] found separation of the commissure without constant lesion of the cusp in all 106 patients examined.

TABLE 58.2. Clinical results in the 13 patients.

No. of patients	Age (years)	Sex	Recurrence	Symptoms (pre-OP/post-OP)			
				Venous engorgement	Calf pain	Tortuous vein	Swelling
1	27	M	+	+/−	−/−	−/−	−/−
2	57	M	−	+/−	−/−	−/−	−/−
3	48	F	−	+/−	−/−	−/−	−/−
4	63	M	−	+/−	−/−	+/−	−/−
5	45	M	−	+/−	+/−	−/−	−/−
6	54	M	−	+/−	+/−	−/−	−/−
7	28	F	−	+/−	−/−	+/−	−/−
8	47	F	−	+/−	−/−	−/−	+/+
9	25	M	−	−/−	−/−	+/−	−/−
10	43	F	−	+/−	−/−	−/−	−/−
11	20	F	−	+/−	+/−	+/−	+/−
12	55	M	−	+/−	−/−	−/−	−/−
13	49	F	−	+/−	−/−	−/−	−/−

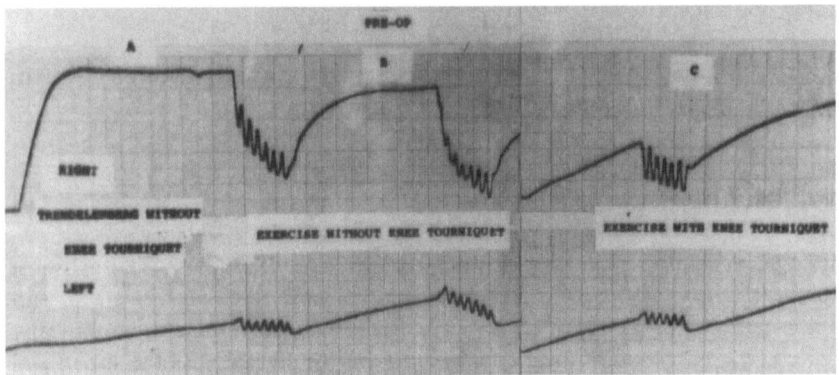

FIGURE 58.5. Preoperative PPG. (A) Trendelenburg test without knee tourniquet; severe back flow was noted in the right leg compared with the left leg. (B) Exercise without knee tourniquet; severe back flow was noted in the right leg. This finding shows insufficient saphenofemoral valvular function. (C) Exercise with knee tourniquet; back flow was not noted in the right leg. This finding shows intact valvular function of the deep and perforating vein.

There are several advantages when using the Venocuff sleeve as treatment for the primary great saphenous varicose vein. First, the procedure is simple and easy. Second, the cuff can be applied on multiple sites of the valve areas. Third, it is a relatively less invasive method. Four, the recurrence rate is low due to the functional restoration of venous valvular competence by reducing the vein circumference. Last, the great saphenous vein can be preserved for

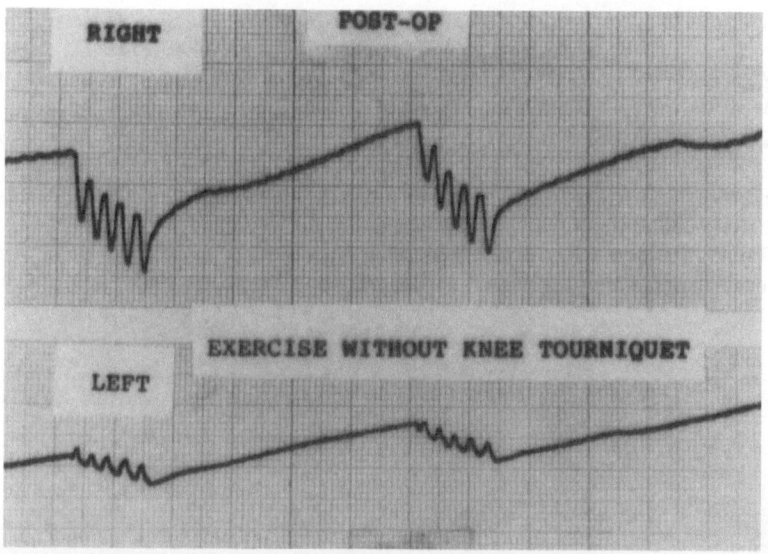

FIGURE 58.6. Postoperative PPG. Exercise without knee tourniquet; venous refilling time was returned to the normal range in the right leg.

further vascular bypass grafts.[4] The disadvantage of using the Venocuff sleeve is the risk of thrombosis due to stenosis or fibrosis and the risk of graft infection.[1]

We did not experience either of these disadvantages. Within 27 months postoperatively, there was only one case of recurrence. There were improvements in venous engorgement, calf pain, and tortuous veins. The swelling of the foot improved in 1 out of 2 patients. All patients were able to return to their normal lifestyles.

Raju et al.[9] reported that the venous refilling time measured by pre- and postoperative venous pressure and PPG test is normally above 22 seconds, but below 10 seconds in chronic venous insufficiency. In almost all of our cases, venous refilling times measured by superficial venous pressure and PPG with foot exercise test returned to normal. In one case the postoperative venous refilling time did not change and this was identified as a recurrence.

References

1. Large J. A conflict in vascular surgery. Aust NZ J Surg 1985;55:373–376.
2. Jessup G, Lane RJ. Repair of incompetent venous valve. J Vasc Surg 1988;8:569–575.
3. Raju S. Valve reconstruction procedures for chronic venous insufficiency. Semin Vasc Surg 1988;1:101–106.
4. Ackroyd JS, Browse NL. The investigation and surgery of postthrombotic syndrome. J Cardiovasc Surg 1986;27:5–16.

5. Sabiston DC, Jr. *Textbook of Surgery: The Biological Basis of Modern Surgical Practice.* 14th ed. Philadelphia: WB Saunders, 1991, pp. 1490–1501.
6. Zoster T, Cronin RFP. Venous distensibility in patients with varicose veins. Can Med Assoc J 1966;94:1293–1297.
7. Cotton LT. Varicose veins. Gross anatomy and development. Br J Surg 1961;48:589–598.
8. Edwards JE, Edwards EA. The saphenous valves in varicose veins. Am Heart J 1940;19:338–351.
9. Raju S, Frederics RK. Valve reconstruction procedures for nonobstructive venous insufficiency. Rationale, techniques and results. J Vasc Surg 1988;7:301–302.

XX
Pulmonary Embolism

59
Genetic Predisposition to Pulmonary Embolism Following Deep Vein Thrombosis

Tomio Kawasaki, Jun-ichi Kambayashi, and Yoshio Uemura

Introduction

Pulmonary embolism (PE) is a common disorder which may be clinically quite silent. Several clinical studies have suggested that PE may be relatively common in especially high-risk hospitalized patients, although many of the patients are asymptomatic.[1-3] A high prevalence of asymptomatic PE, as high as 50%, following deep vein thrombosis (DVT) in the lower limbs has been also proven in several reports.[4-8] Approximately 90% of patients diagnosed with PE have evidence of DVT.[9,10] Thus, PE is frequently associated with DVT. Genetic predisposition to PE and DVT should be taken into account as one of the major pathogenic indicators of PE following DVT. Various congenital thrombotic disorders such as dysplasminogenemia (DPG),[11] antithrombin III deficiency,[12,13] and protein C and protein S deficiency[14-17] have been included as major etiologic factors of DVT. Our aim was to study the involvement of congenital thrombotic disorders in pathogenesis of PE as well as DVT.

Subjects and Methods

Patients

Forty-four consecutive patients with DVT of the lower extremity who were seen at the Department of Surgery II in Osaka University Medical School over a 3-year period extending from January 1, 1989 to December 31, 1991 were reviewed for this study. The diagnosis of DVT was made by a combination of duplex scanning, contrast venography, and radioisotopic (RI) venography. In the present investigation, two groups of patients were studied. One group consisted of 22 patients with PE confirmed by RI lung scanning. The other group consisted of 22 patients who had normal RI lung scanning. All the patients with positive venograms were analyzed in terms of age, diagnosis, symptoms, physical findings, and complications.

Venography and Lung Scanning

RI venography followed by RI perfusion lung scanning was performed after injection of ^{99m}Tc-labeled macroaggregated albumin. Eight views were obtained in the upright position: anterior, posterior, right and left lateral, and right and left anterior and posterior oblique. The perfusion lung scan was considered abnormal if a perfusion defect was present in at least two of the eight views.

Plasma Preparation and Laboratory Test

Blood was collected from antecubital veins into 1/10 volume of 3.8% sodium citrate in a plastic tube and was centrifuged at 2,000 g for 15 minutes to prepare platelet-poor plasma. The plasma was stored at $-80°C$ until use.

Laboratory tests were performed on the fibrinolytic system and regulatory systems of hemostasis to study the thrombotic abnormalities. The activity of plasminogen was assayed by a chromogenic assay using S-2251 (Kabi-Vitrum, Sweden), and the antigenicity was assayed by a single radial immunodiffusion using M-Partigen plates (Behring-werke, Germany). DPG was identified by the dissociation between activity and antigenicity of plasminogen. Antithrombin III activity was assayed by a chromogenic substrate assay kit using S-2238 (Test-zym, Daiichi Pure chemicals, Japan). Protein C activity was assayed also by a chromogenic substrate assay kit using PGPA-MNA (Berichrom, Behring-werke, Germany). Protein S activity was assayed by a clotting assay according to the method described by Comp PC.[18] Antithrombin III deficiency and protein C and S deficiency were strictly diagnosed only in the patients without liver failure and with a negligible amount of protein induced by vitamin K absence (PIVKA), which potentially affects the amount of those proteins.

Antithrombotic Therapy

Patients in the acute stage received a bolus injection of 100 U/kg of unfractionated heparin followed by a continuous infusion of 10–20 U/kg/hr monitored by the activated partial thromboplastin time to be between 50 and 100 seconds, and these patients also received a bolus injection of 4,000 U/kg of urokinase followed by a continuous infusion of 2,000–4,000 U/kg/hr. A subcutaneous injection of concentrated calcium heparin (25,000 U/ml) in a dose of 100 U/kg b.i.d. was given to those patients who were in subacute or chronic stage and who were admitted in our hospital. To some inpatients and to most outpatients, a relatively small dose of warfarin (2–5 mg) was administered to lower their PT value to 30–60%. The efficacy of warfarin therapy was monitored by serial determination of thrombin–antithrombin III complex (TAT).

Results

The average age of the 44 patients with DVT was 51 ± 13 years (ranging 12 to 74). The male/female ratio was 22/22. Twenty-two of these patients had evidence of association of PE identified by RI lung scan. The average age of patients with or without PE was 54 ± 12 and 49 ± 13 years, respectively. The difference was not statistically significant. The primary lesion of DVT in 44 cases is summarized in Table 59.1. The iliofemoral vein was mainly involved in thrombosis in both PE-positive and PE-negative groups. Four of five patients with thrombosis limited to the popliteal/calf vein had PE at admission, and no hematological abnormality was detected in these patients.

Eleven of 14 patients (79%) with DVT present in the right or both limbs were more prone to PE than those with left limb DVT (37%), although the involvement of left limb in DVT is more common (68%) than right (Table 59.2). Two of 9 patients with thrombotic disorders developed DVT in the right or both limbs (22%), and they developed PE. DPG was detected in these 2 patients. Eleven patients with DVT present in the right or both limbs developed PE (25%). The difference was not statistically significant. DPG was involved in the pathogenesis of PE in patients with DVT in the right limb or in both limbs.

As for hematological risk factors of DVT, all the cases were subjected to

TABLE 59.1. Primary lesion of thrombosis.

	PE positive		PE negative		Total	
	No.	Mean age	No.	Mean age	No.	Mean age
Iliac vein	8	55	9	48	17	51
Femoral vein	10	56	12	51	22	53
Popliteal vein	4	46	1	32	5	43
Total	22		22		44	

TABLE 59.2. Laterality of DVT.

	PE positive		PE negative	
	PE	CTD	PE	CTD
Left	11	3	19	4
Right	4	1	0	0
Both	7	1	3	0
Total	22	5	22	4

CTD, Congenital thrombotic disorders.

determination of plasminogen and antithrombin III. The plasma concentration of protein C was also determined in 23 patients who were not receiving warfarin at the time of assay. There were 4 cases of DPG, including one case of homozygote, and 3 cases of protein C deficiency, 1 case of protein S deficiency, and 1 case of antithrombin III deficiency, as summarized in Table 59.3.

The incidence of PE in 4 cases of DPG in this series is shown in Table 59.4. Three of 22 cases in the PE-positive group were DPG (14%), whereas only 1 of 22 cases in the PE-negative group (5%) was DPG. There was no statistically significant difference between the above values, which is probably due to the small number of cases. The age distribution of those patients who had congenital thrombotic disorders is shown in Table 59.5. The average age of

TABLE 59.3. Thrombotic disorders as risk factors for DVT.

Dysplasminogenemia (Aplasminogenemia = 1)	4 (of 44 cases)
Antithrombin III deficiency	1 (of 44 cases)
Protein C deficiency	3 (of 23 cases)
Protein S deficiency	1

TABLE 59.4. Incidence of PE.

	PE positive	PE negative
DPG positive	3	1
DPG negative	19	21
Total	22	22

TABLE 59.5. Age and incidence of PE in patients with congenital thrombotic disorders.

	Age (years)	PE
Dysplasminogenemia	32	−
	46	+
	58	+
Aplasminogenemia	43	+
Antithrombin III deficiency	65	+
Protein C deficiency	36	−
	52	−
	61	+
Protein S deficiency	12	−
Average age of patients:	45 ± 16	
with thrombotic disorders	53 ± 11	
without thrombotic disorders	$(p > 0.05)$	

TABLE 59.6. Other risk factors.

Surgery-related factors	
Pelvis (intestinal, urological, gynecological)	7
Bed rest for a long time (orthopedic, neurosurgical)	5
Restriction of leg movement (orthopedic)	1
Others	
Diabetes mellitus	4
Familial hyperlipidemia	2
Renal failure (nephrosis)	2
Behcet disease	2
Idiopathic thrombocytopenic purpura	1
Pregnancy	1

patients with thrombotic disorders (45 years) was lower than that of patients without any congenital thrombotic disorders (53 years). The overall incidence of congenital thrombotic disorder in the 44 DVT patients and 22 PE-positive patients was 20% and 23%, respectively. There was no statistically significant difference between the above values. Also, it was noteworthy that the incidence of PE in DPG patients was relatively high (75%) compared with that of protein C deficiency (33%). The results indicate that congenital thrombotic disorders are deeply involved in pathogenesis of DVT as well as PE, and that DPG is a predisposing factor for PE.

Other risk factors in this series are summarized in Table 59.6. Among them, surgery-related factors such as pelvic surgery and prolonged bed rest were major factors.

All the patients received antithrombotic therapy as described earlier. Special care was taken to treat the patients with protein C or S deficiency, as synthesis of these factors is vitamin K dependent. Practically, a relatively smaller dose of warfarin or subcutaneous self-injection of heparin was given to these patients seen at the outpatient clinic. By this treatment, the occurrence or exacerbation of DVT or PE was prevented.

Discussion

An unexpectedly high incidence of PE (as high as 50%) following DVT in the lower leg has been shown in several reports.[4-8] Our data support their findings, as 22 out of 44 DVT patients were diagnosed to have PE on lung perfusion study.

Cohen et al.[19] collected 44 cases with DVT and reported that none of 14 cases with thrombosis limited to the popliteal/calf veins developed PE, and only patients with iliofemoral and superficial femoral vein thrombosis developed PE. In contrast, Giachino[20] reported that 13% of fatal pulmonary emboli originated from isolated calf vein thrombosis.[20] Four of five patients with popliteal/calf DVT had PE at admission in our results, and involvement of thrombotic disorder in these patients was ruled out. Kakkar et al.[21,22] reported that clotting initially occurred in the tibial veins and soleal sinuses before extending into the thigh veins.[21,22] The popliteal/calf DVT patients we experienced were in subacute or chronic stages. During the time lag between onset and admission, some part of the thrombus extending from the popliteal/calf veins to the iliofemoral vein might have migrated to the pulmonary artery.

Patients with thrombosis present in the right limb were more prone to be involved in PE than those with left limb DVT in our results. No literature is available to compare with our result in this aspect. We postulated that the presence of physiological compression of the left iliac vein by the right iliac artery may prevent dislodging or migration of thrombi formed in the distal deep veins. It is also postulated that fibrinolytic and thrombotic disorders differently act on dislodging of thrombi, as 2 cases of DPG only were included among these patients.

Deficiencies of anticoagulant proteins and impairment of fibrinolytic proteins predispose patients to thrombotic disorders such as DVT and PE by decreasing either the body's restraints on the coagulation system or the component of fibrinolysis. Congenital deficiency of antithrombin III has an incidence of 0.05%, and over 60% of these patients will develop thrombotic disorders by age 40.[23,24] The incidence of protein C deficiency may be 0.5%, and thrombosis develops in more than half of affected patients.[25,26] Approximately 70% of protein S-deficient patients will have a venous thrombosis by 35 years of age.[27]

Although various thrombotic disorders have been included as major etiologic factors of DVT, the role of DPG in the impairment of fibrinolysis has not been studied in detail. DPG was identified by the dissociation between the amount and activity of plasminogen. This abnormality has autosomal dominant type inheritance and is uncommon, except among Japanese and probably other people of eastern Asian origin. The incidence of DPG in Japanese is relatively high (3.6%) within thrombotic disorders,[11,28] including DVT and visceral vein thrombosis.[29] The incidence of DPG, including aplasminogenemia, in this study was 9.1%, and the incidence of DPG in patients with PE was 13.6% (Table 59.4). Thus, DPG is deeply involved in pathogenesis of PE as well as DVT. As the average age of patients with congenital thrombotic disorders is younger than that of patients without these disorders (Table 59.5), those patients who have congenital thrombotic disorders have a tendency to develop PE as well as DVT at a younger age.

The blood samples were collected from 23 of 44 patients for protein C assay before starting prescription of warfarin, because warfarin inhibits vitamin K-dependent enzymes, including protein C and protein S. Although protein C and protein S deficiencies are rare, they are involved in the pathogenesis of PE as well as DVT. Prescribing warfarin to those patients should be minimized, since warfarin may induce skin necrosis.[30,31]

To evaluate the effectiveness of anticoagulation therapy, the amounts of TAT and fibrinogen degeneration product (d-d) were monitored. In cases when warfarin was administered, prothrombin time (PT) was monitored to the level between 30% and 60%; in such conditions, TAT and d-d were well controlled. The amount of warfarin we prescribed is relatively low compared with other reports. However, our regimen is capable of maintaining a low TAT value, and none of the patients in the present series developed additional DVT or PE. These observation indicated that a low dose of warfarin is sufficient as a treatment and prevention of DVT and/or PE. Recently, bedside monitoring of PT has been performed using a capillary coagulation monitor.[32]

Conclusions

The congenital thrombotic disorders such as DPG, antithrombin III deficiency, protein C deficiency, and protein S deficiency were deeply involved in the pathogenesis of DVT and PE. The average age of those hematologically abnormal patients is younger than normal. As DPG is deeply involved in the occurrence of DVT and pulmonary embolism, it is advisable to screen for the presence of DPG in treating at least Japanese DVT patients (and probably non-Japanese as well).

References

1. Goldhaber SZ. Strategies for diagnosis. In: *Pulmonary Embolism and Deep Vein Thrombosis*. Philadephia: WB Saunders, 1985, p. 79.
2. Rissanen V, Suomalainen O, Karjalainen P, et al. Screening for postoperative pulmonary embolism on the basis of clinical symptomatology routine electrocardiography and plain chest radiography. Acta Med Scand 1984;215:13.
3. Williams JV, Eikman EA, Greenberg S. Asymptomatic pulmonary embolism. A common event in high risk patients. Ann Surg 1982;193:323.
4. Kistner RL, Ball JJ, Nordyke RA, et al. Incidence of pulmonary embolism in the course of thrombophlebitis of the lower extremities. Am J Surg 1972;124:169.
5. Moser KM, LeMoine JR. Is embolic risk conditioned by location of deep venous thrombosis? Ann Intern Med 1981;94:439.
6. Plate G, Einarsson E, Eklof B, Ohlin P. Incidence of pulmonary embolism in acute iliofemoral vein thrombosis. Acta Chir Scand Suppl 1983;506:35.
7. Huisman MV, Buller HR, ten Cate JW, et al. Unexpected high prevalence of silent pulmonary embolism in patients with deep venous thrombosis. Chest 1980;95:498.
8. Monreal M, Barroso CRJ, Manzano JR, et al. Asymptomatic pulmonary embolism in patients with deep vein thrombosis. Is it useful to take a lung scan to rule out this condition? J Cardiovasc Surg 1989;30:104.
9. Hull RD, Hirsh J, Carter CJ, et al. Diagnostic efficacy of impedance plethysmo-

graphy for clinically suspected deep vein thrombosis: A randomized trial. Ann Intern Med 1985;102:21.

10. Huisman MV, Buller HR, ten Cate JW, Vreeken J. Serial impedance plethysmography for suspected deep vein thrombosis in outpatients: The Amsterdam general practitioner study. N Engl J Med 1986;314:823.

11. Aoki N, Moroi M, Sakata Y, et al. Abnormal plasminogen. A hereditary molecular abnormality found in a patient with recurrent thrombosis. J Clin Invest 1978; 61:1186.

12. Thaler E, Lechner K. Antithrombin III deficiency and thromboembolism. Clin Haematol 1981;10:369.

13. Prochownick EW, Antonarakis S, Bauer KA, et al. Molecular heterogeneity of inherited antithrombin III deficiency. N Engl J Med 1983;308:1549.

14. Griffin JH, Evatt B, Zimmerman TS, et al. Deficiency of protein C in congenital thrombotic disease. J Clin Invest 1981;68:1370.

15. Broekmans AW. Hereditary protein C deficiency. Haemostasis 1985;15:233.

16. Walker FJ. Protein S and the regulation of activated protein C. Semin Thromb Haemost 1984;10:131.

17. Bertina RM. Hereditary protein S deficiency. Haemostasis 1985;15:241.

18. Comp PC, Esmon CT. Recurrent venous thromboembolism in patients with a partial deficiency of protein S. N Engl J Med 1984;311:1525.

19. Cohen JR, Tymon R, Pillari G, Johnson H. Regional anatomical difference in the venographic occurrence of deep vein thrombosis and long-term follow-up. J Cardiovasc Surg 1988;29:547.

20. Giachino A. Relationship between deep-vein thrombosis in the calf and fatal pulmonary embolism. Can J Surg 1988;31:129.

21. Kakkar VV, Flang C, Howe CT. Natural history of postoperative deep-vein thrombosis. Lancet 1969;2:30.

22. Kakkar VV, Howe CT, Nicolaides AN, et al. Deep vein thrombosis of leg. Is there a "high risk" group. Am J Surg 1970;120:527.

23. Cosgriff TM, Bishop DT, Hershgold, et al. Familial antithrombin III deficiency: Its natural history, genetics, diagnosis and treatment. Medicine 1983;62:209.

24. Conard J, Horellou MH, Samama M. Incidence of thromboembolism in association with congenital disorders in coagulation and fibrinolysis. Acta Chir Scand (Suppl.) 1988;543:15.

25. Miletich J, Sherman L, Broze G. Absence of thrombosis in subjects with heterozygous protein C deficiency. N Engl J Med 1987;317:991.

26. Broekmans AW, Veltcamp JJ, Bertina RM. Congenital protein C deficiency and venous thromboembolism: A study of three Dutch families. N Engl J Med 1983; 309:340.

27. Engesser KL, Broekmans AW, Briet E, et al. Protein S deficiency: Clinical manifestations. Ann Intern Med 1987;106:677.

28. Aoki N, Terano K, Sakata Y. Differences of frequency distributions of plasminogen phenotypes between Japanese and American populations: New methods for the detection of plasminogen variants. Biochem Genet 1984;22:871.

29. Kawasaki T, Kambayashi J, Sakon M, et al. Portal vein calcification: A review of the last 50 years and report of a case with dysplasminogenemia. Surg Today 1993;23(2):176–181.

30. Faraci PA, Deterling RA, Stein AM, et al. Warfarin-induced necrosis of the skin. Surg Gynecol Obstet 1978;146:695.

31. Goldberg SL, Orthner CL, Yalisove BL, et al. Skin necrosis following prolonged administration of coumarin in a patient with inherited protein S deficiency. Am J Hematol 1991;38:64.
32. Yano Y, Kambayashi J, Murata K, et al. Bedside monitoring of warfarin therapy by a whole blood capillary coagulation monitor. Thromb Res 1992 1;66(5):583–590.

XXI
Portosystemic Shunt

60
Transjugular Intrahepatic Portosystemic Shunt

Jae Hyung Park, Joon Koo Han, Jin Wook Chung, and Man Chung Han

Introduction

In the treatment of esophageal variceal bleeding due to portal hypertension, medical conservative treatment with the Sengstaken-Blackmore tube, endoscopic sclerotherapy, and percutaneous transhepatic embolization for esophageal veins are available.[1,2] Medical conservative treatment enables transient hemostasis, and the aim of endoscopic sclerotherapy and percutaneous transhepatic embolization is to occlude the variceal veins. The surgical portosystemic shunt decompresses portal hypertension in a more radical way. However, the surgical method has its own disadvantages, such as surgical morbidity and hepatic encephalopathy in patients with a large shunt or severe liver cirrhosis.[1,2]

Recent advances in interventional radiology have made possible a new procedure for portal decompression, transjugular intrahepatic portosystemic shunt (TIPS).[3] In this procedure one can approach the hepatic vein via the right internal jugular vein and make a new parenchymal tract by puncture with a long 16 gauge metallic needle. Recent development of metallic stents facilitates long-term patency of this parenchymal tract between the hepatic vein and the portal vein.[3,4] We report our results for TIPS performed in 28 patients with portal hypertension.

Subjects and Methods

A total of 28 patients underwent TIPS in the Department of Radiology, Seoul National University Hospital, from June 1992 to August 1993. There were 21 males and 7 females. Age ranged from 27 to 64 years (mean, 47 y). All patients except one with intractable ascites had been suffering from gastroesophageal bleeding. Four patients had initial bleeding. The others all had recurrent bleeding, even after multiple trials of endoscopic sclerotherapy. Eleven patients had had more than three episodes of bleeding. Endoscopic sclerotherapy was not tried in 6 patients, attempted once in 7 patients, and repeated variable times in 15 patients. One patient received percutaneous transhepatic variceal embolization for recurrent variceal bleeding.

The Child classification was A in 3 patients, B in 8, and C in 17. Esophageal varices were demonstrated endoscopically as grade I or II in 11 patients and as grade III or IV in 17. Gastric varices were present in 16 patients.

Before the procedure, the presence of associated portal vein thrombosis or hepatoma should be checked with ultrasonography. Endoscopic examination demonstrates the severity and extent of esophageal varices, the presence of gastric varices, and other bleeding foci such as gastroduodenal ulcer. To prevent infection due to contamination during the procedure, antibiotic coverage is done 1 day before. We explain the procedure and obtain consent from the patient or the family.

After skin preparation on the right neck with the face toward the left, right internal jugular vein puncture is made with a Seldinger needle, recognizing the pulse of the right common carotid artery with palpation or under the guidance of ultrasonography. Once the venous blood is aspirated, a guide wire is inserted to the superior vena cava down to the inferior vena cava. A 9 Fr long sheath (Cook Inc., Bloomington, USA) follows the guide wire to the inferior vena cava. Through the sheath, a 5 Fr angiographic catheter is inserted to the selected right hepatic vein or middle hepatic vein. After visualizing the hepatic vein, a Colapinto needle (Cook Inc., Bloomington, USA), a 16 gauge long needle for transjugular biopsy, is introduced into the sheath to make the portal vein puncture. We performed blind puncture in the initial stage of our experience. Recently we developed an accurate guiding method to target the portal vein to insert a 0.014" fine guide wire into the main portal vein via the percutaneous transhepatic route. With the guide wire in the right portal vein and the main portal vein, we can easily make sure of the relationship between the hepatic vein and the portal vein with C-arm fluoroscopy. Usually we start the puncture at the hepatic vein 2 cm from the junction of the vena cava to target the right portal vein at its junction with the main portal vein or within 2 to 3 cm from the junction. Blood may be aspirated or contrast may be injected once the portal vein is punctured. Heavy-duty guide wire is inserted down to the superior mesenteric vein. Then the 5 Fr catheter can follow the guide wire to insert in the superior mesenteric vein or splenic vein, where portal venography and pressure measurement are performed.

Along the heavy-duty guide wire, an 8-mm balloon catheter (7 Fr, 4 cm, Cook Inc., Bloomington, USA) is inserted across the puncture site of liver parenchyma to dilate the tract from the hepatic vein to the portal vein. After confirming the disappearance of the balloon waist at the puncture sites of the hepatic vein and the portal vein, a metallic stent is inserted along the dilated shunt (Fig. 60.1). Four different types of stent were used: Wallstent (Schneider, Switzerland), Palmaz stent (Johnson & Johnson, USA), Strecker stent (Meditech, USA), and Gianturco stent (homemade).

After deployment of the stent, we dilate the stent with an 8-mm balloon catheter. The Wallstent may be dilated further up to 10 mm. Pressure mea-

FIGURE 60.1. Schematic drawing of transjugular intrahepatic portosystemic shunt. The metallic stent connects the portal vein to the hepatic vein for portal decompression.

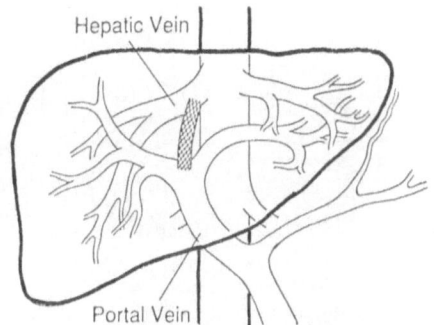

surement and transjugular portal venography are performed again to demonstrate the patency of the stent shunt. After removing the sheath from the right internal jugular vein, the puncture site is compressed manually for hemostasis.

Two days later, complete blood count and endoscopic examination are recommended to evaluate the status of gastroesophageal varices. After 1 month and then every 3 months, duplex sonography or transjugular portal venography and liver function test are recommended.

Results

The procedure was successful in making patent stent shunt in all cases except one patient with portal vein thrombosis. A single metallic stent was used in 24 patients (Fig. 60.2). Among them the Wallstent was used in 21 patients. The diameter of the Wallstent was 8 mm in 18 patients and 10 mm in 10 patients. The length varied from 37 to 91 mm. The Gianturco stent was used in 2 patients. The Strecker stent was used in 1 patient. In 4 patients, a Palmaz or Gianturco stent was used in addition to the Wallstent or Strecker stent. In one of the two cases with a Gianturco stent, recanalization and Wallstent insertion were attempted successfully after recognizing occlusion of the Gianturco shunt after 3 months. The mean ± standard deviation of portal vein pressure decreased from 29.0 ± 8.4 mmHg before the procedure to 22.4 ± 4.7 mmHg after the procedure. The average portosystemic pressure gradient between the main portal vein and the inferior vena cava decreased from 22.4 to 14.5 mmHg after the procedure (Fig. 60.3). In 5 patients, simultaneous embolization for the coronary vein was undertaken with coils. The gastroesophageal collateral varices were identified in all cases before the TIPS shunt. However, they disappeared completely in 20 patients and partially in 7 patients after the shunt.

Blood flow before the procedure was hepatofugal in 4 patients and hepatopedal in 23 patients. After the procedure, all changed to the hepatopedal direction. However, the status of portal perfusion was different. No hepatic

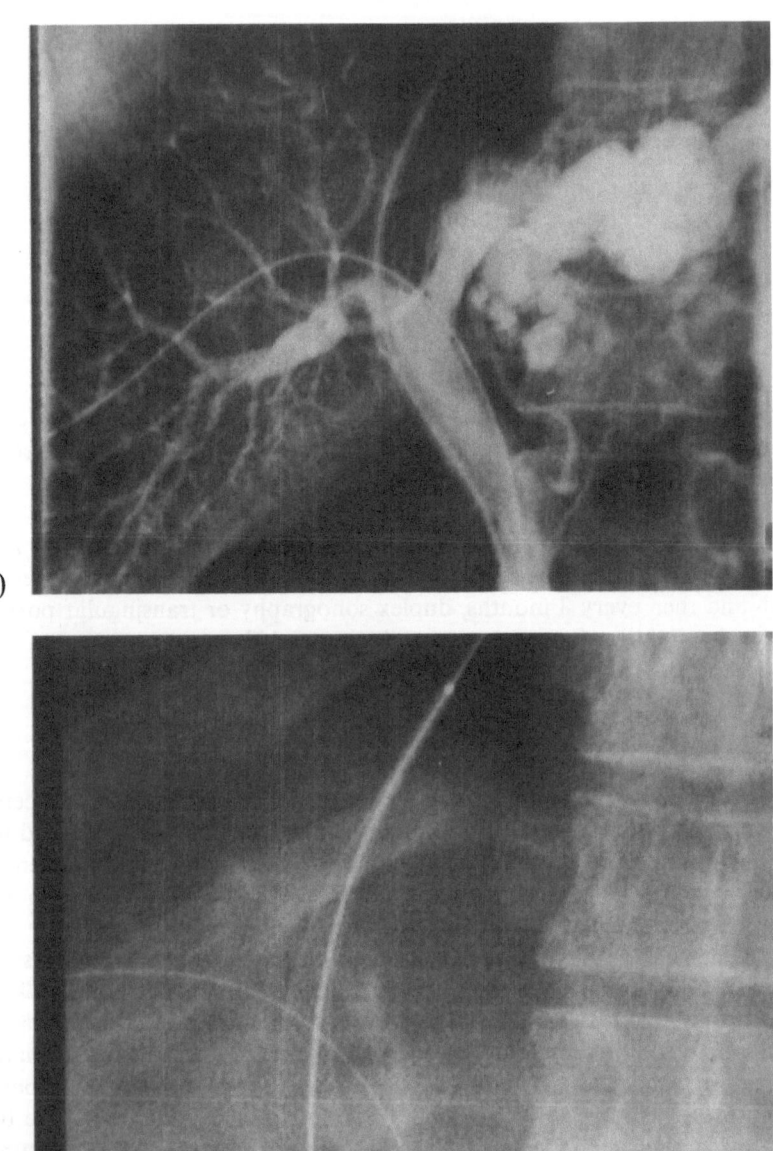

(a)

(b)

parenchymal perfusion was demonstrated in 4 patients. Minimal perfusion with opacification of proximal portal vein was seen in 5 patients. Moderate perfusion with opacification of third order branches of the portal vein and parenchymal staining was seen in 18 patients.

During the follow-up period from 2 to 14 months, rebleeding developed in 10 patients (37%). In 3 patients the bleeding episode could not be controlled, leading to death. During the follow-up period, shunt occlusion occurred in 3

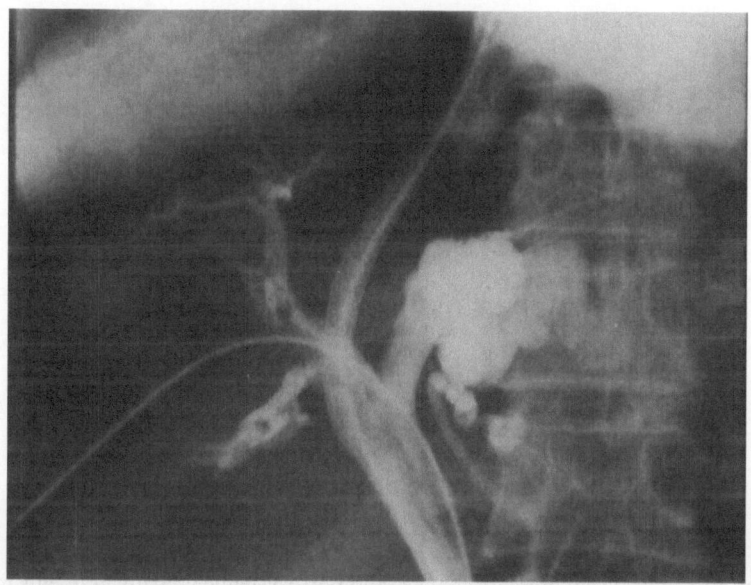

(c)

FIGURE 60.2. Transjugular intrahepatic portosystemic shunt in a 40-year-old female patient. (A) Transjugular portal venography reveals prominent gastroesophageal varices due to portal hypertension. Note the fine guide wire in portal vein from percutaneous transhepatic route. (B) Wallstent is half released from the constraining membrane through the parenchymal tract between hepatic vein and portal vein. (C) Immediate follow-up portal venography after stent installation shows evident decrease of the variceal collaterals and patent communication from portal vein to hepatic vein and right atrium.

patients. Retrial of the TIPS shunt was attempted in 4 patients with redilatation in 2 patients and restenting in 2 patients.

Hepatic encephalopathy was the most serious complication; it was aggravated or newly occurred in 7 patients (26%). Among them, medical management such as lactulose and enema was effective in 2 patients. However, 5 patients failed to recover and died. The overall mortality was 11 of 27 patients (40.7%) during the follow-up period from 2 to 14 months. Other complications were local hematoma in 1 patient and acute renal failure in 2 patients. Duplex sonography showed the patency of the stent shunt in 11 patients during the follow-up period, demonstrating the echogenic metallic stent and Doppler signals in the stent shunt.

Discussion

There are many causes of portal hypertension, such as portal vein thrombosis and hepatic vein occlusion.[1,2] The most frequent cause is liver cirrhosis. The normal pressure of the portal vein is 5 to 10 mmHg, slightly higher than that

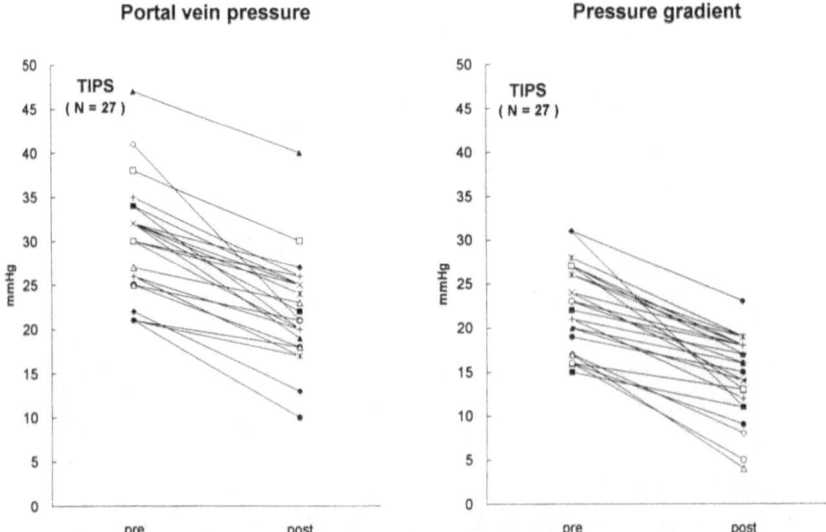

FIGURE 60.3. Portal vein pressure changes and portosystemic pressure gradients in 27 patients with transjugular intrahepatic portosystemic shunt.

of the inferior vena cava. If the difference is greater than 5 mmHg, the condition is defined as portal hypertension. If the pressure difference is greater than 12 mmHg, one can assume variceal rupture due to portal hypertension as the cause of gastrointestinal bleeding.[1,2,5]

Endoscopic sclerotherapy is now popular in the treatment of esophageal varices. The sclerosant is ethanolamine oleate or sodium morrhuate. The primary success rate for bleeding control with sclerotherapy is higher than 90%.[6,7] The disadvantages of sclerotherapy are the relatively high frequency of rebleeding and poor control of gastric varices. Percutaneous transhepatic embolization for the gastroesophageal varices was done extensively after the first report by Lunderquist. However, a relatively high incidence of rebleeding and possible complications due to reflux of embolic material prevent the further application of this procedure.[8-10]

As for the surgical management, there are total portal diversion, nonshunt operation, and selective shunt. The most appropriate surgical method is known to be the selective shunt, such as distal splenorenal shunt in which selective portal decompression of the gastroesophageal varices is undertaken while the main portal blood flow is maintained.[1,2,4] However, the surgical technique is difficult and the long-term patency is yet to be determined.[1,2,11] Johansen[12] reported that the pressure gradient remained 10 mmHg, the rebleeding rate 8%, and encephalopathy only 6% in the cases of 10- to 12-mm small stoma of side-to-side portocaval shunt. Coldwell[13] attempted embolization of the varices in addition to the same surgical technique, resulting in similar good results. Generally speaking, endoscopic sclerotherapy shows a higher rate of recurrent bleeding after the procedure, but the long-term survival is almost the same as or better than that of the surgical shunt operation.[14-16] Warren et al.[17] reported that the rebleeding rate of sclerotherapy was 53% while that of the distal splenorenal shunt was 3%. However, they reported that portal perfusion status was much better in the cases with sclerotherapy.

As treatment of portal hypertension, TIPS has several advantages, such as local anesthesia and minimal damage due to the puncture of the right internal jugular vein. The first attempt at the transjugular approach was reported by Rösch[18] in 1969. Recently the idea was revived for the interventional management of portal hypertension after the advent of metallic stent.[18-20] Among the metallic stent, the Wallstent seems most appropriate for TIPS because of its long length and flexibility, though it has the drawback of shortening during expansion.[21,22]

TIPS as well as surgical shunt may be complicated with hepatic encephalopathy. The hepatic encephalopathy may be induced by the portosystemic shunt or hepatic insufficiency itself or both.[23] The incidence of hepatic encephalopathy after TIPS was reported as from 2.5% to 30%.[24] The optimal size of the stent shunt to minimize the complication and to decompress portal hypertension sufficiently should be investigated with further workup.

Since the periprocedural morbidity of TIPS is low compared with that of surgical shunt, the indications of TIPS are now expanding. It is indicated for intractable ascites and Budd-Chiari syndrome in addition to the previous indications, such as recurrent variceal bleeding after repeated sclerotherapy, gastric varices, and recurrence after surgical shunt.

References

1. Boyer TD. Portal hypertension and bleeding esophageal varices. In: Zakin D, Boyer TD (eds.). *Hepatology*. 2nd ed. Philadelphia: WB Saunders, 1990, pp. 572–615.
2. Skinner DB, Belsey RHR. Management of esophageal disease. 1st ed. Philadelphia: WB Saunders, 1980, pp. 821–856.
3. Richter GM, Noeldge G, Palmaz JC, et al. Transjugular intrahepatic portacaval stent shunt: Preliminary clinical results. Radiology 1990;174:1027–1030.
4. Palmaz JC, Garcia F, Sibbitt RR, et al. Expandable intrahepatic portacaval shunt stents in dogs with chronic portal hypertension. AJR 1986;147:1251–1254.
5. Viallet A, Marleau D, Huet M, et al. Hemodynamic evaluation of patients with intrahepatic portal hypertension. Gastroenterology 1975;69:1297–1300.
6. Chung JM, Choi WK, Yang YS, Kang YH, Choi HJ. A clinical study on esophageal varices bleeding. Korean Intern Med 1985;28:28–35.
7. Kang JK, Hyun JH. The clinical study of endoscopic sclerotherapy in active esophagogastric variceal bleeding. J Korean Med Assoc 1986;29:619–627.
8. Lunderquist A, Simert G, Tylen U, Vang J. Follow-up patients with portal hypertension and esophageal varices treated with percutaneous obliteration of gastric coronary vein. Radiology 1977;122:59–63.

9. Smith-Laing G, Scott J, Long RG, Dick R, Sherlock S. Role of percutaneous transhepatic obliteration of varices in the management of hemorrhage from gastroesophageal varices. Gastroenterology 1981;80:1031–1036.

10. Kim YJ, Suh KJ, Kim TH, Kang DS. Percutaneous transhepatic variceal obliteration of intractable bleeding of gastroesophageal varices. Korean Radiol Soc 1989;25:672–679.

11. Warren WD. Control of variceal bleeding. AM J Surg 1983;145:8–16.

12. Johansen K. Partial portal decompression for variceal hemorrhage. Am J Surg 1989;157:497–482.

13. Coldwell DM, Moore ADA, Ben-Menachem Y, Johansen KH. Bleeding gastroesophageal varices: Gastric vein embolization after partial portal decompression. Radiology 1991;178:249–251.

14. Cello JP, Grendell JH, Crass RA, Weber TE, Trunkey DD. Endoscopic sclerotherapy versus protacaval shunt in patients with severe cirrhosis and acute variceal hemorrhage. N Engl J Med 1987;316:11–15.

15. Rikkers LF, Burnett DA, Volentine GD, Buchi KN, Cormier RA. Shunt surgery versus endoscopic sclerotherapy for long-term treatment for variceal bleeding. Ann Surg 1987;206:261–271.

16. Reynolds TB, Donovan AJ, Mikkelsen WP, Redeker AG, Turrill FL, Weiner JM. Results of a 12 year randomized trial of portacaval shunt in patients with alcoholic liver disease and bleeding varices. Gastroenterology 1981;80:1005–1011.

17. Warren WD, Henderson JM, Millikan WJ, et al. Distal splenorenal shunt versus endoscopic sclerotherapy for long-term management of variceal bleeding. Ann Surg 1986;203:454–462.

18. Rösch J, Hanafee WN, Snow H. Transjugular portal venography and radiologic portacaval shunt: An experimental study. Radiology 1969;92:1112–1114.

19. Rösch J, Antonovic R, Dotter CT. Transjugular approach to the liver biliary system, and portal circulation. AJR 1975;125:602–608.

20. Colapinto RF, Stronell RD, Birch SJ, et al. Creation of an intrahepatic portosystemic shunt with a Gruntzig balloon catheter. Can Med Assoc J 1982;126:267–268.

21. Palmaz JC, Sibbitt RR, Reuter SR, Garchia F, Tio F. Expandable intrahepatic portocaval shunt stents: Early experience in the dog. AJR 1985;145:821–825.

22. Rösch J, Uchida BT, Putnam JS, Buschmann RW, Law RD, Hershey AL. Experimental intrahepatic portacaval anastomosis: Use of expandable Gianturco stents. Radiology 1987;162:481–485.

23. Schafer DF, Jones EA. Manifestations of abnormal liver function. In: Zakin D, Boyer TD (eds.). Hepatology. 2nd ed. Philadelphia: WB Saunders, 1990, pp. 447–460.

24. Proceedings of 17th Annual Scientific Meeting of Society of Cardiovascular and Interventional Radiology, April 4–9, 1992, Washington, DC.

61
Effectiveness of Portal Vein Arterialization During an Emergency Situation in Partial Liver Transplantation

MASAHIKO YAMAGUCHI, KAORU KUMADA, HIROSHI HIGASHIYAMA, TAISUKE MORIMOTO, AND KAZUE OZAWA

Introduction

Portal vein arterialization (PVA) has been used clinically as a hepatic revascularization method to prevent hepatic failure after portocaval shunt operation for portal hypertension since 1952.[1] Recently, this method has been adopted as a temporary technique to prevent hepatic ischemia in liver transplantation[2] and in other forms of liver surgery.[3] In our series of partial liver transplantation which we have performed for pediatric cases using liver grafts obtained from living related donors, it is essential to reduce the ischemic time of the liver graft by smooth and speedy revascularization. In view of the time-consuming nature of this operation, temporary PVA can be a useful method to avoid prolongation of warm ischemic injury to the liver graft. We report here a case of partial liver transplantation using temporary PVA technique and discuss the effects of PVA on liver viability as a theoretical support of this technique.

Case Example

The patient received a right lobectomy of the liver due to hepatoblastoma at the age of 3 months in 1982. Laparoscopy done for postoperative liver dysfunction revealed liver cirrhosis in 1983. Bleeding from the esophageal varices began in 1986. At 9 years of age, he was admitted to our institute on November 13, 1990, with massive bleeding recurring once a month. Preoperative angiography revealed postphlebitic constriction in the portal vein trunk, but it also revealed sufficient diameter for the anastomosis at the confluence of the splenic vein and the portal vein. Liver transplantation was indicated for this patient who had severely deteriorated liver function with massive bleeding. Partial liver transplantation was performed 8 days after admission using a left lobe obtained from his father as a liver graft. After the anastomosis of the hepatic vein, the portal vein of the graft was anastomosed conventionally to the confluence where the diameter was sufficient for anastomosis, although the wall was sclerotic. However, the confluence was barely mobilized, causing the portal vein of the graft to be stretched strongly and become stenotic. Reflow was scarcely obtained due to thrombosis at the anastomosis site. The portal vein was reconstructed again with the insertion of an autogenous vein graft. At reflow, bleeding from the lower site of the anastomosis was detected but was difficult to control because it was located deep behind the plate-hard pancreas. By now, 85 minutes had already passed after putting in the liver graft, and considerable time might be required to

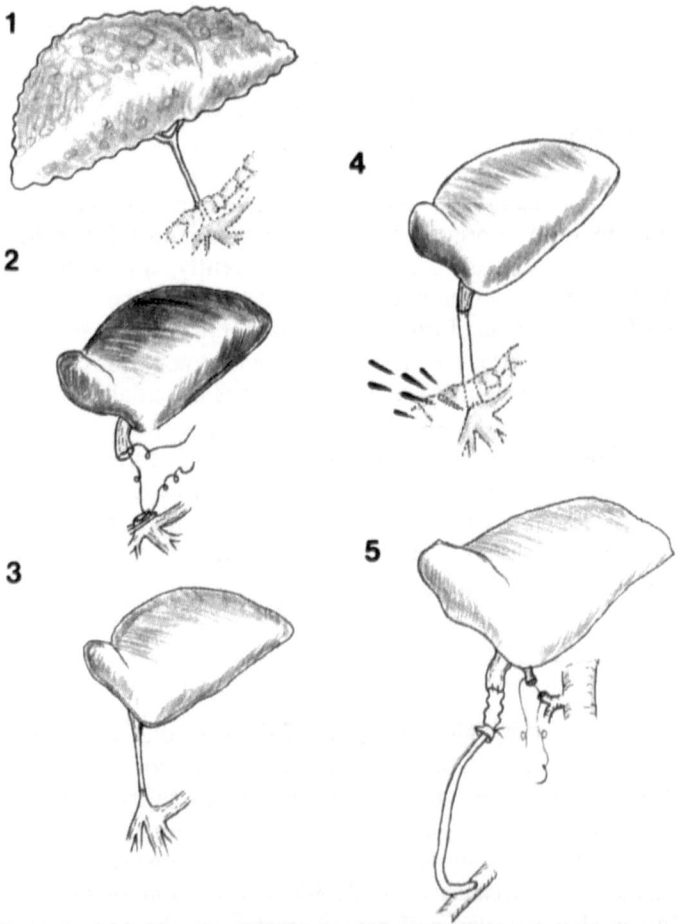

FIGURE 61.1. Portal vein arterialization (PVA) technique used during an emergency situation in partial liver transplantion. 1. Cirrhotic liver and constricted portal vein trunk. 2. Anastomosis performed between the portal vein of the graft and the confluence of the recipient's portal vein. 3. Stretched portal vein of the liver graft, becoming stenotic. 4. Bleeding from lower site of the anastomosis done with the insertion of a vein graft. 5. PVA adopted temporarily during the anastomosis the hepatic artery.

repair the bleeding site. To avoid the impending ischemic crisis, the PVA technique was adopted temporarily for 25 minutes. Anastomosis of the hepatic artery was performed during PVA, followed by the portal vein reanastomosis which was completed safely (Fig. 61.1).

Discussion

PVA is not just a simple revascularization technique but involves the introduction of arterial blood with arterial blood pressure to the portal venous bed. This revascularization technique has been used to prevent hepatic ischemia in liver surgery, although its actual effects on the liver have yet to be clarified. Previously[4,5] we investigated the effects of PVA on liver viability by measuring the levels of the arterial blood ketone body ratio (KBR: acetoacetate/β-hydroxybutyrate in arterial blood), which reflects the hepatic mitochondrial redox state (NAD^+/NADH) that plays an essential role in ATP production in hepatic mitochondria.[6,7] Briefly, the experiments and their results are described as follows:

Seventeen mongrel dogs were used in the experiments. In the operation, a side-to-side mesocaval anastomosis was performed to avoid splanchnic congestion before 60 minutes of hepatic ischemia was administered by clamping the portal vein and hepatic artery. After 60 minutes of hepatic ischemia, PVA was performed by shunting the arterial blood from the femoral artery to the portal vein. The effects of PVA after 60 minutes of hepatic ischemia were

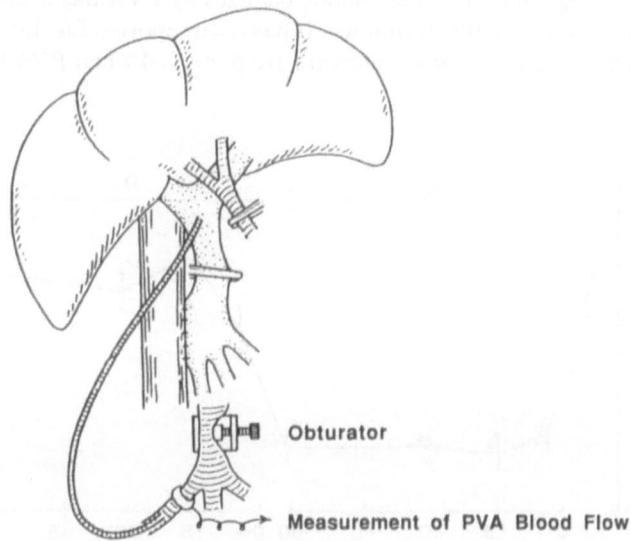

Obturator

Measurement of PVA Blood Flow

FIGURE 61.2. Scheme for changing the blood flow levels of PVA performed by shunting the arterial blood from the femoral artery to the portal vein.

investigated by measuring the KBR. The portal vein pressure and the total hepatic blood flow (THBF) were monitored. Furthermore, the blood flow level of PVA was reduced by constricting the aorta with an obturator, and the KBR was measured at a certain blood flow level of PVA (Fig. 61.2).

The levels of KBR were decreased immediately 5 minutes after clamping the portal vein and the hepatic artery, and remained at low levels throughout hepatic ischemia. PVA, which was done after 60 minutes of hepatic ischemia, rapidly restored the levels of KBR to preclamping levels within 15 minutes, and these levels were maintained during arterialization (Fig. 61.3). The levels of portal vein pressure after PVA were almost the same as the preclamping values. Blood flow levels of PVA without constriction of the aorta were almost 25% of the preclamping total hepatic blood flow (Fig. 61.4). KBR was maintained at high levels when PVA blood flow was reduced to 12% of preclamping THBF. However, the levels of KBR were significantly decreased when the blood flow was reduced to 8% of preclamping THBF (Fig. 61.5).

We showed that the KBR levels, which were decreased by hepatic ischemia, were restored to the preclamping levels by PVA, and that the critical level of PVA blood flow to keep the KBR at high levels was approximately 10% of preclamping THBF in this model. It is essential to keep the KBR at high levels to maintain the functional capacity of the liver because the production of ATP in hepatic mitochondria is inhibited by reduced mitochondrial redox potential, which is reflected by the low levels of KBR.[6,7] The data suggest that temporary PVA is a simple and effective method to restore the liver function from the ischemic state, and that a high blood flow of PVA may not be necessary to maintain liver viability.

Hepatic damage due to hemodynamic changes by PVA has been pointed out as a disadvantage of this technique. It has been reported for this problem that the hepatic function and architecture are preserved when PVA flow and

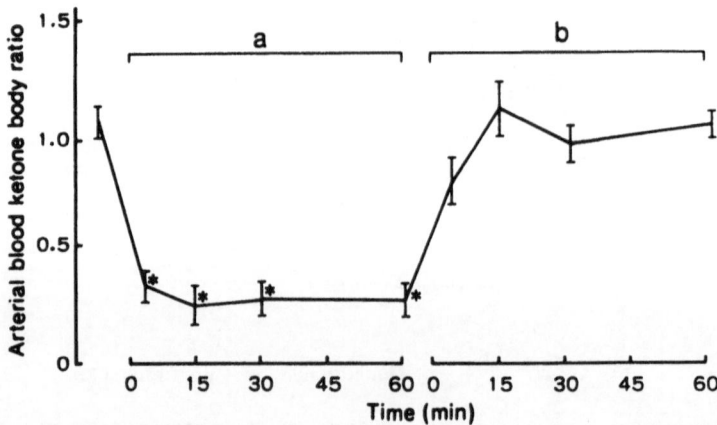

FIGURE 61.3. Changes in the levels of KBR by clamping of hepatic hilar vessels (a) and arterialization of the portal vein (b). *$p < 0.001$ as compared to preclamping value.

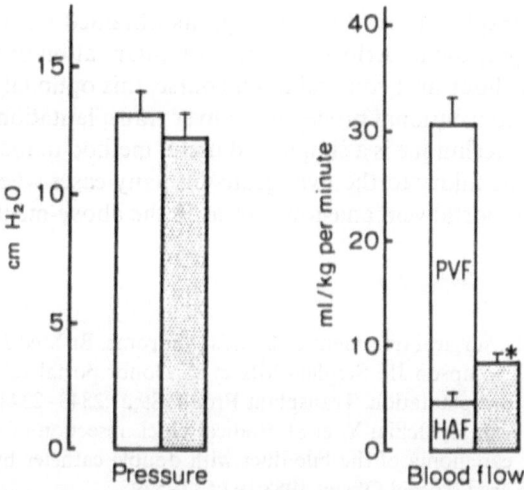

FIGURE 61.4. Portal vein pressure and total hepatic blood flow at preclamping time (white bar) and at PVA time (shaded bar). PVF, Portal vein flow; HAF, hepatic artery flow.

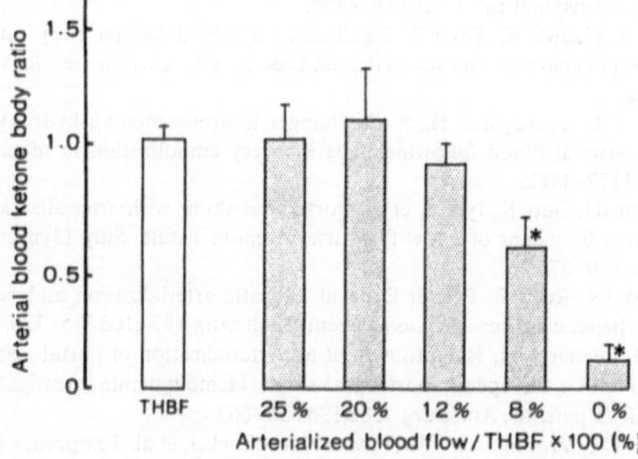

FIGURE 61.5. Changes in the levels of KBR at various blood flow levels of PVA. THBF, preclamping total hepatic blood flow. $*p < 0.01$ as compared to the values at THBF.

pressure in the portal vein are kept within preoperative values.[8-10] On the other hand, damage by superoxides produced when ischemic tissue is exposed to high concentrations of oxygen in arterial blood might be another possible disadvantage of PVA. However, no evidence has been reported to support this theory, at least for short-term PVA.[11]

At our institute, the PVA technique was applied to the first several cases of partial liver transplantation using liver grafts obtained from living related donors for the purpose of performing the revascularization procedures safely and carefully without time constraint. Of course, this optional method is not required in the conventional procedure of liver transplantation. Even so, this temporary PVA technique is a simple and useful method to reduce the period of warm ischemic injury to the liver grafts in many cases where trouble has occurred during portal vein anastomosis, as in the above-mentioned case.

References

1. Hunt AH. The surgical treatment of Banti's syndrome. Br Med J 1952;2:4–9.
2. Sheil AGR, Thompson JF, Stephen MS, et al. Donor portal vein arterialization during liver transplantation. Transplant Proc 1989;21:2343–2344.
3. Mimura H, Kim H, Ochiai Y, et al. Radical block resection of hepatoduodenal ligament for carcinoma of the bile duct with double catheter bypass for portal circulation. Surg Gynecol Obstet 1988;167:527–529.
4. Yamaguchi M, Higashiyama H, Kumada K, et al. Evaluation of portal vein arterialization as a method of liver graft revascularization by blood ketone body ratio. Transplantation 1989;47:514–516.
5. Yamaguchi M, Higashiyama H, Kumada K, et al. Evaluation of temporary portal vein arterialization: The minimum arterialized blood flow for maintaining liver viability. Transplant Int. 1990;3:162–166.
6. Tanaka J, Ozawa K, Tobe T. Significance of blood ketone body ratio as an indicator of hepatic energy status in jaundiced rabbits. Gastroenterology 1979;76:691–696.
7. Tani T, Taki Y, Aoyama H, et al. Changes in acetoacetate/β-hydroxybutyrate ratio in arterial blood following hepatic artery embolization in man. Life Sci 1984;35:1177–1182.
8. Adamson RJ, Butt K, Iyer S, et al. Portacaval shunt with arterialization of the portal vein by means of a low flow arteriovenous fistula. Surg Gynecol Obstet 1978;146:869–876.
9. Maillard JN, Rueff B, Prandi D, et al. Hepatic arterialization and portacaval shunt in hepatic cirrhosis. An assessment. Arch Surg 1974;108:315–320.
10. Otte JB, Reynaert M, HemptinneB, et al. Arterialization of portal vein in conjunction with a therapeutic portacaval shunt. Hemodynamic investigations and results in 75 patients. Ann Surg 1982;196:656–663.
11. Terpstra OT, Vroonhoven TJMV, van Noordhoek J, et al. Temporary beneficial effect of arterialization of the liver in cirrhotic dogs with a portacaval shunt. A preliminary report. Eur Surg Res 1982;14:333–343.

XXII
Angioaccess

62
Factors Influencing the Patency of Arteriovenous Fistulae in Patients with Chronic Renal Failure

W.H. Cho, Y.S. Kim, and H.C. Kim

Introduction

Preservation of an adequate vessel for repeated punctures is essential for hemodialysis, and various efforts have been made for this purpose. Extracorporeal dialysis of blood was introduced by Kolff et al.[1] in 1943. The Scribner external arteriovenous shunt was described by Quinton et al.[2] in 1960, and it became widely adopted as a vascular access for the treatment of end-stage renal diseases. However, several complications, such as catheter-associated infection and sepsis, pulmonary and cerebral emboli, risk of displacement of cannula, pressure necrosis of the overlying skin, and poor prolonged patency, urged surgeons to find a better method of vascular access. In 1966, Brescia et al.[3] described an internal arteriovenous fistula between the radial artery and an adjacent vein with arterialization of that anastomosed vein, and this Cimino fistula has become the method of choice in most hemodialysis centers. Although the result of this arteriovenous fistula formation has been better than that of any other method of vascular access, keeping this vascular access patent for a prolonged period of time is still the most important problem for both patients and surgeons.

To analyze the factors that may influence the patency of the arteriovenous fistulae, we reviewed our experience with the internal arteriovenous fistulae performed over the past 8 years in patients with end-stage renal diseases at Dongsan Hospital, Keimyung University, Taegu, Korea.

Materials and Methods

Between January 1983 and December 1990, a total of 733 arteriovenous fistulae were created in 445 males and 285 females. The ages of patients ranged between 14 and 78 years. These 733 patients included 634 patients with radiocephalic fistulae, 28 patients with ulnobasilic fistulae, and 35 patients who had either synthetic grafts (21 patients) or autografts (19 patients) inserted between the brachial artery and an adjacent vein. Our average observation period for each patient has been 4 years. Age, sex, and laboratory

577

data including blood urea nitrogen (BUN), serum creatinine and cholesterol, blood sugar, hemoglobin, and hematocrit at the time of fistula creation were studied as factors that may influence the patency of their fistulae. The usual systolic blood pressure and the systolic pressure at the time of operation were also evaluated.

The status of fistulated vessels, such as arteriosclerotic changes and perivascular fibrosis, was also examined, and local vascular conditions such as thrill over the fistulae and dilatation of veins distal to the fistulae immediately after the fistula formation were also studied.

All the data were processed in an SPSS survival program. The influence of suspected factors on the dependent variable and duration of patency of the fistula was evaluated by multivariant analysis and actuarial life table computation.

Results

Among the factors suspected to have influence on the patency of fistula construction, age, BUN, blood pressure at the time of operation, serum cholesterol, and creatinine level were statistically significant (Table 62.1). Blood glucose level was found to have no statistical significance in this study, but since many patients were already under the control of oral hypoglycemic agents when the blood sample was obtained, this analysis was expected to have no particular significance, although our previous study showed a statistically significance, although our previous study showed a statistically significant relationship between diabetes and fistula patency.[4] The sites of arteries used for fistula construction also showed significant differences.

The overall fistula patency rates were 59.8% at 1 year and declined to 40.8% at the end of 5 years (Fig. 62.1)

Age

Age was a highly significant factor ($p = 0.0000$) for fistula patency; the patency rate for the group under 30 years of age was 71.4% but for the group of patients over 60 years of age, it was 37.2% at 1 year (Fig. 62.2).

TABLE 62.1. Statistically significant variables on multivariant analysis.

Variables	Wilks' lambda	Significance
Age	.92409	$p < 0.05$
BUN	.90975	$p < 0.05$
Systolic blood pressure at operation	.90206	$p < 0.05$
Serum cholesterol	.89493	$p < 0.05$
Serum creatinine	.89334	$p < 0.05$

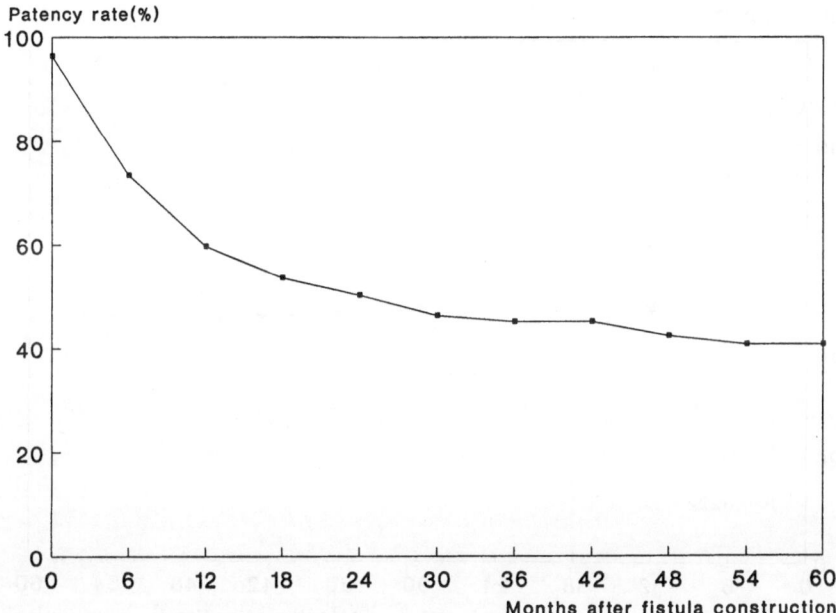

FIGURE 62.1. Overall fistula patency rates.

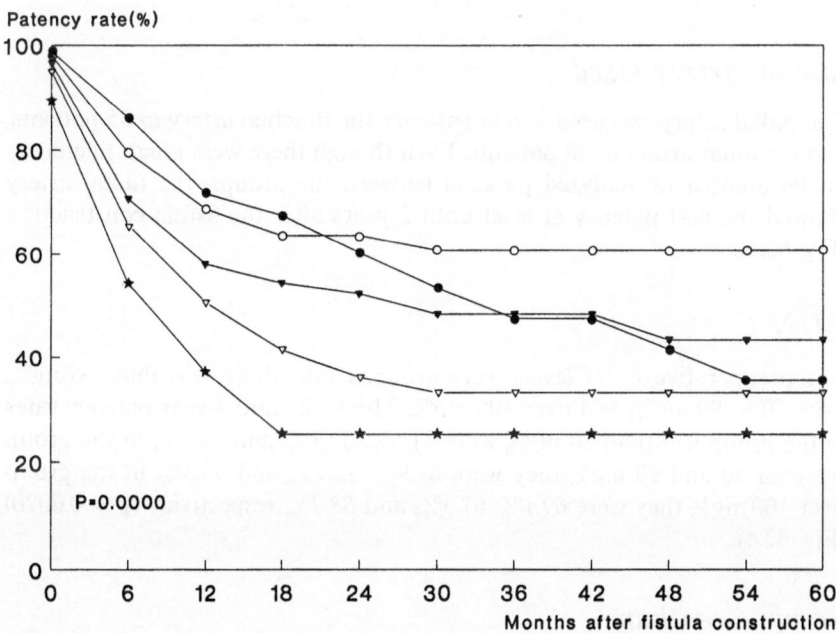

FIGURE 62.2. Fistula patency rates according to the patient's age: less than 30(●), 30 to 39(○), 40 to 49(▼), 50 to 59(▽) and over 60(★) years.

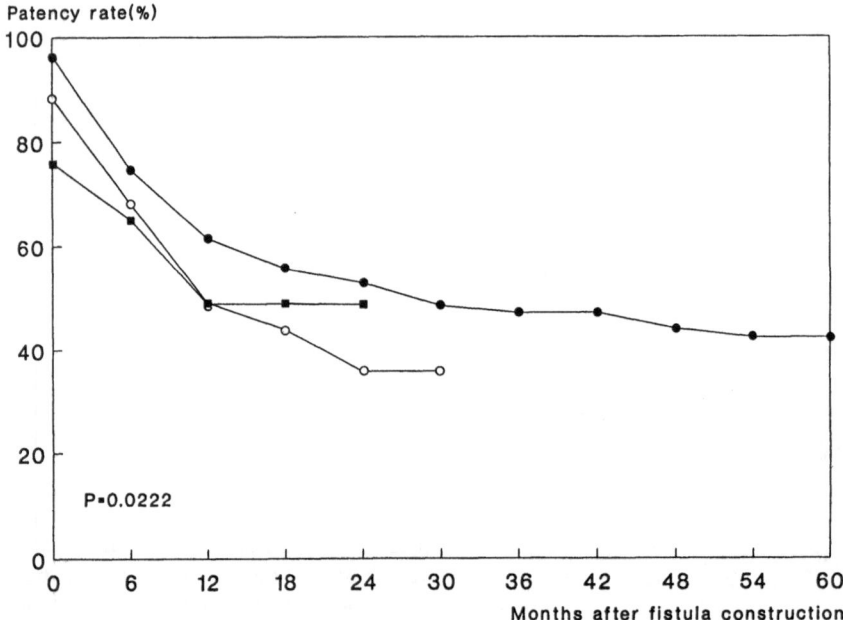

FIGURE 62.3. Fistula patency rates in radial artery(●), ulnar artery(■), and brachial artery(○).

Site of Artery Used

The radial artery was used in 634 patients, the brachial artery in 35 patients, and the ulnar artery in 28 patients. Even though there were great differences in the number of analyzed patients between the groups, the radial artery showed the best patency at least until 2 years after the fistula construction (Fig. 62.3).

BUN

The preoperative BUN levels were grouped into three: less than 50 mg%; from 50 to 99 mg%, and over 100 mg%. The 1-, 2-, and 3-year patency rates in the group less than 50 mg% were 41.5%, 32.1%, and 32.1%; in the group between 50 and 99 mg% they were 61.9%, 52.1%, and 45.8%; in the group over 100 mg% they were 69.1%, 67.3%, and 58.7%, respectively ($p = 0.0020$) (Fig. 62.4).

Serum Creatinine

Serum creatinine levels were available in 642 patients at the time of operation, and these patients were divided according to their serum creatinine levels into 5 groups (Fig. 62.5): less than 5 mg%, from 5 to 9.9 mg%, 10 to

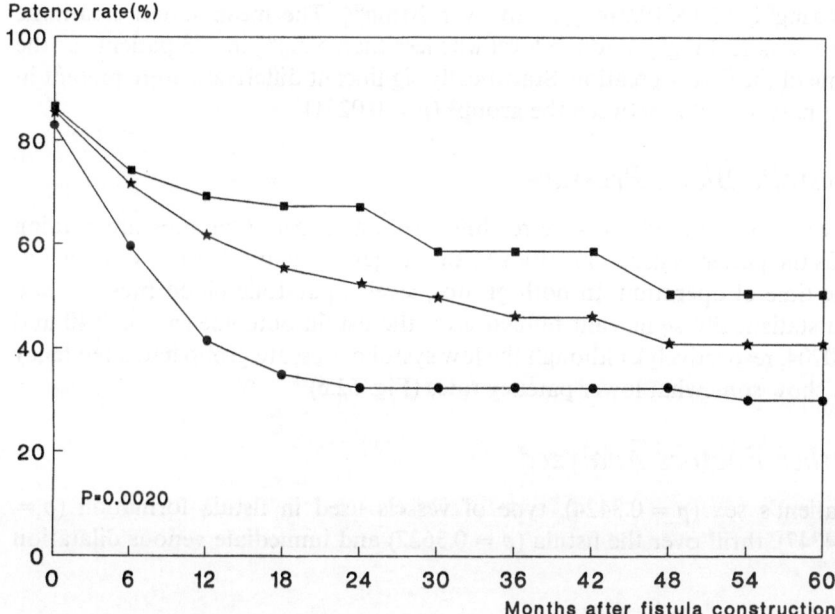

FIGURE 62.4. Fistula patency rates among patients with BUN less than 50 mg%(●), 50–99 mg%(★), and over 100 mg(■).

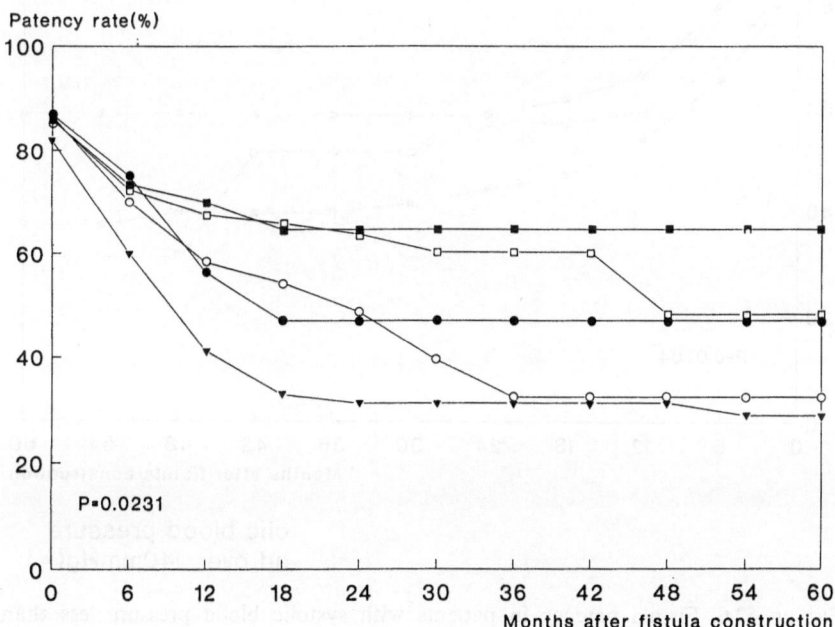

FIGURE 62.5. Fistula patency rates in patients with serum creatinine less than 5 mg%(▼), 5–9.9 mg%(○), 10–14.9 mg%(□), 15–19.9 mg%(■), and over 20 mg%(●).

14.9 mg%, 15 to 19.9 mg%, and over 20 mg%. The mean serum creatinine level was 12.1 mg%, and the level was less than 5 mg% in 173 patients at the time of the fistula creation. Statistically significant differences were present in the patency rates between the groups ($p = 0.0231$).

Systolic Blood Pressure

Two systolic blood pressure readings were analyzed. One pressure reading was the patient's usual one prior to the surgery, and another was obtained at the time of operation. In both groups, levels of systolic blood pressure had no statistically significant influence on the fistula outcome ($p = 0.7640$ and 0.0704, respectively), although the low systolic pressure group had a tendency to show somewhat lower patency rates (Fig. 62.6).

Other Factors Analyzed

Patient's sex ($p = 0.3424$), type of vessels used in fistula formation ($p = 0.4347$), thrill over the fistula ($p = 0.3622$) and immediate venous dilatation

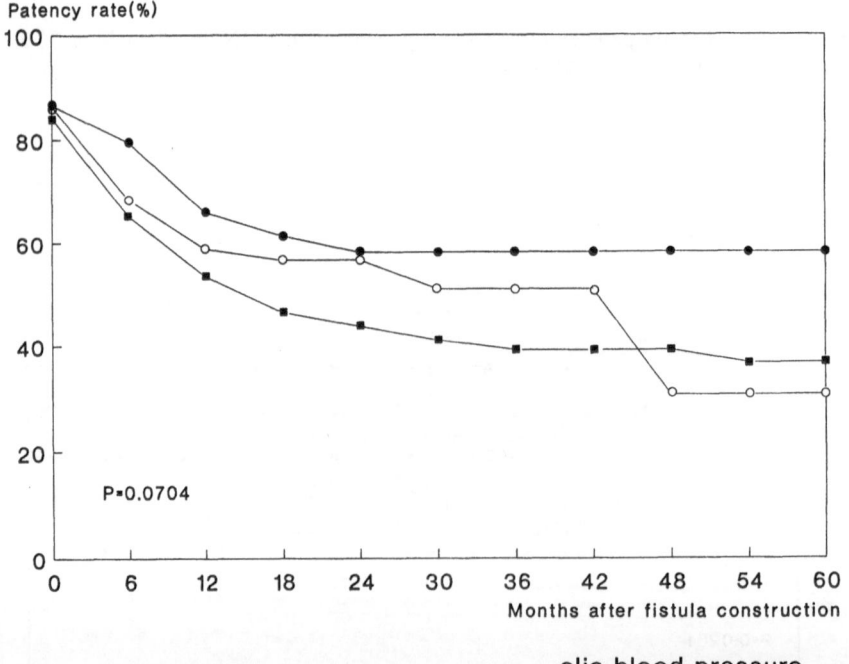

olic blood pressure
nd over 140mmHg(•)

FIGURE 62.6. Fistula patency in patients with systolic blood pressure less than 120 mmHg(■), 120–140 mmHg(o) and over 140 mmHg(•) at the time of fistula construction.

($p = 0.8748$) following fistula creation, hemoglobin ($p = 0.2148$), and cholesterol ($p = 0.5397$) levels had no significant effect on fistula patency.

Discussion

In the treatment of end-stage renal diseases, it is essential to create and preserve a sufficient length of arterialized vein for repeated punctures for hemodialysis. To prepare high-flow, thick-walled vessels, an external arteriovenous shunt using silastic cannula was introduced by Scribner et al. in 1960 and followed by the internal arteriovenous fistula by Cimino et al. in 1966. Beside these procedures, autologous or artificial grafts have been used to create the vascular access. Because of the complications frequently encountered in external shunts, most transplant centers presently use subcutaneous arteriovenous fistula as the first choice for vascular access for hemodialysis. The advantages of the internal fistula as a hemodialysis vascular access are well known: less infectivity, prolonged patency, long distance of usable vein, etc. But the overall reported 4-year patency rates of these arteriovenous fistulae have been about 50% to 60%,[5-7] necessitating repeated fistula creations to be able to continue the hemodialysis.

Vascular injury by needles, prolonged tight compression at the puncture site, and repeated punctures at the same site were all considered causative factors of the obstruction of arterialized vein.[8,9] Early use of unmatured vein may also cause thrombosis and obstruction.[6]

Many important factors that may have a bearing in keeping the arteriovenous fistula patent have been described in the literature. As Haimov[10] pointed out, using a small vein or a thrombectomized vein, especially by surgeons lacking experience, can be a cause of failure. Local vascular conditions, such as perivascular fibrosis and stenosis, and the patient's general condition, such as hypotension and dehydration, at the time of surgery, and the immediate postoperative status of newly formed fistulae are all important in the fate of the created fistulae. Thick layers of subcutaneous fat, obesity, edema of the arm, and small, fragile, thin-walled veins are also conditions unfavorable to the successful outcome of the fistulae.

Microvascular anastomotic techniques have been used for fistula creation. Efforts have been made to avoid obliteration of the lumen during stitches, twisting of the vein, and overtension at the anastomotic site.[11] Failure to adhere to these technical details can cause poor early and late patency of the fistulae.

Thrombectomy, balloon dilation, and/or angioplasty should be performed immediately if decreased fistula function is detected during or soon after the surgery. The usual findings of decreased fistula function due to venous outflow obstruction are loss of bruit, palpable pulsation without thrill or bruit, high venous resistance (150 mmHg or greater) during hemodialysis, prolonged bleeding after withdrawal of the dialysis needle, and excessive fluid loss while on dialysis.[7] Venous angiography is also necessary in such cases for diagnosis and management.[12,13]

Thomsen et al.[14] reported no difference between the age groups and the fistula patency rate, but our result showed a decreasing rate of patency as the age of the patient increased, and this difference in the rate of patency according to age was statistically significant. Increasing rates of arteriosclerosis and serious complications in the aged group may explain our result.

The radial artery was used in the overwhelming majority of patients to create an arteriovenous fistula in this study and the patency rates with the radial artery through the first 5 years following fistula creation have been much better than those with the use of the brachial artery or the ulnar artery. Similar results were reported by Geis and Giacchino.[9] The use of the distal radial artery also gave a satisfactory length of vein available for repeated punctures, and this was found to be a very important advantage. Fistulae using the ulnar artery showed poorer patency than those using the brachial artery, but this difference had no statistical meaning because of the small numbers involved with these arteries. In situations where the brachial artery had to be utilized for fistula formation, especially when the distal artery was not available any more, or in obese patients, a reversal fistula using the basilic vein has been recommended instead of a side-to-side anastomosis with the antecubital vein.[15,16]

Saphenous vein autografts or artificial vascular grafts have also been used in chronic dialysis. Reports about the patency rates with these grafts have not been uniform. Anderson[17] and Kherlakian[5] reported better early patency of the fistulae using artificial grafts than for the Cimino fistulae, but their long-term outcome showed better results in the Cimino group. Although several advantages have been reported with the use of artificial grafts, especially in patients with thick subcutaneous fat layers or with peripheral vascular diseases, frequent development of infections or pseudoaneurysms[18] prevented us from using artificial grafts, at least in the initial stage of the arteriovenous fistula creation.

The immediate postfistula local vascular conditions, such as thrill or venous dilatation, had no relationship with long-term fistula patency, but the possibility of early fistula failure by arterial spasm of anastomosed vessels is still debatable.[8,19] Immediate exploration of the anastomotic site and distal course of the anastomosed vein should be performed whenever decreased fistula functions or fistula failures are suspected.

BUN and serum creatinine levels of the patients had a close relationship with the fistula patency rate, showing better patency rates as both BUN and serum creatinine levels of the patients increased. Most patients with advanced uremia develop hypertension, and increased circulating volume, which facilitate the rate of blood flow and eventually increase the patency rate of the fistula.[14,20] Moreover, decreased coagulability caused by poor platelet aggregation in advanced uremic patients will also have beneficial effects on fistula patency.[21] Because of these physiologic changes, the best time to make an arteriovenous fistula is when the patient's BUN is about 100 mg/dL and creatinine about 10 mg/dL.

As Thomsen et al.[14] and Rohr et al.[22] reported, hypotension from any cause, especially if the systolic pressure is less than 110 mmHg, during or soon after the fistula creation and during hemodialysis, decreases the early and late patency rate of the fistulae. Increasing circulating blood volume by infusing saline preoperatively and during fistula creation could increase the fistula patency.

References

1. Kolff WJ, Berk HThj. The artificial kidney: A dialyser with a great area. Acta Med Scand 1944;117:121–131.
2. Quinton WE, Dillard D, Scribner BH. Cannulation of blood vessels for prolonged hemodialysis. Trans Am Soc Artif Int Organs 1960;6:104–113.
3. Brescia MJ, Cimino JE, Appel K, Hurwich BJ. Chronic hemodialysis using venipuncture and a surgically created arteriovenous fistula. N Engl J Med 1966;275:1089–1092.
4. Cho WH, Park SD, Park YK. Internal arteriovenous fistula for hemodialysis. J Korean Surg Soc 1986;30:408–415.
5. Kherlakian GM, Roedersheimer LR, Arbaugh JJ, Newmark KJ, King LR. Comparison of autogenous fistula versus expanded polytetrafluoroethylene graft fistula for angioaccess in hemodialysis. Am J Surg 1986;152:238–243.
6. Palder SB, Kirkman RL, Whittemore AD, et al. Vascular access for hemodialysis. Ann Surg 1985;202:235–239.
7. Schuman ES, Gross GF, Hayes JK, Standage BA. Long-term patency of polytetrafluoroethylene graft fistulas. Am J Surg 1988;155:644–646.
8. Zerbino VR, Tice DA, Katz LA, Nidus BD. A 6 year clinical experience with arteriovenous fistulas and bypasses for hemodialysis. Surgery 1974;76:1018–1023.
9. Geis WP, Giacchino J. A game plan for vascular access for hemodialysis. Surgical Rounds 1980 (January).
10. Haimov: Vascular access for hemodialysis. New York State J Med 1981 (September): 1490–1496.
11. Dagher FJ. The upper arm AV hemoaccess: Long term follow up. J Cardiovasc Surg 1986;27:447–449.
12. Anderson CB, Gilula LA, Harter HR, et al. Venous angiography and the surgical management of subcutaneous hemodialysis fistulas. Ann Surg 1978;187:194–199.
13. Anderson CB, Gilula LA, Sicard GA, et al. Venous angiography of subcutaneous hemodialysis fistulas. Arch Surg 1979;114:1320–1326.
14. Thomsen MB, Deurell S, Elfstrom J, Alm A. What causes the failure in surgically constructed arteriovenous fistulas? Acta Chir Scand 1982;149:371–376.
15. Thompson BW, Barbour G, Bissett J. Internal arteriovenous fistula for hemodialysis. Am J Surg 1972;124:185–788.
16. Giacchino JL, Geis WP, Buckingham JM, Vertuno LL, Bansal VK. Vascular access: Long-term results, new techniques. Arch Surg 1979;114:403–409.
17. Bergan JJ, Yao JST(eds.). *Evaluation and Treatment of Upper and Lower extremities.* New York: Grune and Stratton, 1983.

18. May J, Harris J, Patrick W. Polytetrafluoroethylene grafts for hemodialysis. Aust NZ J Surg 1979;49:639–644.
19. Elfstrom J, Thomsen M. The prognostic value of blood flow measurements during construction of arteriovenous fistulae. Scand J Urol Nephrol 1981;15:323–326.
20. Ohta K. Twelve chapters for successful creation of A-V fistula. Kidney Dialysis 1976;1:171–176.
21. Larsson SO, Hedner U, Nilsson IM. On coagulation and fibrinolysis in conservatively treated chronic uremia. Acta Med Scand 1971;189:433–441.
22. Rohr MS, Browder W, Frentz GD, McDonald JC. Arteriovenous fistulas for long-term dialysis. Arch Surg 1978;113:153.

63
Arteriovenous Fistula for Hemodialysis: Early Failure or Complications According to Different Criteria for Patient Selection and Surgical Procedures

YU SEUN KIM, SOO HO CHOO, AND KIIL PARK

Introduction

Due to the shortage of donor organs, complicated medical problems, or economic reasons, the number of end-stage renal failure (ESRF) patients requiring maintenance dialysis in Korea has been consistently increasing. By the end of 1990, a total of 4,311 patients were dependent on maintenance hemodialysis (HD), and the intake of new patients was 2,418 in 1990.[1] Despite the rapid growth of renal transplantation (RT), less than 20% of patients have had the privilege of RT. Therefore, the importance of HD as a maintenance or bridging measure until RT should not be overlooked. To improve patient survival and quality of life, comfortably located, well-functioning, potentially permanent angioaccess is mandatory. This review summarizes our 14-year experience with internal vascular access procedures, especially focusing on the importance of early failure (EF) at the Severance Hospital, Yonsei University Medical Center, Seoul, Korea.

Clinical Materials and Methods

Between 1978 and 1991, 681 patients with ESRF had a total of 756 internal vascular access procedures for maintenance HD. For this review, data on 664 procedures in 594 patients were available for analysis, and this constitutes the study population. These 594 patients included 356 men and 238 women, ranging in age from 11 to 80 years. There were 44 (7.41%) diabetic patients. Only 66 patients received two or more repeated multiple-access surgeries, because significant portions of patients with failed access wanted to have alternative renal replacement therapy rather than HD (Table 63.1). The longest survivor with a patent fistula is currently a 56-year-old male with 13 years of HD. During the follow-up period, 126 patients died of diseases complicating ESRF, 76 converted to continuous ambulatory peritoneal dialysis (CAPD) for various reasons, and 82 had RT. Fistulas were considered func-

TABLE 63.1. Procedures for patients with failed primary of secondary access.

	2nd procedures	3rd procedures
New access	68	12
CAPD	52	6
Transplant	48	2
Total	168	20

tional only if they were in use. EF was defined as the access that could not be used for any reason after 30 days from construction. Rates of EF as well as early surgical complications occurring within 1 month after surgery were compared between different types of access surgery groups. Statistical significance among the groups was established using the ANOVA test. Long-term patency rates for various kinds of procedures were estimated by the BMDP 1L statistical program, and significance was assessed by the Mantel-Cox test.

Changing Trend for Vascular Access Procedures

Repeated percutaneous femoral vein puncture or subclavian double lumen catheter was used for temporary or acute HD. We never made the external shunt because the inherent risk of infection or thrombosis. For primary access, we preferred the creation of a radiocephalic fistula (RCF) at the wrist level on the nondominant side. Between 1978 and 1983, formation of side-to-side RCF (SS RCF) according to Brescia[2] was the mainstay of the procedure. After recognizing side effects such as tortuous overgrowth of the venous channel into the hand, edema of the hand, or symptomatic venous hypertension (data not shown), we changed the mode of anastomosis. Instead of SS RCF, we sutured the end of the vein to the side of the artery, that is, side-to-end RCF (SE RCF). This mode was our basic type of access procedure regardless of the size or status of the cephalic vein until the end of 1985. An important technical modification since 1991 has been the use of a venous branch patch in the presence of a small (diameter less than 2 mm) branching cephalic vein according to Whittmore.[3] Using this method, we were able to increase the size of the anastomotic stoma through the elimination of potential constricting effects of running sutures.

From 1986 onward, we abandoned trial of SE RCF as the primary choice in the presence of a small, unsuitable, marginal cephalic vein, because the incidence of EF such as early thrombosis or inadequate venous runoff was unexpectedly high. If the cephalic vein was too small (diameter less than 2 mm), friable, and tortuous, embedded in deep fatty tissue, or damaged by repeated venipuncture, we did not hesitate to make a brachiocephalic fistula (BCF)[4] as the primary procedure at the antecubital fossa. Artificial graft fistula (AGF) was the last choice for the patients with exhausted superficial veins from repeated failed access surgeries. Table 63.2 lists the procedures used in our unit.

Results

Early Complications

Twenty-eight episodes of surgical complication (SC) excluding early thrombosis occurred within 1 month after 664 access surgeries of various kinds (Table 63.3). The SC included arterial bleeding from the suture line or unligated minor branches of vein, wound hematoma of unknown origin, collection of serum or lymph, and wound infection or disruption. The SC rates ranged from 3.74% to 7.32% according to the type of surgery. Surgical problems after AGF were higher than in autogenous RCF or BCF groups ($p <$ 0.05). No fistulas were lost from these SC, but morbidity such as prolonged wound care or hospital stay was evident. We experienced a rare case of active bleeding from a suture line 7 days after SE RCF in a 35-year-old male during severe strain to the wrist. There was no evidence of infection or wound hematoma. On exploration, arterial bleeding from the proximal corner of the

TABLE 63.2. 664 access procedures on 594 patients

Wrist level fistula	$n = 475$
Radial artery-cephalic vein side-to-end	312
Radial artery-cephalic vein side-to-side	158
Radial artery-cephalic vein end-to-end	5
Upper arm fistula	$n = 107$
Brachial artery-cephalic vein side-to-end	106
Brachial artery-basilic vein side-to-end	1
Artificial graft fistula	$n = 82$
Polytetrafluoroethylene loop	65
Polytetrafluoroethylene straight	5
Polytetrafluoroethylene short interposition	6
Polyurethane loop	6

TABLE 63.3. SC within 1 month after various kinds of access procedures ($n = 664$)

Complications	Wrist level fistula ($n = 475$)	Upper arm fistula ($n = 107$)	AGF ($n = 82$)
Bleeding	8 (1.68%)	2 (1.87%)	2 (2.44%)
Wound problems	10 (2.11%)	2 (1.87%)	4 (4.88%)
Total	18 (3.79%)	4 (3.74%)	6 (7.32%)

anastomosis was found. A suture line was reinforced with interrupted 6–0 Prolene sutures, while the fistula was rescued.

Early Failures

EF included thrombosis of vascular access, inadequate venous runoff which made cannulation impossible, or graft removal from infection within 1 month after surgery. A total of 56 events after 664 access surgeries was documented, with a range from 3.7% to 11.0%, according to three representative types of access surgery (Table 63.4). The BCF group had the lowest EF rates ($p < 0.05$) compared to the RCF or AGF group. As a cause of EF, poor venous outflow rather than thrombosis was evident in the RCF group, possibly from the poor condition of the cephalic vein. Two grafts had to be removed due to perigraft infection. If we divided the RCF into four subgroups according to the different criteria for patient selection and types of surgery, we found an interesting result (Table 63.5). As mentioned earlier, there was no exclusion for choosing the RCF as the primary trial until 1985.

Initially 158 SS RCF (A group) and later 72 SE RCF (B group) were carried out at the wrist. With these procedures, rates of early thrombosis were acceptable, less than 7.0%, but incidences of cannulation failure due to poor venous outflow were unexpectedly high, more than 8.0%. After these

TABLE 63.4. EF within 1 month after various kinds of access procedures ($n = 664$)

	Wrist level fistula ($n = 475$)	Upper arm fistula ($n = 107$)	AGF ($n = 82$)
Total	43 (9.1%)	4 (3.7%)	9 (11.0%)
Thrombosis	18 (3.8%)	2 (1.9%)	5 (6.1%)
Poor flow	25 (5.3%)	2 (1.9%)	2 (2.4%)
Infection	0	0	2 (2.4%)

TABLE 63.5. EF According to criteria for patient selection and types of RCF

	SS RCF (A)	SE RCF (B)	SE RCF (C)	SE RCF (D)
Era (year)	1978–1983	1984–1985	1986–1991	1991
Criteria	No exclusion	No exclusion	Vein diam. >2 mm Vein injury (−)	Vein diam. <2 mm Vein injury (−) Branches (+)
Total No.	158	72	192	48
Thrombosis (%)	5.7	6.9	1.6	2.1
Poor flow (%)	8.2	8.3	2.1	4.2
Total EF (%)	13.3	15.3	3.7	6.3

TABLE 63.6. Long-term patency rates according to criteria for patient selection and types of access procedures

Types of access	No. patients	Cumulative patency rate (%)		
		1 yr	2 yr	3 yr
SS RCF (A)	158	72	67	64
SE RCF (B)	72	70	64	62
SE RCF (C)	192	84	78	74
SE RCF (D)	48	82	—	—
SE BCF	106	82	77	76
PTFE	70	70	68	56
Polyurethane	6	67	—	—

findings, we chose SE RCF as the primary procedure only in the case of a suitable cephalic vein, that is, a diameter larger than 2 mm, and no venous sclerosis or damage (C group). Until the end of 1991, 192 cases were selected and we could decrease the EF rate to 3.7%. Recently we tried the venous branch patch technique in 48 cases of RCF when the cephalic vein was small but not damaged and had one or two branches at the wrist level (D group). The rate of EF was acceptable.

Long-Term Patency

In every type of vascular access surgery, there was a major loss within 1 year after surgery, especially within 1 month due to EF. Therefore we considered EF as one of the major determinants affecting the long-term patency, because after 1 year, rates of access failure were slow, steady, and nearly the same regardless of the type of surgery. The BCF or SE RCF (C group) with low EF had superior long-term patency ($p < 0.05$) compared with the RCF (A or B) or AGF group, reflecting the importance of EF (Table 63.6).

Vascular Access in Diabetics

Thirty-two RCF, 10 BCF, and 6 AGF were placed in 44 diabetic patients. When compared to similar types of surgery in nondiabetics, there was no difference in the rates of early complications or EF. The small numbers of diabetics precluded statistical significance for long-term patency.

Conclusion

For successful vascular access during maintenance HD, selection of types of surgery according to the size or status of the vein is important to reduce EF, which is one of the major factors influencing long-term patency. SE RCF at wrist level should be tried initially. But if the cephalic vein is not suitable, there is no reason to explore the wrist, because even after successful anastomosis, venous outflow might be inadequate to prevent cannulation. In this situation, the BCF at the antecubital fossa is preferred as the primary choice. We could achieve more than 70% 3-year success rates with the RCF or BCF if the vein was good. More perfect techniques and careful attention are necessary to reduce early complications such as bleeding or wound problems.

References

1. Kim YS, Bang BK. Combined report on dialysis and transplantation in Korea, 1989–1990. Korean J Nephrol 1991;10:311–323.
2. Brescia MJ, Cimino JE, Appel K, et al. Chronic hemodialysis using venipuncture and a surgically created arteriovenous fistula. N Engl J Med 1966;275:1089–1092.
3. Whittmore A. Vascular access for hemodialysis. In: Tilney NL, Lazarus JM (eds.). *Surgical Care of the Patient with Renal Failure*. Philadelphia: WB Saunders, 1982.
4. Cantelmo NL, LoGerfo FW, Menzoian JO. Brachiobasilic and brachiocephalic fistulas as secondary angioaccess routes. Surg Gynecol Obstet 1982;155:545–548.

Index

Abdominal aortic aneurysm (AAA)
  with aortocaval fistula, 206–211
  comparative incidence in Korea and
      Western countries, 206, 208
  complicating consumption coagulo-
      pathy, 248–255
    Futhan for, 250, 252
  concomitant renal artery reconstruc-
      tion and, 278–284
  incidence of, 257–258
    in Korea vs. in Western countries,
        206, 208
  inflammatory (IAAA), 226–236, 238–
      247
    vs. atherosclerotic AAA, 246
    case reports, 245
    description of, 238
    history of, 236, 238
    operative findings, 241–242
    operative results, 242–245
    pathology, 242
    radiologic findings, 241
    vs. ruptured or expanding AAA,
        239
    signs and symptoms, 231–232, 238–
        239
  management of coronary disease and,
      213–217
  with perianeurysmal fibrosis, 194–
      199
  repair
    acute normovolemic hemodilution
        in, 99, 101
    myocardial infarction and, 52
  ruptured or expanding, vs. IAAA,
      239
  surgical management, 257–264

Abdominal aortic occlusion and bra-
      chial arteriography, 67–68
Abdominal distension and pain in in-
      flammatory AAA and, 231
ABF (aortobifemoral) bypass grafts,
      159, 162–164, 411
ABI, see Ankle-brachial index
Ablative surgery vs. sclerotherapy in
      vein disease, 535–538
ACA (anterior cerebral artery), 202
ACE (angiotensin-converting enzyme),
      30–31
Acidosis, lactic, 528
Activated clotting time (ACT), 99, 102,
      103, 105
Activated partial prothrombin time
      (aPTT), 249, 254
Activated partial thromboplastin ratio
      (APTR), 99, 102, 103, 105–106
Acute normovolemic hemodilution
      (ANH), blood coagulation and,
      99–108
  blood withdrawal technique, 102
  perioperative complications, 106–107
Adjunctive arteriovenous fistula with
      tibial and peroneal reconstruc-
      tion, 461–466
ADP (adenosine diphosphate), 100
ADPFL (aortic dissection with patent
      false lumen), 180
ADTFL (aortic dissection with throm-
      bosed false lumen), 175–182
Age
  deep hypothermia and circulatory ar-
      rest and, 275
  fistula patency and, 578
AGF (Artificial graft fistula), 589–590

AIOD, *see* Aortoiliac occlusive disease
Amicar, 222
Amputation, 441
  in acute arterial occlusion, 472
  chemical sympathectomy prior to,
    477–479
  congenital vascular defects and, 390
ANA (anti-nucleic acid antibody),
    360
Anesthesia and perioperative cardiac
    risk, 51–62
Anesthesia, general or epidural, 60–
    62
Aneurysm(s), 401
  abdominal aortic, *see* Abdominal aor-
    tic aneurysm
  anastomotic, 288
  aortic, evolution of treatment of,
    187–193
  ascending and proximal arch, 189
  descending aorta, 191
  dissecting, 189
  false, 286
  peripheral arterial, in South India,
    347–355
  sacciform, 188
  syphilitic aneurysm, 349, 355
  thoracoabdominal aneurysm, 219–
    224
  transverse arch aneurysms, 191
Aneurysmotomy, 262
Angina, 52, 214–215
Angioaccess, *see* Arteriovenous fistula
Angiodysplasia, 393
Angiography
  brachial approach for lower limb arte-
    riography, 67–76
  profunda femoris artery runoff evalu-
    ation, 77–82
  Seldinger, 370–371
Angioosteohypertrophy, 391
Angioosteohypotrophy, 391
Angiopeptin, 489, 492–493
Angiotensin II, 31, 38
Angiotensin-converting enzyme (ACE),
    30–31
Angiotensin inhibition, 155
ANH, *see* Acute normovolemic hemodi-
    lution
Ankle-brachial index (ABI)
  in acute arterial occlusion, 470–471

  in aortic occlusive disease, 159–160
  aortic surgery and, 292, 319, 320
  femoral popliteal artery disease, 431,
    433
  iliofemoral occlusive disease, 341
  as preoperative indicator, 473
Annuloaortic ectasia, 188, 189
Anterior cerebral artery (ACA), 202
Antiarrhythmic agents, 55
Anticoagulant therapy, 21, 469
Antihypertensive agents, 55
Antiischemic agents, 55
Anti-nucleic acid antibody (ANA),
    360
Antiplatelet drugs, 21, 416, 422
Antithrombin III deficiency, 549, 550,
    554
Antithrombotic therapy, 550
Aorta, difficult aneurysmal problems
    of, 219–224
Aortic aneurysm
  abdominal (AAA)
    aortocaval fistula and, 206–211
    consumption coagulopathy compli-
      cated with, 248–255
    incidence of, 257–258
    inflammatory (IAAA), 226–236,
      238–247
    management of coronary disease
      and, 213–217
    perianeurysmal fibrosis and, 194–
      199
    and surgical management, 257–264
  difficult aneurysmal problems, 219–
    224
  evolution of treatment of, 187–193
  surgical treatment for, 188–193
  thoracoabdominal aneurysm, 219–
    224
  vasospasm and ruptured aneurysmal
    surgery, 201–205
Aortic arch arteritis, 359
Aortic dissection
  with patent false lumen (ADPFL),
    180
  with thrombosed false lumen
    (ADTFL), 175–182
    CT finding of, 175
    surgical indications, 176
Aortic reconstruction, complications
    following, 286–293

Aortic surgery
  in aortoiliac occlusive disease, 306–
    330
  complications following, 286–293
  concomitant renal artery reconstruc-
    tion and, 278–284
  deep hypothermia and circulatory ar-
    rest in, 269–276
  infrarenal aortic cross-clamping, 296–
    305
Aortitis syndrome, 359
Aortoarteritis, 359
Aortobifemoral (ABF) bypass grafts,
  159, 162–164, 411
Aortocaval fistula
  and AAA, 206–211
  etiology of, 209–210
  preoperative diagnosis, 210–211
Aortoenteric fistula, 286, 288
Aortofemoral bypass, 308–316
  retroperitoneal approach, 312–316
  transabdominal approach, 309–312
Aortoiliac disease, types of, 306–307
Aortoiliac endarterectomy, 316–317
Aortoiliac occlusive disease (AIOD)
  axillofemoral and axilloiliac bypass,
    166–172
  chronic, 159–164
  combined infrainguinal and, 317–
    320
  preoperative assessment, 308
  surgical management of, 306–330
Aortoiliac reconstruction in Japan, 413
Aortoiliofemoral bypass, 412
Aplasminogenemia, 554
APTR (activated partial thromboplastin
    ratio), 99, 102, 103, 105–106
Arteria gastrolienalis, 132
Arterial aneurysm, peripheral, in South
    India, 347–355
Arterial bypass reconstruction, 469,
    471, 473
  in femoropopliteal region, 415–422
Arterial hypertension, 214–215
Arterial occlusion, acute, 469–474
Arterial occlusive disease
  peripheral lower limb, 67–68
  surgical treatment of, 409–414
Arterial reconstruction of lower extrem-
    ities, 3–22
Arteries

Takayasu's arteritis, 359–369
thromboangiitis obliterans (TAO),
    370–379
Arteriography, brachial approach, 67–
    76
  abdominal aortic occlusion and, 67–
    68
  vs. axillary or lumbar approach, 71,
    75–76
Arteriosclerosis obliterans (ASO), 278
  arterial reconstruction in, 3–22
  concomitant renal artery reconstruc-
    tion and, 278–284
  femoropopliteal, 415, 417, 420, 422
  in Japan, 412
  tibial peroneal occlusive disease, 455,
    458, 461–462
Arteriosclerotic occlusion, brachial ap-
    proach and, 70–71
Arteriovenous fistula, 401
  adjunctive, with tibial and peroneal
    reconstruction, 461–466
  in chronic renal failure, 577–585
  for hemodialysis, 587–592
Arteriovenous (AV) shunt, 389, 465
Artificial graft fistula (AGF), 589–590
Ascending and proximal arch aneu-
    rysms, 189
Ascending aortofemoral artery bypass,
    329
Ascites, intractable, 561, 566
Asian Vascular Society, 27
ASO, see Arteriosclerosis obliterans
    and Atherosclerosis obliterans
Aspirin, 416
Atherosclerosis, 349, 404–405, 411
Atherosclerosis obliterans (ASO), 167,
    370, 378
Atherosclerotic change in graft, 18
Atherosclerotic occlusion, 401, 402, 407
Auriculoventricular block (AVB), 152
Autogenous vein graft, 9–21, 283
AV (arteriovenous) shunt, 389, 465
Axillary-femoral artery bypass, 326–
    328, 410
Axillofemoral bypass, 166–172, 412
Axilloiliac bypass, 166–172

Balloon angioplasty, 306, 307, 320–325
Balloon dilatation, 410–411, 412

Barbiturate coma, 223
Batroxobin, 412
BCF (brachiocephalic fistula), 588–592
Beck's triad, 126
Beta antagonists, 55
BIMA, *see* Bovine internal mammary
    artery
Biograft in arterial reconstruction, 5–8
Blood glucose levels during surgery, 221
Blood pressure (BP), 43–44
Blood sugar, 578
Blood urea nitrogen (BUN), 578, 580,
    584–585
Blood volume, total (TBV), 118
Bovine internal mammary artery
    (BIMA), compliance of, 495–
    502
  elasticity, 498
  graft healing, 498–500
  patency rate, 500
  wall stability, 501
BP (blood pressure), 43–44
Brachial approach for lower limb arteri-
    ography, 67–76
  vs. axillary or lumbar approach, 71,
    75–76
Brachial artery, 577, 580, 584
Brachiocephalic fistula (BCF), 588–
    592
Brewster's classification, 159
Bronchospasm, 54
Budd-Chiari syndrome, 566
Buerger's disease, 401, 402, 405–406,
    407, 412, 415
  brachial approach and, 71
  in Korea, 25
BUN (blood urea nitrogen), 578, 580,
    584–585

C-reactive protein (CRP), 226, 227,
    231, 239, 360
CABG, *see* Coronary artery bypass
    graft
Calcium-activated neutral protease, 41–
    46
Calcium channel blockers, 55
Calf pump failure, 523
Calpain, 41–46

Calpeptin, 41, 43, 44, 46
Cannula, 111
CAPD (continuous ambulatory perito-
    neal dialysis), 587
Captopril, 151, 152, 155
Cardiac contractility, 296–305
Cardiac events, postoperative, 215
Cardiac hemodynamics
  acute normovolemic hemodilution
    (ANH), 99–108
  cardiac tamponade, 118–130
  coronary artery bypass graft CABG
    with inferior epigastric artery, 145–
    148
    with right gastroepiploic artery,
    138–143
  percutaneous bidirectional femoral
    artery cannulation, 110–116
  posterior gastric artery, incidence and
    anatomy and surgical impor-
    tance of, 132–136
  vasodilators in surgery for ventricular
    septal defect (VSD) with serious
    pulmonary hypertension (SPH),
    150–155
Cardiac tamponade, radiographic as-
    sessment of, 118–130
Cardiopulmonary bypass for ventricu-
    lar septal defect (VSD), 151
Cardiovascular changes after infrarenal
    aortic cross-clamping,
    296–305
Cardiovascular risk factors, 214–215
Carotid artery surgery, 85–94
Carotid bifurcation for DEA technique,
    86–87
Catheters, Zeon-1 and Zeon-2, 68–
    70
Causal treatment for congenital vascu-
    lar defects, 384
CBC (complete blood count), 360
CCA (common carotid artery), 86
Cefalosporin, 485
Central venous pressure (CVP), 151
Cerebrospinal fluid (CSF) pressure,
    221, 222–223
Childhood and congenital vascular de-
    fects, 384
Cholecystitis, 441
Cholesterol, 578, 583

Chronic aortoiliac occlusive disease, 159–164

Chronic obstructive pulmonary disease, 441, 462

Chronic renal failure, 577–585

Cilazipril, 30, 38

Cilostazol, 412

Circulatory arrest and deep hypothermia in aortic surgery, 269–276

Citrate phosphate dextrose solution (CPD), 102

Claudication, 231, 405

Clonidine, 55

Clotting time, activated (ACT), 99, 102, 103, 105

CMMR (cumulative mortality-morbidity rate), 93

Coagulopathy in acute normovolemic hemodilution (ANH), 107, 108

Colonic ischemia, 260–261

Common carotid artery (CCA), 86

Complete blood count (CBC), 360

Compliance
arterial, 498
radial, defined, 495

Composite graft, 410

Congestive heart failure, 154

Consumption coagulopathy complicated with AAA, 248–255

Continuous ambulatory peritoneal dialysis (CAPD), 587

Contractility, cardiac, 296–305

Convulsion after deep hypothermia and circulatory arrest, 273

Coronary artery bypass graft (CABG)
with inferior epigastric artery, 145–148
with right gastroepiploic artery, 138–143

Coronary artery disease, 51

Coronary disease, AAA in, 213–217

Coronary steal phenomenon, 56

CPD (Citrate phosphate dextrose solution), 102

CRP (C-reactive protein), 226, 227, 231, 239, 360

CSF (cerebrospinal fluid) pressure, 221, 222–223

CT (computed tomography) scan, 199

Cumulative mortality-morbidity rate (CMMR), 93

CVP (central venous pressure), 151

Cystic medionecrosis, 235

Dacron graft, 4, 25, 292, 312
gelatin sealed, 483–486

Dacron mesh, 447

Dacron patch, 283

DEA, see Division-endarterectomy-anastomosis technique

Declamp shock, 304

Deep femoral artery (DFA), 319

Deep hypothermia and circulatory arrest in aortic surgery, 269–276

Deep vein thrombosis (DVT), 549–555

Deep venous postthrombotic disease, 515–521

Delayed ischemic neurologic deficit (DIND), 201–205

Delayed onset paraplegia, 219, 224

Descending aorta aneurysms, 191

Descending thoracic aortofemoral bypass graft, 320

Devascularization for congenital vascular defects, 387–389

Dextran, 406

DFA (deep femoral artery), 319

Diabetes, 52, 214–215, 307, 415, 441, 455, 462, 477

DIC (disseminated intravascular coagulation), 169, 248, 263

Digital subtraction angiography (DSA), 308

Digitalis, 152, 154

Digoxin, 52

Dihydralazine, 151

DIND (delayed ischemic neurologic deficit), 201–205

Dipyramidamole-thallium scintigraphy, 56–57

Dipyridamole, 341, 416

Dissecting aneurysms, 189

Disseminated intravascular coagulation (DIC), 169, 248, 263

Distal thrombosis, 287, 290

Diuresis, 154

Diuretics, 55, 152

Division-endarterectomy-anastomosis
    (DEA) technique, 85, 86–92
  pilot study, 92–93
  prospective randomized comparative
    study, 93–94
  special problems, 89–92
  standard technique, 87–89
Dopamine, 154
DSA (digital subtraction angiography),
    308
DVT (deep vein thrombosis), 549–555
Dysplasminogenemia (DPG), 549, 551
Dysrhythmia, 52

ECA (external carotid artery), 87
EGF (epidermal growth factor), 488
Eisenmenger's syndrome, 154
Elastic property of artery wall, defined,
    495
Electrocardiography (ECG), 57, 99, 102
  detection of intraoperative myocar-
    dial ischemia, 57
  postoperative myocardial ischemia
    and, 51–52, 54
Electrocerebral silence (ECS), 275
Electroencephalography (EEG), 86
Embolectomy, 469, 471
Embolism
  in acute arterial occlusion, 469–470
  multiple organ, 473
  pulmonary, genetic predisposition to,
    549–555
Embolization, 287
Embryonal vein, 391
Enalapril to inhibit smooth muscle cell
    (SMC) migration, 28–38
  antihypertensive effect of, 34
  SMC proliferation and, 34–37
End-stage renal failure (ESRF), 587
Endarterectomy, 412
  and reimplantation for carotid steno-
    sis, 85–94
  vs. synthetic bypass graft, 410
Endocarditis, bacteria-infective, 154
Endoscopy
  fasciotomy by, 536
  sclerotherapy, 566
Endovascular procedures, 320–325

Epidermal growth factor (EGF), 488
EPTFE (expanded PTFE) vascular
    grafts, 416, 417, 419
  vs. saphenous vein, 420–421
Erdheim's cystic medial necrosis, 189
Erythrocyte sedimentation rate (ESR),
    360, 364
  inflammatory AAA and, 226, 227,
    231, 239
ESRF (end-stage renal failure), 587
Ethanol intoxication and cardiac tam-
    ponade, 128
Ethanolamine oleate, 566
Eversion endarterectomy, 90–91
Exclusion technique for AAA, 262–263
Expandable metallic stents, 337–342
External carotid artery (ECA), 87
Extraanatomic bypasses, 325–330, 410

False aneurysm, 286
Fasciotomy by endoscopy, 536
FBNG (fibrinogen), 102, 105
FDP (fibrin/fibrinogen degradation
    products), 249, 254
Femoral artery, percutaneous bidirec-
    tional cannulation, 110–116
Femoral popliteal artery disease
  arterial bypass in femoropopliteal re-
    gion, 415–422
  arterial occlusive disease, chronic,
    409–414
  femoropopliteal occlusions, percuta-
    neous transluminal angioplasty
    (PTA) and segmentally enclosed
    thrombolysis (SET) for, 430–438
  lower limb
    ischemic disease, 401–451
    multivessel disease of, 441–444
  popliteal artery entrapment syndrome
    (PAES), 445–451
  Warfarin as antithrombotic therapy,
    424–428
Femorofemoral artery bypass graft,
    328–329, 410, 411
Femorofemoral crossover bypass, 412
Femoropopliteal bypass with in situ sa-
    phenous vein, 416
Femoropopliteotibial bypass, 412, 413

Fibrin/fibrinogen degradation products
    (FDP), 249, 254
Fibrinogen (FBNG or Fbg), 102, 105,
    249, 254
Fibrinopeptide A (FPA), 430, 437
Fibroblast(s)
    growth factor (FGF), 488, 493
    in pseudointimal hyperplasia (PH),
        488, 492
Fibrosis, perianeurysmal (PF), 194–
    199
Fistula
    adjunctive arteriovenous with tibial
        and peroneal reconstruction,
        461–466
    artificial graft (AGF), 589–590
Fogarty thrombectomy, 366
Foot gangrene, 477–479
Frank-Starling relationship, 298, 300,
    302
Fusiform aneurysmal lesions, 188
Futhan, 250, 252

Gabexate mesilate, 255
Gas analysis in venous ulcers, 523–
    527
Gastrectomy, subtotal, 132
Gastric remnant, ischemic necrosis of,
    132
Gastrocnemius muscle involvement in
    PAES, 446–449, 450
Gastrocnemius vein division, 536
Gastroepiploic artery (GEAR or GEA)
    in CABG, 138–143
    vs. IEA, 145–148
Gastroesophageal bleeding, 561
Gelatin solutions in acute normovo-
    lemic hemodilution (ANH), 100
Gelofusine, 102, 103
Genetic predisposition to pulmonary
    embolism, 549–555
GH (growth hormone), 488, 493
Gianturco stent, 562, 563
    modified, 337–342
Graft(s)
    aortobifemoral (ABF) bypass, 159,
        162–164, 411
    atherosclerotic change in, 18

autogenous vein, 9–21, 283
    PGE$_1$ and PGI$_2$ (prostaglandin E$_1$
        and I$_2$) in, 14, 21
    biograft in arterial reconstruction, 5–
        8
    composite, 410
    coronary artery bypass graft (CABG)
        with inferior epigastric artery, 145–
            148
        with right gastroepiploic artery,
            138–143
    Dacron graft, 4, 25, 283, 292, 312, 447
        gelatin sealed, 483–486
    descending thoracic aortofemoral by-
        pass, 320
    endarterectomy vs. synthetic bypass,
        410
    EPTFE (expanded PTFE) vascular
        grafts, 416, 417, 419
        vs. saphenous vein, 420–421
    femoral-femoral artery bypass, 328–
        329, 410, 411
    homolateral long saphenous vein as
        valvulated, 515–521
    illofemoral artery bypass, 329
    infection, 286, 287–288
    occlusion, 289–290
    patency, 77–82
    PTFE (polytetrafluorethylene) graft
        in AAA with aortocaval fistula,
            211, 292, 312, 327, 330, 362–363,
            442, 464
        vs. autogenous vein, 413–414
        vs. BIMA, 495–502
    saphenous vein, in situ vs. reversed,
        419, 420–421
    sequential bypass graft, 410
    synthetic bypass graft vs. endarterec-
        tomy, 410
    thrombectomy, 289
    thrombosis and graft occlusion, 286,
        287
    valvulated, 515–521
    vascular
        in pseudointimal hyperplasia, 488–
            492
        Rifampicin to increase resistance to
            staphylococcal infection, 483–486
Graft-enteric fistula, 286

Great saphenous vein
    vs. gastroepiploic artery (GEAR) in
        CABG, 138–143
    stripping, 536
    varicose, 539–545
Groin exploration in recurrent varicose
    veins, 536
Growth hormone (GH), 488, 493
Gunshot wounds and cardiac tampon-
    ade, 126

Hallucination after deep hypothermia
    and circulatory arrest, 272
Heart failure, 53–54
Hematocrit, 42, 44, 578
Hematuria, 231
Hemiparesis after deep hypothermia
    and circulatory arrest, 273
Hemodialysis (HD)
    arteriovenous fistula for, 587–592
    vascular access for, 583
Hemodilution, acute normovolemic
    (ANH), blood coagulation and,
    99–108
Hemodynamic nonradical surgery,
    389
Hemodynamics, cardiac, see Cardiac
    hemodynamics
Hemoglobin, 42–43, 578, 583
Hemolymphatic malformations, 389
Hemothorax, 119, 124, 128, 129
Heparin, 255, 433, 435–437, 469
Hepatic encephalopathy, 565, 567
Hepatic mitochondrial redox potential,
    571, 572
Hepatic revascularization, portal vein
    arterialization, 569–574
Hepatic vein occlusion, 565
Holter monitor, 56
Homolateral long saphenous vein as val-
    vulated graft, 515–521
Hormonal contraceptives, 530
Human lymphocyte antigen (HLA), 405
Hydralazine, 38, 152, 154, 155
Hydroureter, 231
Hydroxyethyl starch, 100
Hypatoblastoma, 569

Hypercoagulability, 287, 426
Hyperfibrinolysis, 426
Hyperglycemia, 223–224
Hyperlipidemia, 415
Hyperoxic ulcers, 526
Hyperplasia, pseudointimal (PH), 488–
    493
Hypertension, 52, 55, 214–215, 307,
    349, 415, 441, 455, 462
Hypertrophy, 52
Hypotension, 224
Hypothermia, 213
Hypovolemia, 287
Hypoxic ulcers, 525–526

IAAA, see Abdominal aortic aneurysm,
    inflammatory
ICA (internal carotid artery), 87, 202
IEA (inferior epigastric artery), 145–
    148
IGH (insulin-like growth factor), 488
IH (intimal hyperplasia), 488, 492
IIA (internal iliac artery) reconstruc-
    tion, 260, 261–262
Iliofemoral artery bypass graft, 329
Iliofemoral occlusive disease, 337–342
IMA (inferior mesenteric artery), 42,
    43, 260–261
Impotence, 307
India, peripheral arterial aneurysm in,
    347–355
Inferior epigastric artery (IEA), 145–
    148
Inferior mesenteric artery (IMA), 42,
    43, 260–261
Inferior vena cava (IVC), 42, 489
Inflammatory AAA (IAAA), see Ab-
    dominal aortic aneurysm, in-
    flammatory
Inflammatory bowel disease, 409
Infrainguinal occlusive disease, com-
    bined aortoiliac and, 317–320
Infrarenal aortic cross-clamping, 296–
    305
Inositol niacinate, 406
Insulin-like growth factor (IGH), 488
Internal carotid artery (ICA), 87, 202

Internal iliac artery (IIA) reconstruction, 260, 261–262
Internal thoracic artery (ITA), 145–148
International normalized ratio coagulation study (INR), 99, 102, 103, 105
Intimal hyperplasia (IH), 488, 492
Intoxication, cardiac tamponade and, 128
Intractable ascites, 561, 566
Intrapleural route of axillofemoral and axilloiliac bypass, 166–172
Ischemia
  chronic critical lower limb, 441–444
  colonic, 260–261
  lower extremity, 159, 161–162, 166–172
    chemical sympathectomy to preserve knee joint, 477–479
  myocardial, 51–52
    clinical risk factors of perioperative, 53–55
    intraoperative monitoring for, 57–59
    patients at risk for perioperative, 56–57
    postoperative, 51–52, 54
    pulmonary artery (PA) catheter to detect intraoperative, 57, 58
    transesophageal echocardiographic (TEE) detection of, 57, 58–59
Ischemia reperfusion injury (IRI), 41, 43, 45
Ischemic heart disease, 349
Ischemic leg ulcer, 412
Ischemic necrosis of gastric remnant, 132
Isoprenaline, 152
Isoproterenol, 154–155
ITA (internal thoracic artery), 145–148
IVC (inferior vena cava), 42, 489

Japan, surgical treatment of chronic arterial occlusive disease in, 409–414
Juvenile vascular disease (JVD), 53–54

Kallikrein, 255
Ketone body ratio (KBR), 571, 572
Korean Vascular Surgery Society, 26–27

Lactate dehydrogenase (LDH), 528
Lactate values after shearing operation for venous ulcers, 528–534
Lactic acidosis, 528
Laser angioplasty, 421
Laser Doppler flowmetry (LDF), 477–478
LC (local communication) between aortic true lumen and clotted false lumen, 175, 177, 180
LE, see Lower extremity
Left internal mammary artery (LIMA), 138–143
Leriche's syndrome, 307
Light microscopy (LM), 43, 45, 489, 491
Lipo-PGE$_1$, 416
Lipodermatosclerosis, 529
Liver cirrhosis, 565
Liver function test (LFT), 360
Liver transplantation, partial, 569–574
LM (light microscopy), 43, 45, 489, 491
Local communication (LC) between aortic true lumen and clotted false lumen, 175, 177, 180
Long saphenous vein (LSV), 515–517
  homolateral transplantation of, 517–519
Lower extremity (LE)
  ischemia, 159, 161–162, 166–172
    chemical sympathectomy to preserve knee joint, 477–479
  ischemic disease, clinical review, 401–451
  length discrepancy, 384, 387, 389
  multivessel disease, 441–444
  occlusive disease, 159–164
    arterial, 461–466
  stasis syndrome, 507
  tibial and peroneal reconstruction, 461–466
  tibial revascularization, 455–459
Lower limb, see Lower extremity

LSV (long saphenous vein), 515–517
  homolateral transplantation of, 517–519
Lumbago, 231
Lumbar sympathectomy, 406
Lung scanning, 550
Lymphangiectasias, malformed, 389
Lymphangiectomy, 389
Lymphovenous anastomoses, 389

Mannitol, 222, 224
Mantle sign, 225, 232
Marfan's syndrome, 189, 269
Memory loss after deep hypothermia and circulatory arrest, 273
Methylene blue, 133–134, 135, 146
Methylprednisolone sodium succinate, 271
Microvascular surgery, in Korea, 26
Middle cerebral artery (MCA), 202
MNMS (myonephropathic metabolic syndrome), 41–46, 116, 472–473, 474
Molecular markers, 424
Multiple organ embolism, 473
Multiple uptake gated acquisition (MUGA) scan, 213, 214
Multivessel disease of lower limb, 441–444
Myocardial infarction, 52, 214–215
Myocardial ischemia, 51–52
  clinical risk factors of, 53–55
  intraoperative monitoring for, 57–59
  patients at risk for, 56–57
Myoglobinuria, 44, 46
Myonephropathic metabolic syndrome (MNMS), 41–46, 116, 472–473, 474

Nafamostat mesilate, 248–255, 251, 252, 255
  vs. gabexate mesilate, 255
NAG (N-acetyl-β-D-glucosaminidase), 43, 44, 46
Necrosis, ischemic, of gastric remnant, 132

Nifedipine, 403
Nitrates, 55
Nitroprusside, 151, 152, 154
  vs. phentolamine, 155

Obliterative aneurysmorrhaphy, 187
Obstruction-reflux, 515
Obstruction syndrome, 515
Occlusive disease
  chronic and acute, 401
  multilevel, 317–320
Occlusive thromboaortopathy, 359
OSFA (occluded superficial femoral arteries), 78
Oxygen balance, myocardial, 60–61

PA (pulmonary artery) catheter, 57, 58
Pacemaker, 152, 154
Packed cell volume (PCV), 99, 101, 102, 103–104, 105
PAES (popliteal artery entrapment syndrome), 445–451
Palmaz stent, 324–325, 341, 562, 563
Pancreatectomy, 136
Pancreatitis, 255
Pancreatoduodenectomy, 136
PAP (peroxidase-antiperoxidase) stain in scanning electron microscopy, 17
Paraparesis, 219, 223
Paraplegia, 191, 219
Paraprosthetic sinus, 288
Parasitic circulation, 389, 391
Paroxysmal ventricular complex (PVC), 54
PBS (phosphate-buffered saline), 33
PC (platelet concentrates), 100
PCNA (proliferating cell nuclear antigen), 32, 34
PCV (packed cell volume), 99, 101, 102, 103–104, 105
PDGF (platelet-derived growth factor), 29–30, 488, 493
PE (pulmonary embolism), 549–555
Pentoxifylline, 412
Percutaneous bidirectional femoral artery cannulation, 110–116

cannula design, 111
distal femoral artery flow, 113–114
distal femoral artery pressure, 114
femoral venous oxygen saturation (SVO₂), 114–115
Percutaneous transluminal angioplasty (PTA), 159, 320–325, 410–411, 412, 421
  with modified Gianturco expandable metallic stents, 337–342
  and segmentally enclosed thrombolysis (SET), 430–438
Perforators discission, 530
Peripheral vascular disease, 214–215
Peritonitis, 409
Peroneal reconstruction, 461–466
Peroxidase-antiperoxidase (PAP) stain in scanning electron microscopy, 17
Personality change after deep hypothermia and circulatory arrest, 272
PF (perianeurysmal fibrosis), 194–199
PGA₁ (prostaglandin A₁), 406
PGE₁ (prostaglandin E₁), 21, 403, 412, 416, 422, 469
PGI₂ (prostaglandin I₂), 14
PH (pseudointimal hyperplasia), 488–493
Phentolamine, 155
Phenylbutazone, 406
Phlebectasias, malformed, 387
Phosphate-buffered saline, 33
Photoplethysmography (PPG) test, 539–541, 543
Pigeon breast deformity, 150
Plasmin, 255
Plasminogen activity (Plg), 249
Platelet concentrates (PC), 100
Platelet (PLT) count, 42, 44, 249, 253–254
Platelet-derived growth factor (PDGF), 29–30, 488, 493
Pneumomediastinum, 119, 124
Pneumothorax, 119, 124
Popliteal artery entrapment syndrome (PAES), 445–451
Portal decompression, 561
Portal hypertension, 565

Portal vein arterialization (PVA) in partial liver transplantation, 569–574
Portosystemic shunt
  portal vein arterialization (PVA), 569–574
  transjugular intrahepatic (TIPS), 561–567
Positioning of surgical patient, 314
Posterior gastric artery, 132–136
Postphlebitic syndrome, 507
PPCI (profunda-popliteal collateral index), 78–80
PPG (photoplethysmography) test, 539–541, 543
Prednisone, 246
Preperitoneal route of axillofemoral and axilloiliac bypass, 166–172
Pressure, mean right atrial, 118
Profunda femoris artery
  in multilevel occlusive disease, 317–320
  runoff evaluation, 77–82
Profundaplasty, 412, 469
Profunda-popliteal collateral index (PPCI), 78–80
Proliferating cell nuclear antigen (PCNA), 32, 34
Propranolol, 38
Prostaglandin A₁ (PGA₁), 406
Prostaglandin E₁ (PGE₁), 21, 403, 412, 416, 422, 469
Prostaglandin I₂ (PGI₂), 14
Protease inhibitor, 248–255
Protein C and S deficiency, 549, 550, 552, 553
Prothrombin time (PT), 249, 254, 425, 426–428
Prourokinase, 407
Proximal arch aneurysms, 189
Pseudo-occlusion, 17
Pseudointimal hyperplasia (PH), 488–493
PSFA (patent superficial femoral arteries), 78
Psychosis after deep hypothermia and circulatory arrest, 272
PT (prothrombin time), 249, 254, 425, 426–428

PTA, *see* Percutaneous transluminal angioplasty

PTFE (polytetrafluorethylene) graft, 292, 312, 327, 330, 362–363, 442, 464
  in AAA with aortocaval fistula, 211
  vs. autogenous vein in Japan, 413–414
  vs. BIMA, 495–502

Pulmonary artery (PA) catheter, 57, 58

Pulmonary contusion, 119, 124, 129

Pulmonary embolism (PE), 549–555

Pulmonary hypertension, serious (SPH), 151

Pulseless disease, 359

PVA (portal vein arterialization) in partial liver transplantation, 569–574

PVC (paroxysmal ventricular complex), 54

Pyridinol-carbamate, 406

Pyruvate values after shearing operation for venous ulcers, 528–534

Radial artery, 580, 584

Radial compliance, defined, 495

Radioisotopic (RI) venography, 549, 550

Radocephalic fistula (RCF), 588–591

Ramus gastricus, 132

Raynaud's phenomenon, 147

Reconstruction, tibial and peroneal reconstruction, 461–466

Reconstructive endoaneurysmorrhaphy, 188

Reconstructive surgery for congenital vascular defects, 386

Recurrent varices, 537

Red blood cell (RBC) count, 42, 44

Redistribution phenomenon, 56

Reflux, deep venous, 515

Regitine, 151

Reinfarction rates, postoperative, 53

Renal failure, 349

Renal transplantation (RT), 587
  early experience in Korea, 25–26

Residual A-V fistula detection, 421–422

Resorcinol glue, 189

Respiratory failure, 54

Rethrombosis following PTA, 430–433

Revascularization
  for congenital vascular defects, 386
  tibial revascularization, 455–459
    adjunctive arteriovenous fistula with, 461–466

RI (radioisotopic) venography, 549, 550

Rifampicin to increase resistance to staphylococcal graft infection, 483–486

RT (renal transplantation), 25–26, 587

Runoff
  resistance values (RRV), 78–80
  in tibial revascularization, 456–457, 459

Sacciform aneurysms, 188

Sandostatin, 489, 492–493

Saphenous vein graft, in situ vs. reversed, 419, 420–421

SBV (systemic blood volume), 118

Scanning electron microscopy (SEM), 489

Sclerotherapy
  vs. ablative surgery in vein disease, 535–538
  endoscopic, 566

Segmentally enclosed thrombosis (SET), 433
  adjunctive therapy for PTA, 437–438
  procedure, 433

Seldinger angiography, 370–371

Sequential bypass graft, 410, 419–420

Serum creatinine, 578, 580–582, 584

SFA (superficial femoral artery), 78, 320

Short stripping, 536

Shower embolism, 473

Shunt
  arteriovenous (AV), 389, 465
  indwelling, in DEA technique, 91–92
  portosystemic
    portal vein arterialization (PVA), 569–574
    transjugular intrahepatic (TIPS), 561–567

SMA (superior mesenteric artery), 315

Small saphenous vein division, 535

Smoking, 378, 402, 403, 406

Smooth muscle cell (SMC) migration in intimal hyperplasia, 28–38

Sodium morrhuate, 566

SPH (serious pulmonary hypertension), 151

Spinal cord blood supply, 220–221

Splenectomy, 136

Stab wounds and cardiac tamponade, 125–126

Staphylococcus aureus, 483–486

Staphylococcus epidermidis, 483–486

Stenosis, 71

Stent(s)
    expandable metallic stents, 337–342
    Gianturco stent, 562, 563
        modified, 337–342
    Palmaz stent, 324–325, 341, 562, 563
    Strecker stent, 341, 562, 563
    Wallstent, 562, 563, 567

Steroids, 221, 224, 236

Strecker stent, 341, 562, 563

Streptokinase, 406

Subarachnoid hemorrhage, 201–205

Subcutaneous emphysema, 119, 124

Subfascial shearing operation for venous ulcers, 529, 530

Superficial femoral artery (SFA), 320
    occluded (OSFA), 78
    patent (PSFA), 78

Superior mesenteric artery (SMA), 315

Surgical technique
    axillofemoral or axilloiliac bypass by intrapleural and preperitoneal route, 167–169
    femoropopliteal bypass with in situ saphenous vein, surgical technique, 416
    retroperitoneal approach for aortofemoral bypass, 312–316
    transabdominal approach for aortofemoral bypass, 309–312
    valvuloplasty for primary deep venous insufficiency, 509–510

Surgical treatment for aortic aneurysm, 188–193

SVO$_2$ (venous oxygen saturation), 114–115, 116

Synthetic bypass graft vs. endarterectomy, 410

Syphilitic aneurysm, 349, 355

Systemic blood volume (SBV), 118

Systolic blood pressure, 578, 582

Takayasu's arteritis, 359–368

Tangential excision with lateral aortorrhaphy, 199

TAO, see Thromboangiitis obliterans

TAT (thrombin-antithrombin III) complex, 424, 425–426, 550, 554

TBI (thigh-brachial index), 320

TBV (total blood volume), 118

TEA (thromboendarterectomy), 445, 469

TEE (transesophageal echocardiography), 57, 58–59

TEM (transmission electron microscopy), 489, 492

Thigh-brachial index (TBI), 320

Thiopental, 222, 223

Thiopental sodium, 271

Thoracoabdominal aneurysm, 219–224
    perioperative protocol, 221–222

Thrombectomy, 469
    Fogarty thrombectomy, 366

Thrombin, 255

Thrombin-antithrombin III (TAT) complex, 424, 425–426, 550, 554

Thromboangiitis obliterans (TAO), 405, 415, 417, 420, 455, 461
    arterial reconstruction in, 3–22
    in Korea, 370–379
    obstructive patterns and collateral circulation, 374, 378, 379

Thromboembolectomy, 473

Thromboembolism, 401, 402
    brachial approach and, 71

Thromboendarterectomy (TEA), 445, 469

Thrombolytic therapy, 469

Thrombosis
    in acute arterial occlusion, 469–470
    deep vein, 549–555
    and graft occlusion, 286, 287

Thrombus, recanalization of, 378, 379

Tibial peroneal occlusive disease
  adjunctive arteriovenous fistula with
    reconstruction, 461–466
  revascularization under transmicro-
    scopic technique, 455–459
Ticlopidine, 412, 416, 422
TIPS (transjugular intrahepatic porto-
    systemic shunt), 561–567
Tissue plasminogen activator (TPA),
    406–407, 431
Total blood volume (TBV), 118
Transesophageal echocardiography
    (TEE), 57, 58–59
Transjugular intrahepatic portosystemic
    shunt (TIPS), 561–567
Transmicroscopic technique for tibial
    revascularization, 456
Transmission electron microscopy
    (TEM), 489, 492
Transverse arch aneurysms, 191
Trauma, brachial approach and, 71
Trendelenburg test, 543
Tricarboxylic acid cycle, 528, 534
Trypsin, 255
Tuberculosis, 349

Ulcers, venous
  gas analysis in, 523–527
  lactate and pyruvate values, 528–534
Ulnar artery, 580, 584
Ureterolysis in surgery for AAA with
    PF, 194, 198
Urokinase, 341, 342, 406, 410, 416,
    469

Valvular incompetence, 421
Valvulated graft, homolateral long sa-
    phenous vein as, 515–521
Valvuloplasty for primary deep venous
    insufficiency, 507–514
  surgical technique, 509–510
Varices, recurrent, 537
Varicose vein(s)
  groin exploration in, 536
  primary great saphenous, 539–545
Vascular access procedures, 588–589
  for hemodialysis, 583
Vascular defects, congenital

surgical treatment of, 383–396
  conventionally inoperable condi-
    tions, 390–394
  tactics, 385–390
  therapeutic strategy, 384–385
Vascular grafts
  bovine internal mammary artery
    (BIMA), 495–502
  pseudointimal hyperplasia (PH), 488–
    493
  Rifampicin to increase resistance to
    staphylococcal graft infection,
    483–486
Vascular pedicle
  defined, 118
  width (VPW) in radiographic assess-
    ment of cardiac tamponade,
    118–130
  measurement, 119–121, 128
Vascular surgery
  anesthesia and perioperative cardiac
    risk, 51–62
  arteriosclerosis obliterans (ASO), ar-
    terial reconstruction in, 3–22
  in Korea, development of modern,
    24–27
  myonephropathic metabolic syn-
    drome (MNMS), 41–46
  smooth muscle cell (SMC) migration
    in intimal hyperplasia, 28–38
Vasodilators in surgery for ventricular
    septal defect (VSD) with serious
    pulmonary hypertension (SPH),
    150–155
  after surgery, 151–152
  before surgery, 151
  indications for surgery, 153–154
Vasomotor disturbance, 401
Vasospasm and ruptured aneurysmal
    surgery, 201–205
Vein disease, ablative surgery vs. sclero-
    therapy in, 535–538
Vein patch angioplasty compared to
    DEA technique, 93–94
Venocuff sleeve in primary great
    saphenous varicose vein, 539–
    545
Venostasis, reduction of, 392–393
Venous oxygen saturation (SVO_2), 114–
    115, 116

Venous system
  ablative surgery vs sclerotherapy in
    vein disease, 535–538
  gas analysis in venous ulcers, 523–
    527
  homolateral long saphenous vein as
    valvulated graft, 515–521
  lactate and pyruvate values in venous
    ulcers, 528–534
  valvuloplasty for primary deep ve-
    nous insufficiency, 507–514
  Venocuff sleeve in primary great sa-
    phenous varicose vein, 539–545
Venous ulcers
  gas analysis in, 523–527
  lactate and pyruvate values, 528–534
Ventricular arrhythmia, 54–55

Ventricular septal defect (VSD), 150–
  155
Ventricular tachycardia, 54
VPW (vascular pedicle width) in radiographic assessment of cardiac
  tamponade, 118–130
  measurement, 119–121, 128

Wallstent, 562, 563, 567
Warfarin, 469, 550, 553, 554
  low-dose, as antithrombotic therapy,
    424–428
White blood cell (WBC) count, 42, 44

Y fistula, 464